OXFORD MEDICAL PUBLICATIONS

Precancerous states

Precancerous states

Edited by R. L. Carter

Reader in Pathology, Institute of Cancer Research, and Consultant Pathologist, Royal Marsden Hospital, Sutton, U.K.

London New York Toronto
OXFORD UNIVERSITY PRESS
1984

Oxford University Press, Walton Street, Oxford OX2 6DP
London Glasgow New York Toronto
Delhi Bombay Calcutta Madras Karachi
Kuala Lumpur Singapore Hong Kong Tokyo
Nairobi Dar es Salaam Cape Town
Melbourne Auckland
and associates in
Beirut Berlin Ibadan Mexico City Nicosia

Oxford is a trade mark of Oxford University Press

British Library Cataloguing in Publication Data
Precancerous states.—(Oxford medical publications)
1. Tumors 2. Precancerous conditions
I. Carter, R.L.
616.99'4 RC262
ISBN 0-19-261279-4

Library of Congress Cataloging in Publication Data
Main entry under title:
Precancerous states.
(Oxford medical publications)
Bibliography: p.
Includes index.
1. Precancerous conditions—Addresses, essays, lectures. I. Carter, R. L. (Richard Lawrance), 1934- II. Series.
RC262.P68 1983 616.99'4071 83-12149
ISBN 0-19-261279-4

Set by DMB (Typesetting), Oxford.
Printed in Hong Kong.

Foreword

by Sir Thomas Symington

Lately Director, Institute of Cancer Research, and Professor of Pathology, University of London; formerly St. Mungo-Notman Professor of Pathology, University of Glasgow.

If we exclude cancers of the skin and cervix uteri, it is generally recognized that for every six patients in the Western World who develop cancer today, only two of them will be alive in five years' time. If cancer at any site could be diagnosed while the disease was still localized, the survival rate would be immeasurably improved using the modes of treatment that are available today. But many of the potentially lethal cancers will unfortunately have already spread when the patient is first seen, and metastatic disease continues to pose the greatest challenges to both clinician and experimentalist.

In the absence of some unforeseen spectacular advance in the treatment of cancer, it is logical to focus attention on prevention and early recognition of malignancy. It has been proposed that perhaps 80 per cent of human cancers are due to environmental or extrinsic factors, and much effort has been directed to identifying and eliminating such agents. Advances have been made in relation to certain occupational carcinogens, but characterizing non-occupational carcinogenic hazards is extremely difficult. The association between lung cancer and cigarette smoking is massively documented, but our knowledge of other extrinsic causes of the common human malignancies—stomach, large bowel, breast, prostate, pancreas—is rudimentary. Identification of chemical, physical, and viral agents as human carcinogens is essential for cancer prevention, but the time-scale of such work is inevitably slow. Early recognition of human cancers and their antecedants—the precancerous states—illustrates another approach. Precancerous states provide insight into the development of human cancer, and they carry therapeutic implications for the control and prognosis of malignant disease. This book provides an extensive and authoritative account of the subject, and some of the important topics that are discussed merit brief comment here.

Nomenclature is notoriously difficult in this field, and there is much to commend Ming's proposal, in his chapter on the oesophagus and stomach, that a useful distinction can be drawn between precancerous conditions and precancerous changes. It is, however, clear that rigid separation along these lines is not feasible at all sites. Calman also reminds us, in his concise concluding section, of the confusion that may arise from even standard pathological terms used by different individuals in different contexts. The examples cited—preneoplasia, dysplasia, intraepithelial and *in situ* carcinoma, low-grade malignancy, early invasive cancer—will all be familiar.

The emphasis in most sections is on evolving morphological lesions, and Mostofi's chapter on the prostate reminds us that there is still much to be learnt from conventional histopathology; but it is stimulating to see the diversity of both morphological and non-morphological techniques that are being used to study precancerous states in man. The point is made particularly clearly in the chapters dealing with cancers of the head and neck (Michaels), bladder (Cohen and colleagues), and uterus (Spriggs; Ferenczy and Gelfand). The histogenesis and interrelationships of *normal* cells in several target sites are—perhaps surprisingly—still disputed, and Gusterson considers recent developments in the origin of mucosal cells in the bronchopulmonary tree and points out their implications in the development of lung cancers. The adenoma→carcinoma sequence in the large intestine is ably discussed by Whitehead. Detailed investigations of precancerous states in man are inevitably limited by ethical and therapeutic constraints, and supplementary studies in laboratory animals have been widely used. A good deal of experimental work is reviewed in this book, notably in relation to the breast (Sloane), bladder, and liver (Weinbren). Opportunities for controlled, sequential observations are obviously wider and more diverse techniques can be employed. Extrapolation to the clinical situation is, however, often difficult. Most of the chapters discuss epidemiological data, often with particular reference to population screening, and the book begins with a chapter by Alderson devoted to the general epidemiology of precancerous states which provides a useful setting for the more detailed appraisals that follow. Genetic aspects are dealt with in a similar fashion: specific topics are considered in each chapter, particularly in relation to the skin (Sanderson) and large bowel (Whitehead), but there is also a more general review of the subject by Harnden in which possible integrative action of a host of aetiological factors—genetic, immunological, hormonal, chemical, viral, and physical—is discussed.

Preface

The synonymous terms 'precancerous states' and 'precancerous lesions' are widely used in oncology, but there is still a large measure of disagreement over the actual changes that these terms connote. Some authors have, indeed, argued that they should be abandoned altogether. Dr. Leslie Foulds, writing in Volume 1 of his *Neoplastic development* (Academic Press 1969), considered that '... these terms have been troublemakers for half a century or more and are best avoided. Without being accurately descriptive, they are unreliably prophetic' (p.79). It is not clear whether Foulds was objecting to the terms themselves or, more fundamentally, to the underlying concept. It is certainly true that, within the field of experimental carcinogenesis, precancerous states and precancerous lesions are very difficult to characterize at the present time—and it was primarily as an experimentalist that Foulds was writing. Seen in the more pragmatic context of clinical practice, however, there is every justification for retaining the concept of precancerous states: there are several well-documented examples, they provide direct information about the natural history of some forms of malignant disease in man, and, above all, they have therapeutic implications in the identification of particular high-risk groups of patients, the introduction of screening procedures, and early prophylaxis.

What is beyond dispute is that precancerous states are still poorly characterized, and one of the main aims of this book is to review the common precancerous lesions in a critical manner and to consider some of the newer techniques that may help to identify them more accurately in the future. The subject matter is presented on a conventional systemic basis, together with general chapters on genetic aspects and epidemiology and a final section dealing with broad principles of clinical management. Experimental studies are included whenever they contribute to the argument.

It is hoped that the book will provide an up-to-date interim appraisal of precancerous states which will be of interest to clinical oncologists, pathologists, and to investigators concerned with experimental aspects of the development and growth of tumours.

It has been a difficult text to compile, and we are more conscious of questions asked than questions answered. I am indebted to the contributors, to Professor Sir Thomas Symington for writing a Foreword, and to the staff of the Oxford University Press for their help and co-operation.

Sutton, Surrey
March 1983

R.L.C.

Acknowledgements

The author of Chapter 5 gratefully acknowledges the assistance of Dr K.E.K. Rowson in preparing the section on nasopharyngeal carcinoma.

The authors of Chapter 10 gratefully acknowledge the comments and photographs provided by Dr George K. Nagy and the assistance of Susan Perrone, Cecile Mosher, and Dorothy Morrissey in preparing the manuscript. Work reported in this chapter from the authors' laboratory was supported in part by USPHS Grants CA15940 and CA15945 from the National Cancer Institute through the National Bladder Cancer Project.

The author of Chapter 12 is grateful to the Librarian of the Royal Society of Medicine for Figs 12.1 and 12.2. He also thanks Dr Ralph M. Richart for supplying Figs 12.4-12.7 and for giving permission to reproduce them. He is grateful to Dr M. Coppleson for Fig. 12.9 which is reproduced with the permission of the publisher and authors. He also thanks Dr Dulcie Coleman for the hitherto unpublished electron micrograph reproduced in Fig. 12.18.

The work reported in Chapter 13 was supported by Grant 3751 from the Medical Research Council of Canada and a grant from the Montreal Cancer Society, Inc.

Contents

To David and Penelope

List of contributors

M.R. Alderson, Formerly Professor of Epidemiology, Institute of Cancer Research, Sutton, UK.

K.C. Calman, Professor of Oncology, University of Glasgow, UK.

R.L. Carter (ed.), Reader in Pathology, Institute of Cancer Research and Consultant Pathologist, Royal Marsden Hospital, Sutton, UK.

S.M. Cohen, Professor of Pathology and Laboratory Medicine, University of Nebraska, Omaha, USA.

A. Ferenczy, Professor of Pathology and Obstetrics and Gynaecology, The Sir Mortimer B. Davis Jewish General Hospital and McGill University, Montreal, Canada.

G.H. Friedell, Medical Director, St. Vincent Hospital, Worcester, Massachusetts, USA.

M.M. Gelfand, Associate Professor of Obstetrics and Gynaecology, Sir Mortimer B. Davis Jewish General Hospital and McGill University, Montreal, Canada.

R.E. Greenfield, Professor of Pathology, St. Vincent Hospital, Worcester, Massachusetts, USA.

B.A. Gusterson, Clinical Scientist, Ludwig Institute for Cancer Research (London Branch), Royal Marsden Hospital, Sutton, UK.

D.G. Harnden, Professor of Cancer Studies, Cancer Research Campaign Laboratories, University of Birmingham, UK.

J.B. Jacobs, Director, Electron Microscopy Laboratory, St. Vincent Hospital, Worcester, Massachusetts, USA.

L. Michaels, Professor of Pathology, Institute of Laryngology and Otology, University of London, UK.

S-C Ming, Professor of Pathology, Temple University School of Medicine, Philadelphia, Pennsylvania, USA.

F.K. Mostofi, Chairman, Department of Genitourinary Pathology, Armed Forces Institute of Pathology, Washington, D.C., USA.

K.V. Sanderson, Consultant Dermatologist, St. George's and Royal Marsden Hospitals, London and Surrey, UK.

J.P. Sloane, Consultant Pathologist, Royal Marsden Hospital, Sutton, UK.

A.I. Spriggs, Consultant Cytologist, The Churchill Hospital, Oxford, UK.

K. Weinbren, Professor of Experimental Pathology, Royal Postgraduate Medical School, London, UK.

R. Whitehead, Professor of Pathology, The Flinders University of South Australia, Bedford Park, South Australia.

Introduction

R.L. Carter

The original concepts of precancerous states and lesions were derived from clinical studies and were based on morphological changes, developing in an organ or tissue, which were later shown to be associated with an increased risk of malignant tumours developing in the same site in the future. The precancerous states and their corresponding tumours shared a common histogenesis, and it was concluded that in most instances the malignancies developed directly from their precancerous precursors. The clinical importance of precancerous states which can be identified and treated needs little emphasis, but it is important to consider some of the difficulties which the notion of precancerous states presents.

There are no pathognomonic histological features which, taken in strict isolation and considered on an individual basis, can be construed as indicating an unequivocally increased risk of cancer. Mucosal and parenchymal changes such as metaplasia, hyperplasia, and atrophy are easily recognized and are, *in defined clinical contexts*, associated with a quantifiable risk of cancer. This is, however, an association which cannot be rigidly described. Even when appropriate lesions occur in an appropriate clinical setting, the cancer risk that they represent can be expressed only in general terms. Accurate prediction for an individual patient is hardly ever possible, and the reasons are clear. Some of the morphological changes may remain static for many years, some may regress, and multifocal lesions are rarely associated with a corresponding number of multiple tumours. More florid dysplasias are less likely to regress and they carry a justifiably higher index of suspicion as far as their precancerous potential is concerned. The problem that arises here is that dysplasias, in contrast to the changes noted earlier, are sometimes difficult to interpret and may be confused with carcinoma *in situ*—a preinvasive cancer rather than a precancerous lesion. Most authors would also include benign tumours among precancerous lesions. They sometimes constitute an obvious identifiable stage in the evolution of malignancy, and valuable information has accrued from studies of the adenoma→carcinoma sequence in certain tissues. Malignant transformation in benign tumours is, however, uncommon in most sites in man and the clinical context in which benign tumours develop is (once again) of paramount importance when assessing their likely precancerous potential. Malignant change in benign tumours appears to be commoner in experimental animals. The demonstration of some co-existing precancerous lesion and a malignant tumour provides presumptive (albeit indirect) evidence for the origin of that tumour. Such evidence may be difficult to obtain, as growing neoplasms tend to efface previous local changes. No antecedent lesions have been identified for several malignant tumours. Confronted with these essentially morphological difficulties, it is scarcely surprising that quantitative estimates of the cancer risks associated with particular precancerous states are usually imprecise, at least in the context of the individual patient. It must, however, be pointed out that the prediction of clinical behaviour based on morphological appearances alone is, in any circumstance, no more than approximate in an individual case. Precancerous lesions, despite the criticisms that can be brought against them, retain their clinical importance; what is needed is to define them with greater precision.

'Lesions' have so far been considered mainly in terms of conventional histology and cytology, and it is important to examine other morphological techniques which may provide more effective ways of describing and analysing these changes. Procedures which are readily applicable to clinical biopsies include qualitative and quantitative histochemistry, transmission and scanning electron microscopy, autoradiography, and immunopathology; and some of their applications are illustrated in this book. Another approach is to broaden the term 'lesion' so that it applies to certain non-morphological changes as well. It is, indeed, essential to do this in order to include the growing number of genetic defects which are known to be associated with an increased risk of cancer at one or more sites. Such defects may be manifested as chromosome aberrations, specific enzyme defects, or systemic dysfunctions such as the immune deficiency syndromes. There are many other circumstances where genetic factors appear to contribute to general states which predispose to the development of cancer at a particular site. Knowledge of such associations is descriptive and, in certain situations, enough information is available for quantitative estimates of risk factors to be made. What is lacking in almost all instances is any understanding of the underlying mechanisms. The critical distinction between genetic and extrinsic factors is often impossible to make, and the nature of their interaction is obscure—either in terms of local structural alterations in the target tissue(s) at risk or as systemic biochemical or endocrine changes. It seems sensible, whenever possible, to distinguish between these general predisposing states and the more specific precancerous states where there are identifiable lesions (morphological or non-morphological) which can be directly related, albeit with varying degrees of precision, to the process of tumour development in one or more target structures.

A major limitation of using clinical material to study precancerous states is the difficulty in following changes as they evolve. Recent advances in endoscopic techniques and the growing practice of repeated endoscopic biopsy go some way to ease the situation, but the inevitable constraints of treatment are such that it is still difficult to elucidate the natural history of most precancerous lesions in man. At a more fundamental level it is hard to evaluate human precancerous lesions in terms of the underlying carcinogenic process because so much of our knowledge of tumour development in man is indirect and inferential. Many aspects of the carcinogenic process have, on the other hand, been analysed in experimental animals in systems where the sequential development of tumours can, at least in theory, be more closely followed.

Based mainly on studies with chemical carcinogens, the phases of initiation and promotion are gradually being characterized in terms of biochemistry and molecular biology. Initiation is generally regarded as a short-lived process which results in an irreversible, heritable change in DNA in the target tissue. Important advances have been made in clarifying the metabolic activation of potential carcinogens, their interaction with cellular macromolecules, and the range of DNA repair. The phase of promotion runs over a longer time-scale, is not primarily associated with genomic change, and may be reversible. Some information on the mode of action of chemically pure promoting agents is now available but many aspects of promotion remain obscure, particularly during the later stages of the 'latent period' before tumours can be recognized. No promoting phase has been identified in some carcinogenic systems and it would be over-simple to regard the initiation/promotion sequence, as defined at present, as the only mechanisms of carcinogenesis.

A disconcertingly wide hiatus exists between what is known of the chemical changes associated with tumour induction and their structural concomitants. No techniques, for example, are available whereby intact initiated cells can be recognized within target tissues. Morphological changes may indeed be present, but so far they are indistinguishable from those associated with non-specific toxic effects in the organ or tissue in question. Promotion is frequently associated with epithelial or parenchymal hyperplasia, but there are major problems of interpretation. First, such changes may be indistinguishable from those evoked by stimuli which lack any kind of tumour-inducing activity. Second, events during the promotion phase are variable: in any group of histologically identical lesions produced by a given promoting agent, some will give rise to tumour while others remain unchanged or regress. Histological similarity is clearly misleading, and the implied functional heterogeneity among such lesions may only be demonstrated by more refined techniques. Examples include histochemistry, analyses of karyotypes and antigenic determinants, biosynthetic activity, and responses to mitogens. Sustained cell proliferation is an essential component in the promotion phase, but two provisos should be noted. First, it appears that initiation and promotion are widespread processes within a particular target tissue. The eventual yield of tumours is, by comparison, small and it is difficult to avoid the notion of some kind of selective growth advantage enjoyed by only a part of an altered cell population. The basis for any such selective advantage is wholly obscure but might include the capacity of certain cells to respond to a particular growth stimulus or to resist destruction by immune and other host surveillance mechanisms. Secondly, experience with clinical material indicates the importance of atrophy in certain target tissues. It is true that patterns of proliferative activity both before and after the atrophic phase have not been characterized, but the part played by atrophy as a precancerous lesion in certain contexts remains to be clarified.

Certain differences thus emerge between clinical and experimental material. In man, various morphological and other changes can be identified which, in appropriate clinical contexts, carry a significantly increased risk of future cancer. Such changes are rarely specific, they have a variable natural history, and they do not (on their own) provide a basis for predicting the development of cancer in an individual patient. Their functional interpretation *vis-à-vis* underlying carcinogenic mechanisms is not yet possible. In experimental animals, some of the phases of tumour development can be characterized in terms of biochemistry and molecular biology, but many of their (presumed) structural concomitants are inapparent. The morphologist cannot identify lesions in 'initiated' target tissues, and the appearances associated with promotion may be uninterpretable. Certain common factors may be discerned between precancerous lesions in man and the promotion phase of carcinogenesis in animals, but it would be premature to draw analogies between them at the present time.

1 Epidemiological aspects of precancerous states

M.R. Alderson

In an early and extensive review of the mortality from cancer, Hoffman (1915) described a number of conditions which he designated as precancerous. Examples included chronic inflammation and ulceration, scars, prolonged irritation, and certain benign tumours. Though opinions have changed on the lesions that should be considered 'precancerous' the reference indicates a longstanding interest in this topic. Sound knowledge of the natural history of any form of malignant disease has a number of obvious applications: it may, for example, help to clarify prognosis for individual patients, provide a guide to the appropriate treatment of premalignant lesions, consolidate information on aetiology, and lead to improved methods of primary prevention.

This chapter discusses various 'epidemiological' ways of studying the topic of precancerous states, reviews very briefly each site of malignancy, and ends with conclusions about the various precancerous states. In designing a satisfactory epidemiological study it is important to have some idea about the possible stages in the development of cancer. The design of the study and the range of items collected will vary, depending in part on the type of hypothesis being tested. For example: do all patients with a malignancy at a particular site pass through a precancerous state, or do only a proportion, and, if the latter, what are the determining factors? Fig. 1.1, which is highly schematic, indicates various stages and pathways of the carcinogenic process; the following notes indicate the various limitations of different approaches to studying such issues.

Some information about the occurrence of precancerous states is derived from case reports of double pathology—for example, of patients with benign and malignant lesions of the breasts—but such material is extremely difficult to interpret. Without knowing the prevalence of each of the two conditions and the degree to which the referral pattern has distorted the identification of each of the conditions (separately and combined), it is not possible to calculate the likely occurrence of any such double pathology. The situation is made still more complex by not knowing the factors which determine the recognition and reporting of the two putatively linked conditions. Having observed such an association in clinical practice, it is

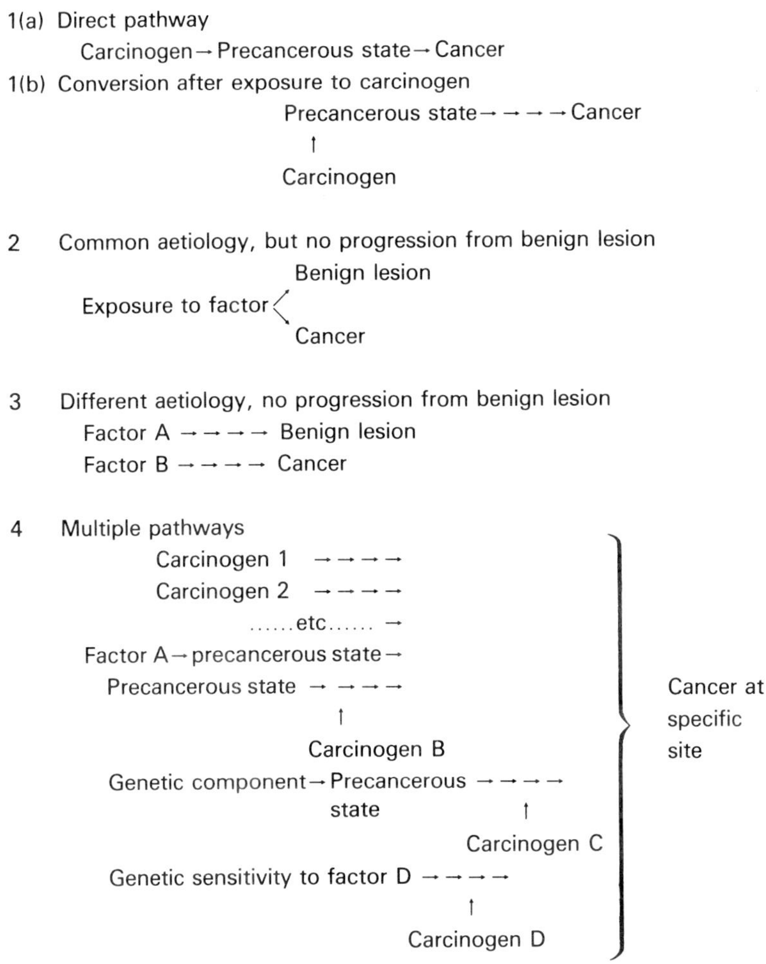

Fig. 1.1. Schematic representation of various pathways in the development of cancer, indicating the possible roles of precancerous states

impossible to place a probability level on the chance—or rarity—of the event. The calculation of the probability of double pathology only becomes feasible where such cases are identified in a defined population and the incidence of each of the two conditions is also available.

Rather different information can be obtained from a detailed analysis following examination of surgical or autopsy specimens. This is the preserve of the hisopathologist; but such material is of limited value without comparing the frequency of the various abnormalities in some sample of 'control' patients. The selection of a control group and consideration of the biases that may arise in the separate steps, (1) hospital referral, (2) decision to operate, or (3) death and performance of an autopsy, raise many issues of an epidemiological nature. Any valid interpretation requires a judicious combination of awareness of the inherent biological plausibility of any proposed chain of events and of the external factors that may have resulted in the specimens coming from a highly selected and biased group of patients. It must also be borne in mind that any such study will provide no direct evidence that the 'premalignant' lesion antedates the invasive cancer, nor that the focus of 'premalignant disease' eventually became invasive cancer.

There are five rather different ways in which this type of material may be supported or refuted on epidemiological grounds. Not all the approaches are possible to implement for every site of malignancy, and there is a striking lack of definitive studies from some of the specific issues discussed later in this chapter. The following notes briefly illustrate the five approaches. They are presented in the form of questions and they are ranked in order of the quality of information that each provides about the occurrence of precancerous states.

Is there an association between mortality from the precancerous state and from the corresponding cancer in different populations?

Examination of the relative mortality rates from benign or other precancerous conditions and from malignant disease of the same organ can be easily carried out—for example, between mortality from goitre and from thyroid cancer (see p. 30). One immediate limitation of such a study is that it can only be considered for those sites of malignancy that have a relatively high mortality. Where there is particular concern about the inaccuracy of mortality statistics, there will obviously be major doubts about the suitability of such an enquiry. If the survival for the two conditions varies considerably between different countries, this would enhance bias in the results. Analysis of routine mortality statistics will thus provide only very limited answers to this problem.

What is the prevalence of premalignant lesions in populations with high and low cancer incidence?

Many countries now have established cancer registries, and it is possible to select countries with very different age-adjusted incidences for a specific malignancy such as gastric cancer. If there was then interest in determining whether there was a relationship with peptic ulcer, statistics on the frequency of this condition would be required. This information may not be directly available from routine statistics but a special enquiry using hospital records of referrals to a gastrointestinal clinic, operation records, and histology reports might generate some comparative data. In certain circumstances, it might be appropriate to mount a special survey to determine the prevalence of the putative premalignant condition in a given population.

Such data obviously require to be interpreted with considerable caution. Because there is an association in different populations of the frequency of the two conditions being studied, it does not follow that individuals who develop one of the conditions are at high risk of the malignancy. (If the same environmental factor independently caused the two conditions—as in pathway 2 of Fig. 1.1—populations would be found with high or low rates for the two conditions, but there would be no direct effect of the benign condition increasing the risk of developing the malignancy.) This limitation would not be overcome by restricting the project to an investigation of the prevalence of the premalignant state in persons with and without exposure to known risk factors for the malignancy.

Do patients with the putative premalignant state and those with the cancer have the same characteristics?

Such an investigation would be concerned with the frequency in reported exposure to a range of known and suspect risk factors and would also examine the general demographic characteristics of the two groups of patients. As with the previous type of study, common exposure to a carcinogen does not demonstrate that the benign condition is more likely to be followed by the cancer. An enquiry along these lines can, however, be used to demonstrate that the relationship is *unlikely* to occur—and thus almost rule out any proposed link between given 'premalignant' lesions and cancer. An extreme example may be considered: if there was only one specific cause of a particular cancer, and none of the subjects with the premalignant state had been exposed to this agent, then pathway 1(a) of Fig. 1.1 could not represent the chain of events, i.e.

exposure to carcinogen → premalignant lesions → cancer.

Furthermore, positive results could not distinguish between pathway 1(a) and pathway 2, i.e.

exposure to carcinogen ↗ benign lesion
exposure to carcinogen ↘ cancer

Do patients with proven cancer have a positive history of antecedent 'premalignant lesions' more frequently than controls?

This type of standard case-control investigation illustrates a number of important points about study design. The two main issues that are of concern in designing an enquiry that will provide a usable answer are the validity of the data obtained from the cases and controls (including both accuracy and bias), and the suitability of the controls to provide an appropriate comparison group. Space does not permit full description of all aspects of these problems (see Alderson (1977) for a fuller discussion) but some of the examples in the following sections illustrate the main points.

On follow-up of patients with histologically proven 'premalignant' lesions, is the incidence of cancer greater than expected?

This is a particular example of a prospective or cohort study; again there are certain points of design that have to be borne in mind in order to achieve valid and interpretable results. Some idea of the latent interval of development of the cancer must be held in order to determine what length of follow-up is required in order to rule out an increased risk of cancer. If the preliminary treatment of the premalignant condition completely extirpates the lesion and effectively prevents progression of the disease, then no controlled trial involving random allocation to an appropriate treatment group and to a watched group can be ethical. But if the proposed treatment has some harmful side-effects—for example, from oestrogen therapy for microscopic carcinomas of the prostate—it may be appropriate to undertake a follow-up study of an untreated group. Obviously, if some form of 'effective' treatment is used for the 'premalignant' lesion, the assessment of the likelihood of subsequent cancer becomes difficult. Use of individuals who refuse treatment may be a partial solution. It is sometimes questioned whether the intensive follow-up that such patients may receive alters the chance of a subsequent malignancy being detected; if this is so, it may create bias. This may occur especially if no comparison group is included, and expected figures for incidence of cancer are derived from national rates. No definite evidence on this point has been published, though Feinstein (1979) maintains that it can be a major source of error in some epidemiological studies.

One needs to bear in mind the influence of multiple factors that might be associated with variation in the risk of cancer, the errors of recognition of the various events, and the biases in the probability of diagnosis occurring in different categories of patients. Where attempts are made to adjust in a statistical analysis for the influence of confounding or other risk factors, one must also bear in mind the validity of the documentation of such risk factors, and the appropriateness of the statistical analysis itself. Finally, because some of these conditions or events are relatively rare and few cases are available, there will be the problem of the continual play of chance.

Koss (1975) defined precancerous epithelial lesions as morphological abnormalities with microscopic characteristics of cancer confined to the epithelium of origin. This restriction to microscopic *'in situ'* lesions is not a very fruitful field of enquiry for the epidemiologist except in the rather special context of the evaluation of population screening such as cytology for cancer of the uterine cervix. A rather wide range of problems is therefore considered in the notes that follow. These have been set out by site of malignancy and follow the order adopted by the *WHO international classification of disease.* In addition to histological or macroscopic epithelial changes, there are comments about a number of chronic non-malignant diseases where there is evidence of an increased risk of malignancy. In general, virus diseases have been excluded apart from some of the evidence on the association between infective hepatitis and hepatocellular carcinoma. No consideration is given to the range of congenital or hereditary syndromes with increased risk of cancers, cancer families, or cancer syndromes affecting multiple sites which are discussed in Chapter 2.

Oral cavity

In a case-control study, Wynder and Bross (1957) concluded that there was an excess of leukoplakia in their cases, 19 per cent of whom had evidence of this ill-defined condition—see Chapter 5. This inquiry has an obvious limitation as patients with leukoplakia were deliberately excluded from the control groups, so that no specific estimate of the prevalence of leukoplakia in the general population could be made. Graham *et al.* (1977) found evidence of an association between poor dentition and an increased risk of oral cancer, but they did not refer to the presence of leukoplakia or other local lesions. On the basis of a case-control study of head and neck cancers, Vogler *et al.* (1962) suggested that snuff placed in the oral cavity acts as an irritant, inducing leukoplakia and (subsequently) low-grade squamous carcinomas.

Pharynx

Larsson *et al.* (1975) reviewed the literature on the association between sideropenic anaemia with or without the Plummer-Vinson syndrome and carcinomas of the upper alimentary tract. These authors accepted the earlier suggestions that both conditions were precancerous. They presented Swedish mortality statistics showing a decline in pharyngeal cancer (with or without oral cancer) in females and a rise in males over the period 1951-70—and hence a marked decrease in the female/male ratio. Female patients attending an oncology department in northern Sweden from 1959 to 1974 included a high proportion with sideropenic anaemia (75 per cent of pharyngeal and 25 per cent of oral cancer); the majority also showed the manifestations of the Plummer-Vinson syndrome. In a case-control study of patients from the Radium Hospital in Stockholm (Wynder *et al.* 1957), the groups of women with oral, pharyngeal, and upper oesophageal cancers and men with lower hypopharyngeal cancer included significantly more cases with symptoms of Plummer-Vinson syndrome than control patients. The women, in particular, gave long histories of this complaint and many cutaneous and other manifestations.

Oesophagus

As a result of examining surgical specimens of oesophageal cancer and autopsy tissues, it has been suggested that epithelial dysplasia is a precancerous condition (Co-ordinating Group 1975). The United States, with a low incidence of oesophageal cancer, has a low prevalence of oesophageal dysplasia (Postlethwait and Musser 1974). High rates of dysplasia were recorded in higher cancer risk areas in China (Co-ordinating Group 1975). Evidence for even earlier lesions comes from Northern Iran where the results of an endoscopy survey were reported by Crespi *et al.* (1979). Oesophagoscopy and biopsies were performed on 430 subjects aged between 15 and 70 years. Chronic oesophagitis accompanied by proliferation and dilatation of submucosal blood vessels was observed in 85 per cent of the individuals examined, even in the younger age groups. No difference by sex was observed in the prevalence of oesophagitis, but the lesions were slightly more severe in men. In 90 per cent of the cases the chronic oesophagitis involved the middle and lower thirds of the oesophagus—the sites most commonly affected by oesophageal cancer in Iran. Even when the lower third was affected by oesophagitis, the precardial region was normal in 94 per cent of the cases. On endoscopy the oesophageal mucosa appeared irregular, swollen, friable, and hyperaemic with scattered or confluent regions of leukoplakia but without ulceration; the precardial mucosa appeared macroscopically normal. Convincing evidence for the malignant potential of such lesions comes from a follow-up study of 184 subjects with mucosal dysplasia. Of 79 cases with severe dysplasia, the lesions regressed in 41 per cent and remained unchanged in 33 per cent; oesophageal cancers developed in 26 per cent. A more recent study from another high-risk area in North West China has also shown a high incidence of oesophagitis accompanied by dysplasia which in some instances regressed and in others appeared to progress to invasive carcinoma (Muñoz *et al.* 1982). Day and Muñoz (1981) have proposed that the chain of events leading to oesophageal cancer begins with chronic inflammation and some epithelial hyperplasia which evolves in some patients to dysplasia and finally to cancer; but the precancerous nature of chronic oesophagitis needs to be established by more detailed studies, particularly in different geographical areas where difference incidence rates for oesophageal cancer are recorded.

Stomach

Using data from the cancer registry and organ bank in Cali, Colombia for the years 1962 to 1966, Correa *et al.* (1970) examined the incidence rates for different histological types of gastric carcinoma in relation to the prevalence of intestinal metaplasia in persons born in Cali and in the main immigrant groups. A positive association between the prevalence of intestinal metaplasia of the stomach and an increased risk of gastric cancer was found. These authors suggest that the prevalence of intestinal metaplasia could be used as an index of gastric cancer risk, and that the lesion itself is probably premalignant. Imai *et al.* (1971) compared the histology of 260 ostensibly healthy stomachs obtained at autopsy in Japan with 350 apparently comparable stomachs in the United States. They found that gastritis was particularly marked in the antrum and strikingly more prevalent in Japan than America—that is, in the country with a high mortality from gastric cancer. The authors also examined stomachs which had been resected either for gastric cancer or for peptic ulcer in the two countries and found appreciable differences in the prevalence of mucosal changes in surgical material from the two population groups. Haenszel *et al.* (1976) carried out endoscopy surveys in certain regions in Colombia and showed that individuals living in areas of very high risk for gastric cancer had a high prevalence of atrophic gastritis and intestinal metaplasia compared with persons born in other parts of Colombia. In a more detailed examination of this issue in Colombia, Correa *et al.* (1976) found that, in the areas of high risk of gastric cancer, 75 per cent of the population had developed some type of gastritis by the age of 45 years, whereas in low- or intermediate-risk areas the proportion of such lesions did not exceed 50 per cent in people examined.

Hirohata and Kuratsune (1969) used national data to examine the age-standardized mortality rates for gastric ulcer and gastric carcinoma throughout Japan in the periods 1949-51 and 1959-61. The two causes of death had entirely different distributions across the country and there was no positive correlation between them. (Various other studies on the long-term trends of mortality from these two conditions also show rather dissimilar patterns.) Hirohata (1968) followed up a large number of patients who had been treated for benign gastric ulcers in nine medical institutions in the Boston area. Data were obtained for 1928 patients who had been treated between 1944 and 1955, and followed until the end of 1963. Primarily a search was made in the state death certificate file, and more direct follow-up was car-

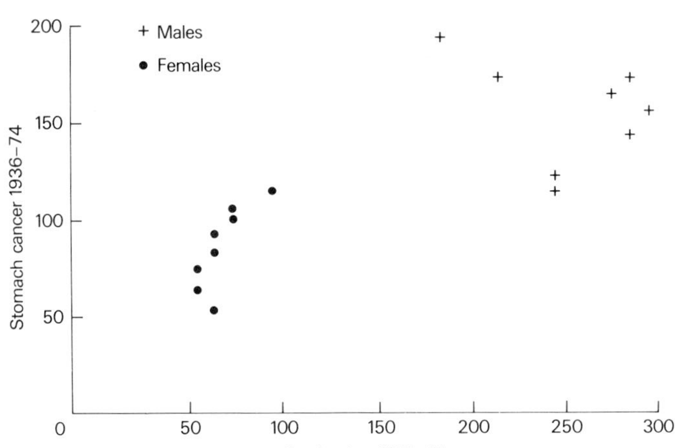

Fig. 1.2. Standardized mortality ratios for peptic ulcer and gastric cancer for males and females in England and Wales.

ried out in a 10 per cent sample. 1038 patients who were treated medically had no excess mortality from gastric cancer five years or more after entry into the study; the 890 patients treated surgically showed no deviation from the normal expectancy of death from gastric cancer. The excess of gastric cancer in the first five years of follow-up of the medical patients was thought to be a reflection of patients in whom the lesion had initially been wrongly diagnosed as benign. Another consideration was whether the regular follow-up of patients treated for benign ulcer might influence the detection of early gastric cancer (should it occur) and thus lead to improved survival from such cancer; but the mortality of gastric cancer among patients identified on follow-up appeared to be as high as that for general patients.

Stalsberg and Taksdal (1971) assembled data for 630 patients with gastric cancer in whom an autopsy was performed, together with material for control subjects. The frequency of previous gastric surgery for benign conditions was lower among matched controls for patients operated on less than 15 years before death, but was higher among controls for patients operated on 25 years or more before death. There was no evidence for a difference in this respect between patients operated on for gastric or duodenal ulcers. The over-representation of previous operations amongst gastric cancer patients in relation to the length of interval since operation was highly significant. Since the 1940s, data have been collected on all patients undergoing intestinal surgery at St. James's Hospital, Balham, in London. Nicholls (1974) found that 22 out of 36 patients presenting with carcinoma in a gastric remnant had been previously operated on for a gastric ulcer. Approximately one in 76 patients undergoing partial gastrectomy for gastric ulcer had developed cancer on follow-up and it was suggested that this was a considerably greater excess than for those patients who had been treated for duodenal ulcer—though a complete analysis of person years at risk by age and calendar period with expected mortality was not carried out. Armijo *et al.* (1981), in a case-control study of 360 patients with gastric cancer and age/sex matched controls in Santiago found no difference in any previous history of peptic ulcer. In a review of the aetiology of stomach cancer, Wynder *et al.* (1966) concluded that there was no consensus over the role of gastric ulcer as a precursor lesion for carcinoma. More recently, an editorial in the *British Medical Journal* (1981) stated that 'neoplastic change in a benign gastric ulcer is now thought to be exceedingly rare'. In attempting to reconcile these conflicting findings it must be remembered that

1. the mortality statistics may be inaccurate;
2. bias can occur in selection of patients for autopsy;
3. retrospective inquiry of past illnesses may produce spurious responses;
4. follow-up may be too short to identify a cancer risk.

The primary condition itself may affect the degree of supervision and likelihood of a cancer being detected.

Hakkinen *et al.* (1980) used an antigen screening test to detect gastric cancer in an adult population of 50 000 people in Finland. Of 3508 tests which were positive, investigation by endoscopy, biopsy, and follow-up identified 36 gastric cancers and 10 patients with tubular adenomas. The latter were thought to represent a precancerous state though the data provided do not support this view.

Large intestine

Polyposis coli (juvenile, familial); single polyps and the adenoma→carcinoma sequence

Veale *et al.* (1966) reported the small number of patients with '*juvenile* polyposis coli' known to St. Mark's Hospital in London and concluded that there was no evidence that it was a precancerous condition.

Bussey (1975) presented data for 617 patients with *familial* polyposis coli of whom 412 (66.8 per cent) were known to have developed colorectal cancer. Some of these patients had had elective prophylactic surgery which would have prevented the development of cancer. In the remaining subjects presenting with symptoms, there were 394 malignancies among 500 patients (78.8 per cent). Bussey points out that it is difficult to believe that the other 20 per cent of polyposis patients would not have developed cancer as well if they had lived long enough without undergoing panproctocolectomy. He indicated that for the general run of patients with colorectal cancer the average age at diagnosis was about 60 years, but for patients with polyposis it was under 40 years. Bussey also presented data on the mean age of death showing that this was about 30 years below the mean age of death of all patients with colorectal cancer in England and Wales.

In a study of possible mechanisms, Reddy *et al.* (1976) analysed faecal samples from patients with familial polyposis, their relatives, and from healthy unrelated controls. There was no difference in the total faecal natural sterols, but the polyposis patients excreted higher levels of cholesterol and lower levels of coprostanol and coprostanone than the other groups.

In an earlier survey Bussey *et al.* (1967) followed up over 3000 patients with colorectal carcinoma treated at St. Mark's Hospital in the period 1928-57. When no polyp was initially present 1.14 per cent patients had subsequently developed a further cancer; where a polyp was initially present 2.67 per cent of the subjects subsequently developed a further colon cancer. Heald and Bussey (1975) examined records of nearly 5000 patients surviving operation for large bowel cancer in the period 1928-70. Of these patients, 157 were found to have synchronous neoplasms, 75 per cent of them associated with the presence of benign neoplasms elsewhere in the large intestine.

Correa (1978) drew attention to a very close parallel in the epidemiology of colonic cancer and adenomatous polyps. Both lesions are strongly related with respect to geographic distribution, socio-economic class, migration experience and time trends, and anatomical location. He suggested that the strength of the association favoured the notion of a direct positive correlation between multiple tumours, size and weight of the other polyps, and cancer risks; these were equivalent to dose-effects. Hill (1981) proposed a hypothesis to account for the aetiology of colorectal cancer, suggesting that adenomas are initially caused by an environmental agent acting on the colorectal epithelium of adenoma-prone persons. Exposure to a further environmental agent causes small adenomas to grow, and exposure to a carcinogen induces malignancy in a high proportion of large adenomas. Hill (1981) later elaborated on this hypothesis, and suggested that an environmental factor would only result in small adenomas in individuals who possessed a recessive gene conferring 'adenoma-prone' status. A further environmental factor would cause such adenomas to grow. A carcinogen would be responsible for the progression of an adenoma to carcinoma, and possibly the *de novo* production of carcinoma from normal cells. A very small proportion (perhaps 1 per cent) of small adenomas might become carcinomatous without passing through the large-adenoma phase.

Shepherd (1971) suggested that regression of rectal polyps might follow a one-stage subtotal colectomy with ileo-rectal anastomosis. Gilbertsen (1974) reported on follow-up of about 18 000 men and women initially aged 45 and over who had had an annual proctosigmoidoscopy. Benign polyps and adenomatous lesions were removed on detection. Only 11 rectal (lower bowel) cancers had occurred, when he estimated that 75-80 were expected. The findings were construed as evidence of the efficiency of screening, but the data are not presented in sufficient detail to assess adequately. The distribution of years of follow-up by age are not given, and there is no discussion of the biases in the study population or the appropriateness of the expected cancer incidence.

Utsunomiya *et al.* (1980) applied a multi-hit model of the age distribution of cancer prevalence in the general population to subjects with polyposis coli. They concluded that in younger patients genetic predisposition was the main determinant, with environment being much more influential in the older patients.

In a study of the mechanisms, Mastromarino *et al.* (1978) found no appreciable difference in faecal flora (anaerobic or aerobic) between a small sample of patients with large bowel cancer, non-hereditary polyps, and healthy controls.

Crohn's disease

Prior *et al.* (1970) followed up 295 patients with Crohn's disease for 1-38 years and observed 6 deaths from cancer of the digestive organs when only 1.8 were expected. Though based on small numbers this significant excess was due to small-intestine and pancreas malignancies, with no demonstrable excess of colon or rectal cancer (Fielding *et al.* 1972). Darke *et al.* (1973) reviewed data on Crohn's disease and the risk of small-intestine and large-bowel cancer. Using the known prevalence of Crohn's disease and incidence of these malignancies, they contrasted the 'expected' number of patients with those observed. They concluded that patients with Crohn's disease had a small but significant risk of carcinoma developing in both the small and the large intestine. Prior (1973) criticized this paper on the grounds that the method used to estimate the risk of occurrence of cancer in the patients from different series gave a very imprecise indication of the actual hazard. Medical records of all patients aged under 22 treated for inflammatory bowel disease at the Mayo Clinic between 1919 and 1965 were reviewed by Weedon *et al.* (1973). It was considered that 449 of them had Crohn's disease and they were followed up until 1972; seven were lost to follow-up and others having a colectomy for benign disease were excluded. Eight colorectal cancers occurred, with only 0.3 expected ($p<0.001$); all occurred in patients who initially had colonic involvement by Crohn's disease. One man with extensive enteritis developed a jejunal carcinoma 24 years after initial diagnosis. Gyde *et al.* (1980) followed up 513 patients with Crohn's disease diagnosed between 1944 and 1976; nine were lost to follow-up. The Birmingham region incidence rates were used to calculate expected cancers. Adjustment was made for the 17.3 per cent of patients having a panprocto-colectomy and the 9.4 per cent of cases who had a colectomy. There was a significant excess of both upper and lower gastrointestinal-tract cancers; the risk for colorectal cancers occurred in those patients who initially had extensive colonic disease (observed 5; expected 0.21; $p<0.001$).

Ulcerative colitis

Edwards and Truelove (1964) reported the follow-up of 624 patients treated at the Radcliffe Infirmary in Oxford between 1936 and 1962 for ulcerative colitis; 22 of the cases had developed cancer of the large bowel (3.5 per cent). This figure was much higher than the expected value applying population estimates to the numbers at risk. An actuarial analysis suggested that the risk of cancer rose with increasing duration of follow-up; it was only 1.6 per cent after 8 years of follow-up, but at 20 years was 12.6 per cent. MacDougall (1964) followed all patients with ulcerative colitis treated at the Gordon Hospital in London between 1947 and 1963 until the end of 1963. Of 196 with total colitis nine developed colorectal cancer (0.3 expected). Of 237 patients with colitis treated by colectomy with preservation of the rectum, five developed cancer of the rectum (0.074 expected). However, with distal colitis and proctitis the cancer risk was not appreciably increased. Hinton (1966) reported 32 large-bowel cancers occurring in patients with ulcerative colitis attending St. Mark's Hospital between 1947 and 1964. No estimate of risk is possible from this paper. Bonnevie *et al.* (1974) followed 332 patients for between 1 and 11 years. No case of cancer was observed on this relatively limited follow-up. Lennard-Jones *et al.* (1977) report on the follow-up of 229 patients with extensive ulcerative colitis observed between 1966 and 1976. Five patients had developed carcinoma, the risk of developing cancer again rising with the length of the follow-up period. Relating this to the initial year of diagnosis, they suggested that in the third decade after diagnosis cancer would develop once in every 60 patient-years of experience. The case records of 267 patients treated for ulcerative colitis at the Mount Sinai hospital in New York were reviewed by Greenstein *et al.* (1979). The risk in those with an intact colon of subsequently developing cancer was considerably higher in those with universal rather than left-sided disease; it rose with duration from onset of colitis of more than 10 years; and it was independent of age of onset of colitis. Life-tables analysis indicated a probability of developing cancer of 0.6 with a duration of disease of 40 years.

In a study of mechanisms, stool specimens were collected from 15 patients with ulcerative colitis, 15 patients with other digestive disease, 15 household relatives of the ulcerative colitis patients, and 40 healthy controls. The patients with ulcerative colitis excreted higher levels of cholesterol and its metabolites but the same levels of faecal bile acids as the other groups of subjects (Reddy *et al.* 1977).

Coeliac disease

Three case reports of patients with idiopathic steatorrhea who subsequently developed lymphomas of the small intestine were published by Gough *et al.* (1962). The authors suggested that the malignancy might be a complication of the initial bowel disease. More recently, Whorwell *et al.* (1976) examined the proportional mortality of members of the Coeliac Society in England and Wales. Due to small numbers they aggregated cancers from the stomach to colon inclusive, and showed a small excess (6 observed and 2.6 expected). This is in line with results from other investigations suggesting an excess of alimentary tract cancers (O'Brien *et al.* 1983). There are no specific data indicating a clear excess of colorectal cancers.

A genetic component to this condition was indicated by Shipman *et al.* (1975), who studied the families of 32 patients with coeliac disease; autopsies were performed on 142 relatives and 15 had diagnostic evidence of coeliac disease.

Schistosomiasis

A number of case reports have drawn attention to an association between schistosomiasis and colorectal cancer. The results are difficult to interpret as the prevalence of the infection in the general community has to be considered. Ch'en *et al.* (1965) described 90 such cases, which represented 27 per cent of the carcinomas seen in a 14-year period; they emphasized that the cancers develop at the site of chronic schistosome polyps or pseudopolyps and in the epithelial proliferation associated with polyps. More recently, Ch'en *et al.* (1981) reviewed records from 60 patients having surgery for schistosomal disease of the large bowel; they did not explain how these cases had been selected from a larger series. The patients had symptoms for 2 to 20 years before surgery. Epithelial dysplasia was present in 36 specimens and *in situ* carcinoma was found in four of them. The authors suggested that this was part of the sequence leading to the known high risk of invasive carcinoma of the large intestine in patients with chronic schistosomiasis. Cheever (1981) pointed out that such findings differed from results reported from Egypt, where chronic polyposis but not cancer cancer is associated with schistosomiasis. He questioned whether there might be a difference in the influence of S. *mansoni* and S. *haematobium* from S. *japonicum*. He emphasized that better data are required to estimate the risks of colon cancer in these three categories of patient.

Liver

Hepatitis

Vogel *et al.* (1970) found that an increased proportion of Ugandan patients with hepatocellular carcinoma had a positive complement-fixation test for hepatitis-associated antigen (HAA) compared with controls (40 per cent compared with 3 per cent). Two patients had either a history of hepatitis or serological evidence but no cirrhosis, suggesting that the hepatitis virus might initiate neoplasia directly without necessarily inducing chronic parenchymal liver disease first. Anthony *et al.* (1972) investigated 91 Ugandan Africans with cirrhosis, 32 of whom had primary hepatocellular cancer. HAA was present in significant excess in cirrhotics compared with controls, except in those with micro-nodular cirrhosis—a condition which is associated with a history of excessive consumption of alcohol. The study of the liver cancer patients was based on relatively small numbers; there was a non-significant increase in hepatitis-associated antigen carriers and a deficiency in those with anti-HAA among the cancer patients compared with controls. Sera from primary hepatic cancer patients in Hong Kong, West Africa, and the United States contained considerably higher titres of antibody to hepatitis B core antigen than controls (Maupas *et al.* 1975). Larouze *et al.* (1976) examined 28 patients with primary hepatic cancer and controls (matched for age, sex, and neighbourhood) in Senegal, West Africa. They investigated the presence of hepatitis B in the cases, in controls, and also in relatives of the index patients. The authors found that mothers of the cases were more likely to be chronic carriers of hepatitis B virus (mothers of 71 per cent of cases compared with 14 per cent of the controls). No fathers of cases had detectable anti-HBs Ag in contrast to 48 per cent of fathers of controls. Larouze and his colleagues suggested that their results were consistent with the hypothesis that the cancer patients were infected with hepatitis B virus by their mothers, and that there was also an environmental factor which influenced the immunological response of all family members to hepatitis B virus. Serological evidence of hepatitis B infection was found in West African and US patients with primary hepatocellular cancer (Tabor *et al.* 1977); this was identified as active on the grounds that HBsAg and Anti-HBc were more frequently positive in patients than in the control group. Turbitt *et al.* (1977) used an immunoperoxidase technique for staining HBsAg in histological sections of liver tissue from biopsies or autopsies carried out in south-west Scotland. This procedure revealed that the surface antigen was present in eight out of 81 cases of primary hepatocellular cancer (10 per cent) but in only four out of 82 cases of cirrhosis (5 per cent). No positive staining was found in 112 controls without overt liver disease who were matched for age and sex. Though the percentage positive was higher than in the controls, the differences were not statistically significant. The authors discussed the various explanations and emphasized that their finding could equally occur if the tumour activated latent virus B.

Trichopoulos *et al.* (1978) studied 80 Greek patients with primary hepatocellular cancer and various controls. They found that the cancer patients more often shared evidence of active infection with hepatitis B virus (presence of HBsAg or anti-HBc without anti-HBs) than the controls; the relative risk was 10.4 ($p<0.001$). Similar findings were not reported in patients with metastatic cancer of the liver, and the authors concluded that variation in the prevalence of virus did not seem to be a consequence of cancer of the liver *per se.* They also noted that the prevalence of active infection was higher in patients with primary liver cancer who also had cirrhosis. Bassendine *et al.* (1979) studied 24 patients in the United Kingdom with primary liver cell cancer. In 16 (67 per cent) there was evidence (from presence of HBcAb) for past or present hepatitis virus infection. The techniques used did not discriminate between patients with and without persisting infection, but the proportion of positive cases was much greater than that usually reported in Britain in ostensibly healthy subjects. McCaughan *et al.* (1979) described 30 patients seen with hepatocellular carcinoma at an Australian Hospital. Using radioimmunoassay for detecting HBsAg, these authors found that six patients had evidence of hepatitis B infection.

An editorial in the *British Medical Journal* (1978) suggested that hepatitis B acts synergistically with aflatoxin to produce liver cancer. Such neoplasms might be a late manifestation of cirrhosis, or the virus may have direct oncogenic properties. It was pointed out that a lower proportion of patients with hepatocellular carcinoma from the United States and France are positive for hepatitis B, but the incidence of pure carriers in the population is also low. By contrast, Egypt has a high prevalence of hepatitis B infection but hepatocellular carcinoma is relatively rare; it would be extremely interesting to know if there was a much lower contamination of food with aflatoxin in Egypt compared with some other African countries.

Schistosomiasis

There is conflicting evidence on the contribution of schistosomiasis to an increased risk of liver cancer. Steiner (1960) in an extensive study of liver cancer in Africa found no evidence to support an aetiological relationship.

Clonorchis sinensis *and* Opisthorchis viverrini *infestations*

Hou (1956) reported 200 autopsies of patients with primary carcinoma of the liver in Hong Kong. He concluded that 30 of the cases showed evidence of 'causation' by the liver fluke *Clonorchis sinensis.* No control series was provided, and the claim remains difficult to evaluate. Sonakul *et al.* (1978) reviewed 154 cases of *opisthorchis* infestation identified over a 17-year period in Bangkok University Hospital. The authors described 87 cases of primary hepatic carcinoma in these 154 patients, the majority (77 per cent) being the relatively rare cholangiocarcinoma. It was concluded that liver fluke infection is a cause of cholangiocarcinoma, but its role in hepatocellular cancer was uncertain. Gibson (1971) has suggested that *Clonorchis sinensis* infection may be partly responsible for the high rates of intrahepatic bile-duct cancer in the Far East.

Cirrhosis

Edmondson and Steiner (1954) reviewed 100 liver cancers (three-quarters of which were hepatocellular carcinomas) identified in 48 900 necropsies in Los Angeles. The commonest associated lesion was cirrhosis; although the prevalence of cirrhosis was the same in both sexes in all the material, liver cancer was associated with Laennec's cirrhosis in 47 men and only 3 women. A similar study was reported by Parker (1957) who analysed 17 732 autopsies carried out over the period 1919-55 at the London Hospital. There were 53 patients with primary hepatic cancer and 184 with cirrhosis. Of these 184, primary cancer was present in 30 (16.3 per cent). There were various estimates of the proportion of patients with cirrhosis who developed a fatal primary cancer of the liver; Parker concluded that it was possible that different criteria for identifying cirrhosis led to quite different statistics. He suggested that there might be geographical differences in the liability of progression of cirrhosis to cancer, but no evidence was provided to substantiate this suggestion.

In a major review of 904 primary liver cancers, 943 patients with cirrhosis, and 1000 cases of other liver disease examined in Africa, Steiner (1960) found that the distribution of various histological patterns was different from that seen in the United States, with hepatocellular cancer occurring most frequently. The prevalence seemed to vary throughout Africa, being commonest in Dakar (as was cirrhosis)—a Moslem area with no alcohol use. There was no major racial variation, though adjacent tribes sometimes had quite different frequencies. The relation with cirrhosis was variable; the natives in the Transvaal had an eightfold increase in liver cancer compared with Europeans, but no difference in the prevalence of cirrhosis. Cancer was much more common in natives with cirrhosis than in European cirrhotics, but there did not appear to be any relationship with the severity of cirrhosis. There appeared to be a negative correlation between frequency of schistosomiasis and cancer of the liver. Mori (1967) emphasized that differences in histological classification could result in widely varying estimates of prevalence of cirrhosis and concomitant liver cancer. Using comparable criteria to Gall (1960), he indicated that the prevalence of various types of cirrhosis at autopsy was similar in Tokyo and Cincinnati, and that the ratio of hepatocellular carcinoma with and without cirrhosis was similar in the two cities. Compared to Cincinnati, there was a much higher prevalence of liver cancer in Tokyo and the tumour was more frequently associated with posthepatic cirrhosis. Nutritional cirrhosis was very uncommon in Tokyo and in both cities rarely occurred in combination with carcinoma.

Cirrhosis and alcohol

Lee (1966), using autopsy material from the London Hospital for the period 1914-63, observed that hepatocellular carcinoma occurred in 24 out of 84 subjects with alcoholic cirrhosis but in only 11 out of 98 with non-alcoholic cirrhosis. This conclusion formed only a small part of his paper, and provided no firm indication of the relative contribution of alcohol to cirrhosis or to the risk of developing liver cancer. Keller (1977) used data from admission to the Veterans Hospitals throughout the United States in 1969 and 1970. He identified all the patients discharged with cirrhosis, and all the cases discharged with cirrhosis who subsequently developed cancer at any site—a group identified by means of an automated retrieval system. The author deliberately excluded cases with cancer followed by cirrhosis. Hospital records of smoking and alcohol consumption were available. There was a significant excess of mouth and liver cancer occurring among the cirrhotics, even within smoking and drinking groups—suggesting that cirrhosis may be a risk factor in its own right, other than through the association with smoking and drinking. Keller's study which is based on relatively large numbers of patients (286 males with liver cirrhosis, and 374 with cancer) is not easy to interpret due to the rather novel study design—but it provided no evidence whatsoever of an association between alcohol, cirrhosis, and risk of liver cancer. Leevy *et al.* (1964) identified 310 patients with alcoholic cirrhosis who came to autopsy; 26 (8.4 per cent) were found to have a primary cancer of the liver. A subset of the patients had serial liver biopsies; there were 8 with moderate cirrhosis of whom one developed hepatoma. No information is given about why these 16 patients were selected, though the authors suggested that there was a direct relationship between the severity of cirrhosis and the risk of developing hepatocellular carcinoma. The apparent association here could be indirect if there was a close relationship between alcohol intake and severity of cirrhosis with—quite separately—a direct relationship between the level of alcohol intake and liver cancer. The Third National Cancer Survey (William and Horn 1977) produced a very different type of study in which 7518 patients in the United States were interviewed in 1969. There was only a 57 per cent response from all the patients approached, although the authors claim there was no appreciable bias from non-response. A detailed interview included a lifetime assessment of drinking, smoking, and socio-economic status derived from years in fulltime education and salary. The data were used as a general exploration (or 'fishing expedition') to look for known and fresh associations between these factors and the risk of cancer. The authors identified the cancers with known associations with drinking and smoking, and used the remaining cancers to generate control statistics in multiple comparisons. They showed an excess risk of liver cancer with intake of alcohol, and an association of prior cirrhosis with liver cancer which did not reach the conventional level of significance. A recent survey by Saunders *et al.* (1982) suggests that genetic determinants linked to HLA-B8 might enhance the rate of development of liver damage in individuals drinking potentially hepatotoxic amounts of alcohol.

A number of investigations have been established where groups drinking excessive amount of alcohol have been followed up to examine their patterns of mortality. The results are summarized in Table 1.1.

Gall bladder

Hospital diagnostic listings and cancer registry records were used by Hart *et al.* (1972) to identify patients with gall-bladder and biliary-tract neoplasms in Israel between 1960 and 1965. European-born women had a higher incidence of gall-bladder cancer than those from Africa and Asia. A significantly higher proportion of males and females with gall-bladder cancer had gallstones, compared with patients with biliary-tract neoplasms. As over half the patients with gall-bladder cancer had a 5-year history of biliary disease, the stones were thought to precede the cancers. Maram *et al.* (1979) examined hospital records from all patients with cancers of the gall-bladder and extra-hepatic biliary tract in Rochester, Minnesota from 1935

Table 1.1. *Observed and expected deaths from liver cancer in prospective studies of various groups with excess alcohol intake*

Author	Liver deaths		Source of subjects
	Observed	Expected	
Sundy (1967)[a]	27	21.1	Psychiatric patients, Oslo
Schmidt and de Lint (1972)	(0)	?	Alcoholics, Toronto Clinic
Pell and d'Alonzo (1973)	0	0	Alcoholics in US company
Costello and Schneider (1974)	—	—	Alcoholics in US rehabilitation clinic
Hakulinen *et al.* (1974)	66	44.3	Registered misusers, Finland
	2	0.8	'Skid-row alcoholics', Finland
Nicholls *et al.* (1974)	(2)	?	Psychiatric patients, England
Monson and Lyon (1975)	4	4.2	Psychiatric patients, Massachusetts
Adelstein and White (1976)	5	1.1	Psychiatric patients, England and Wales
Dean *et al.* (1979)	7	5.5	Brewery workers, Dublin
Jensen (1979)	42	28.2	Brewery workers, Denmark
Robinette *et al.* (1979)[b]	2	0	Hospitalized US servicemen
Thorarinsson (1979)	3	?	Hospital patients, Iceland
Schmidt and Popham (1981)	—	—	Alcoholics, Ontario clinics
Total (excluding numbers in parentheses)	155	105.2	

[a] Liver plus intestine. [b] Liver primary plus secondary.

to 1971. The prevalence of gallstones was compared with an expected figure, derived from the age distribution of these patients and the age-specific incidence of gallstones for the population. For males there were 10 observed and 3 expected in 16 cancers, for females 27 observed and 12 expected in 36 cancers; both these differences were statistically significant. The authors do not clearly indicate how they align prevalence in the cancer patients to calculated 'incidence', and no comment is made as to the likely duration of cholelithiasis before surgery.

Pancreas

Gall-bladder disease

Wynder *et al.* (1973) in a case-control study found that more women with carcinoma of the pancreas gave a history of previous cholecystectomy. Though this did not reach the conventional level of statistical significance, the authors consider it suggestive of a true relationship to risk of cancer of the pancreas.

Diabetes

Karmody and Kyle (1969) investigated the details of 265 proven cancers of the pancreas. Fifty-one of the patients had been diagnosed as diabetic, but in only 6 of them had the diagnosis been made for more than 2 years before their cancer was identified. Using population statistics, the authors calculate that 3.9 might have been expected. Statistics from four other surveys are presented, all of which support the contention that diabetics are at increased risk of developing cancer of the pancreas. Clark and Mitchell (1961) examined the detailed records for 65 patients treated at their hospital with primary cancer of the pancreas. Ten were identified as diabetic at the time of diagnosis of their primary cancer, but for nine of these patients it was a recent or concurrent diagnosis. The exception was a 70-year old male with unstable diabetes for a number of years. The authors suggest that it is individuals over the age of 40 with unstable diabetes who are probably at higher risk of developing cancer of the pancreas. Wynder *et al.* (1973), in a case-control study, found a significant association with early-onset diabetes among women but not among men. Kessler (1970) examined the mortality of 21 447 diabetics registered at a large diabetic clinic in Boston in the period 1930-56. All the patients were followed until the end of 1959. No individuals were included in the survey until at least one year after their diabetes had been diagnosed. Calculating person-years at risk by age, sex, and calendar period, the expected mortality was compared with the observed mortality. A significant increase of observed deaths from pancreatic cancer was found. There was an increased risk of dying from cancer of the pancreas relatively soon after diagnosis of the diabetes which was more pronounced among males than females; after excluding those cases where there was any likelihood of overlap of the two conditions, a significant excess of cancers remained among women.

Pancreatitis

Bartholomew *et al.* (1958) reported two patients with pancreatic cancer 14 and 21 years after developing well-documented chronic relapsing pancreatitis. Robinson *et al.* (1970) described a similar patient developing cancer nine years after pancreatitis, while Gambill (1971) recorded the history of a woman with symptoms of chronic pancreatitis from the age of 15 who had a pancreatic carcinoma at 54. Such case reports are very difficult to evaluate. Ishii *et al.* (1973) compared the data on 150 patients with chronic pancreatitis and over 1000 patients with cancer of the pancreas. For the majority of the analyses they examined data for 42 patients with pancreatitis age-matched with 311 cancer patients. They found considerable similarity in the recorded data for occupation, smoking, and food consumption. The predominant difference was the higher alcohol intake in patients with chronic pancreatitis compared with cases of pancreatic cancer, although both categories of patients had a higher alcohol intake than age-matched controls from the general population. Wynder *et al.* (1973) in their case-control study of pancreatic cancer reported a possible association with previous pancreatitis in males. What is not clear from these case reports and case-control studies is whether a common aetiological factor such as alcohol might *directly* increase the risk of both conditions; this is different from the suggestion that chronic fibrosis due to chronic pancreatitis might lead indirectly to an increased risk of cancer.

Sommers *et al.* (1954) used autopsy material to determine the prevalence of pancreatic duct hyperplasia in various groups of patients, the results of which are tabulated below.

Cause of death	Number of patients	Per cent with duct hyperplasia
Pancreatic cancer	141	41
Diabetes	100	28
Other cancers: single	581	23
multiple	284	28
Other conditions, excluding cancer and pancreatic disease	150	9

These findings were interpreted as circumstantial evidence that pancreatic cancers develop as a consequence of the duct hyperlasia.

Larynx

In a study of laryngeal cancer in India, Sweden, and the United States, patients were matched with controls according to age, hospital status, religion, sex, and education. Evidence of sideropenic dysphagia was found in a majority of the Swedish women with extrinsic laryngeal cancer (Wynder *et al.* 1956*a*). There was no evidence of an association with Plummer-Vinson syndrome in the US males or females (Wynder *et al.* 1956*b*).

Lung

Chronic bronchitis

Finke (1956), Campbell and Lee (1963), and Van der Wal *et al.* (1966) have all found a higher prevalence of chronic bronchitis among lung cancer patients compared with controls. A hint of this association had come from from original case-control study on smoking reported by Doll and Hill (1952). By contrast, Damon and McClung (1967) found no evidence of significant previous pulmonary disease in lung cancer patients compared with controls; reviewing the topic, McClung (1967) pointed out that there were discrepant findings from a number of studies. More recent investigations continue to be in conflict. Stavraky (1971) examined the detailed histories of patients with lung cancer and controls; in the 12-year period before developing cancer there was no difference in illness patterns compared with controls. More conclusive evidence comes from studies based on mass X-ray schemes. Rimington (1968) observed a much higher prevalence of persistent productive cough in those taking part in such a survey who were found to have lung cancer on X-ray. A subsequent study (Rimington 1971) followed up individuals whose X-ray was initially clear, identifying those who subsequently developed lung cancer. Such patients had a far higher prevalence of chronic bronchitis at least five years before developing lung cancer, which was independent of the numbers of cigarettes the subjects reported smoking. There may, however, be some subtle difference in the way of smoking that influences the risk of both conditions; alternatively those who develop chronic bronchitis and subsequently lung cancer may be particularly sensitive to the effects of combustion products from their cigarettes. No definitive study has explored this issue.

Tuberculosis

Haybittle (1962, 1963) suggested that there was in inverse relationship between mortality trends in England and Wales for tuberculosis and lung cancer. A review of this work (Editorial, *British Medical Journal* 1963) concluded that it was much more likely that rising standards of living and improved treatment for tuberculosis coincided with the extension of cigarette smoking, so that chance had resulted in opposite trends for these two diseases; at the same time a number of reports had occurred of an association between tuberculosis and lung cancer in patients. More recently, Springett (1977) suggested that men aged 35 and over with tuberculosis have a higher than expected death rate from cancer of the bronchus.

Melanoma

McGovern and Mackie (1958-9) reviewed the case records of 229 melanoma patients treated in Sydney between 1950 and 1957. They noted the recording of pronounced skin changes from solar radiation, pigmented moles, and subsequent development of melanoma where no preliminary changes had been evident prior to the age of 20. A syndrome of precursor lesions in *familial* melanoma has been reported by Clark and his colleagues (see for example, Reimer *et al.* (1978). Seven families were reported, in each of which at least two members had melanoma; in 18 of the 20 melanoma patients and 24 of 43 first-degree relatives, pigmented lesions with distinctive clinical and histological characteristics were identified. The authors suggested that this was due to an autosomal dominant trait, which could serve as a cutaneous marker to identify persons at high risk of developing melanoma. Frichot *et al.* (1977) independently reported a comparable family; the cutaneous phenotype was different from xeroderma pigmentosum, in which there is an increased risk of melanoma and other cancers. Holman *et al.* (1980) investigated the characteristics of patients developing pre-invasive melanoma and invasive malignant melanoma in Western Australia in 1975-6. Both lesions were more common in females and their age-incidence curves were similar. The incidence rates were higher in native-born Australians than immigrants, in those in professional social classes, and in individuals living in Perth and the South West part of the state. These similarities suggested a common aetiology and that the lesions represent two components of the same disease.

Skin

The classic paper on scrotal cancer in chimney sweeps (Pott 1775) acknowledged that cancers were preceded by 'warts'. Subsequent studies on the influence of oil, pitch, and tar on the development of scrotal and skin cancers all refer to the occurrence of multiple hyperkeratoses before the cancers develop (see Southam and Wilson 1922; Henry 1946; Cruickshank and Squire 1950). Other precancerous states in the skin are listed in Table 1.2. Koss (1975) acknowledged the precancerous nature of lesions such as Bowen's disease,* but emphasized that only a small proportion progressed to invasive cancer. He also pointed out that exposure to the sun may result in actinic keratosis, which is a precursor lesion for skin cancer. It is now accepted that arsenic exposure can lead to skin cancer. A number of studies of different groups have demonstrated the high incidence of arsenic-associated, multiple skin keratoses and the subsequence development of skin cancer:

1. after medicinal use (Hutchinson 1888; Neubauer 1947; Regelson *et al.* 1968);
2. occupational exposure (Hill and Faning 1948; Braun 1958);
3. water contamination (Tseng *et al.* 1968).

Chronic bacterial infection that results in extensive fibrosis and persistent regenerative stress may be associated with an increased risk of malignancy. As far as skin tumours are concerned these may follow osteomyelitis,

Table 1.2. *Various aetiological agents and precancerous states that may precede skin cancer*

Aetiological agent	Precancerous state
Oil Pitch Tar	Hyperkeratoses
Ultraviolet light	Actinic keratoses
Arsenic	Multiple keratoses
Chronic bacterial infection Osteomyelitis Tropical ulcer Varicose ulcer	Fibrosis
Bites Corrosive burns Thermal burns	Scars
Irradiation	Radiodermatitis, multiple keratoses

* Most authors would, however, regard Bowen's disease as *in situ* carcinoma rather than a precancerous lesion.

varicose ulcers, or tropical ulcers (Templeton 1975). The importance of such predisposing factors in African natives has been stressed by Davies (1975). Similarly, scars which also result in protracted regeneration may be associated with increased risk of malignancy, and it has been suggested that skin cancer—usually squamous carcinomas—may follow lesions of the skin from burns, bites, infections, and corrosive damage (Templeton 1975).

Breast

Previous benign breast disease

An editorial in the *Lancet* (1972) drew attention to the importance of defining the relationship between benign and malignant breast disease, but suggested that no acceptable epidemiological studies had yet been carried out. Devitt (1976) presented results from over 1000 patients seen with breast lesions: he reported that only about 11 per cent of breast cancer patients had had a previous benign biopsy, and that 9 per cent of patients with a previous benign breast biopsy were found to have breast cancer compared with 13 per cent of women with breast cancer who had not been previously biopsied. He concluded that benign breast disorders did not predispose patients to cancer. Some of the limitations of this work were pointed out by Weiss (1976) who emphasized the need to follow up groups with benign disorders in order to identify the subsequent incidence of cancer and compare this with the expected figures. Patients treated at the Mayo Clinic in Rochester between 1935 and 1949 with benign breast lesions were followed by Donnelly *et al.* (1975) to identify the incidence of breast cancer and compare it with the local incidence rates. The average follow-up period was 13.5 years; 14 cancers developed in Rochester residents compared with 8.5 expected. These cancers seemed to occur within ten years, particularly in women aged between 40 and 49 with an initial diagnosis of chronic cystitic mastitis—though these findings are based on rather small numbers. Monson *et al.* (1976) followed 733 women indentified as having 'chronic mastitis' before 1940 until 1975. They found that 49 had died from breast cancer compared with 18.8 expected (this figure was not corrected for factors such as social class and parity). The authors suggested it was unlikely that the observed association, existing for over 30 years after the initial biopsy, could have been the result of incorrect initial diagnosis although the increased breast cancer mortality rate in the first ten years of follow-up may indicate that some benign cases might have been misdiagnosed. Levene (1976) commented that despite the long interval of follow-up, this result might still be a reflection of failure to identify intraductal or intralobular carcinoma. The records from the Kaiser Permanente facility in Oakland, San Francisco were used by Kodlin *et al.* (1977) to identify 2931 women found to have benign breast disease in the period 1948-73. The nominal roll was checked against the cancer files. A significant excess of breast cancers occurred, with variation in the risk with different benign conditions. The overall relative risk was 2.7, but 7.0 for fibroadenoma and 5.0 for adenosis. The cancers occurred on average seven years after the diagnosis of benign disease. Possible biases in the study are not discussed. Page *et al.* (1978) reviewed case records at Vanderbilt University Hospital in 1952 to 1959 and identified 1127 women with a histologically proven benign breast lesion. The cases were followed until the end of 1976, and 925 women were suitable for analysis. Breast cancer occurred in 31 (expected 22.6; $p<0.01$). Cancer appeared to occur most frequently in those with atypical lobular hyperplasia at the time of initial biopsy.

Hutchinson *et al.* (1980) followed 1441 women treated in private practice between 1940 and 1975 for benign breast disease until 1976. Complete follow-up information was only available on 85 per cent of the sample. The average follow-up period was 12.9 years. Sixty-six women developed breast cancer and their original histology was reviewed; expected figures were calculated, based upon person-years-at-risk and the national incidence inflated by 17 per cent to allow for differences in the area in which the patients lived. It was estimated that the incidence was 2.1-fold greater than that expected, and this was related to initial fibrocystic disease; fibroadenomas *per se* were not associated with increased risk unless there was concomitant fibrocystic disease in the breast. Because the women in this study were those seeking private care it is not clear whether their innate risk of breast cancer was different from the population incidence, thus distorting the comparison between observed and expected cancers.

A rather different approach to the problem comes from a case-control study by Sartwell *et al.* (1978) who investigated patients with breast cancer and three types of benign breast disease—cystic disease of the breast, fibroadenoma, and 'miscellaneous breast conditions'. Controls were matched for age, race, marital status, hospitalization, and pay status. For the three types of benign breast disease they found a general similarity in deviations from the normal patterns of reproductive history which were comparable to those observed in breast cancer: the factors in question were pre-menopausal status, age at first pregnancy, and numbers of total pregnancies. It was concluded that patients with benign breast disease share some of the demonstrated risk factors of breast cancer.

Parenchymal patterns in mammograms

Wolfe (1976) has described a classification of breast parenchymal patterns based on radiological appearances at mammography: prominent duct patterns in dense parenchyma appeared to indicate an increased risk of breast cancer. Over 5000 mammograms from symptomatic women were reviewed without knowing the subsequent events and classified into four groups; cancer incidence, at least six months after X-ray, was different in these groups. This finding has been supported by other groups such as

Krook *et al.* (1978) who found similar differences though of a lesser magnitude. The observations of Egan and Mosteller (1977) indicate a rather different relationship with increased risk in fatty breasts and those with ductal hyperlasia. Further work on women who were related (sisters and daughters) compared with controls matched for age, parity, and family history of breast cancer, suggested that the high-risk parenchymal patterns occurred more frequently within families than in controls (Wolfe *et al.* 1980).

Cervix uteri

Information was compared for 4738 women attending a cancer detection centre in Los Angeles who had normal cervical smears, with 77 having dysplasia, 128 with *in situ* cancer, and 60 with clinically invasive cancer (Stern and Dixon 1961). Using a multivariate analysis, multiple changes in marital status emerged as the main risk factor while race, religion, nationality, and circumcision of spouse were of secondary importance. Age appeared to be the dominant feature distinguishing subjects with dysplasia from those with more advanced lesions. More recently, Evans *et al.* (1981) reported results from screening over 45000 women aged between 25 and 69 living in Cardiff in 1965-71. Follow-up smears were requested 2 to 3 years later for women with normal initial cytology, and earlier for those with various cytological abnormalities. Details are provided for about 254 women with dyskaryosis: two years later 20 per cent had carcinoma *in situ* or microinvasive tumours and 3 per cent occult or clinical invasion; 6 per cent had persistent dyskaryotic cells and 4 per cent were subsequently found to have *in situ* cancer. Fasal *et al.* (1981) examined data from cervical screening of over 30000 women in California in 1975-9; 560 women with abnormal smears were investigated further, although no additional information was available for 181. Biopsy results identified 108 with dysplasia, 49 with *in situ* cancer, and 9 with invasive cervical cancer. The findings were compared with those for 2771 women with negative smears. An increased risk of malignancy was associated with the women being poor, separated, widowed, or divorced. A decreased risk was associated with nulliparity, use of a diaphragm, and oestrogen therapy for menopausal symptoms. The authors found no effect from ethnicity; age at marriage, first pregnancy, or birth of first child; mean number of children, or the use of oral contraceptives.

Prostate

Although it is conceivable that benign prostatic hypertrophy predisposes to malignant disease or that a factor is responsible for increasing the risk of both benign and malignant disease of the prostate, the trends in mortality of these two conditions have been quite different in England and Wales since 1911. Armenian *et al.* (1974) found in a case-control study that there was a relative risk of 5.1 ($p<0.001$) when prior benign prostatic hypertrophy was reported. They also followed up to 345 patients with benign prostatic hypertrophy and observed that the death rates from prostate cancer were 3.7 times greater following benign disease of the prostate than among the controls. These findings have been disputed. Franks (1974) suggested that benign hypertrophy was so common that it could not be directly responsible for the risk of cancer. Both Williams and Blackard (1974) and Rotkin (1975) concluded that the selection of cases and controls introduced bias in the quality of diagnosis and criticized the use of death certificates. Greenwald *et al.* (1974) followed over 800 patients with benign prostatic hyperplasia and failed to find any difference in the proportion of patients with benign hyperplasia and controls who subsequently developed prostate cancer. An editorial in the *British Medical Journal* (1975) concluded that there was little reason to doubt the validity of the findings. Higgins (1975) suggested that latent cancers were likely to be eliminated in benign cases treated by prostatectomy and would remain in untreated controls, but the argument is fallacious as resection for hyperplasia does not include the lateral lobes in which cancer tends to occur.

Testis

Mumps orchitis

Gilbert (1944) recorded a patient with a tumour of the testis following a previous attack of mumps orchitis. A review of the literature indicated that out of over 5000 records of patients with testicular tumours only 24 were reported to have had mumps. Gilbert suggested that this figure was unexpectedly small in view of the general incidence of mumps orchitis. Ehrengut and Schwartau (1977) questioned nearly 300 patients with testicular tumours and found only two examples in whom unilateral mumps orchitis had previously occurred. They also followed up 87 patients who had had mumps orchitis, none of whom developed testicular tumours up to seven years after infection.

Cryptorchism

For a long while it has been suggested that an undescended testicle increased the risk of tumour development. Campbell (1942) concluded that the risk of malignancy in the undescended testicle was statistically higher, and that this was particularly related to abdominal non-descent (he suggested that 1 in 20 abdominal testicles and 1 in 80 inguinal testicles showed malignant change). Some disagreement ensued, and Carroll (1949) concluded that statistics 'proving' this higher incidence of malignancy were unacceptable. Further reviews (Campbell, 1959; Altman and Malament 1967) disputed Carroll's conclusions and reaffirmed the belief that cryptorchism did increase the risk of testicular tumours. Many studies have been carried out but the source of patients and the way the statistics have been collated and presented continue to create problems in interpretation. To illustrate the range of findings, Gilbert and Hamilton (1940) suggested that crytorchism was a factor in 11 per cent of over 7000 patients with testicular cancer; Gehring *et al.* (1974) in 7 per cent of 529 patients; and Morrison (1976) in 2.9 per cent of 596 patients. These associations are higher than the estimated prevalence of undescended testicle, but there are difficulties in interpreting the data because the findings depend on the age at which the estimate of testicular maldescent is made. In a survey of English schoolchildren, Ward and Hunter (1960) found a prevalence of under 5 per cent of children up to the age of 11, falling to 0.3 per cent in children aged between 14 and 17. Li and Fraumeni (1972), in a limited study of 70 patients with testicular tumours, reported that 15 of them had inguinal hernia, undescended testis, or some other genito-urinary defect—a frequency which they refer to as 'excessive'. In an investigation concerned primarily with *early* detection of testicular neoplasms, Krabbe *et al.* (1979) invited 180 men aged between 18 and 35 with a history of cryptorchism to attend for investigation; 76 came to hospital and 50 of them agreed to have a testicular biopsy. In this group, two had evidence of an invasive cancer and two had carcinoma *in situ*. Only one of these four patients showed any symptoms—an enlarged testicle in a man with an embryonal carcinoma. Conceding the selection in the patients that were investigated, the authors concluded that their results confirmed the risk of testicular malignancy in cryptorchism.

Carcinoma in situ

Skakkebaek (1972) described two infertile males, referred for testicular biopsy, who had abnormal seminiferous epithelium and subsequently developed carcinomas. In a further study of carcinoma *in situ* occurring in fifteen men aged between 26 and 36, nine of them developed invasive germ-cell tumours within six years (Skakkebaek and Berthelsen 1978). Detailed histological examination of orchidectomy specimens from 105 cases of testicular germ-cell tumours showed *in situ* tumour in adjacent regions in 88.6 per cent of seminomas and in 99.2 per cent of other tumours.

Kidney

Association with upper urinary tract diseases

Longstanding urinary stones may predispose to cancer of the renal pelvis (MacLean and Fowler 1965), and the lesions of Balkan nephropathy are associated with a high frequency of tumours of the renal pelvis and other parts of the urothelium. Several studies have shown an aggregation of the two different lesion in the same population as well as the two conditions in the same subjects (Petković *et al.* 1966; Chernozemsky *et al.* 1977).

Renal papillary necrosis

Case reports from Sweden identified an assocation between renal papillary necrosis and cancer of the renal pelvis (see, for example, Hultengren *et al.* 1965). It was subsequently observed in three different locations in Sweden that such patients had been consuming large quantities of phenacetin-containing drugs. Bengtsson and Angervall (1970) presented data on 14 cases showing appreciable consumption of phenacetin-containing analgesics, varying between a total of one and twenty-five kilograms with an average exposure of over 15 years. Johansson *et al.* (1974) reviewed the histories of patients coming from a variety of localities in Sweden; data were available for 62 cases with detailed information of phenacetin consumption in 38. All these subjects met the same criteria of grossly excess consumption, defined by the authors as either more than one gram per day for more than one year or a total of at least one kilogram. There was evidence that the other subjects had all consumed excess amounts, though this could not be quantified. No evidence of any confounding environmental factors was found in the survey; the occupations and localities of the patients were very different and the only common theme was abuse of phenacetin-containing analgesics.

Bladder

In situ *lesions*

Melamed and his colleagues (1960) studied urine cytology in over 500 men exposed to the potent carcinogen, 4-aminobiphenyl xenylamine. Follow-up of these men (Koss *et al.* 1969) confirmed an increased risk for bladder cancer. The authors noted that abnormal cells were shed prior to development of invasive cancer, and biopsies of bladder mucosa indicated that they were derived from *in situ* cancers.

Schistosomiasis

Nasr *et al.* (1962) reviewed a personal series of Egyptian patients with bladder cancer and found that only 3 per cent showed no evidence of bilharzial infestation. There is, however, no description of the patterns of referral nor of the prevalence of bilharzia in appropriate controls. Gelfand *et al.* (1967) compared a consecutive series of patients with bladder cancer admitted to an African hospital in Rhodesia with age-, sex-, and race-matched controls. A significant excess of the patients with bladder cancer had calcification of the bladder (a sign of severe and longstanding schistosoma infestation) and positive rectal biopsies for S. *haematobium.* The diagnosis in the control groups were not stated. In a discussion on the role of bilharziasis, Elsebai (1977) suggested that cancer of the bladder in association with this infestation has the following features: it occurs where bilharziasis is frequent, it is more common in males than females, younger age groups are affected, the tumour is frequently a squamous-cell carcinoma, and it presents at an advanced stage with pelvic infiltration but limited lymphatic and haematogenous metastatic spread. Morrison and Cole (1976) emphasized that no adequate epidemiological investigation had been reported, although they concluded that there were no grounds to refute the general suspected association between the two conditions.

Thyroid

Thyroiditis

Hirabayashi and Lindsay (1965) reported a statistically significant association between papillary carcinoma of the thyroid and chronic thyroiditis, although they point out that the latter may be secondary to the presence of thyroid cancer. The specific association of Hashimoto's thyroiditis and lymphoma of the thyroid is beyond the scope of this chapter.

Goitre

As long ago as 1928, Wegelin pointed out that the percentage of autopsies which identified a thyroid carcinoma was related to the known prevalence of goitre in the locality (see Table 1.3). A number of studies have involved the parallel examination of national or regional data. Clements (1954) presented Australian findings that showed no relationship between mortality from thyroid cancer and either mortality from thyrotoxicosis or the incidence of goitre in the different states. Saxén and Saxén (1954) also found no association between the distribution of deaths from thyroid cancer and either the known prevalence of goitre or deaths from exophthalmic and toxic goitre. Smithers (1959) reviewed published material and was satisfied that reduction of goitre by the introduction of iodized salt had lowered thyroid cancer mortality. Prendergast *et al.* (1961) found no association between the prevalence of goitre and thyroid cancer in the United States, while Correa *et al.* (1969) noted major differences in these indices

Table 1.3. *Percentage of autopsies identifying carcinoma of the thyroid in relation to estimated goitre prevalence in different localities (after Wegelin 1928)*

	Per cent of thyroid cancers found at autopsy	Goitre prevalence
Bern	1.04	Highly endemic
Vienna	0.27	Mildly endemic
Prague	0.22	Mildly endemic
USA	0.11	Variable
Berlin	0.09	Rare

for a number of different countries. However, these latter authors suggested that anaplastic carcinoma might predominate in areas with known endemic goitre. Ramalingaswami (1969) discussed a number of problems associated with such studies and suggested that detailed analysis of the literature was futile.

A rather different approach is based on the histological examination of surgical and autopsy material. Beahrs *et al.* (1951) presented extensive data from the Mayo Clinic, based on over 13 000 examinations. Thyroid cancer was found in 0.5 per cent of patients with exophthalmic goitre, 1.0 per cent with adenomatous goitre with hyperthyroidism, 4.8 per cent with nodular goitre, and 7.5 per cent with adenomatous goitre without hyperthyroidism. Olen and Klinck (1966) found thyroid cancer in 2.5 per cent of specimens from over 2000 patients with thyrotoxicosis, which they considered demonstrated a relationship—rather extraordinary conclusion since they acknowledged that a higher prevalence of thyroid cancer had been reported from an unselected series of autopsies. Winship (1967) suggested that fetal adenomas are the only lesions in the thyroid which can be regarded as precancerous. He indicated that they appear most frequently in women, predominantly in the age range 40-60, and are extremely rare in children. In a relatively small series of 172 patients treated surgically for thyrotoxicosis, Shapiro *et al.* (1970) found 15 (9 per cent) with unsuspected carcinoma. They suggested that the relationship of the two conditions might be underestimated in the literature, although their findings could be a reflection of chance variation.

These two approaches can be profitably combined in studies of geographic pathology. Wahner *et al.* (1966) examined the relationship of thyroid cancer to goitre in Cali, Columbia—a known endemic goitre area. They showed that the age-adjusted incidence was higher than in Puerto Rico or New York State and that follicular and anaplastic carcinomas, but not papillary carcinomas, were associated with nodular parenchymatous goitre. The foci of carcinoma were, however, found more frequently in tissue *outside* the thyroid nodules. These results are compatible with a common aetiological agent and it is not necessary to involve a sequential process from normality to benign thyroid disease which subsequently becomes malignant. Bondeson and Ljungberg (1981) studied thyroid glands from 500 consecutive autopsies in Malmo in 1979; ten cases were excluded due to previous thyroid surgery. One- to two-mm slices of the fixed glands were scrutinized for macroscopic lesions and were then examined histologically. Fifty-nine per cent of the patients were aged between 61 and 80. A total of 43 primary thyroid carcinomas were found—32 papillary, 7 follicular, 4 medullary—giving a prevalence of 8.6 per cent. All but three follicular tumours were less than 1 cm in diameter; five papillary tumours occurred in multinodular goitres; six papillary and one follicular tumour occurred together with chronic thyroiditis. The authors reviewed other series and suggested that follicular and medullary carcinomas were more frequent in their Swedish study.

Brain

Brain trauma

Walsh *et al.* (1969) reported two cases of meningioma which developed at the site of head injury. Such reports are extremely difficult to evaluate, even if there is good evidence that the tumour is close to the site of documented injury, and case-control studies (such as Choi *et al.* 1970) have failed to substantiate a hazard from trauma.

Toxoplasma infection

Schuman *et al.* (1967) tested sera for *Toxoplasma gondii* infection from 157 patients with cerebral tumours and controls matched for age, sex, race, area, and type of residence. The cases were drawn from four Minnesota-St. Pauls hospitals in 1963-4, and histological information was available in 80 per cent of cases. The controls had attended the same hospitals for any condition except neoplasms at any site or neurological, psychiatric, ophthalmic, or lymphatic disorders. A significant excess of the patients with brain tumour had a positive serological test, particularly for gliomas of all types. There was no significant difference for glioblastomas, meningiomas, and non-verified tumours. There was no evidence that previous transfusion would account for this association, nor that patients with toxoplasmosis were susceptible to cerebral neoplasms or developed a secondary infection.

Leukaemia

In addition to genetic conditions with excess chromosome fragility, there is now good evidence that chromosome abnormalities may be associated with an enhanced risk of leukaemia. The excess of leukaemia developing in subjects with Down's syndrome (Carter 1956; Stewart *et al.* 1958) had been recognized before the chromosomal abnormalities that accompany this condition were elucidated. Other work has demonstrated that patients with chronic myeloid leukaemia may have a deletion of the Philadelphia chromosome (Nowell and Hungerford 1960) and that translocation of this to another autosome may occur (Rowley 1973). A number of reports have indicated an excess of leukaemia cases or deaths in workers exposed to benzene (e.g. McMichael *et al.* 1976*a,b*; Rushton and Alderson 1981). There is some indication that subjects exposed to high levels of benzene have depressed haematopoiesis before leukaemia develops.

References

Adelstein, A. and White, G. (1976). Alcoholism and mortality. *Pop. Trends* **6**, 7.
Alderson, M.R. (1977). *An introduction to epidemiology*. Macmillan, London.

Altman, B.L. and Malament, M. (1967). Carcinoma of the testis following orchiopexy. *J. Urol.* **97**, 498.

Anthony, P.P., Vogel, C.L., Sadikali, F., Barker, L.F., and Peterson, M.R. (1972). Hepatitis associated antigen and antibody in Uganda : correlation of serological testing with histopathology. *Brit. med. J.* **1**, 403.

Armenian, H.K., Lilienfeld, A.M., Diamond, E.L., and Bross, I.D.J. (1974). Relation between benign cancer, prostatic hyperplasia and cancer of the prostate. *Lancet* **2**, 115.

Armijo, R., Orellana, M., Medina, E., Coulson, A.H., Sayre, J.W., and Detels, R. (1981). Epidemiology of gastric cancer in Chile : 1 - case-control study. *Int. J. Epidemiol.* **10**, 53.

Bartholomew, L.G., Gross, J.B., and Comfort, M.W. (1958). Carcinoma of the pancreas associated with chronic relapsing pancreatitis. *Gastroenterol.* **35**, 473.

Bassendine, M.F., Chadwick, R.G., Lyssiotis, T., Thomas, H.C., Sherlock, S., and Cohen, B.J. (1979). Primary liver cell cancer in Britain—a viral aetiology. *Brit. med. J.* **1**, 166.

Beahrs, O.H., Pemberton, J.de J., and Black, B.B. (1951). Nodular goitre and malignant lesions of the thyroid gland. *J. clin. Endocrin. Metab.* **11**, 1157.

Bengtsson, U. and Angervall, L. (1970). Analgesic abuse and tumours of renal pelvis. *Lancet* **1**, 305.

Bondeson, L. and Ljungberg, O. (1981). Occult thyroid carcinoma at autopsy in Malmo, Sweden. *Cancer* **47**, 319.

Bonnevie, O., Binder, V., Anthonisen, P., and Riis, P. (1974). The prognosis of ulcerative colitis. *Scand. J. Gastroenterol.* **9**, 81.

Braun, W. (1958). Carcinoma of the skin and the internal organs caused by arsenic : delayed occupational lesions due to arsenic. *Ger. med. Monthly* **3**, 321.

British Medical Journal (1963). Tuberculosis and cancer. *Brit. med. J.* **1**, 1430.

—— (1975). Benign hyperplasia and cancer of the prostate. *Brit. med. J.* **1**, 2.

—— (1978). Link between hepatoma and hepatitis B. *Brit. med. J.* **2**, 718.

—— (1981). Gastric ulcer : benign or malignant. *Brit. med. J.* **282**, 843.

Bussey, H.J.R. (1975). *Familial polyposis coli.* Johns Hopkins University Press, Baltimore.

——, Wallace, M.H., and Morson, B.C. (1967). Metachronous carcinoma of the large intestine and intestinal polyps. *Proc. R. Soc. Med.* **60**, 208.

Campbell, H.E. (1942). Incidence of malignant growth of the undescended testicle : a critical and statistical study. *Arch. Surg.* **44**, 353.

—— (1959). The incidence of malignant growth of the undescended testicle : a reply and re-evaluation. *J. Urol.* **81**, 663.

Campbell, A.H. and Lee, E.J. (1963). The relationship between lung cancer and chronic bronchitis. *Brit. J. Dis. Chest* **57**, 113.

Carroll, W.A. (1949). Malignancy and cryptorchidism. *J. Urol.* **61**, 396.

Carter, C.O. (1956). Challenge of mongolism. *Brit. med. J.* **2**, 993.

Cheever, A.W. (1981). Schistosomiasis and colon cancer. *Lancet* **1**, 1369.

Ch'en, M-C., Hu, J-C., Chang, P-Y., Chuang, C-Y., Ts'ao, P.F., Chang, S-H., Wang, F.P., Ch'en, T.L., and Chou, S.C. (1965). Pathogenesis of carcinoma of the colon and rectum in *Schistosomiasis Japonica* : a study of 90 cases. *Chinese med. J.* **84**, 513.

——, Chang, P-Y., Chuang, C-Y., Chen, Y-J., Wang, F.P., Tang, Y-C., and Chou, S-C. (1981). Colo-rectal cancer and schistosomiasis. *Lancet* **1**, 971.

Chernozemsky, I.N., Stojanov, I.S., Petkova-Bocharova, T.K., Nicolov, I.G., Dragonov, I.V., Stokker, I.I., Tanchev, Y., Naidenov, D., and Kalcheva, H.D. (1977). Geographic correlation between the occurrence of endemic nephropathy and urinary tract tumours in Vratza district, Bulgaria. *Int. J. Cancer* **19**, 1.

Choi, N.W., Schuman, L.M., and Gullen, W.H. (1970). Epidemiology of primary central nervous system neoplasms. *Amer. J. Epidemiol.* **91**, 467.

Clark, G.G. and Mitchell, P.E.G. (1961). Diabetes mellitus and primary carcinoma of the pancreas. *Brit. med. J.* **2**, 1259.

Clements, F.W. (1954). The relationship of thyrotoxicosis and carcinoma of the thyroid to endemic goitre. *Med. J. Australia* **2**, 894.

The Coordinating Group for Research on Aetiology of Oesophageal Cancer in North China (1975). The epidemiology of oesophageal cancer in North China. *Chinese med. J.* **1**, 167.

Correa, P. (1978). Epidemiology of polyps and cancer. In *The pathogenesis of colo-rectal cancer* (ed. B.C. Morson), pp. 126-52. Saunders, Philadelphia.

——, Cuello, C., and Eisenberg, H. (1969). Epidemiology of different types of thyroid cancer. In *Thyroid cancer* (ed. C.E. Hedinger), pp. 81-93. Heinemann, London.

—— ——, and Duque, E. (1970). Carcinoma and intestinal metaplasia of the stomach in Columbian migrants. *J. Nat. Cancer Inst.* **44**, 297.

—— —— ——, Burbano, L.C., Garcia, F.T., Bolanos, O., Brown, C., and Haenszell, W. (1976). Gastric cancer in Columbia. III. Natural history of precursor lesions. *J. Nat. Cancer Inst.* **57**, 1027.

Costello, R.M. and Schneider, S.L. (1974). Mortality in an alcoholic cohort. *Int. J. Addict.* **9**, 355.

Crespi, M., Muñoz, N., Grassi, A., Aramesh, B., Amiri, G., Mojtabai, A., and Casale, V. (1979). Oesophageal lesions in Northern Iran : a premalignant condition? *Lancet* **2**, 217.

Cruickshank, C.N.D. and Squire, J.R. (1950). Skin cancer in the engineering industry from the use of mineral oil. *Brit. J. indust. Med.* **7**, 1.

Damon, A. and McClung, J.P. (1967). Previous pulmonary disease and lung cancer : a case-control study. *J. chron. Dis.* **20**, 59.

Darke, S.G., Parks, A.G., Grogono, J.L., and Pollock, D.J. (1973). Adenocarcinoma and Crohn's disease. *Brit. J. Surg.* **60**, 169.

Davies, J.N.P. (1975). Overview : geographic opportunities and demographic leads. In *Persons at high risk of cancer* (ed. J.F. Fraumeni), pp. 373-81. Academic Press, New York.

Day, N.E. and Muñoz, N. (1980). *Cancer of the oesophagus.* In *Cancer epidemiology and prevention* (ed. D. Schottenfeld and J.F. Fraumani). Saunders, New York.

Dean, G., MacLennan, R., McLoughlin, H., and Shelley, E. (1979). Cause of death of blue-collar workers at a Dublin brewery, 1954-73. *Brit. J. Cancer* **40**, 581.

Devitt, J.E. (1976). Breast cancer and preceding clinical benign breast disorders. A chance association. *Lancet* **1**, 793.

Doll, R. and Hill, A.B. (1952). Aetiology of carcinoma of the lung. *Brit. med. J.* **2**, 1271.

Donnelly, P.K., Baker, K.W., Carney, J.A., and O'Fallon, W.M. (1975). Benign breast lesions and subsequent breast carcinoma in Rochester. *Mayo Clin. Proc.* **50**, 650.

Edmondson, H.A. and Steiner, P.E. (1954). Primary carcinoma of the liver. A study of 100 cases among 48,900 necropsies. *Cancer* **7**, 462.

Edwards, F.C. and Truelove, S.C. (1964). The course and prognosis of ulcerative colitis, part IV. *Gut* **5**, 15.

Egan, R.L. and Mosteller, R.C. (1977). Breast cancer and mammography patterns. *Cancer* **40**, 2087.

Ehrengut, W. and Schwartau, M. (1977). Mumps orchitis and testicular tumours. *Brit. med. J.* **2**, 191.

Elsebai, J. (1977). Parasites in the etiology of cancer—bilharziasis and bladder cancer. *CA* **29**, 100.
Evans, D.M.D., Hibbard, B.M., Jones, J.M., and Sweetnam, P. (1981). The Cardiff cervical cytology study: prevalence of findings of cytological grades and initial histological findings. *Brit. med. J.* **1**, 689.
Fasal, E. Simmonds, M.E., and Kampert, J.B.(1981). Factors associated with high and low risk of cervical neoplasia. *J. Nat. Cancer Inst.* **66**, 631.
Feinstein, A.R. (1979). Methodologic problems and standards in case-control research. *J. chron. Dis.* **32**, 35.
Fielding, J.F., Prior, P., Waterhouse, J.A.H., and Cooke, W.T. (1972). Malignancy in Crohn's disease. *Scand. J. Gastroenterol.* **7**, 3.
Finke, W. (1956). Chronic pulmonary disease as a possible aetiologic factor in lung cancer. *Int. Rec. Med.* **169**, 61.
Franks, L.M. (1974). Benign prostate hyperplasia. *Lancet* **2**, 293.
Frichot, B.C., Lynch, H.T., Guirgus, H.A., Harris, R.E., and Lynch, J.F. (1977). A new cutaneous phenotype in familial malignant melanoma. *Lancet* **1**, 864.
Gall, E.A. (1960). Post necrotic, post hepatitic, and nutritional cirrhosis. *Amer. J. Pathol.* **36**, 241.
Gambill, E.E. (1971). Pancreatitis associated with pancreatic carcinoma : a study of 26 cases. *Mayo Clin. Proc.* **46**, 174.
Gehring, G.G., Rodriguez, F.R., and Woodhead, D.M. (1974). Malignant degeneration of cryptorchid testes following orchiopexy. *J. Urol.* **112**, 354.
Gelfand, M., Weinberg, R.W., and Castle, W.M. (1967). Relation between carcinoma of the bladder and infestation with *Schistosoma haematobium*. *Lancet* **2**, 1249.
Gibson, R.B. (1971). *Parasites, liver disease, and liver cancer.* IARC Sci. Publ. No.1., Lyon.
Gilbert, J.B.(1944). Tumors of testis following mumps orchitis. *J. Urol.* **51**, 296.
—— and Hamilton, J.B. (1940). Studies in malignant testis tumors : III incidence and nature of tumors in ectopic testes. *Surg. Gynaecol. Obstet.* **71**, 731.
Gilbertsen, V.A. (1974). Proctosigmoidoscopy and polypectomy in reducing the incidence of rectal cancer. *Cancer* **34**, 936.
Gough, K.R., Read, A.E., and Nash, J.M. (1962). Intestinal reticulosis as a complication of idiopathic steatorrhoea. *Gut* **3**, 232.
Graham, S., Dayal, H., Rohrer, T., Swanson, M., Sultz, H., Shedd, D., and Fischman, S. (1977). Dentition, diet, tobacco, and alcohol in the epidemiology of oral cancer. *J. Nat. Cancer Inst.* **59**, 1611.
Greenstein, A.J., Sachar, D.B., Smith, H., Pucillo, A., Papatestas, A.E., Kreel, I., Geller, S.A., Janowitz, H.D., and Aufses, A.H. (1979). Cancer in universal and left-sided ulcerative colitis: factors determining risk. *Gastroenterol.* **77**, 290.
Greenwald, P., Kirmss, V., Polan, A.K., and Dick, V.S. (1974). Cancer of the prostate among men with benign prostatic hyperplasia. *J. Nat. Cancer Inst.* **53**, 335.
Gyde, S.N., Prior, P., Macartney, J.C., Thompson, H., Waterhouse, J.A.H., and Allan, R.M. (1980). Malignancy and Crohn's disease. *Gut* **21**, 1024.
Haenszel, W., Kurihara, M., Locke, F.B., Shimuzu, K., and Segi, M. (1976). Stomach cancer in Japan. *J. Nat. Cancer Inst.* **56**, 265.
Hakkinen, I.P.T., Heinonen, R., Inberg, M.V., Jarvia, O.H., Vaajalahti, P., and Viikari, S. (1980). Clinicopathological study of gastric cancers and precancerous states detected by fetal sulfaglycoprotein antigen screening. *Cancer Res.* **40**, 4308.
Hakulinen, T., Lehtimäki, L., Lehtonen, M., and Teppo, L. (1974). Cancer morbidity among two male cohorts with increased alcohol consumption in Finland. *J. nat. Cancer Inst.* **52**, 1711.

Hart, J., Shani, M., and Modan, B. (1972). Epidemiological aspects of gallbladder and biliary tract neoplasms. *Amer. J. publ. Hlth.* **62**, 36.

Haybittle, J.L. (1962). Study of cancer mortality in England and Wales using birth standardised populations. *Brit. J. preven. Soc. Med.* **16**, 93.

—— (1963). Mortality rates from cancer and tuberculosis. *Brit. J. preven. Soc. Med.* **17**, 23.

Heald, R.J. and Bussey, H.J.R. (1975). Clinical experiences at St. Marks Hospital with multiple synchronous cancers of the colon and rectum. *Dis. Colon Rectum* **18**, 6.

Henry, S.A. (1946). *Cancer of the scrotum in relation to occupation.* Oxford University Press, London.

Higgins, I.T.T. (1975). The epidemiology of cancer of the prostate. *J. chron. Dis.* **28**, 343.

Hill, A.B. and Faning, E.L. (1948). Studies in the incidence of cancer in a factory handling inorganic compounds of arsenic. *Brit. J. indust. Med.* **5**, 1.

Hill, M. (1981). Etiology of the adenoma-carcinoma sequence. In *The pathogenesis of colo-rectal cancer* (ed. B.C. Morson), pp. 153-62. Saunders, Philadelphia.

——, Morson, B.C., and Bussey, H.J.R. (1978). Aetiology of adenoma-carcinoma sequence in large bowel. *Lancet* **1**, 245.

Hinton, J.M. (1966). Risk of malignant change in ulcerative colitis. *Gut* **7**, 427.

Hirabayashi, R.N. and Lindsay, S. (1965). The relationship of thyroid carcinoma and chronic thyroiditis. *Surg. Gynaecol. Obstet.* **121**, 243.

Hirohata, T. (1968). Mortality from gastric cancer and other causes after medical or surgical treatment for gastric ulcer. *J. Nat. Cancer Inst.* **41**, 895.

—— and Kuratsune, M. (1969). The geographical comparison of mortality from cancer of the stomach and ulcer of the stomach in Japan. *Cancer* **23**, 465.

Hoffman, F.L. (1915). The mortality from cancer throughout the world. Prudential Press, Newark, New Jersey.

Holman, C.D.J., Mulroney, C.D., and Armstrong, B.K. (1980). Epidemiology of pre-invasive and invasive malignant melanoma in Western Australia. *Int. J. Cancer* **25**, 317.

Hou, P.C. (1956). The relationship between primary carcinoma of the liver and infestation with Clonorchis sinensis. *J. Path. Bact.* **LXXII**, 239.

Hultengren, N., Lagergren, C., and Ljungquist, A. (1965). Carcinoma of the renal pelvis in renal papillary necrosis. *Acta Chir. Scand.* **130**, 314.

Hutchinson, J. (1888). On some examples of arsenic keratosis of the skin and of arsenic cancer. *Trans. Path. Soc. Lond.* **39**, 352.

Hutchinson, W.B., Thomas, D.B., Hamlin, W.B., Roth, G.J., Peterson, A.V., and Williams, B. (1980). Risk of breast cancer in women with benign breast disease. *J. Nat. Cancer Inst.* **65**, 13.

Imai, T., Kubo, T., and Watanabe, H. (1971). Chronic gastritis in Japanese with reference to high incidence of gastric carcinoma. *J. Nat. Cancer Inst.* **47**, 179.

Ishii, K., Nakamura, K., Takeuchi, T., and Hirayama, T. (1973). Chronic calcifying pancreatitis and pancreatic carcinoma in Japan. *Digestion* **9**, 429.

Jensen, O.M. (1980). Cancer morbidity and causes of death among Danish Brewery workers. International Agency for Research in Cancer. Lyon.

Johansson, S., Angervall, L., Bengtsson, U., and Wahlquist, L. (1974). Uroepithelial tumors of the renal pelvis associated with abuse of phenacetin-containing analgesics. *Cancer* **33**, 743.

Karmody, A.J. and Kyle, J. (1969). The association between carcinoma of the pancreas and diabetes mellitus. *Brit. J. Surg.* **56**, 363.

Keller, A.Z. (1977). Alcohol, tobacco and age factors in the relative frequency of cancer among males with and without liver cirrhosis. *Amer. J. Epid.* **106**, 194.

Kessler, I.I. (1970). Cancer mortality among diabetics. *J. Nat. Cancer Inst.* **44**, 673.
Kodlin, D., Winger, E.E., Morgenstern, N.L., and Chen, I.J. (1977). Chronic mastopathy and breast cancer : a follow-up study. *Cancer* **39**, 2603.
Koss, L.G. (1975). Precancerous lesions. In *Persons at high risk of cancer* (ed. J.F. Fraumeni), pp. 85-101. Academic Press, New York.
——, Melamed, M.R., and Kelly, R.E. (1969). Further cytologic and histologic studies of bladder lesions in workers exposed to para-aminodiphenyl : progress report. *J. Nat. Cancer Inst.* **43**, 233.
Krabbe, S., Skakkebaek, N.E., Berthelsen, J.G., Eyben, F.V., Volsted, P., Mauritzen, K., Eldrup, J., and Nielsen, A.H. (1979). High incidence of undetected neoplasia in maldescent of testes. *Lancet* **1**, 999.
Krook, P.M., Carlile, T., Bush, W., and Hall, M.H. (1978). Mammographic parenchymal patterns as a risk indicator for prevalent and incident cancer. *Cancer* **41**, 1093.
Lancet (1972). Benign and malignant breasts. *Lancet* **2**, 218.
Larouze, B., London, W.T., Saimot, G., Werner, B.G., Lustbader, E.C., Payet, M., and Blumberg, B.S. (1976). Host responses to hepatitis-B infection in patients with primary hepatic carcinoma and their families: a case/control study in Senegal, West Africa. *Lancet* **2**, 534.
Larsson, L., Sandstrom, A., and Westling, P. (1975). Relationship of Plummer-Vinson disease to cancer of the upper alimentary tract in Sweden. *Cancer Res.* **35**, 3308.
Lee, F. (1966). Cirrhosis and hepatoma in alcoholics. *Gut* **7**, 77.
Leevy, C.M., Gellener, R., and Ning, M. (1964). Primary liver cancer in cirrhosis of the alcoholic. *Ann. NY Acad. Sci.* **114**, 1026.
Lennard-Jones, J.E., Morson, B.C., Ritchie, J.K., Shove, D.C., and Williams, C.B. (1977). Cancer in colitis : assessment of the individual risk by clinical and histological criteria. *Gastroenterol.* **73**, 1280.
Levene, A. (1976). Chronic mastitis and carcinoma of the breast. *Lancet* **2**, 475.
Li, F.P. and Fraumeni, J.F. (1972). Testicular cancers in children : epidemiologic characteristics. *J. Nat. Cancer Inst.* **48**, 1575.
MacDougall, I.P.M. (1964). The cancer risk in ulcerative colitis. *Lancet* **2**, 655.
MacLean, J.T. and Fowler, V.B.(1965). Pathology of tumours of the renal pelvis and ureter. *J. Urol.* **75**, 384.
Maram, E.S., Ludwig, J., and Kurland, L.T. (1979). Carcinoma of the gallbladder and extrahepatic biliary ducts in Rochester, Minnesota, 1935-1971. *Amer. J. Epidemiol.* **109**, 152.
Mastromarino, A.J., Reddy, B.S., and Wynder, E.L. (1978). Fecal profiles of anaerobic microflora of large bowel cancer patients and patients with non-hereditary large bowel polyps. *Cancer Res.* **38**, 4458.
Maupas, P., Werner, B., Larouze, B., Millman, I., London, W.T., O'Connell, A., and Blumberg, B.S. (1975). Antibody to hepatitis-B core antigen in patients with primary hepatic carcinoma. *Lancet* **2**, 9.
McCaughan, G., Parsons, C., and Gallagher, N.D. (1979). Primary hepatocellular carcinoma in Australia : aetiological considerations. *Med. J. Aust.* **1**, 304.
McClung, J.P. (1967). Previous pulmonary infection in lung cancer : a review. *J. chron. Dis.* **20**, 65.
McGovern, V.J. and Mackie, B.S. (1958-9). The relationship of solar radiation to melanoblastoma. *Aust. New Zealand J. Surg.* **28**, 257.
McMichael, A.J., Andjelkovic, D.A., and Tyroler, H.A. (1967*a*). Cancer mortality among rubber workers : an epidemiologic study. In *Occupational carcinogens* (ed. U. Saffiotti and J.K. Wagoner), pp. 125-37. *Ann. NY Acad. Sci.* **271**.

——, Spirtas, R., Gamble, J.F., and Toosey, P.M. (1976*b*). Mortality among rubber workers : relationship to specific jobs. *J. occup. Med.* **18**, 178.

Melamed, M.R., Koss, L.G., Ricci, A., and Whitmore, W.F. (1960). Cytohistological observations on developing carcinoma of the urinary bladder in man. *Cancer* **13**, 67.

Monson, R.R. and Lyon, J.L. (1975). Proportional mortality among alcoholics. *Cancer* **36**, 1077.

——, Yen, S., MacMahon, B., and Warren, S. (1976). Chronic mastitis and carcinoma of the breast. *Lancet* **2**, 224.

Mori, W. (1967). Cirrhosis and primary cancer of the liver. Comparative study in Tokyo and Cincinnati. *Cancer* **20**, 627.

Morrison, A.S. (1976). Cryptorchidism, hernia, and cancer of the testis. *J. Nat. Cancer Inst.* **56**, 731.

—— and Cole, P. (1976). Epidemiology of bladder cancer. *Urol. Clin. N. Amer.* **3**, 13.

Muñoz, N., Crespi, M., Grassi, A., Qing, W.G., Qiong, S., and Cai, L.Z. (1982). Precursor lesions of oesophageal cancer in high-risk populations in Iran and China. *Lancet* **i**, 876.

Nasr, A., Gazayerli, M.E., Fawzi, R.M., and Elsebai, A.I. (1962). Epidemiology and pathology of cancer of the bladder in Egypt. *Acta Un. Int. Cancer.* **18**, 528.

Neubauer, O. (1947). Arsenical cancer : a review. *Brit. J. Cancer* **1**, 192.

Nicholls, J.C. (1974). Carcinoma of the stomach following partial gastrectomy for benign gastroduodenal lesions. *Brit. J. Surg.* **61**, 244.

Nicholls, P., Edwards, G., and Kyle, E. (1974). Alcoholics admitted to 4 hospitals in England. II General and cause specific mortality. *Quart. J. Stud. Alcohol* **35**, 841.

Nowell, P.C. and Hungerford, D.A. (1960). Chromosome studies in normal and leukemic human leucocytes. *J. Nat. Cancer Inst.* **25**, 85.

O'Brien, C.J., Saverymuttu, S., Hodgson, H.F.J., and Evans, D.J. (1983). Coeliac disease, adenocarcinoma of jejunum and in situ squamous carcinoma of oesophagus. *J. clin. Path.* **36**, 62.

Olen, E. and Klinck, G.H. (1966). Hyperthyroidism and thyroid cancer. *Arch. Pathol.* **81**, 531.

Page, D.L., Vanderzwaag, R., Rogers, L.W., Williams, T.L., Walker, W.E., and Hartmann, W.H. (1978). Relation between component parts of fibrocystic disease complex and breast cancer. *J. Nat. Cancer Inst.* **61**, 1055.

Parker, R.G.F. (1957). The incidence of primary hepatic carcinoma in cirrhosis. *Proc. R. Soc. Med.* **50**, 145.

Pell, S. and D'Alonzo, C.A. (1973). A five year mortality study of alcoholics. *J. occup. Med.* **15**, 120.

Petković, S., Tomić, M., and Mutavozić, M. (1966). Quelques considerations sur l'étiologie et le clinique du cancer du bassinet. *J. Urol. Néphrol.* **72**, 429.

Postlethwait, R.W. and Musser, A.W. (1974). Changes in the esophagus in 1,000 autopsy specimens. *J. thorac. cardiovasc. Surg.* **68**, 953.

Pott, P. (1775). *Chirurgical observations relative to the cateract, the polypus of the nose, the cancer of the scrotum, the different kinds of ruptures, and the mortification of the toes and feet.* Hawse Clark and Collins, London.

Prendergast, W.J., Milmore, B.K., and Marcus, S.C. (1961). Thyroid cancer and thyrotoxicosis in the U.S. Their relation to endemic goitre. *J. chron. Dis.* **13**, 22.

Prior, P. (1973). Crohn's disease and intestinal cancer. *Brit. med. J.* **2**, 358.

——, Fielding, J.F., Waterhouse, J.A., and Cooke, W.T. (1970). Mortality in Crohn's disease. *Lancet* **1**, 1135.

Ramalingaswami, V. (1969). Iodine and thyroid cancer in man. In *Thyroid carcinoma* (ed. C.E. Hedinger), pp. 111-23. Heinemann, London.
Reddy, B.S., Mastomarino, A., Gustafson, C., Lipkin, M., and Wynder, E.L. (1976). Fecal bile acids and neutral sterols in patients with familial polyposis. *Cancer* **38**, 1694.
——, Martin, C.W., and Wynder, E.L. (1977). Fecal bile acids and cholesterol metabolites of patients with ulcerative colitis, a high-risk group for development of colon cancer. *Cancer Res.* **37**, 1697.
Regelson, W., Kim, U., Ospina, J., and Hollan, J.F. (1968). Hemangioendothelial sarcoma of liver from chronic arsenic intoxication by Fowler's solution. *Cancer* **21**, 514.
Reimer, R.R., Clark, W.H., Greene, M.H., Ainsworth, A.M., and Fraumeni, J.F. (1978). Precursor lesions in familial melanoma. *J. Amer. Med. Assoc.* **239**, 744.
Rimington, J. (1968). Smoking, sputum, and lung cancer. *Brit. med. J.* **1**, 732.
—— (1971). Smoking, chronic bronchitis, and lung cancer. *Brit. med. J.* **2**, 373.
Robinette, C.D., Hrubec, Z., and Fraumeni, J.F. (1979). Chronic alcoholism and subsequent mortality in World War II veterans. *Amer. J. Epidemiol.* **109**, 687.
Robinson, A., Scott, J., and Rosenfeld, D.D. (1970). The occurrence of carcinoma of the pancreas in chronic pancreatitis. *Radiology* **94**, 289.
Rotkin, I.D. (1975). Benign prostatic hyperplasia, prostatic cancer, and carcinogenesis. *Lancet* **2**, 359.
Rowley, J.D. (1973). Chromosomal patterns in myelocytic leukemia. *New Engl. J. Med.* **289**, 220.
Rushton, L. and Alderson, M.R. (1981). A case-control study to investigate the association between exposure to benzene and deaths from leukaemia in oil refinery workers. *Brit. J. Cancer* **43**, 77.
Sartwell, P.E., Arthes, F.G., and Tonascia, J.A. (1978). Benign and malignant breast tumours : epidemiological similarities. *Int. J. Epidemiol.* **7**, 217.
Saunders, J.B., Wodak, A.D., Haines, A., Powell-Jackson, P.R., Portmann, B., Davis, M., and Williams, R. (1982). Accelerated development of alcoholic cirrhosis in patients with HLA-B8. *Lancet* **i**, 1381.
Saxén, E.A. and Saxén, L.O. (1954). Mortality from thyroid disease in an endemic goitre area in Finland. *Docum. med. geogr. et. trop. Amst.* **6**, 335.
Schmidt, W. and de Lint, J. (1972). Causes of death of alcoholics. *Quart. J Stud. Alcohol* **33**, 171.
—— and Popham, R.E. (1981). The role of drinking and smoking in mortality from cancer and other causes in male alcoholics. *Cancer* **47**, 1031.
Schuman, L.M., Choi, N.W., and Gullen, W.H. (1967). Relationship of central nervous system neoplasms to *Toxoplasma gondii* infection. *Amer. J. publ. Hlth.* **57**, 848.
Shapiro, S.J., Friedman, N.B., Perzik, S.L., and Catz, B. (1970). Incidence of thyroid disease in Graves' disease. *Cancer* **26**, 1261.
Shepherd, J.A. (1971). Familial polyposis of the colon with special reference to regression of rectal polyposes after subtotal colectomy. *Brit. J. Surg.* **58**, 85.
Shipman, R.T., Williams, A.L., Kay, R., and Townley, R.R.Q. (1975). A familial study of coeliac disease. *Aust. New Zealand J. Med.* **5**, 250.
Skakkebaek, N.E. (1972). Possible carcinoma-in-situ of the testis. *Lancet* **2**, 516.
—— and Berthelsen, J.G. (1978). Carcinona-in-situ of testis and orchiectomy. *Lancet* **1**, 204.
Smithers, D.W. (1959). Tumours of the thyroid gland in relation to some general concepts of neoplasia. *J. Fac. Rad.* **X**, 3.
Sommers, S.C., Murphy, S.A., and Warren, S. (1954). Pancreatic duct hyperplasia and cancer. *Gastroenterol.* **27**, 629.

Sonakul, D., Koompirochana, C., Chinda, K., and Stitnimankarn, T. (1978). Hepatic carcinoma with opisthorchiasis. *SE Asian J. trop Med. publ. Hlth.* **9**, 215.

Southam, A.H. and Wilson, S.T. (1922). Cancer of the scrotum. *Brit. med. J.* **2**, 971.

Springett, V.H. (1971). Ten-year results during the introduction of chemotherapy for tuberculosis. *Tubercle* **52**, 73.

Stalsberg, H. and Taksdal, S. (1971). Stomach cancer following gastric surgery for benign conditions. *Lancet* **2**, 1175.

Stavraky, K.M. (1971). A study of precursor illness in lung cancer patients. *J. chron. Dis.* **23**, 691.

Steiner, P.E. (1960). Cancer of the liver and cirrhosis in trans-saharan Africa and the United States of America. *Cancer* **13**, 1085.

—— and Davies, J.N.P. (1957). Cirrhosis and primary liver carcinoma in Ugandan Africans. *Brit. J. Cancer* **11**, 523.

Stern, E. and Dixon, W.J. (1961). Cancer of the cervix—a biometric approach to etiology. *Cancer* **14**, 153.

Stewart, A., Webb, J., and Hewitt, D., (1958). A survey of childhood malignancies. *Brit. med. J.* **1**, 1495.

Sundby, P. (1967). *Alcoholism and mortality.* Universitetsforlaget, Oslo.

Tabor, E., Gerety, R.J., Vogel, C.L., Bayley, A.C., Anthony, P.P., Chan, C.H., and Barker, L.F. (1977). Hepatitis B virus infection and primary hepatocellular carcinoma. *J. Nat. Cancer Inst.* **58**, 1197.

Templeton, A.C. (1975). Acquired diseases. In *Persons at high risk of cancer* (ed. J.F. Fraumeni), pp. 69-83. Academic Press, New York.

Thorarinsson, A.A. (1979). Mortality among men alcoholics in Iceland, 1951-74. *J. Studies Alcohol* **40**, 704.

Trichopoulos, D., Tabor, E., Gerety, R.J., Xirouchaxi, E., Sparros, L., Muñoz, N., and Linsell, C.A. (1978). Hepatitis B and primary hepatocellular carcinoma in a European population. *Lancet* **2**, 1217.

Tseng, W.P., Chu, H.M., How, S.W., Fong, J.M., Lin, C.S., and Yeh, S. (1968). Prevalence of skin cancer in an endemic area of chronic arsenicism in Taiwan. *J. Nat. Cancer Inst.* **40**, 453.

Turbitt, M.L., Patrick, R.S., Goudie, R.B., and Buchanan, W.M. (1977). Incidence in South-west Scotland of Hepatitis B surface antigen in the liver of patients with hepatocellular carcinoma. *J. clin. Pathol.* **30**, 1124.

Utsunomiya, J., Murata, M., and Tanimura, M. (1980). An analysis of the age distribution of colon cancer in adenomatosis coli. *Cancer* **45**, 198.

Van der Wal, A.M. Huizinga, E., Orie, N.G.M., Slutter, H.J., and Vries, K.de (1966). Cancer and chronic non-specific lung disease (CNSLD). *Scand. J. resp. Dis.* **47**, 161.

Veale, A.M.O., McColl, I., Bussey, H.J.R., and Morson, B.C. (1966). Juvenile polyposis col. *J. Med. Genet.* **3**, 5.

Vogel, C.L., Anthony, P.P., Mody, N., and Barker, L.F. (1970). Hepatitis-associated antigen in Ugandan patients with hepatocellular carcinoma. *Lancet* **2**, 621.

Vogler, W.R., Lloyd, J.W., and Milmore, B.K. (1962). A retrospective study of etiological factors in cancer of the mouth, pharynx, and larynx. *Cancer* **15**, 246.

Wahner, H.W., Cuello, C., Correa, P., Uribe, L.F., and Gaitan, E. (1966). Thyroid carcinoma in an endemic goitre area, Cali, Columbia. *Amer. J. Med.* ***40***, 58.

Walsh, J., Gye, R., and Connelley, T.J. (1969). Meningioma: a late complication of head injury. *Med. J. Aust.* **1**, 906.

Ward, B. and Hunter, W.M. (1960). The absent testicle : a report of a survey carried out among schoolboys in Nottingham. *Brit. med. J.* **1**, 1110.

Weedon, D.D., Shorter, R.G., Ilstrup, D.M., Huizenga, K.A., and Taylor, W.F. (1973). Crohn's disease and malignancy. *New Engl. J. Med.* **289**, 1099.

Wegelin, C. (1928). Malignant disease of the thyroid gland and its relations to goitre in man and animals. *The Cancer Review III*, 297.

Weiss, N.S. (1976). Breast cancer and preceding breast disease. *Lancet* **1**, 1076.

Whorwell, P.J., Foster, K.J., Alderson, M.R., and Wright, R. (1976). Death from ischaemic heart disease and malignancy in adult patients with coeliac disease. *Lancet* **2**, 113.

Williams, R.D. and Blackard, C.E. (1974). Benign prostatic hyperplasia and cancer of the prostate. *Lancet* **2**, 1265.

Williams, R.R. and Horn, J.W. (1977). Association of cancer sites with tobacco and alcohol consumption and socio-economic status of patients. Interview study from the 3rd National Cancer Survey. *J. Nat. Cancer Inst.* **58**, 525.

Winship, T. (1967). Cancer of the thyroid gland. In *The prevention of cancer* (ed. R.W. Raven and F.J.C. Roe), pp. 319-21. Butterworths, London.

Wolfe, J.N. (1976). Risk for breast cancer development determined by mammographic parenchymal pattern. *Cancer* **37**, 2486.

——, Albert, S., Belle, S., and Salene, M. (1980). Familial influences on breast parenchymal patterns. *Cancer* **46**, 2433.

Wynder, E.L., Bross, I.J., and Day, E. (1956*a*). Study of environmental factors in cancer of the larynx. *Cancer* **9**, 86.

—— —— —— (1956*b*). Epidemiological approach to the etiology of cancer of the larynx. *J. Amer. med. Assoc.* **160**, 1384.

—— —— (1957). Aetiological factors in mouth cancer. *Brit. med. J.* **1**, 1137.

——, Hultberg, S., Jacobsson, F., and Bross, I.J. (1957). Environmental factors in cancer of the upper alimentary tract. *Cancer* **10**, 470.

——, Graham, S., and Eisenberg, H. (1966). Conference on the etiology of cancer of the gastro-intestinal tract. *Cancer* **19**, 1561.

——, Mabuchi, K., Maruchi, N., and Fortner, J.G. (1973). A case-control study of cancer of the pancreas. *Cancer* **31**, 641.

2 The genetics of precancerous lesions

D.G. Harnden

The development of cancer is a multistep process that involves not only an initial cellular event resulting from an alteration in the expression of the cellular genome (which may or may not be the result of a structural change in the DNA) but also the response of other tissues of the body to the abnormal cells. In considering the genetics of neoplasia it is important to appreciate that genetic susceptibility may reside at several different levels. For example, susceptibility could result from an unusual liability of cells to undergo the initial event (initiation) either because they are inherently unstable or because they are unusually sensitive to the carcinogenic action of specific environmental stimuli. We also know from animal experiments that initiated cells may not always progress towards malignancy unless they are exposed to a second 'promoting' stimulus. Susceptibility could reside at this level because of an unusual, genetically determined response to the action of promoting chemicals. For some cancers, immunological controls are important; for others, the precise hormone balance is critical in determining progression. Thus genetically determined changes in immune or endocrine function may be associated with susceptibility to neoplasia.

In some cases of inherited susceptibility to cancer, perhaps the majority, we do not know precisely the nature of the mechanism that leads to susceptibility to cancer. In the following discussion therefore no attempt is made to separate the various conditions according to mechanisms, but where we have some understanding of mechanisms these will be dealt with briefly.

For this consideration of the genetics of premalignant lesions it is convenient to define a premalignant lesion as a clinical situation which should alert the clinician to the possibility that cancer or leukaemia may follow, and, since we are considering the genetics of the situation, we must extend the definition to mean that neoplasia will follow in that patient or in other members of the immediate family. For example, the presence of multiple colonic polyps is clearly associated with a risk of carcinoma of the colon in that patient; but it also makes it imperative that other family members are examined for the presence of colonic polyps because the known mode of inheritance suggests that other family members will also be at risk of colonic carcinoma. If we adopt this definition, two quite distinct categories of lesion emerge:

1. Those where the lesion is itself precancerous;
2. Those which signal that there is a high probability that malignancy may arise elsewhere either in another tissue or another individual.

Polyposis coli would fall into the first category whereas the presence of a deleted chromosome 11 in a child with aniridia and genitourinary anomalies must be considered as a signal that the patient is at a high risk of developing Wilms' tumour. This definition is rather wide and could perhaps be extended to include the whole of cancer genetics and it will therefore be necessary to be somewhat selective, using examples to illustrate the main principles. Attention will be focused on Category 1 disorders, and Category 2 will be considered more briefly.

While in some cases the mode of inheritance is clear, in others there is an undoubted familial incidence but no overt inheritance pattern. Familial examples of this type are considered as are situations where there may be no familial occurrence of neoplasia but where studies of the genetic material of the cell (most often the chromosomes) may help in the elucidation of the problem.

Lesions which are themselves precancerous

Leukoplakia

While this term is correctly applied to lesions occurring in a number of different sites it is commonly used to refer to any white lesion within the oral cavity. The gross appearance is not always a good guide to the potential seriousness of the lesion. In a study of 3256 oral leukoplakias Waldron and Shafer (1975) found severe epithelial dysplasia or carcinoma *in situ* in 4.5 per cent of the specimens while 3.1 per cent showed infiltrating squamous-cell carcinoma. Serial follow-up has shown that only about 5 per cent of cases of simple oral leukoplakia progress to invasive cancer. There are some differences in the overall incidence of leukoplakia and in its sex ratio in different states of the USA. More striking, however, is that in material from Georgia, Florida, and Tennessee, the incidence of epithelial dysplasia was 26.6 per cent while only 7.4 per cent of the specimens from Indiana, Ohio, and Illinois showed evidence of epithelial dysplasia. Similarly, differences in regional incidence of leukoplakia and oral carcinoma have also been shown in studies in India (Mehta *et al.*, 1971), but it seems probable that these differences are more likely to be related to environmental factors such as the chewing of tobacco or betel quid rather than to hereditary differences in the population (Mehta *et al.* 1972).

The one clear instance of inheritance of leukoplakia occurs in the X-linked syndrome, dyskeratosis congenita (Zinsser-Cole-Engman syndrome).

In addition to oral leukoplakia these patients show abnormal cutaneous pigmentation, dystrophy of the nails, atresia of the lacrimal ducts, thrombocytopenia, anaemia, and in some cases testicular atrophy (McKusick 1978). They may also have leukoplakia at other sites including the urethra, glans penis, vagina, and anorectal region.

Sirinavin and Trowbridge (1975) review 50 cases including four patients from a family showing clear X-linked inheritance which they describe in detail. Eight patients had malignant disease. One patient developed three separate malignancies (squamous carcinomas of the tongue and nasopharynx and an adenocarcinoma of the rectum). A second had an epidermoid carcinoma of the buccal mucosa and a mucinous carcinoma of the rectum. The remaining patients had squamous-cell carcinoma of hand, cervix and vagina, buccal mucosa (three cases), and oesophagus. In three cases the carcinoma clearly originated in the pre-existing leukoplakia though the time interval between the recognition of the leukoplakia and the development of carcinoma ranged from 10 to 27 years.

There are some similarities between dyskeratosis congenita and Fanconi's pancytopenia, but, since the latter is inherited as an autosomal recessive condition, there is clearly no direct connection between the two diseases. This is confirmed by the fact that Fanconi patients are unusually susceptible to *in vitro* cell killing and the induction of chromosome change by mitomycin-C and other DNA cross-linking agents. Patients with dyskeratosis congenita do not show this sensitivity (Kano and Fujiwara 1982; Dr A.M.R. Taylor, personal communication). There have been suggestions that spontaneous chromosome aberrations occur in dyskeratosis congenita but most reports find the chromosome to be normal.

Although the evidence of sex linkage is quite clear in some families (Sirinavin and Trowbridge 1975; Cheesebrough and Kinmont 1978), symptoms resembling dyskeratosis congenita have been described in female relatives in some families and they may also develop squamous carcinoma. In these families the mode of inheritance is not clear and the possibility that autosomal forms of the disease exist cannot at present be ruled out.

Warts

Human warts and papillomas are not normally considered to be precancerous lesions. However there are several situations in which cancers do, or appear to, arise out of warts or wart-like lesions. These are (1) condylomata acuminata, which occasionally progress to malignancy; (2) warts in patients with immunodeficiency; (3) warty lesions of the uterine cervix; and (4) warts in patients with the genetically determined disease epidermodysplasia verruciformis (EV).

While there is considerable current interest in the role of papilloma viruses in the aetiology of both condylomata acuminata and warty lesions of the cervix, there is no specific information to suggest that genetic factors are important in either of these diseases. However, in view of the complex interaction between different aetiological factors which is being revealed by a study of EV, it would be prudent to consider that a genetic component may yet prove to be important in determining the progression of these benign lesions to neoplasia.

In individuals with induced immunodeficiency, such as renal homograft patients, the occurrence of multiple warts and *in situ* cancers is associated with the presence of human papilloma virus type 5 (HPV5) which had previously only been associated with EV; this observation prompted the suggestion that HPV5 may have a wide role in the aetiology of skin cancers in immunosuppressed patients (Lutzner *et al.* 1980). In most individuals with the classical inherited immunodeficiency syndromes there does not appear to be an increased incidence of warts or of skin cancers.

Epidermodysplasia verruciformis (Lewandowsky and Lutz 1922) is a familial disease which is probably inherited in an autosomal recessive manner. McKusick (1978) does not consider the mode of inheritance to be demonstrated beyond doubt, but the occurrence of four consanguineous marriages in 16 families reported in one study strongly suggests that inheritance is autosomal recessive. It is possible that there may be more than one mode of inheritance. The disease is characterized by the widespread occurrence of wart-like lesions over all parts of the body, usually starting during childhood. The warts are of two types, flat and pityriaform (resembling the lesions of pityriasis versicolor). The pityriaform warts tend to develop into malignant lesions (about 30 per cent), especially in the sun-exposed areas of the skin. Human papilloma viruses types 3 and 5 (HPV3 and HPV5) have been recovered from EV patients and it appears that HPV5 is especially associated with the pityriaform lesions and hence with malignant change. HPV5 DNA has been demonstrated to be present in the carcinomas of these patients as free unintegrated DNA within the cell nucleus (Ostrow *et al.* 1982). Other HPV types have also been recovered from EV lesions, but these may be subtypes of HPV5 (Yutsudo *et al.* 1982). EV patients have a depressed cell-mediated immunity and also in some cases a deficient antibody response against HPV (Pyrhonen *et al.* 1980). It is clear that patients with immune deficiency are unusually liable to have problems with warts (Bunney 1982). Morrison (1975) in a study of secondary immune deficiency concludes that such problems are most acute in individuals with deficient cell-mediated immunity rather than in those with humoral immune deficiencies. It is curious therefore that no information is available to suggest that patients with inherited immune deficiencies are prone to develop warts. In our own studies on ataxia-telangiectasia (A-T) patients, all of whom have a defect of cell-mediated immunity, we have not found any mention of an increased incidence of warts. If immune deficiency were the critical factor in EV, A-T patients should also have problems with warts. There is, however, one interesting report of a single patient with Fanconi's anaemia and depressed cell-mediated immunity who developed recalcitrant viral warts (Johansson *et al.* 1982). Depressed cellular immunity is not however a regular feature of Fanconi's anaemia, but the authors conclude that the treatment the patient had received could not reasonably account for his depressed immunity. It seems probable that the neoplasia in EV patients results from a complex interaction between a specific HPV serotype, the defective immunity of the patient, exposure to sunlight, and possibly some other genetically determined factor as yet unrecognized.

Interaction between papilloma viruses and the genotype of the host in determining the benign or malignant nature of the lesion has been recognized for many years in animals. The classic work of Shope (1933) showed that rabbit papilloma virus produced benign lesions in the natural host (the cottontail rabbit) while inoculation into domestic rabbits often led to malignant tumours from which the virus could not be recovered.

Dysplastic naevus syndrome

It has been recognized for many years that a proportion (about 1-6 per cent) of malignant melanoma patients had affected relatives. Anderson *et al.* (1967*a*, 1971) documented several examples and showed that familial cases tended to occur earlier, that there was a preponderance of males and that the course of the disease was less aggressive. Clark *et al.* (1977) found 3 per cent of their cases to be familial, confirmed the early onset, but noted that for any given type of lesion the natural history was the same in familial and non-familial cases. About this time several different groups recognized that some of the families with malignant melanoma, perhaps the majority, could be recognized because of the occurrence, even before the appearance of melanoma, of large atypical dysplastic naevi. Different names were proposed. Clark *et al.* (1978) first suggested the name 'B-K mole syndrome' but in later papers this entity is referred to as either the large atypical naevus syndrome (LANS) or the dysplastic naevus syndrome (Green *et al.* 1980; Elder *et al.* 1980). It seems clear that this is the same syndrome described by Lynch *et al.* (1978) as the familial atypical multiple mole melanoma syndrome (FAMMMS). The nomenclature is unimportant—though dysplastic naevus syndrome seems to be fairly widely accepted (*Journal of the American Medical Association* 1981)—but it is of great interest that a new and relatively frequent syndrome involving preneoplastic lesions which signal the probable occurrence of malignant melanoma should now be clearly recognized. The affected patients may have fewer than ten or more than 100 moles. The moles may occur on any part of the body, though they are less frequent on non-exposed surfaces. The pattern of moles may be similar in different members of the same family. The moles vary greatly in size, shape, and colour. They typically range in size from less than 5 mm in diameter to well over 10 mm; they are irregular in outline and often show a mixture of colours in the same mole from pink through various shades of brown (Clark *et al.* 1978). Malignant progression within individual moles has been well documented and it seems certain that close scrutiny of the moles by the subject together with prophylactic treatment in certain instances (Bondi *et al.* 1981) may aid in the prevention of melanoma in some cases. From the studies of Clark *et al.* (1978) and Lynch *et al.* (1978) the mode of inheritance is clearly autosomal dominant with a high degree of penetrance. This was confirmed in a recent report by Greene (1982) who studied 400 members of 14 families prone to the development of cutaneous malignant melanoma (CMM). He confirms that over 90 per cent of familial malignant melanoma patients and 40 per cent of their first relatives show dysplastic naevi. Within these families 31 new primary CMM developed over a 5-year period, all in patients with the dysplastic naevus syndrome (DNS). Family members with DNS are 100 times more likely to develop CMM than persons in the general population.

In patients with melanoma, therefore, the presence of dysplastic naevi should be considered as a high risk factor for the development of multiple primary tumours and also as a risk factor for other family members.

Basal-cell naevus syndrome (BCNS)

This rare disease, also known as Gorlin's syndrome (Gorlin and Goltz 1960), is characterized by the presence of multiple basal-cell naevi and a number of other systemic abnormalities. The commonest are odontogenic keratocysts, bifid rib, and palmar and plantar pits. The patients may also have a very wide range of other minor anomalies of the skin, the skeleton, and other systems. There is often a characteristic facies sometimes described as 'cherubic' because of the presence of jaw cysts, hyperteleorism, and the mild mandibular prognathism seen in most patients. There is a very high susceptibility to the development of basal-cell carcinomas while the occurrence of both medulloblastomas (Gorlin and Sedano 1971) and uterine and ovarian fibromas (Southwick and Schwartz 1979) is so common that susceptibility to these neoplasms must be considered part of the syndrome.

Gorlin and Goltz (1960) originally proposed that this was a single-gene, autosomal dominant condition, a view that has been borne out by the majority of subsequent studies summarized by Gorlin and Sedano (1971). It has been suggested that BCNS is an X-linked trait (Block and Clendenning 1963) but clear examples of male to male transmission seems to rule this out (Anderson *et al.* 1967*b*).

Though there have been rare reports of constitutional chromosome aberrations in BCNS patients it is now agreed that the basic karyotype is normal. Happle *et al.* (1971) and Happle and Kupferschmid (1972) suggest that there may be a higher proportion of chromosome aberrations in both lymphocytes and cultured fibroblasts from patients with BCNS. These and other studies led Hecht and McCaw (1977) to classify BCNS as a chromosomal instability syndrome. However, Featherstone (1981) in a careful study of cultured lymphocytes from eight control subjects and nine BCNS patients (three being members of the same family) concluded that there was no indication of a raised level of spontaneous unstable aberrations in BCNS patients. While the number of stable aberrations in the BCNS patients was greater than in the controls, the difference was not significantly different. Studies on cultured fibroblasts from five BCNS patients again showed no excess of chromosome aberrations as compared with six control subjects. Spontaneous chromosome abnormalities are not, therefore, an important feature of this disease.

Much recent interest has focused on the observation that these patients are unusually sensitive to the induction of basal-cell carcinomas by ionizing radiation. In particular, following radiation to the cranium and spinal axis for the treatment of medulloblastoma in children with BCNS, very large numbers of basal-cell carcinoma have developed within the irradiation field (Strong 1977*a, b*). It seems quite clear, from the number of tumours that arise and their very short latent period (sometimes less than 1 year), that the response of these patients to ionizing radiation is quite unlike that of normal subjects. However *in vitro* studies on cell survival have shown that cells from BCNS patients are normally sensitive to ionizing radiation (Taylor *et al.* 1975; Featherstone 1981) and that they are capable of repair of potential lethal damage. They may be slightly sensitive to the induction of chromosome damage by ionizing radiation (Featherstone *et al.* 1983) but this is not marked compared with the sensitivity of patients with ataxia telangiectasia (Taylor *et al.* 1976).

Xeroderma pigmentosum (*XP*)

The incidence of XP is estimated at between 1 and 4 per million of the population. Of all the premalignant conditions XP has probably been studied more thoroughly from the genetic point of view than any of the others. It is clear that it is inherited in an autosomal recessive manner but studies at the cellular and molecular level strongly suggest that it is not a single abnormal allele that is responsible for all cases of the disease (Giannelli 1976; Kraemer 1980).

The disease is characterized by extreme sun sensitivity. Exposed skin shows extensive freckling with different sizes and colours of freckles. Depigmented areas and regions of telangiectasia are also found. Histological changes in the skin are characteristic of actinic keratosis. As the patients get older multiple skin cancers—basal-cell and squamous carcinomas and melanomas—occur. Some patients show neurological abnormalities and these may be severe (de Sanctis-Cacchione syndrome). It is clear that the skin anomalies are a direct result of sun exposure since if patients with XP are protected from sunlight neither the skin changes nor the neoplasms occur. There are reports of tumours in other tissues in XP patients but it seems unlikely that these are more common than would be expected by chance (Kraemer 1980).

It was shown many years ago by Cleaver (1969) that XP patients are defective in repair of DNA damage caused by ultraviolet light, and it has subsequently been demonstrated that cells from XP patients are also defective in the repair of DNA damage caused by many chemical agents which cause 'u.v.-like' DNA damage and which require 'long patch' excision repair. XP cells are therefore unusually sensitive to cell killing and to the induction of chromosome damage by u.v. light and by certain chemicals such as 4 nitroquinoline-1-oxide (NQO), *N*-acetoxy-2 acetylaminofluorene, and aflatoxin B1. They are not sensitive to other carcinogens and mutagens such as *N*-methyl-*N'*-nitro-*N*-nitrosoguanidine, methyl methane sulfonate, and methyl nitrosourea. XP cells are also more sensitive than are normal cells to the induction of mutations by u.v. light, 4NQO and 2-acetylaminofluorene. The situation is clearly one of great complexity. If, for example, cells from one XP patient are fused with the cells of some (but not all) other XP patients, the hybrids so formed are able to repair u.v.-induced damage (Giannelli 1976; Matsukuma *et al.* 1981). Extensive studies of this kind have revealed seven different complementation groups (A-G). Within each complementation group the characteristics of the individual patients tend to be similar. Thus, Group A patients have a very profound defect of DNA repair (2-5 per cent of normal), show the most severe neurological abnormalities, and include the de Sanctis-Cacchione group. Group E patients have about 50 per cent of the normal capacity for excision repair of u.v.-induced DNA lesions and show less neurological disorder.

In addition to these seven groups some XP patients have been discovered who have normal levels of excision repair of u.v. light-induced lesions and who are deficient in the process of post-replication repair of DNA damage. These XP 'variants' have the usual skin manifestations including cancer but show no neurological abnormalities.

Groups A, C, and the variants are very much commoner overall than the other groups. There are, however, considerable differences in incidence of the various complementation groups in different parts of the world. Group A is the commonest subtype in Japan and substantial numbers of Group A also occur in other parts of the world. Group C cases are very rare in Japan but common in other parts of the world. Of the other types, variants are about twice as frequent in Japan as in other areas (Kraemer 1980). The other groups are represented by only very small numbers of cases, B by only one and E and G by only two families.

The implications of this subdivision of a rare disease into eight subtypes are important for both theoretical and practical reasons. Since complementation in hybrid cells suggests intergenic rather than intragenic complementation, it seems clear that mutation at eight different loci can lead to the phenotype that we call xeroderma pigmentosum. This conclusion suggests that simple deficiency of a site-specific endonuclease is not an adequate explanation. Excision repair probably involves both a glycosylase and an apurinic site endonuclease. Furthermore there is evidence which suggests that XP cells do contain an enzymatic activity which can recognize pyrimidine dimers in DNA but not in chromatin. Thus what at one time seemed a simple enzyme defect is now known to be complex and is still not fully understood.

From the counselling point of view the existence of multiple forms has interesting consequences which would hold equally in other recessive conditions which are comprised of several complementation groups. The probability of a mating between heterozygotes of any one type is considerably decreased so that the total frequency of all heterozygotes in the population must be greater to give the observed frequency of homozygotes than if only one mutant allele existed.

Antenatal diagnosis has been shown to be possible but of course this will only be of potential value to second and subsequent pregnancies in any family.

Neurofibromas

Isolated non-familial neurofibromas rarely, if ever, show malignant change. Indeed the development of a neurofibrosarcoma would suggest that the patient has a significant family history. Multiple neurofibromatosis, or von Recklinghausen's disease (Fig. 2.1), is a clear-cut autosomal dominant inherited disease (Fig. 2.2) whose main features are a variable number of neurofibromas (from one to two to many hundreds) and the presence of multiple *'café-au-lait'* spots. The incidence is about 1 in 3000. In addition to the very obvious skin fibromas, tumours of nerve sheaths may be palpable. Though several forms of this disease have been suggested it seems likely that they form one single entity (Schimke 1977). Bilateral acoustic neuroma is probably a separate autosomal dominant disorder. A variety of other disorders occur irregularly in neurofibromatosis patients including mental retardation, pseudoarthritis of the tibia, and a whole variety of neoplasms such as phaeochromocytomas, meningiomas, gliomas, and optic neuromas. Malignant degeneration of the neurofibromas to give neurofibrosarcomas or fibrosarcomas is estimated to occur in between 3 and 15 per cent of the cases. The precise cellular origin of these malignant tumours is still a matter of discussion among pathologists. While it is often argued that all the cancers seen in neurofibromatosis patients are of neural crest origin, Hope and Mulvihill (1981) have stressed that some of the tumours occurring in excess in these patients, such as Wilms' tumours and leukaemias, are clearly not of neural crest origin while cancers of known neural crest origin, such as melanoma, do not appear to occur in excess. Hope and Mulvihill however point out that accurate information on cancer

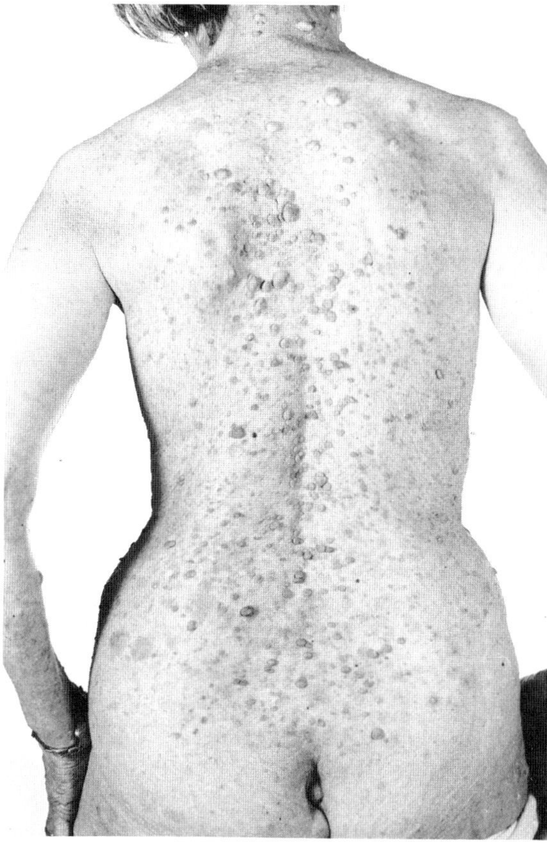

Fig. 2.1. Neurofibromatosis, showing multiple cutaneous neurofibromas (courtesy of Dr. John Hallam).

in neurofibromatosis is hard to obtain because of haphazard reporting of cases.

Polyps and polyposis

Adenomatous polyps of the colon and rectum are usually accepted as potentially precancerous lesions. The risk of malignancy increases as the size and number of the lesions increase. The risk of malignant change is also signalled by the accumulation of cells in the mucosa which fail to repress DNA synthesis so that actively dividing cells are found not only in the proliferation zone of the crypts but also on the surface of flat mucosa and on the villi (Lipkin and Deschner 1977). It has been suggested that some cases with isolated polyps show a familial occurrence and that such families represent an entity discrete from the multiple polyposis syndromes. It seems more likely however, since the variation in number of polyps observed in different

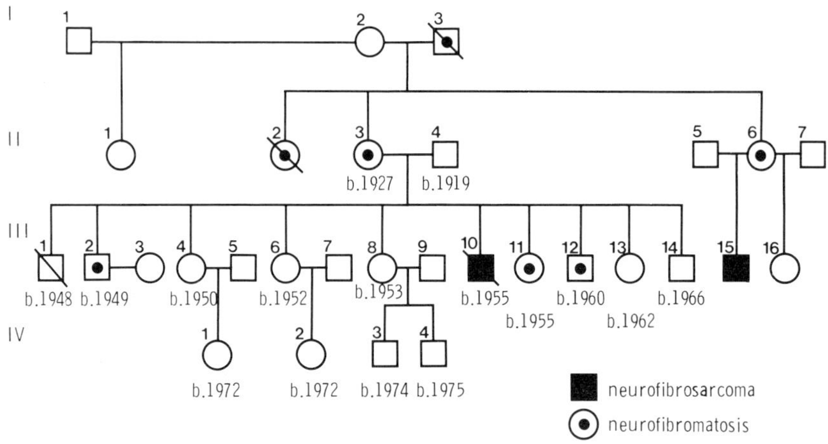

Fig. 2.2. Pedigree of family with neurofibromatosis. The brother (III 10) of the propositus (III 12) and a maternal cousin (III 15) both developed neurofibrosarcoma. III 10 has now died while III 15 is alive and well after amputation of a lower limb.

individuals in polyposis families is very great, that these cases represent extreme variants of the polyposis genes.

There are several distinct familial syndromes involving polyposis of the intestine. Classical familial polyposis coli (FPC), also known as adenomatosis of the colon and rectum (ACR) or intestinal polyposis type I, is characterized by extremely numerous adenomatous polyps of the colon and rectum. The probability of development of carcinomatous change is very high indeed and virtually all affected members of these families eventually develop carcinomas if left untreated (Muto, Bussey, and Morson 1976). The age of onset of malignancy may vary considerably. Some very young cases of cancer have been reported though some families with 'juvenile polyposis' have hamartomatous polyps which are probably not precancerous (Veale *et al.* 1966). The average age for detection of carcinomas in polyposis families is reported to be 30 years (Anderson and Romsdahl 1977). It is clear that familial polyposis coli is inherited in an autosomal dominant manner and, while the expressivity may vary in terms of the number of polyps, the penetrance is close to 100 per cent.

It is usual to restrict the term familial polyposis coli to patients whose polyps are confined to the colon and rectum and who do not show any other intestinal abnormalities. There are however two other conditions characterized by intestinal polyps which are also inherited in an autosomal dominant fashion. These are the Peutz-Jegher syndrome and the Gardner syndrome which McKusick (1978) classifies as intestinal polyposis types II and III respectively. In the Peutz-Jegher syndrome polyps may occur in any part of the gastro-intestinal tract though jejunal polyps are always present. The probability of progression to malignancy is less than in FPC but may occur in any part of the gastrointestinal tract (Dodds *et al.* 1972). Polyps may also occur at other sites such as the bladder, bronchus, and nose. The patients are, in addition, characterized by the presence of melanized spots on the lips, face, and hands. This disease does seem to be a distinctive entity. On the other hand the division between the Gardner syndrome and FPC is by no means a sharp one. In the Gardner syndrome polyps may occur primarily in the colon but also in the small intestine and also the stomach. Like those of FPC, the polyps frequently undergo malignant change. The distinguishing feature is the presence of benign tumours of other tissues such as fibromas (on the face) and sebaceous or epidermal tumours (of the back); fibromas are also common, especially following surgery.

While these conditions are clearly determined by single genes, there has been considerable discussion of the role of chromosome changes in these disorders. Danes *et al.* (1977) reported increased tetraploidy in 'epithelial derived cells' from patients with the Gardner syndrome. Later studies reported increased tetraploidy also in skin cells from familial polyposis coli patients (Danes and Alm 1979; Delhanty *et al.* 1980). It seems probable that in both cases the cells being studied were fibroblasts. More recently Gardner *et al.* (1980) and Delhanty *et al.* (1983) have reported the occurrence of chromosome abnormalities of many different kinds in lymphocytes and in fibroblasts cultured from both the skin and colonic tissue from polyposis patients. Delhanty *et al.* record tetraploidy in skin fibroblast cultures from only some patients and even then not in all cultures. Tetraploidy levels tended to be high in fibroblasts derived from colon biopsies. All classes of chromosome aberration rings, dicentrics, fragments, breaks, and nonclonal rearrangements were approximately threefold higher in FPC cultures than in control cultures. Delhanty *et al.* comment particularly on the formation of clones of cells with stable chromosome rearrangements. Seven out of 23 cultures showed clones and in several cultures a very high proportion of the cells (in two cases, 100 per cent) showed a clonal rearrangement even at an early stage in the culture. This could mean that the clones either have a considerable proliferative advantage or were present *in vivo.* While cytogenetically abnormal clones do occur in fibroblasts cultured from normal subjects (Harnden *et al.* 1976), it is suggested that they occur more commonly at an early culture stage in FPC patients.

Whether or not these observations have any bearing on the development of benign and malignant tumours in these patients is not known. Mitelman *et al.* (1974) have, however, demonstrated chromosome aberrations in polyps from both polyposis patients and from non-familial cases.

Carcinoma in situ

Carcinoma *in situ* may occur in many different tissues. The majority of cases do not show any familial pattern. In some cases however a pattern of genetic interest is noted and a few examples are given below.

(*a*) *Breast.* The relationship between benign breast disease and mammary carcinoma is a complex issue which is discussed in Chapter 4. But it does seem clear that in patients with lobular neoplasia (lobular carcinoma *in situ*) of the breast the risk of developing breast carcinoma is increased if there is a significant family history. Lattes (1980) report that in a series of 209 patients with lobular disease of the breast the ratio of patients observed to develop breast carcinoma compared with the expected number was approximately 6:1 for patients with no mother or sister with breast carcinoma but 13.8:1 for those who did have an affected mother or sister. This observation may be of special interest since Black and Kwon (1980) suggest that progression to malignancy may be promoted by oral contraceptives in those cases of carcinoma *in situ* of the breast with a family history but that they may be protective in patients with no affected relatives. It is quite unclear, however, whether or not these familial cases are genetically determined and further study of this situation should prove to be interesting.

(*b*) *Endometrium.* Carcinoma of the endometrium is uncommon in young women though Ostor *et al.* (1982) have described four cases in women under 40, all of whom were found to have abnormal chromosome compliments (45,X or 45,X mosaicism). In two patients extensive areas of adenocarcinoma *in situ* of the endometrium were observed. While the role of hormone therapy complicates the discussion in three cases (see Chapter 13), in one case no hormone therapy had been given.

(*c*) *Cervix.* There are several reports of carcinoma *in situ* of the uterine cervix occurring in mother and daughter (Andrews *et al.* 1981; Chiemchanya 1982). It is of considerable interest that in some of these families the carcinoma *in situ* was recognized at a very early age (17 years in one of Andrews' cases and 21 years in the family described by Chiemchanya). While both authors are cautious in ascribing the familial occurrence to heredity it seems possible that such family groupings could be due to genetic factors.

Hydatidiform mole

The incidence of hydatidiform mole varies widely in different parts of the world from 1 in 200 in parts of south-east Asia to 1 in 2000 in Europe and North America (Bagshawe and Lawler 1982*a*). About 10 per cent of molar pregnancies lead on to invasive mole or the development of choriocarcinoma (Bagshawe and Lawler 1982*b*). While approximately 70 per cent of all moles are partial moles (Jacobs *et al.* 1982) about 70 per cent of those moles that have serious sequelae are complete moles (Stone and Bagshawe 1976).

There is little evidence to suggest that the occurrence of a molar pregnancy is a familial trait. It appears to be determined more by environmental factors since Japanese migrants living in Hawaii do not have the high incidence found among Japanese in Japan (Jacobs *et al.* 1982). Age too is a predisposing factor, complete molar pregnancies being commoner in both younger and older mothers (Jacobs *et al.* 1982).

The cytogenetic findings are of considerable interest, and these are reviewed concisely by Bagshawe and Lawler (1982*b*). It has been known for many years that the chromosomes in a complete hydatiform mole were indistinguishable from those of a normal female by classical cytogenetic techniques (Harnden 1961). However it soon became apparent that moles could be divided by both pathologists and cytogeneticists into two groups: (i) classical complete moles with absence of embryo and a 46, XX karyotype; (ii) partial moles where only some of the villi show hydatidiform change, where an embryo is normally present and where most, if not all, cases have a triploid chromosome composition. Kajii and Ohama (1977) showed, using chromosomal heteromorphic markers, that for complete moles the 46, XX karyotype was derived by diandry in the majority of cases. This has been confirmed by Bagshawe and Lawler (1982*a*) and by Jacobs *et al.* (1980, 1982). It seems most likely that an enucleate ovum is fertilized by a normal sperm which then divides to restore the diploid number; subsequent parthenogenetic development leads to a molar pregnancy in which there is widespread if not complete homozygosity. The possibility of fertilization of an enucleate ovum by a diploid sperm is ruled out in most instances but the recognition of cases of 46, XY moles by Jacobs *et al.* and by others suggests that this is another possible origin of molar pregnancies. The earlier observations that most partial moles are triploid is borne out by recent studies. Jacobs *et al.* (1982) found 75 out of 80 partial moles in which cytogenetic results were obtained to be triploid. Four out of the five remaining cases had chromosome abnormalities of other kinds (three with trisomy 16, and one with monosomy X). Lawler *et al.* (1982) showed that out of 15 cases of partial mole studied, diandry was the mechanism in six cases. In all cases studied dispermy was possible and this was considered proven in four cases.

It is particularly interesting that the highest risk of malignancy should be associated with the complete moles which are uniformly homozygous, since there have been many suggestions that malignancy may be the result of sequential mutations either inherited or acquired which result in homozygosity at a specific and critical locus (Knudson 1973).

Benign ovarian teratomas

There is now some evidence that ovarian teratomas may also show substantial regions of homozygosity suggesting an origin in a cell in which the second meiotic division has failed giving rise to a parthenogenetic development. In one remarkable patient described by Carritt, Parrington, West, and Povey (1982) seven benign ovarian teratomas (five in the right ovary and two in the left) were all found to have independent origins by studying chromosomal polymorphisms and enzyme markers. In three of the cysts the degree of homozygosity suggested failure of meiosis II or possibly endoreduplication of a triploid gamete. The other cysts all showed quite extensive heterozygosity more compatible with failure of the first meiotic division. These findings confirm the germ cell origin of these tumours.

Preleukaemia

Preleukaemia is a heterogeneous group of blood disorders in which neither the clinical picture nor the haematological findings justify the designation leukaemia but where experience has shown that a proportion of them (about 25 per cent) will develop into acute non-lymphocytic leukaemia (ANLL). Several groups have shown that a proportion of patients with 'preleukaemia' may have chromosome abnormalities in direct preparations made from bone marrow. A review of 224 such patients is presented in the report of the Second International Workshop on Chromosomes in Leukaemia (1980). While most of these abnormalities are random, certain types of aberration such as trisomy 8, monsomy 7, and 7q- monsomy 5 and 5p- occur more frequently than would be expected by chance. These abnormalities tend to resemble the kind of aberration found in the fully developed acute non-lymphocytic leukaemia, suggesting that some of the chromosomal events can occur at an early stage of the disease. The specific translocations associated with acute leukaemia were not found in the preleukaemias. Of the cases with entirely normal chromosomes 15 per cent progressed to ANLL while, in those with either some or all of the cells with abnormal chromosomes, roughly 27 per cent progressed to ANLL.

Nowell (1982) divides the preleukaemias into three groups: (1) the dysmyelopoietic syndromes where there is a very high (50-75 per cent) risk of progressing to leukaemia; (2) the myeloproliferative disorders with a 5-15 per cent risk of ANLL; and (3) an ill-defined group including the chromosome breakage syndromes (*vide infra*) and unexplained marrow hypoplasias and dysplasias. Nowell agrees that certain specific aberrations are observed in addition to random changes. He concludes however that only in the dysmyelopoietic syndromes is an abnormal chromosome complement of prognostic value. In the myeloproliferative disorders the presence of a cytogenetically abnormal clone does not necessarily indicate imminent progression to leukaemia.

Disorders associated with a high incidence of neoplasia

In this group of diseases the lesions observed may not themselves be premalignant (though they may affect the tissue in which malignancy ultimately arises), but the association with malignant disease is so strong that they can be considered precancerous.

Chromosome disorders

(*a*) *Chromosome breakage syndromes.* While many diseases have been designated as chromosome breakage syndromes such as scleroderma, porokeratosis of Mibelli, and incontinentia pigmenti, only the three diseases where there is widespread agreement about chromosome changes and susceptibility to malignancy will be considered here. These are Fanconi's anaemia, ataxia-telangiectasia, and Bloom's syndrome. Each has its own characteristic pattern of chromosome damage and its own spectrum of malignant disease. All three are, however, quite clearly inherited in an autosomal recessive manner.

Ataxia-telangiectasia (A-T) has recently been reviewed (Bridges and Harnden 1982) and is described only briefly here. In A-T a progressive cerebellar ataxia is associated with telangiectasia of the conjunctivae (Fig. 2.3),

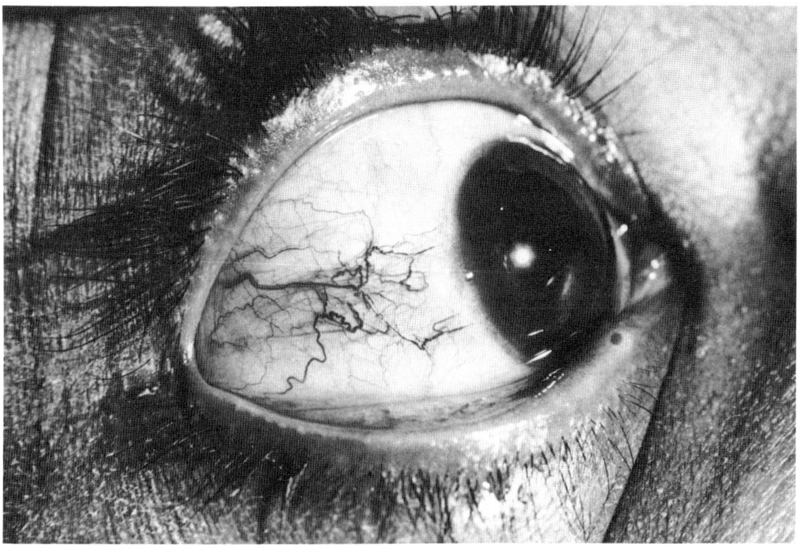

Fig. 2.3. Right eye of a patient with ataxia-telangiectasia to show the characteristic telangiectasia which differentiates A-T from other ataxias.

butterfly area of the face, ears, and possibly hands and feet. The telangiectasia may be quite inconspicuous in early life and differential diagnosis may be difficult. These patients are all unusually sensitive to ionizing radiation and the demonstration of the radio-sensitivity at cellular and chromosomal level can form the basis of a firm diagnosis in early childhood, or even antenatally. Most cases show spontaneous chromosome breakages in cultured peripheral blood lymphocytes (Taylor 1982). There appears to be no particular pattern of aberration except that many patients develop cytogenetically marked clones of lymphocytes which expand with time. Many of the clones have specific aberrations (Fig. 2.4) often involving translocation between chromosome band 14q12 and a small number of other locations, notably the short or long arms of chromosome 7, the long arm of the X chromosome, and the end of the other chromosome 14 (14q32). All patients show a defect of cell-mediated immunity, a consequent susceptibility to infection, and raised levels of serum alpha-fetoprotein (AFP). Some patients have a specific deficiency of IgA or IgE. It is generally agreed that cells from A-T patients show a defect of repair of DNA damage caused by ionizing radiation or radiomimetic chemicals such as bleomycin and neocarzinostatin. In particular, the repair of potentially lethal damage is defective but there is no consensus on the nature of the defect. Further, following exposure to ionizing radiation, A-T cells do not reduce replication synthesis of DNA to the same extent as do normal cells. These techniques have been used to demonstrate that, as in XP, several different complementation groups of A-T exist.

Interest has focused on A-T patients because of their undoubted susceptibility to malignant disease (Spector *et al.* 1982). Most of the malignancies are lymphomas or lymphocytic leukaemias but tumours of the brain,

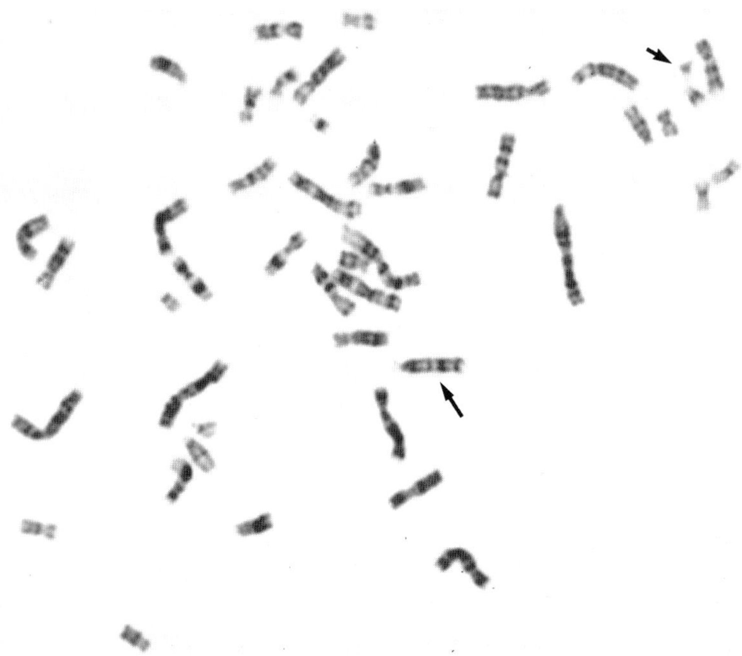

Fig. 2.4. G-banded chromosomes of a peripheral blood lymphocyte from a patient with ataxia-telangiectasia. The spontaneously occurring chromosome translocation between two chromosomes 14 results in one abnormally short acrocentric chromosome (small arrow) and one abnormally long acrocentric chromosome (long arrow); (courtesy of Dr. Malcolm Taylor).

ovary, stomach, skin, parotid, liver, and breast have also been reported. The early onset of carcinoma of the stomach is particularly striking. It has been suggested that the unusual sensitivity to radiation or the immunodeficiency may be important factors in the onset of cancer, but the cancer pattern does not resemble exactly either that seen in irradiated subjects or in other immune-deficient patients.

There is some evidence that the lymphoid neoplasms arise within the pre-existing lymphoid clones (Kaiser-McCaw and Hecht 1982) but this is not always so. Nevertheless, the parallel between the specific chromosome aberrations in A-T and those that have been reported in B cell lymphomas is close, and it is tempting to speculate that these translocations may represent rearrangements of the genome which bring together activated promoting regions and cellular oncogenes.

Epidemiological studies suggest that cancer incidence may be increased in A-T heterozygotes (Swift 1982). If confirmed, this could have far-reaching consequences, since the incidence of A-T in the population is estimated at 1 in 40 000 so that 1 per cent of the population are heterozygotes.

Bloom's syndrome is another rare autosomal recessive disease where there is a high probability of development of cancer. The features of the disease are short stature, a sun-sensitive erythema, and a characteristic 'bird-like' facies. Patients are particularly liable to respiratory and gastro-intestinal infections, and defects of both humoral and cell-mediated immunity have been described. Spontaneous chromosome aberrations are found regularly in cultured lymphocytes. In particular, chromatid interchanges involving symmetrical exchanges between homologous chromosomes are regularly observed in these patients. The resulting quadriradial figures are quite characteristic of this disease. In addition there is an unusually high frequency of sister chromatid exchanges (SCE) though in some patients there appear to be two populations—one with and one without increased numbers of SCEs (German *et al.* 1977). There is no clear evidence of any abnormality of DNA repair in cells from Bloom's patients but there are several indications that the cells are sensitive to u.v. light and that DNA replication may be abnormal (Giannelli *et al.* 1977).

Patients with Bloom's syndrome have an unusually high incidence of many different kinds of cancer. Like A-T there is a preponderance of reticuloendothelial neoplasms but cancers of many other tissues such as skin, colon, and oesophagus have also been reported to occur at unusually early ages (German *et al.* 1979).

Patients with Fanconi's anaemia, another autosomal recessive disease (Schroeder *et al.* 1976), typically show marked growth retardation and a range of other abnormalities of which aplasia or hypoplasia of thumb and radius are the most common. There is a progressive panmyelopathy leading to anaemia, leucopenia, and thrombocytopenia. The age of onset of anaemia varies, and it may not be obvious till late childhood in some cases.

There is a high incidence of spontaneous chromosome aberrations in cultured lymphocytes and (in particular) of non-symmetrical, non-homologous chromatid interchanges (Fig. 2.5) giving rise to quadriradial or triradial configurations, the patterns being quite unlike those seen in Bloom's syndrome (Schroeder and German 1974). The cells do not have elevated SCE levels.

Cultured cells from Fanconi patients are unusually sensitive to mitomycin-C (Sasaki 1975) and to other DNA cross-linking agents such as diepoxybutane (Auerbach *et al.* 1981). This may be demonstrated either by cell killing or by the induction of chromosome aberrations. Once again the pattern is characteristic and is of considerable help in early and antenatal diagnosis.

It has been recognized for some time that there is an unusual risk of leukaemia, especially acute myelomonocytic leukaemia, in these patients. There are also several reports of hepatoma though there is some evidence to suggest that these may, at least in some cases, be the consequence of treatment with drugs such as oxymetholone (Obeid *et al.* 1980). There seems no doubt, however, that neoplasms other than leukaemia do occur more often than expected in Fanconi patients. A report that there is an increased cancer risk in relatives has not been confirmed by more recent studies (Swift 1982).

(*b*) *Constitutional chromosome aberrations.* While chromosome aberrations are relatively common as causes of congenital malformations, there is

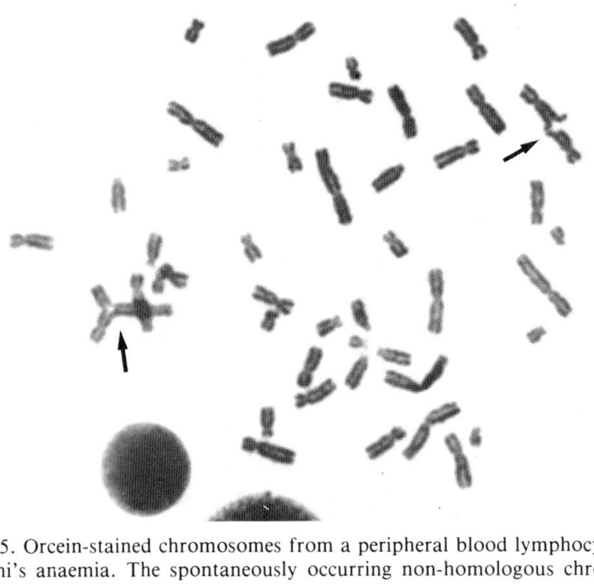

Fig. 2.5. Orcein-stained chromosomes from a peripheral blood lymphocyte of a patient with Fanconi's anaemia. The spontaneously occurring non-homologous chromatid interchanges which are characteristic of this syndrome are arrowed (courtesy of Dr. Gillian Duckworth).

no evidence that there is an overall increased incidence of chromosome aberrations in a population of cancer patients (O'Riordan *et al.* 1972). The presence of certain specific chromosome aberrations does, however, indicate an increased probability that particular cancers or leukaemias may occur. Interest in this area has recently increased quite dramatically with the recognition that cellular homologues of viral oncogenes are present in human cells and moreover that they can be precisely localized on specific chromosomes (Sakaguchi *et al.* 1982). Most attention has focused so far on acquired specific chromosome aberrations, but constitutional chromosome abnormalities associated with specific neoplasms are also now under close scrutiny. The increased incidence of leukaemia in patients with Down's syndrome (trisomy 21) which has been recognized for many years (Miller 1970) together with the common occurrence of an extra chromosome 21 in leukaemia patients has led to the suggestion that specific genes on chromosome 21 may be important in the development of both lymphocytic and non-lymphocytic leukaemias (Rowley 1981). The increased incidence of carcinoma of the breast in males (47, XXY) with Klinefelter's syndrome (Harnden *et al.* 1971) may, however, be due to the hormonal imbalance which occurs in these patients rather than to the activation of specific genes caused by the chromosome abnormality.

More recently, several highly specific chromosome rearrangements have been associated with particular cancers. A remarkable family reported by Cohen *et al.* (1979) shows a clear association between a translocation involving chromosomes 3 and 8 (46, XX or XY, t (3;8) (p21;q24)) and renal-cell carcinoma, but so far this family is unique. Nevertheless, the presence of such a translocation should immediately suggest the possibility of kidney carcinoma. Similarly, two other abnormalities, deletion of the short arm of chromosome 11 (including band 11p13) and deletion of the long arm of chromosome 13 (including band 13q14), clearly indicate an increased risk of Wilms' tumour and retinoblastoma respectively (see review by Harnden and Herbert 1982). In both instances the deletion is associated with a malformation syndrome, the severity of which depends on the extent of the deletion. In the case of the deletions of the short arm of 11 (Fig. 2.6) the main anomalies are aniridia, genitourinary abnormalities (Fig. 2.7), and mental retardation (Riccardi *et al.* 1978). While children with this group of malformations and the deleted 11 are very likely to develop Wilms' tumour not all such cases do so. Francke *et al.* (1978) report apparently monozygotic twins with aniridia and a deletion of the short arms of chromosome 11, of whom only one developed Wilms' tumour. It is important to remember that the majority of children with Wilms' tumours have normal chromosomes and the group with a deleted 11 form a special sub-group.

Children with a deletion of the long arm of chromosome 13 have a variety of different abnormalities, but several show anomalies of eye development (Hittner *et al.* 1980). Such patients are at an increased risk of developing

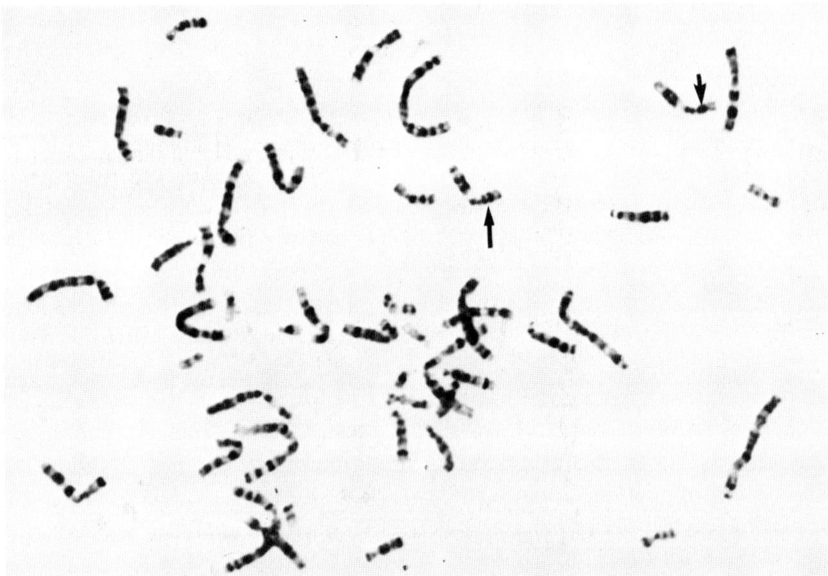

Fig. 2.6. G-banded chromosomes of a peripheral blood lymphocyte from a patient with Wilms' tumour and aniridia. A small deletion of the pale band 11p13 (small arrow) brings the two dark bands 11p12 and 11p14 much closer together than they are on the normal chromosome 11 (large arrow).

retinoblastoma. The reported deletions vary in extent and the only segment common to all the retinoblastoma patients is band 13q14. Indeed the case of Yunis and Ramsay (1978) suggests that deletion of only a part of the band 13q14 may be necessary. Once again the deletion cases of retinoblastoma are only a small proportion of all cases of retinoblastoma, probably not more than 5 per cent; but two recent reports describe mosaicism for deletions of chromosome 13 in patients with retinoblastoma and it is therefore possible that this may play an important role in the genesis of this tumour in nonfamilial cases (Motegi 1982; Orye *et al.* 1982).

There have been suggestions that other specific chromosome abnormalities are associated with particular cancers—for example, the association of the multiple endocrine neoplasia type 2 (MEN II) syndrome with a deletion of chromosome 20 p12.2 (van Dyke *et al.* 1981)—but there is as yet no general agreement about such cases.

(*c*) *Inappropriate sex chromosomes.* While not strictly chromosome abnormalities these cases are usually confirmed by chromosome techniques. Briefly, the presence of a Y chromosome in a patient with a female phenotype is associated with an increased risk of both dysgerminoma and gonadoblastoma (Teter 1976). Patients with testicular feminization seem to have little or no increase in risk and patients with 46, XX gonadal dysgenesis have no increased risk. In Teter's series, out of 25 gonadal dysgenesis patients with a 46,XY complement or who were mosaic with one line at least having

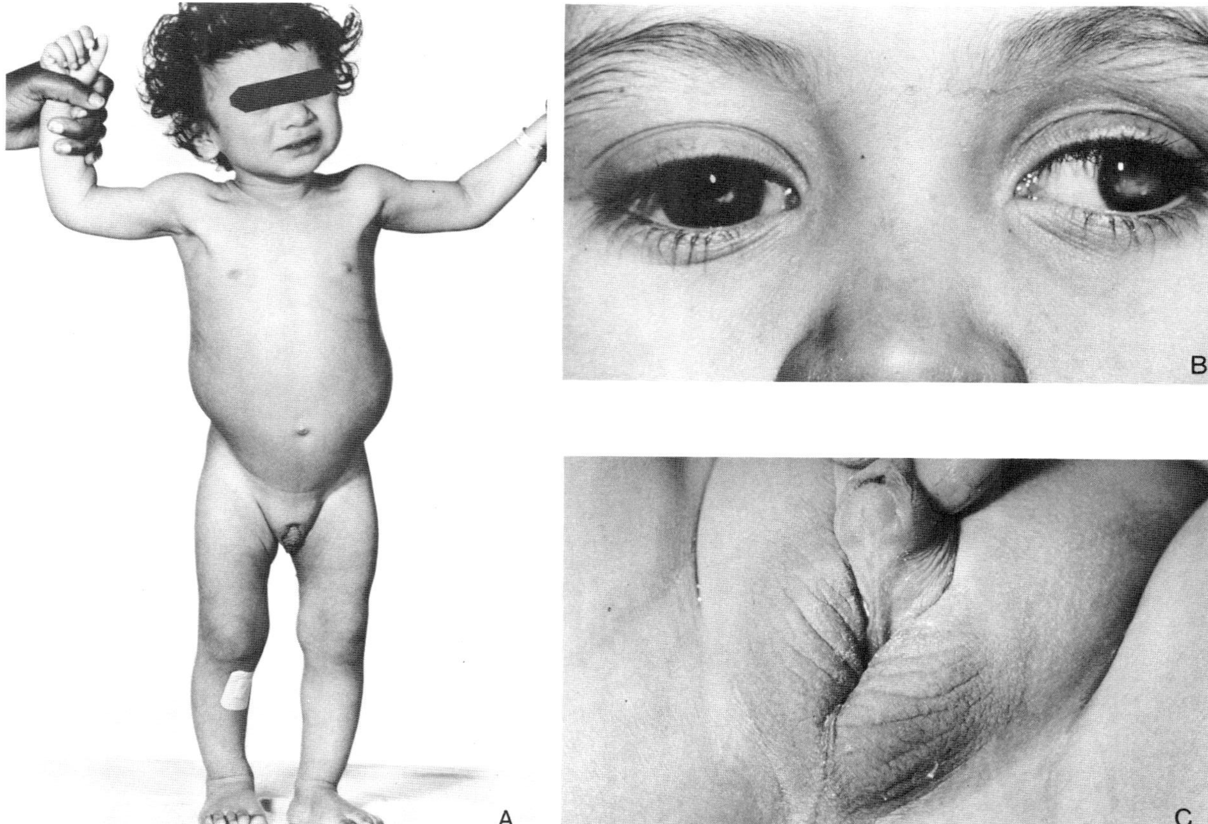

Fig. 2.7. Wilms' aniridia syndrome showing (A) abdominal swelling at diagnosis indicating bilateral Wilms' tumours, (B) aniridia, and (C) abnormal external genitalia (courtesy of Dr. J.R. Mann).

a Y chromosome, 14 developed tumours, while none of his 24 patients with testicular feminization developed tumours. This exceptionally high risk of malignancy in gonadal dysgenesis appears even more marked in familial cases. Mann *et al.* (1982) report a family in which five phenotypic females with a 46, XY karyotype all had gonadal tumours. The trait is inherited within the family in an X-linked fashion. The index case, a 14-year-old girl, died of a yolk sac tumour arising in a dysgenetic pelvic gonad, while her two sisters were shown to have bilateral gonadoblastomas when their gonads were removed prophylactically. A maternal aunt and a maternal cousin also had gonadal tumours.

There is no question that in such cases the chromosomal sex is a dramatic indicator of high cancer risk and this can lead to the removal of cancers or precancerous lesions before clinical problems have arisen.

Genetically determined immunodeficiency diseases (GDID)

It would not be appropriate to consider the immune deficiency diseases in detail here but they unquestionably fall within the definitions given at the beginning of this chapter. Much of the information except for individual case reports comes from the work of the Immune Deficiency Cancer Registry in the University of Minnesota, Minneapolis. In a series of reports, Kersey, Spector, and their colleagues record cases that have been reported to them of cancer occurring in patients with a prior diagnosis of GDID (Spector *et al.* 1978; Filipovich *et al.* 1980). They list the patients according to the WHO classification criteria for immunological disorders. The principal categories are ataxia-telangiectasia (A-T), Wiskott-Aldrich syndrome (WAS); common variable immunodeficiency (CVI), selective IgA deficiency, X-linked (Bruton) agammaglobulinaemia, severe combined immunodeficiency, selective IgM deficiency, immunodeficiency with normal or elevated immunoglobulins, and a miscellaneous group. In the most recent report A-T, WAS, and CVI account for 101, 52, and 74 out of a total of 292 cases recorded as having cancer and far outnumber the other types. The general conclusions are that there is a considerable excess of cancer amongst all the groups of patients. While each type of immunodeficiency has its own characteristic pattern of cancer occurrence (including age of onset and histological type), certain generalities can be stated. Lymphomas account for 58 per cent of all malignancies, leukaemias 17 per cent, epithelial tumours 23 per cent, and others 2 per cent. In children the most likely tumour is non-Hodgkin lymphoma while in adult patients non-Hodgkin lymphomas and carcinomas occur in almost equal proportions.

The genetics and cytogenetics of A-T have already been considered (p. 57). Wiskott-Aldrich syndrome, characterized by eczema, thrombocytopenia, proneness to infection, and bloody diarrhoea is clearly an X-linked recessive disease. The vast majority of neoplasms which occur in WAS are lymphoid while epithelial tumours are rare. The other immunodeficiency diseases are conveniently grouped according to the WHO system for clinical and diagnostic purposes but they may not represent discrete, homogeneous entities from the genetic point of view. One form of agammaglobulinaemia, Bruton-type, which is due to a defect of B-cells is inherited in an X-linked manner. However, severe combined immunodeficiency may have both X-linked and autosomal recessive forms. Even the autosomal recessive form may be due to several different genes since one form is clearly associated with deficiency of adenosine deaminase while others are not.

The genetics of selective immunoglobulin deficiencies may be even more complex. Selective IgA deficiency is relatively common, but only a proportion of cases will be genetically determined and even amongst those that appear to be familial there is no general agreement about the mode of inheritance. A useful brief summary of the genetics of the immune deficiency diseases is given by Kirkpatrick (1979).

Other single gene disorders

There are several other conditions which have neither chromosomal abnormalities nor inherited immune deficiency but which clearly indicate patients at risk of developing malignancy. A few examples are given below.

(*a*) *Tylosis.* This condition, also known as keratosis palmaris et plantaris familiaris, is a dominantly inherited disorder which probably exists in two forms. In one form diffuse keratosis of the palms of the hands and soles of the feet with very eary age of onset is the only problem. In several families first described by Howel-Evans *et al.* (1958) a late onset tylosis is associated with a moderately high risk of developing oesophageal carcinoma at a mean age of 45 years. This form of the disease seems to be confined geographically to a small area around Liverpool, England and several of the families which have been described may be related.

(*b*) *Retinoblastoma.* Though itself a malignant neoplasm, retinoblastoma should be included here since it is clear that gene carriers in families with retinoblastoma are at risk of developing apparently unrelated neoplasms (Fig. 2.8), namely osteosarcoma and other sarcomas (Kitchin and Ellsworth 1974; Francois 1977). Some of these tumours appear to be the result of prior irradiation for treatment of retinoblastoma (Strong 1977*b*), but since osteosarcomas may develop in sites distant from the irradiation field (notably the long bones) it is probable that their occurrence is in some cases an independent result of the dominantly inherited retinoblastoma gene.

(*c*) *Albinism.* There are probably several different forms of albinism but the mode of inheritance is autosomal recessive in all types. Albinos are at an unusual risk of developing skin cancers but it seems probable that this is one extreme of the well recognized range of risk for people with different degrees of skin pigmentation (Lutzner 1977). It does not seem to be the result of any specific sensitivity to skin cancer such as is seen in xeroderma pigmentosum.

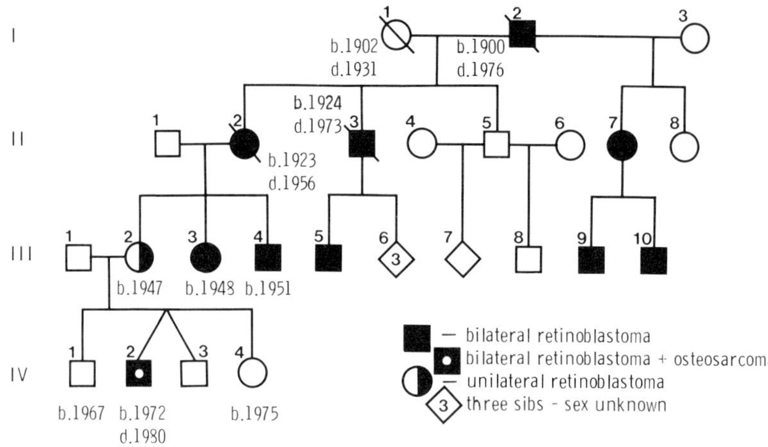

Fig. 2.8. Pedigree of a family with retinoblastoma. The propositus (IV 2) died at eight years of age after developing an osteogenic sarcoma of the orbit. The occurrence of other cancers in this family is also noteworthy—I 2 (carcinoma of the colon at age 76); II 2 (carcinoma of the ovary at age 33); II 3 (carcinoma of the lung at age 49).

(*d*) *Rothmund-Thomson syndrome* (poikiloderma atrophicans and cataract) is another rare, recessively inherited disorder with atrophy, hyperpigmentation, and telangiectasia of the skin associated with juvenile cataract and possibly a number of other skeletal and soft tissue defects. These patients have a high risk of developing cutaneous squamous carcinoma (Reed *et al.* 1974).

(*e*) *Beckwith-Wiedemann syndrome* (*exomphalos-macroglossia-gigantism syndrome*). In this autosomal recessive disease, the enlarged tongue and omphalocoele usually permit diagnosis at birth. Other features are neonatal hypoglycaemia, visceromegaly, adrenocortical cytomegaly, and dysplasia of the renal medulla. Patients with this disease have an unusual risk of developing Wilms' tumour (Miller 1976). There has been some discussion that the mode of inheritance may not be the same in all cases and that a dominant inheritance with 'delayed mutation' may explain some unusual families (McKusick 1978).

Conclusions

In many of the cases discussed here, there is no hint of the nature of the role of the genetic factor in the premalignant lesion or signal which leads on to malignancy. Particularly baffling is the association between familial tylosis and oesophageal cancer. In other cases, however, there are indications of what is happening and several different types of concept emerge. First, if one considers cancer as a multistage process the genetic susceptibility may facilitate one of the stages in the process. In xeroderma pigmentosum the susceptibility to u.v. light may enhance the probability of the first (initiation) step occurring. This general idea has been propounded most succinctly in Knudson's two-mutation hypothesis (Knudson 1973). The author proposes that cancers are due essentially to two sequential mutations and that in the case of familial cancers one of the significant mutations is inherited and the second is acquired. It follows that any circumstance which enhances the probability of somatic mutation will predispose to cancer. In Wiskott-Aldrich syndrome the impaired immunity, or in Klinefelter's syndrome the hormone imbalance, may in some manner facilitate the later stages of progression to malignancy. For this to be correct, however, it is necessary to assume that there is a stage in the development of a neoplasm when progression to malignancy is not inevitable and that there are altered cell states whose further development depends on either the response of the body to their presence or simply to the physiological state of the body at a particular moment in time. This seems not unreasonable, but the logical extension is that, since these factors are under genetic control, all tumours will have a genetic component: in other words, Wiskott-Aldrich syndrome, Klinefelter's syndrome, and similar conditions are only extreme examples of a general phenomenon.

A second consideration is the interaction of different factors in carcinogenesis. In epidermodysplasia verruciformis we apparently have an interaction between four factors: genetic constitution, papilloma virus, depressed immunity, and exposure to u.v. in sunlight. While this is perhaps an extreme example it is clear that in many other cases interaction between environmental factors and genetic constitution is important in determining the progression of preneoplastic lesions to malignancy—for example, u.v. light in xeroderma pigmentosum and ionizing radiation in the basal-cell carcinoma syndrome. When considering premalignant lesions, therefore, the possibility must always be considered that there is a subgroup (perhaps a small subgroup) in which genetic susceptibility to some other environmental or endogenous factor may make progression to malignancy more probable.

Lastly, in some cases it seems that genetic factors which in some way disrupt either normal development or differentiation may be important in determining the occurrence of preneoplastic lesions. In familial polyposis coli the normal differentiation of the colonic mucosa is disrupted creating a situation in which multiple adenomatous polyps are formed, each one of which (from our knowledge of isolated polyps) has a malignant potential, making cancerous change almost inevitable by sheer weight of numbers. The association of overt developmental abnormalities of the eye with retinoblastoma is not common, but the age of onset of the disease and the synchrony between the eyes in the onset of the disease in bilateral cases (Matsunga 1980) strongly suggest that a defect in a critical stage in the development of the eye may be important in the origin of retinoblastoma.

References

Anderson, D.E. (1971). Clinical characteristics of the genetic variety of cutaneous melanoma in man. *Cancer* **28**, 721.

—— and Romsdahl, M.M. (1977). Family history: a criterion for selective screening. In *Genetics of human Cancer* (ed. J.J. Mulvihill, R.W. Miller, and J.F. Fraumeni), p. 257. Raven Press, New York.

——, Smith, J.L., and McBride, C.M. (1967*a*). Hereditary aspects of malignant melanoma. *J. Am. med. Ass.* **200**, 741.

——, Taylor, W.B., Falls, H.F., and Davidson, R.T. (1967*b*). The nevoid basal cell carcinoma syndrome. *Am. J. hum. Genet.* **19**, 12.

Andrews, F.J., Linehan, J.J., and Melcher, D.H. (1981). Cervical carcinoma in both mother and daughter. *Acta Cytologica* **25**, 3.

Auerbach, A.D., Adler, B., and Chaganti, R.S.K. (1981). Prenatal diagnosis and carrier detection of Fanconi anemia by a cytogenetic method. *Pediatrics* **67**, 128.

Bagshawe, K.D. and Lawler, S.D. (1982*a*). Choriocarcinoma. In *Cancer epidemiology and prevention* (ed. D. Schottenfeld and J. Fraumeni). W.B. Saunders, Eastbourne.

—— —— (1982*b*). Unmasking moles. *Br. J. Obstet. Gynaecol.* **89**, 255.

Black, M.M. and Kwon, S. (1980). Precancerous mastopathy: structural and biological considerations. *Path. Res. Pract.* **166**, 491.

Block, J.B. and Clendenning, W.E. (1963). Parathyroid hormone hyporesponsiveness in patients with basal cell nevi and bone defects. *New Engl. J. Med.* **268**, 1157.

Bondi, E.E., Clark, W.H., Elder, D., Guerry, D., and Greene, M.H. (1981). Topical chemotherapy of dysplastic melanocytic nevi with 5% fluorouracil. *Arch. Dermatol.* **117**, 89.

Bridges, B.A. and Harnden, D.G. (1982). *Ataxia telangiectasia: A cellular and molecular link between cancer, neuropathology and immune deficiency.* Wiley, Chichester.

Bunney, M.H. (1982). *Viral warts: their biology and treatment.* Oxford University Press.

Carritt, B., Parrington, J., West, L., and Povey, S. (1982). Linkage phase in multiple heterozygous ovarian teratomas revealed by somatic cell hybridization. Human Gene Mapping 6. *Cytogenetics Cell Genetics* **32**, 256.

Cheesebrough, M.J. and Kinmont, P.D.C. (1978). Dyskeratosis congenita. *Br. J. Dermatol.* **99** (suppl. 16), 29.

Chiemchanya, S. (1982). Cervical carcinoma in both mother and daughter. *Acta Cytologica* **26**, 379.

Clark, W.H., Mastrangelo, M.J., Ainsworth, A.M., Berd, D., Bellet, R.E., and Bernardino, E.A. (1977). Current concepts of the biology of human cutaneous malignant melanoma. *Adv. Cancer Res.* **24**, 267.

——, Reimer, R.R., Greene, M., Ainsworth, A.M., and Mastrangelo, M.J. (1978). Origin of familial malignant melanoma from heritable melanotic lesions. The B-K mole syndrome. *Arch. Dermatol.* **114**, 732.

Cleaver, J.E. (1969). Xeroderma pigmentosum: a human disease in which an initial stage of DNA repair is defective. *Proc. Nat. Acad. Sci. USA* **63**, 428.

Cohen, A.J., Li, F.P., Berg, S., Marchetto, D.J., Tsai, S., Jacobs, S.C., and Brown, R.S. (1979). Hereditary renal cell carcinoma associated with chromosomal translocation. *New Engl. J. Med.* **301**, 592.

Danes, B.S. and Alm, T. (1979). *In vitro* studies in adenomatoses of the colon and rectum. *J. Med. Genet.* **16**, 417.

——, Krush, A.J., and Gardner, E.J. (1977). Is Gardner syndrome a distinct genetic disorder? *Lancet* **ii**, 925.

Delhanty, J.D.A., Davis, M.B., and Wood, J. (1983). Chromosome instability in lymphocytes, fibroblasts and colon epithelial like cells from patients with familial polyposis coli. *Cancer Genet. Cytogenet.* **8**, 27.

——, Pritchard, M.B., Bussey, H.J.R., and Morson, B.C. (1980). Tetraploid fibroblasts and familial polyposis coli. *Lancet* **i**, 1365.

Dodds, W.J., Schulte, W.J., Hensley, G.T., and Hogan, W.J. (1972). Peutz-Jeghers syndrome and gastrointestinal malignancy. *Am. J. Roentgen.* **115**, 374.

Elder, D.E., Goldman, L.I., Goldman, S.C., Greene, M.H., and Clark, W.H. (1980). The large atypical nevus syndrome: a phenotype association of malignant melanoma. *Cancer* **46**, 1787.

Featherstone, T. (1981). Ph.D. thesis. University of Birmingham.

——, Harnden, D.G., and Taylor, A.M.R. (1983). Studies on the radiosensitivity of cells from patients with basal cell naevus syndrome. *Am. J. hum. Genet.* **35**, 58.

Filipovich, A.H., Spector, B.D., and Kersey, J.H. (1980). Immunodeficiency in humans as a risk factor in the development of malignancy. *Prevent. Med.* **9**, 252.

Francke, U., Riccardi, V.M., Hittner, H.M., and Borges, W. (1978). Interstitial del(11p) as a cause of the aniridia-Wilms' tumor association: band localisation and a heritable basis. *Am. J. hum. Genet.* **30**, 81A.

Francois, J. (1977). Retinoblastoma and osteogenic sarcoma. *Ophthalmologica* **175**, 185.

Gardner, E.J., Rogers, S.W., Woodward, S.R., Neff, L.K., Burt, R.W., and Moon, R.G. (1980). Diagnosis of the Gardner syndrome at the cellular level. *Encyclia* **57**, 48.

German, J., Bloom, D., and Passarge, E. (1979). Bloom's syndrome. VII. Progress report for 1978. *Clin. Genet.* **15**, 361.

——, Schonberg, S., Louie, E., and Chaganti, R.S.K. (1977). Bloom's syndrome. IV. Sister chromatid exchanges in lymphocytes. *Am. J. hum. Genet.* **29**, 248.

Gianelli, F. (1976). Xeroderma pigmentosum. In *Scientific foundations of oncology* (ed. T. Symington and R.L. Carter), p. 476. Heinemann Medical Publications, London.

——, Benson, P.F., Pawsey, S.A., and Polani, P.E. (1977). Ultraviolet light sensitivity and delayed DNA chain maturation in Bloom's syndrome fibroblasts. *Nature* **265**, 466.

Gorlin, R.J. and Goltz, R.W. (1960). Multiple nevoid basal cell epithelioma, jaw cysts and bifid rib, a syndrome. *New Engl. J. Med.* **262**, 908.

—— and Sedano, H.O. (1971). The multiple nevoid basal cell carcinoma syndrome revisited. *Birth defects*, original article series Vol. VII, No. 8, p. 140.

Greene, M.H. (1982). The dysplastic nevus syndrome: a model for human neoplastic traits. *Proc. 13th Int. Cancer Congr.*, Seattle, Washington, p. 364.

——, Clark, W.H., and Kraemer, K.H. (1980). New observations in heritable melanoma. *Cancer Res.* **21**, 323.

Happle, R. and Kupferschmid, A. (1972). A further case of BCNS and structural chromosome abnormalities. *Humangenetik* **15**, 287.

——, Mehrle, G., Sanden, L.Z., and Hohn, H. (1971). Basal cell naevus syndrome with pigmented retinopathy, recurrent intravitreous bleeding and chromosome aberrations. *Arch. Derm. Forsch.* **241**, 96.

Harnden, D.G. (1961). Congenital abnormalities with an apparently normal chromosome complement. In *Human chromosomal abnormalities*. Staples Press, London.

——, Benn, P.A., Oxford, J.M., Taylor, A.M.R., and Webb, T.P. (1976). Cytogenetically marked clones in human fibroblasts cultured from normal subjects. *Somatic cell Genet.* **2**, 35.

—— and Herbert, A. (1982). Association of constitutional chromosome rearrangements and neoplasia. *Cancer Surv.* **1**, 150.

——, Maclean, N., and Langlands, A.O. (1971). Carcinoma of the breast and Klinefelter's syndrome. *J. Med. Genet.* **8**, 460.

Hecht, F. and McCaw, B.K. (1977). Chromosome instability syndromes. In *Genetics of human cancer* (ed. J.J. Mulvihill, R.W. Miller, and J.F. Fraumeni Jr), p. 105. Raven Press, New York.

Hittner, H.M., Riccardi, V.M., Kretzer, F.L., Levy, C.H., and Moura, R.A. (1980). Two-step mutation theory for retinoblastoma: ultrastructural support. *Documenta Ophthalmol.* **48**, 345.

Hope, D.G. and Mulvihill, J.J. (1981). Malignancy in neurofibromatosis. In *Advances in neurology*, Vol. 29, Neurofibromatosis (von Recklinghausen's Disease) (ed. V.M. Riccardi and J.J. Mulvihill), p. 33. Raven Press, New York.

Howel-Evans, W., McConnell, R.B., Clarke, C.A., and Sheppard, P.M. (1958). Carcinoma of the oesophagus with keratosis palmaris et plantaris (tylosis): a study of two families. *Quart. J. Med.* **27**, 413.

Jacobs, P.A., Hunt, P.A., Matsuura, J.S., Wilson, C.C., and Szulman, A.E. (1982). Complete and partial hydatidiform mole in Hawaii: cytogenetics, morphology and epidemiology. *Brit. J. Obstet. Gynaecol.* **89**, 258.

——, Wilson, C.M., Sprenkle, J.A., Rosenshein, N.B., and Migeon, B.R. (1980). Mechanism of origin of complete hydatidiform moles. *Nature* **286**, 714.

Johansson, E., Niemi, K-M, Siimes, M., and Pyrhonen, S. (1982). Fanconi's anemia: Tumor-like warts, hyperpigmentation associated with deranged keratinocytes and depressed cell-mediated immunity. *Arch. Dermatol.* **118**, 249.

Journal of the American Medical Association (1981). Editorial: Dysplastic nevus syndrome may herald melanoma. *J. Am. med. Ass.* **245**, 2277.

Kaiser-McCaw, B. and Hecht, F. (1982). Ataxia telangiectasia: chromosomes and cancer. In *Ataxia telangiectasia—a cellular and molecular link between cancer, neuropathology and immune deficiency* (ed. B.A. Bridges and D.G. Harnden), p. 243. Wiley, Chichester.

Kajii, T. and Ohama, K. (1977). Androgenetic origin of hyatidiform moles. *Nature (Lond.)* **268**, 633.

Kano, Y. and Fujiwara, Y. (1982). Dyskeratosis congenita: survival, sister chromatid exchange and repair following treatments with cross linking agents. *Mutation Res.* **103**, 327.

Kirkpatrick, C.H. (1979). Genetic disorders of the immune system. In *Clinical genetics—a source book for physicians* (ed. L.G. Jackson and R.N. Schimke), p. 121. Wiley, New York.

Kitchin, F.D. and Ellsworth, R.M. (1974). Pleiotropic effects of the gene for retinoblastoma. *J. med. Genet.* **11**, 244.

Knudson, A.G. (1973). Mutation and human cancer. *Adv. Cancer Res.* **17**, 317.

Kraemer, K.H. (1980). Xeroderma pigmentosum. In *Clinical dermatology* (ed. D.J. Demis, R.L. Dobson, and J. McGuire), Unit 19-7, p. 1. Harper Row, New York.

Lattes, R. (1980). Lobular neoplasia (lobular carcinoma *in situ*) of the breast—a histological entity of controversial clinical significance. *Path. Res. Pract.* **166**, 415.

Lawler, S.D., Fisher, R.A., Pickthall, V.J., Povey, S., and Evans, M.W. (1982). Genetic studies on hydatidiform moles. 1. The origin of partial moles. *Cancer Genet. Cytogenet.* **5**, 309.

Lewandowsky, F. and Lutz, W. (1922). Ein Fall einer Bisher nicht beschriebenen Hanterktankung (Epidermodysplasia verruciformis). *Arch. Dermatol. Syphilol.* **141**, 193.

Lipkin, M. and Deschner, E.E. (1977). Gastrointestinal neoplasia: an investigative approach. In *Genetics of human cancer* (ed. J.J. Mulvihill, R.W. Miller and J.F. Fraumeni), p. 369. Raven Press, New York.

Lutzner, M.A. (1977). Nosology among the neoplastic genodermatoses. In *Genetics of human cancer* (ed. J.J. Mulvihill, R.W. Miller, and J.F. Fraumeni), p. 145. Raven Press, New York.

——, Croissant, O., Ducasse, M-F, Kreis, H., Crosnier, J., and Orth, G. (1980). A potentially oncogenic human papilloma virus (HPV-5) found in two renal allograft patients. *J. Invest. Dermatol.* **80**, 353.

Lynch, H.T., Frichot, B.C., and Lynch, J.F. (1978). Familial atypical multiple mole-melanoma syndrome. *J. Med. Genet.* **15**, 352.

Mann, J.R., Corkery, J.J., Fisher, H., Cameron, A.H., Wooley, V., Mayerova, A., Wolf, U., and Sanger, R. (1982). The X-linked form of gonadal dysgenesis: investigation of a family with a high incidence of gonadal tumours, including cytogenetic, dermatoglyphic and blood group studies and measurement of H-Y antigen. UK Childhood Cancer Study Group Meeting, Manchester, November 1982.

Matsukuma, S., Zelle, B., Keijzer, W., Berends, F., and Bootsma, D. (1981). Different rates of restoration of the repair capacity in complementing xeroderma pigmentosum cells after fusion. *Exp. cell Res.* **134**, 103.

Matsunaga, E. (1980). Retinoblastoma: host resistance and 13q-chromosomal deletion. *Human Genet.* **56**, 53.

McKusick, V.A. (1978). *Mendelian inheritance in man*, (5th ed.). Johns Hopkins University Press, Baltimore.

Mehta, F.S., Pindborg, J.J., and Hamner, J.E. (1971). *Oral cancer and precancerous conditions in India.* Munksgaard, Copenhagen.

——, Shroff, B.C., Gupta, P.C., and Daftary, D.K. (1972). Oral leukoplakia in relation to tobacco habits. *Oral Surg.* **34**, 426.

Miller, R.W. (1970). Neoplasia and Down's syndrome. *Ann. NY Acad. Sci.* **171**, 637.

—— (1976). Cancer and congenital malformations: another view. In *Genetics of human cancer* (ed. J.J. Mulvihill, R.W. Miller, and J.F. Fraumeni), p. 77. Raven Press, New York.

Mitelman, F., Mark, J., Nilsson, P.G., Denker, H., Norryd, C., and Tranberg, K-G. (1974). Chromosome banding patterns in human colonic polyps. *Hereditas* **78**, 63.

Morrison, W.L. (1975). Viral warts, herpes simplex and herpes zoster in patients with secondary immune deficiencies. *Brit. J. Dermatol.* **92**, 625.

Motegi, T. (1982). High rate of detection of 13q14 deletion mosaicism among retinoblastoma patients (using more extensive methods). *Human Genet.* **61**, 85.

Muto, T., Bussey, H.J.R., and Morson, B.C. (1976). The evolution of cancer of the colon and rectum. *Cancer* **36**, 2251.

Nowell, P.C. (1982). Cytogenetics of preleukemia. *Cancer Genet. Cytogenet.* **5**, 265.

Obeid, D.A., Hill, F.G.H., Harnden, D.G., Mann, J.R., and Wood, B.S.B. (1980). Fanconi anemia-oxymetholone hepatic tumours and chromosome aberrations associated with leukemic transition. *Cancer* **46**, 1401.

O'Riordan, M.L., Langlands, A.O., and Harnden, D.G. (1972). Further studies on the frequency of constitutional chromosome aberrations in patients with malignant disease. *Eur. J. Cancer* **8**, 373.

Orye, E., Benoit, Y., Coppieters, R., Jeannin, P., Vercruysse, C., Delaey, J., and Delbeke, M-J. (1982). A case of retinoblastoma associated with histiocytosis X and mosaicism of a deleted D-group chromosome (13q14→q31). *Clin. Genet.* **22**, 37.

Ostor, A.G., Adam, R., Guttridge, B.H., and Fortune, D.W. (1982). Endometrial carcinoma in young women. *Aust. N.Z. J. Obstet. Gynaecol.* **22**, 38.
Ostrow, R.S., Bender, M., Nimura, M., Seki, T., Kawashima, M., Pass, F., and Faras, A.J. (1982). Human papillomavirus DNA in cutaneous primary and metastasized squamous cell carcinomas from patients with epidermodysplasia verruciformis. *Proc. Nat. Acad. Sci. USA* **79**, 1634.
Pyrhonen, S., Jablonska, S., Obaley, S., and Kuismanen, E. (1980). Immune reactions in epidermodysplasia verruciformis. *Brit. J. Dermatol.* **102**, 247.
Reed, W.B., Boder, E., and Gardner, M. (1974). Congenital and genetic skin disorders with tumor formation. *Birth Defects* **10**, 265.
Riccardi, V.M., Sujansky, E., Smith, A.C., and Francke, U. (1978). Chromosomal imbalance in the aniridia-Wilms' tumor association: 11p interstitial deletion. *Pediatrics* **61**, 604.
Rowley, J.D. (1981). Down's syndrome and acute leukaemia: increased risk may be due to trisomy 21. *Lancet* **ii**, 1020.
Sakaguchi, A.Y., Naylor, S.L., and Shows, T.B. (1982). A human gene homologous to RSV v-src on chromosome 20. *Proc. 13th Int. Cancer Cong.*, Seattle, Washington, p. 584.
Sasaki, M.S. (1975). Is Fanconi's anaemia defective in a process essential to the repair of DNA cross links.? *Nature* **257**, 501.
Schimke, R.N. (1977). Tumors of the neural crest system. In *Genetics of human cancer* (ed. J.J. Mulvihill, R.W. Miller, and J.F. Fraumeni), p. 179. Raven Press, New York.
Schroeder, T.M. and German, J. (1974). Bloom's syndrome and Fanconi's anemia: demonstration of two distinctive patterns of chromosome disruption and rearrangements. *Human Genetik* **25**, 299.
——, Tilgen, D., Kruger, J., and Vogel, F. (1976). Formal genetics of Fanconi's anemia. *Hum. Genet.* **32**, 257.
Second International Workshop on Chromosomes in Leukaemia (1980). *Cancer Genet. Cytogenet.* **2**, 93.
Shope, R.E. (1933). Infectious papillomatosis in rabbits. *J. exp. med.* **58**, 607.
Sirinavin, C. and Trowbridge, A.A. (1975). Dyskeratosis congenita: clinical features and genetic aspects: report of a family and review of the literature. *J. med. Genet.* **12**, 339.
Southwick, G.J. and Schwartz, R.A. (1979). Basal cell nevus syndrome disasters occurring among a series of 36 patients. *Cancer* **44**, 2294.
Spector, B.D., Filipovich, A.H., Perry, B.S., and Kersey, J.H. (1982). Epidemiology of cancer in ataxia telangiectasia. In *Ataxia-telangiectasia—a cellular and molecular link between cancer, neuropathology and immune deficiency* (ed. B.A. Bridges and D.G. Harnden), P. 103. Wiley, Chichester.
——, Perry, B.S., and Kersey, J.H. (1978). Genetically determined immunodeficiency diseases (GDID) and malignancy: report from the immunodeficiency—Cancer Registry. *Clin. Immunol. Immunopathol.* **11**, 12.
Stone, M. and Bagshawe, K.D. (1976). Hydatidiform mole: two entities. *Lancet* **i**, 535.
Strong, L.C. (1977*a*). Genetic and environmental interaction in the development of multiple primary tumours. *Cancer* **40**, 1861.
—— (1977*b*). Theories of pathogenesis: mutation and cancer. In *Genetics of human cancer* (ed. J.J. Mulvihill, R.W. Miller, and J.F. Fraumeni), p. 401. Raven Press, New York.
Swift, M. (1982). Disease predisposition of ataxia telangiectasia heterozygotes. In *Ataxia-telangiectasia—a cellular and molecular link between cancer, neuropath-*

ology and immune deficiency (ed. B.A. Bridges and D.G. Harnden), p. 353. Wiley, Chichester.

Taylor, A.M.R. (1982). Cytogenetics of ataxia-telangiectasia. In *Ataxia-telangiectasia—a cellular and molecular link between cancer, neuropathology and immune deficiency* (ed. B.A. Bridges and D.G. Harnden), P. 53. Wiley, Chichester.

——, Harnden, D.G., Arlett, C.F., Harcourt, S.A., Lehmann, A.R., Stevens, S., and Bridges, B.A. (1975). Ataxia telangiectasia: a human mutation with abnormal radiation sensitivity. *Nature* **258**, 427.

——, Metcalfe, J.A., Oxford, J.M., and Harnden, D.G. (1976). Is chromatid-type damage in ataxia-telangiectasia after irradiation at G_0 a consequence of defective repair? *Nature* **260**, 441.

Teter, J. (1976). Cytogenetics with reference to gonadoblastoma and gonocytomas. In *Cancer genetics* (ed. H.T. Lynch), p. 146. C.C. Thomas, Springfield, Illinois.

van Dyke, D.L., Jackson, C.E., and Babu, V.R. (1981). Possible chromosome 20 deletion in multiple endocrine neoplasia type 2 (MEN-2). *Proc. 6th Int. Cong. Human Genetics*, p. 159.

Veale, A.M., McColl, I., Bussey, H.J.R., and Morson, B.C. (1966). Juvenile polyposis coli. *J. med. Genet.* **3**, 5.

Waldron, C.A. and Shafer, W.G. (1975). Leukoplakia revisited: a clinicopathotopic study of 3256 oral leukoplakias. *Cancer* **36**, 1386.

Yunis, J.J. and Ramsay, N. (1978). Retinoblastoma and sub-band deletion of chromosome 13. *Am. J. Dis. Childhood* **132**, 161.

Yutsudo, M., Tanigaki, T., Tsumori, T., Watanabe, S., and Hakura, A. (1982). New human papillomavirus isolated from epidermodysplasia verruciformis lesions. *Cancer Res.* **42**, 2440.

3 Precancerous conditions of the skin

K.V. Sanderson

The skin, both of man and experimental animals, tends to be more exposed to prevailing carcinogenic agents than most other tissues. The published work on skin carcinogenesis in animals is of questionable relevance to the premalignant disorders of human skin for several reasons. The classical experiments were performed on hair-bearing rodents whose skin behaves in a different way from human skin and, furthermore, the investigators were concerned more to elucidate the range and potency of carcinogens and their mode of action than to demonstrate the patterns of response in the skin. The appearance of a wart in the painted area, which was the indicator of a skin response to a carcinogen used by the earlier experimenters, seems to have been a premalignant phenomenon. Only a proportion of the warts became invasive if allowed to run their natural course and some would shrivel and disappear. This behaviour paralleled that of some lesions seen in the clinic. The two-stage hypothesis of carcinogenesis, also advanced on the basis of changes in mouse skin, is relevant to understanding the induction of human skin cancer in which, however, the clear-cut distinction drawn between initiating and promoting agents in the original experiments cannot be made. The idea that a promoting agent, which can be voluntarily avoided, may be the determining factor in causing a precancerous lesion is particularly important in cancer education. The erroneous belief that cancer is an essentially random and irreversible event over which the individual has little control is still widely prevalent and used as an excuse for persisting with carcinogenic habits. The evidence that there are repair mechanisms for damaged DNA and immunological responses to transformed cells disposes of the view that carcinogenesis is irreversible. The phenomenon of promotion, whatever its mechanism may be, destroys the idea of a random or predestined quality to the process.

There are now reliable data on the incidence of human-skin malignancy in a number of areas derived from well conducted epidemiological surveys, and rather less reliable information for particular occupational hazards. The data on the incidence of premalignant changes are much more difficult to obtain. They are, however, of considerable interest—both as a measure of the reaction of the skin to carcinogenic influences and as a means of determining the probability that any single premalignant lesion will become invasive and of establishing the time course of such transformation. It might be thought that it would be easier to obtain prevalence rates from workers exposed to industrial hazards than from the population in general, but the tendency for workers to move from job to job and the long latent interval of such lesions make the tracing and regular examining of all those exposed to a particular hazard at work almost impossible. Further, when a class of workers, such as those in the coal-gas industry who were exposed to known carcinogens, are studied, the initial question of what constitutes a premalignant lesion may be a source of uncertainty.

Premalignant skin lesions

A possible biological definition of a premalignant lesion might be that it is a lesion which becomes an invasive tumour sufficiently frequently for its behaviour to be statistically predictable. This definition does not rule out the possibility of an indefinitely prolonged pre-invasive period or indeed of spontaneous remission in some of the lesions. It does presuppose distinctive clinical and microscopical features which separate the lesion from other conditions, and it requires proof that the lesions of the defined class have a calculable probability of becoming malignant.

Those who work with tar and pitch may develop warty plaques, especially on the hands and face, which have the microscopical features of benign acanthomata (Fig. 3.1); the lesions do not become malignant and they may regress when the exposure to tar ceases. These workers also develop

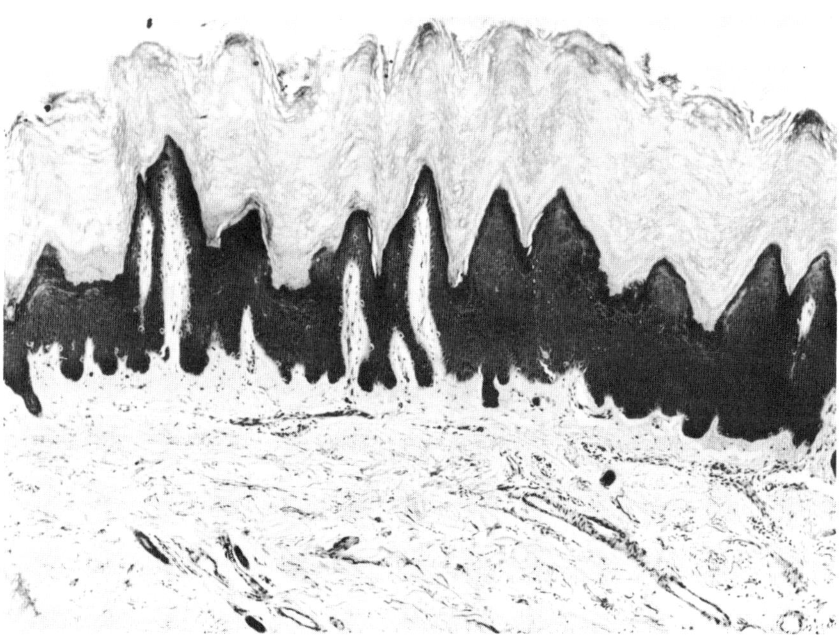

Fig. 3.1. A benign tar acanthoma, showing hyperplastic, normally maturing epidermis supported by elongated papillae and producing hyperkeratosis ×35. H & E.

keratoses which show cellular atypia and which may, more often on the face than the hands, develop into invasive squamous-cell carcinomas in the fullness of time. A third type of lesion resembles an indolent keratoacanthoma whose course is, to some extent, dependent on the region where it erupts. Scrotal lesions of this type have a more sinister behaviour than those appearing on (say) the face or hands, which may regress.

This brief summary does not do justice to the changes caused in the skin by contact with tar, which have been well described by Götz (1976), but it is introduced to illustrate that a variable proportion of precancerous lesions are validated by becoming invasive tumours and that the region of the skin on which they occur is an important factor determining the likelihood of this event. Other factors include the characteristics of the coal, which determine the composition of the distillate, and the intensity and duration of the exposure. The photosensitizing action of tar and pitch is another feature to be considered. Thus, even in the human situation which most resembles the classical experiments in skin carcinogenesis, the factors are so numerous that prevalence rates of premalignant conditions and the probability of their malignant change have not been established.

The one carcinogen in which a reasonable assessment of the response of the human skin has been obtained is inorganic arsenic. It is interesting that man is the only animal in which arsenic has been shown to be carcinogenic. The data were obtained from Taiwan where, for about 45 years, an area occupied mainly by a static community of fishermen was supplied from wells with water containing arsenic in solution. Epidemiological surveys (Tseng *et al.* 1968; Yeh *et al.* 1968) of 37 villages where the water supply contained different amounts of arsenic showed a prevalence of skin cancer which increased with age to a figure of more than 10 per cent in people over the age of 59. The prevalence also increased in proportion to the degree of contamination of the water. A control population whose water was arsenic-free showed none of the signs seen in those exposed to arsenic. The comparison of these data with those of other published series is made rather difficult because the authors separated keratoses from Bowen's disease, classifying the former as benign and the latter as carcinoma.

It has been known for many decades that those individuals most likely to develop premalignant lesions after chronic damage from sunlight possess easily recognizable physical features of skin, hair, and iris colouring. Their distribution within the population is genetically determined, and those possessing them experience a burning reaction without effective tanning after sun exposure. An even more sensitive indicator occurs in xeroderma pigmentosum in which an enzyme defect allows the prediction of future precancerous lesions whilst the fetus is *in utero* (Ramsay *et al.* 1974). The features of this disease and its biochemical basis will be considered later in the chapter, but it raises several general points which can be considered in this introduction. The defects in enzymic excision and repair of damaged

DNA in this condition occur in all somatic cells and, as might be expected, a range of premalignant and malignant tumours arise at areas where nuclei are exposed to damage by ultraviolet radiation. There is no difficulty in recognizing clinically the keratoses due to intra-epidermal transformation, and the aberrant melanocytes show their presence by pigmentary changes before developing into malignant melanoma. Basal-cell carcinoma and a variety of connective-tissue tumours may also develop. The nosology of all forms of basal-cell carcinoma has been disputed in the past and doubts have been expressed about its malignant potential. Its ability to organize its stroma and the interaction between tumour and stroma, its rather meagre evidence of differentiation, the rapid rate of cell division but slow rate of growth, and its very low capacity to metastasize are features which remain puzzling and are as yet incompletely explained. The present view is that there is no clinically recognizable pre-invasive stage of basal-cell carcinoma and that actinic keratoses, despite their basaloid budding, only transform into squamous-cell carcinoma. The converse idea that squamous-cell carcinoma (or, for that matter, malignant melanoma) always develop from a precancerous lesion is not substantiated by clinical evidence, as a significant proportion of both tumours arise *de novo*. This view has a bearing on the attempt to prevent malignant tumours by screening for and treating their pre-invasive stage, although it is, of course, not an argument against such a policy. The profusion of keratoses and pigmented lesions in xeroderma pigmentosum presents the clinician with a very difficult problem in pursuing this policy.

Patients in sunny areas like Australia may, if they are astute observers, report that some keratoses disappear spontaneously. These observations are supported by a shred of experimental evidence (Gerstein and Freeman 1963). Transpositional full-thickness grafts were exchanged between the exposed and sun-damaged skin of the neck and the unexposed inner aspect of the forearm. Over a period of months both the gross and microscopic changes of collagen degeneration were reduced in the graft transposed on to the forearm and epidermal changes, of a type which could not be regarded as precancerous but might amount to early dysplasia, also reverted to normal. Over the period of the experiment the forearm skin transferred to the neck did not show actinic damage and no improvement occurred in skin grafts taken from and then replaced on the neck. There is no doubt that the actinically damaged dermis in the transplants persisted because hair follicles in the centre of the graft survived and continued to produce hair.

Premalignant states

There is some virtue in separating the premalignant lesion, the gross evidence that transformation has occurred, from the premalignant state in which a propensity for precancerous change exists without, as yet, visible lesions. Xeroderma pigmentosum *in utero* is the epitome of the premalignant state but there may be less well-defined circumstances where the concept is valuable. The following case history illustrates this point.

A 55 year-old man who had worked as a furnaceman for 27 years sustained a burn to his left upper eyelid by a hot flying fragment while smelting iron. During the course of his daily work he had been exposed to radiation from the hot metal in the furnace for 4-6 hours a day, and although his scalp and arms were protected from hot metal and radiation, the protection of the eyes was with tinted spectacles which were worn on the end of the nose, so that they did not have to be removed when not looking into the furnace. The upper lids were thus unprotected. Following the burn to the eyelid he had no symptoms for two days and then developed purulent left-sided conjunctivitis. Two weeks after the injury a crack developed on the surface of the eyelid which grew rapidly into a destructive tumour. When excised a few weeks later this proved to be a rather poorly differentiated squamous-cell carcinoma (Fig. 3.2). His claim for industrial benefit was contested by the insurance company on the grounds that there were authoritative published statements that physical injury did not cause cancer. The patient's account of the train of events was explained when the sections of his eyelid were re-examined. Deeply embedded below the carcinoma and quite close to the palpebral conjunctiva there were small fragments of mineral matter (Fig. 3.3). There was a foreign-body reaction to this material and it contained doubly refractile crystalline particles and stained as if containing basic ions. The microscopic evidence therefore suggested that it was slag, and its presence had caused inflammation of the palpebral conjunctiva.

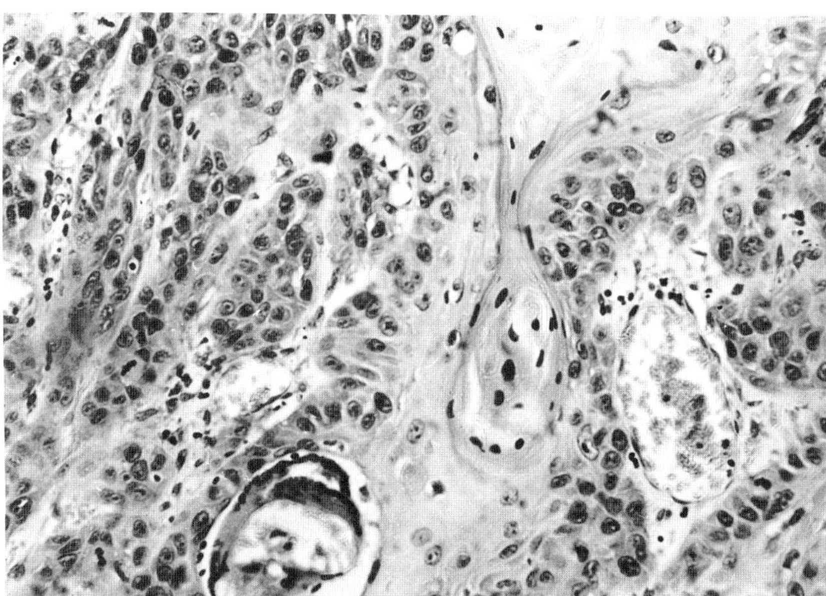

Fig. 3.2. Squamous-cell carcinoma of the eyelid occurring at the site of a recent burn. × 280. H & E.

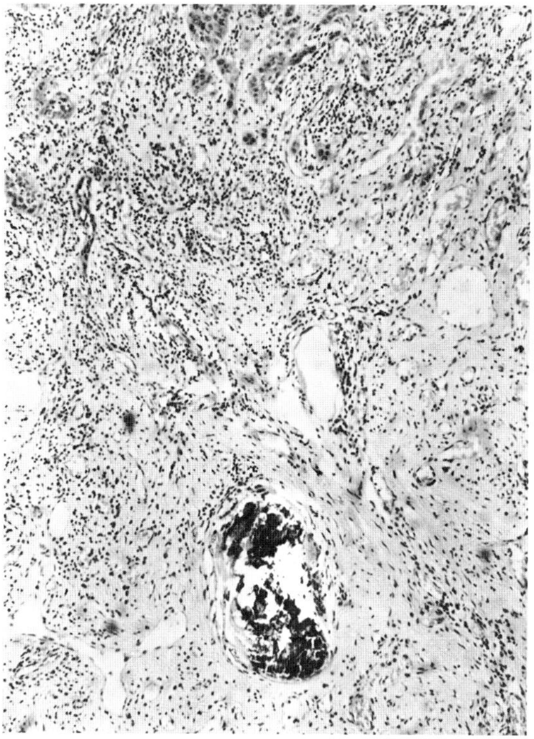

Fig. 3.3. Lower edge of squamous-cell carcinoma of eyelid situated directly above a foreign body. × 135. H & E.

There is thus no doubt that an aggressive squamous-cell carcinoma arose in this patient directly after and at the exact site of the injury. Presumably the long exposure to radiant energy from the furnace had initiated the premalignant state which was activated by the injury. It is unusual to have confirmation of a patient's story of injury in this fashion, but I also have in my collection two squamous-cell carcinomas from Australians, each with a splinter of wood embedded beneath the tumour. The localizing effect of injury on the tumours arising in carcinogen-treated rodent skin was an early finding of experimental cancer research (Deelmann 1923), so the documented cases of trauma inducing cancer should not cause surprise if the skin is in a premalignant state due to previous exposure to a carcinogen. It is only difficult to comprehend a case like the above if one has a fixed idea of an orderly progression of change from normal skin, through cytological atypia to a recognizable premalignant lesion and thence to invasive carcinoma. Such a progression may be usual but it is by no means invariable in squamous-cell carcinoma of the skin.

There is a group of disorders in which a premalignant state appears to follow damage to the junctional zone between the epidermis and the dermis.

This group includes the various chronic granulomas and accidental injuries which leave scars. In most such scars there is the possibility that either treatment or the primary agent itself may have exerted a carcinogenic effect on the epithelium. Examples include radiotherapy, which was frequently used by a previous generation of clinicians to treat chronic inflammatory states, and arsenic. In lichen sclerosus of the vulva, however, such effects are unlikely and the primary pathological process is unquestionably in the upper dermis. Leukoplakia of the epithelium is a frequent event in the course of lichen sclerosus of the vulva and there would seem to be at least a one in ten probability of squamous carcinoma occurring. Other dermatoses which cause precancerous scarring are discoid lupus erythematosus, lichen planus of mucosal surfaces, dystrophic epidermolysis bullosa, porokeratosis of Mibelli, and poikiloderma congenitale. The common feature of these disorders is replacement of the normal papillary structure by a scarred papillary layer with a flattened dermo-epidermal junction. Epithelial carcinogenesis is thus influenced by dermo-epidermal interactions. There are longstanding experimental studies showing the same effect of dermal scarring in rodent skin (Orr 1938).

Causes of precancerous skin lesions

Ultraviolet light is the most important cause of precancerous skin lesions. The adaptation of skin colour to climatic conditions has been greatly disturbed by European colonization during the last five centuries with the result that fair-skinned people in Australasia, East Africa, and the south-western states of the United States of America, to mention only some conspicuous examples, have a high incidence of skin cancer. Premalignant lesions are even more common. Actinic keratoses, for example, are said to occur in more than half the inhabitants of rural Queensland who reach the age of 70. Individual susceptibility has been related to hair and iris colouring, and to the tendency to suffer sunburn and to become freckled. Red-headed, blue- or green-eyed frecklers are particularly prone to develop skin tumours of various sorts and premalignant changes. This complexion is common among the Scots and Irish. The susceptibility of the Irish is revealed in the statistics from the Republic of Ireland where skin malignancy (and of necessity the unrecorded premalignant states) are quite prevalent among rural and outdoor workers. Ultraviolet carcinogenesis is likely to be a continuing problem in all areas where fair-skinned individuals are living in an inappropriately sunny area. The current obsession with acquiring a suntanned skin will ensure a plentiful supply of premalignant keratoses for the next half century as the latent period varies from 20 years upward.

The other recognized skin carcinogens have been very largely eliminated. Industrial and occupational causes from fossil fuels and their derivatives are now well-recognized, and in general the premalignant changes of the skin due to mineral oils and tar derivatives are rarely seen. This is certainly true of the larger factories, although isolated cases are still observed in older workers who have been employed in small 'backyard' factories where there are no medical advisers. The same is true for ionizing radiation. The prevention of skin premalignancies thus depends upon changing popular attitudes among fair-skinned people to the value of a suntan. There seems to be little hope for improvement in countries like Australia unless for instance a lesson is taken from the traditional mode of dress of the Arab races or unless effective sunscreens are regularly used by all susceptible individuals. The commercial pressures acting against a healthy undamaged skin are widespread and powerful.

In this brief review of the aetiology of skin precancers mention must be made of the hazards of medical practice. It is only in the last three decades that the degree of danger from ionizing radiation has been generally recognized and measures have been taken to protect patients and medical personnel. Both in the case of X-rays and of another medically used carcinogen, potassium arsenite (Fowler's solution), there was a delay of half a century or more between the earliest description of the skin malignancies caused by the agents and the modification of their use to avoid ill effects. The practice of medicine is still beset with potential carcinogenic influences, and notable examples are provided by some of the cytotoxic drugs used for immunosuppression and the recent introduction of photochemotherapy for psoriasis and some other skin disorders. Immunosuppressed patients and those whose Hodgkin's disease is in remission have already begun to show multiple premalignancies. Photochemotherapy, in which UV-A radiation (320-400 nm) is potentiated by a photo-active psoralen either previously ingested or applied to the skin, has also begun to produce accelerated actinic damage.

Evidence for viral oncogenesis in the human skin has been slow in coming. An earlier claim that herpes infection preceded squamous-cell carcinoma (Wyburn-Mason 1957) has not been confirmed, although it accords with epidemiological evidence concerning the cause of carcinoma of the cervix uteri. There is now an accumulating body of data favouring the human papilloma virus (HPV) as the cause for some unusual anogenital precancerous lesions, and, rarely, of invasive tumours. A case of carcinoma *in situ* adjacent to anal warts in which virus particles were demonstrated has been reported by Oriel and Whimster (1971). Three further examples of malignant transformation of condylomata acuminata are recorded with electron microscopic demonstration of virus particles in one case, but only in the wart and not in the transformed tissue (Kovo *et al.* 1974). There are a number of other reports in which the evidence of association between genital warts and malignancy is clinical and not supported by demonstration of the virus. The virtual disappearance of the virus from transformed tissue, mentioned above, has also been noticed in the rare disorder epidermodysplasia verruciformis. In this autosomal, recessively inherited disease, profuse and intractable viral warts, mainly of the planar type, are present from an early age and a considerable proportion of patients eventually develop intra-epidermal or squamous-cell carcinoma (Lutzner 1978). The disease is thus a very good model for observing serial changes, and has been carefully studied. A defect of cell-mediated immunity has been demonstrated which may be relevant both to the intractable nature of the warts and to their transformation. Recent techniques have allowed the recognition of at least seven types of human papilloma virus of which two, HPV-3 and HPV-5, have been found in epidermodysplasia verruciformis. The malignant transformation, however, is specifically associated with HPV-5 (Orth *et al.* 1979).

Two other conditions in the anogenital region, multicentric pigmented Bowen's disease (Lloyd 1970) and bowenoid papulosis of the penis (Wade *et al.* 1978), may show evidence of an association with virus warts or of virus particles in the affected area (Kimura *et al.* 1978). An aetiological relationship between virus plantar warts and carcinoma cuniculatum has been proposed by McKee *et al.* (1981). The difficulty in establishing the relationship in these cases is partly due to technical problems in culturing human papilloma virus and in its typing and in part arises from the disappearance of virus particles at the stage of malignant transformation. Serial clinical and microscopic observations are thus required to show the association; such observations are more likely to be undertaken in rare disorders like epidermodysplasia verruciformis than the banal condyloma acuminatum.

Clinicopathological aspects

The precancerous response of the epidermis to a carcinogen, whether it be physical or chemical, is to undergo dysplasia in one or more patches, forming a more or less imperfect horny layer which is clinically recognizable as a keratosis (sometimes called a hyperkeratosis by clinicians). The range of cellular deviation from the normal varies from very minor, as for example in most palmo-plantar keratoses due to arsenic, to the frank carcinoma *in situ* of Bowen's disease—which is also a post-arsenical manifestation in many instances. A similar range of microscopic appearance is found in actinic keratoses. The response to ultraviolet radiation seems to be partly determined by the anatomical region affected. The dorsum of the hand, one of the commonest sites, generally shows less atypia than the face, lip, or ear. The microscopic character of the premalignant lesion correlates with the likelihood of metastasis from squamous carcinomas in the different regions. Metastasis from tumours on the dorsum of the hand, for instance, is very uncommon. There is also a variation in response between individuals. Some persons who sunburn easily develop greater dysplasia at an earlier age, and the tumours will invade much sooner than the average. This individual variation is partly explicable in terms of the heavier dose of ultraviolet radiation received by the lower layer of the epidermis and partly in terms of the relative effectiveness of the cellular DNA repair mechanisms.

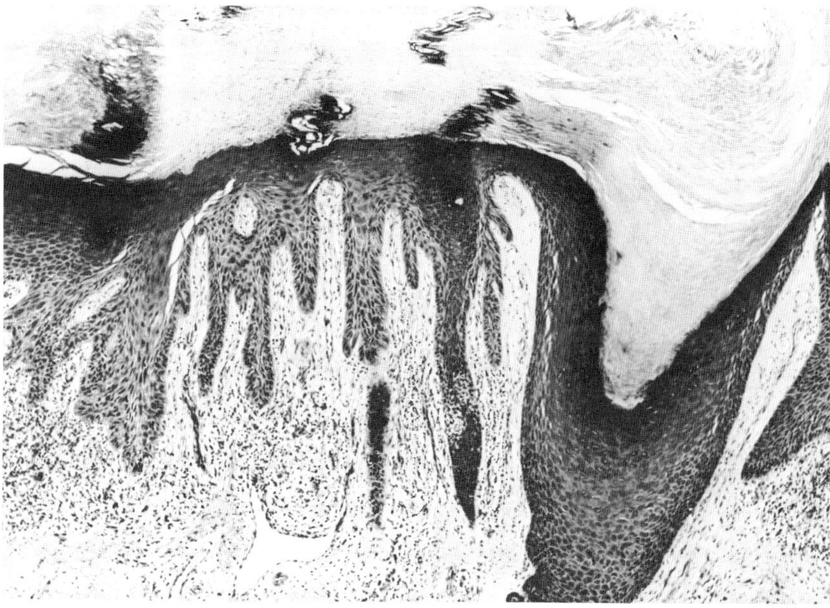

Fig. 3.4. Actinic keratosis. The dysplastic epidermis has provoked an inflammatory reaction and produced a parakeratotic surface. The sweat and follicle ducts are spared and are covered by columns of orthokeratosis. ×56. H & E.

The classical description of the microscopic appearance of actinic ('senile') keratosis by Freudenthal (1926) drew attention to alternating columns of hyperkeratosis and parakeratosis on the surface. It was later shown by Pinkus (1958) that skin appendage ducts emerging through the epidermis were unaffected by the dysplastic process and retained the normal deeper tinctorial quality and the ability to mature to an orthokeratotic horny layer. The microscopic appearance of the surface is thus that of a parakeratotic sheet penetrated by columns of hyperkeratosis arising from the sweat and pilosebaceous ducts like plumes of smoke from chimneys (Fig. 3.4). Sparing of sweat ducts is found in most cases of Bowen's disease and the phenomenon clearly demonstrates the heterogeneous character of the skin surface, the epidermis being shot through by small discs of appendage epithelium capable of reacting differently. The dysplastic cells usually extend down for a short distance around appendage ducts (Fig. 3.5) and also tend to undermine the normal marginal epidermis, providing a sharp diagonal line of junction.

The blood vessels of the papillary dermis are invariably altered by overlying epidermal changes and, indeed, visible changes in the skin vessels may be one of the earliest clinical indications of an impending actinic keratosis. Many keratoses appear to be inflamed and superficial ones may closely simulate inflammatory skin diseases such as discoid lupus erythematosus. Histologically a band of chronic inflammatory cells usually occupies the altered papillary dermis. Elastotic degeneration of the collagen of the

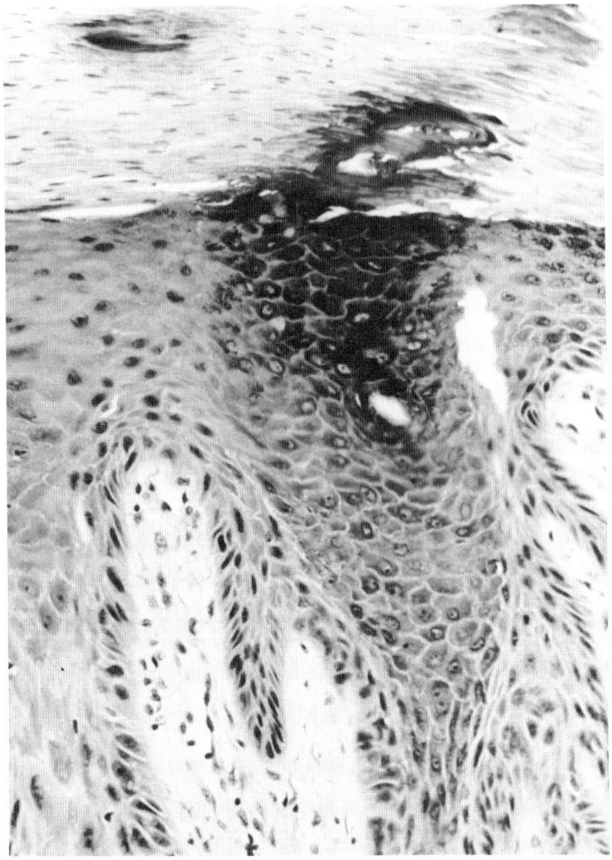

Fig. 3.5. Detail of the sweat duct showing normal sweat duct sharply outlined from dysplastic epidermis. ×220. H & E.

papillary and upper reticular dermis is invariably seen, although the border zone immediately beneath the basal-cell layer usually shows evidence of normal collagen production.

The lower levels of the epidermis of an actinic keratosis may show focal accumulation of immature keratinocytes ('basaloid buds'), which indent the dermo-epidermal junction (Fig. 3.6). A similar accumulation, perhaps as the main pathological feature, sometimes occurs in arsenical keratosis or Bowen's disease (Fig. 3.7), and such lesions may be confused with superficial basal-cell carcinoma. To use the term 'superficial epitheliomatosis' for such lesions, as has been done in the past, may sidestep the microscopist's problem but leaves the clinician uncertain about possible future developments. The distinction can often be made by examining the way the epidermis matures over the affected area. The surface keratin is usually orthokeratotic over a superficial basal cell carcinoma (Fig. 3.8) but shows patchy or confluent parakeratosis over an arsenical keratosis or Bowen's disease.

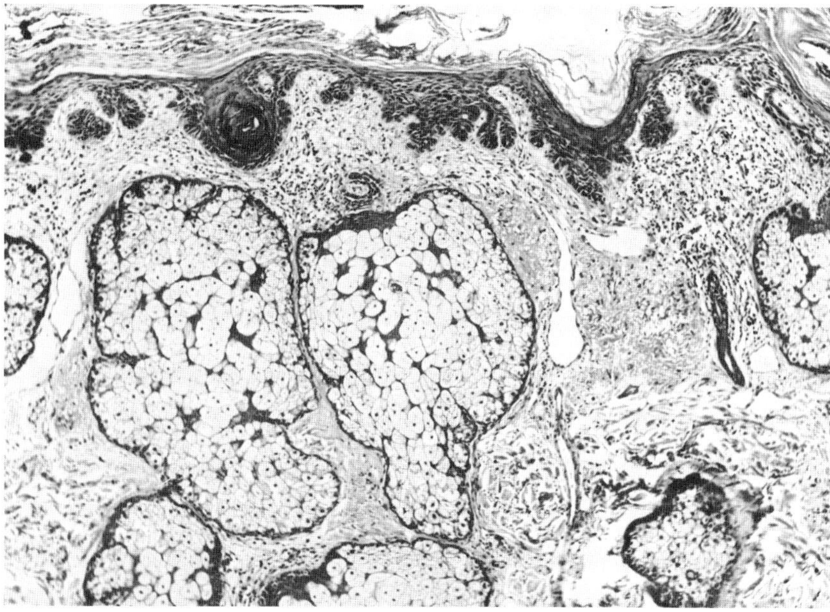

Fig. 3.6. Superficial actinic keratosis of the cheek. The epidermis shows basaloid buds of immature atypical cells. ×56. H & E.

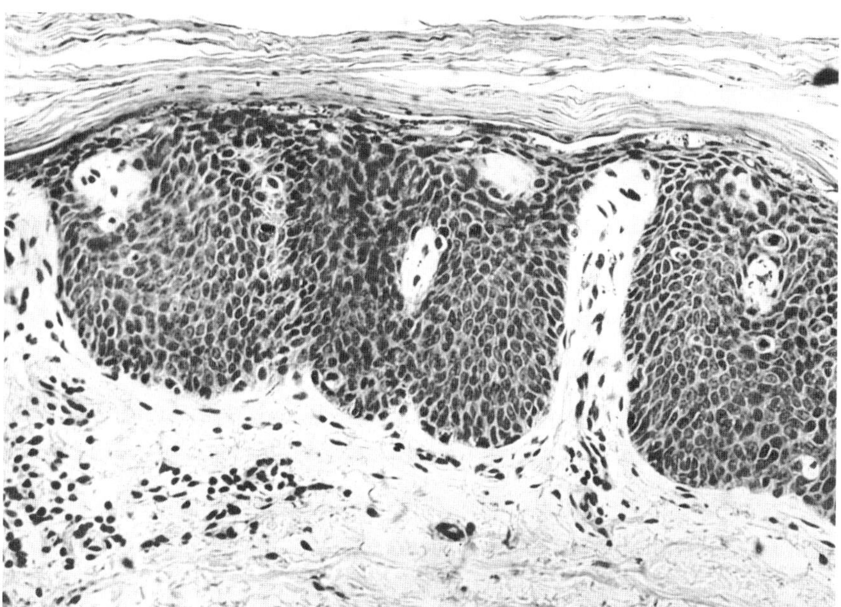

Fig. 3.7. Bowen's disease of the finger. The majority of the epidermal cells show little evidence of maturation. The surface is parakeratotic. ×175. H & E.

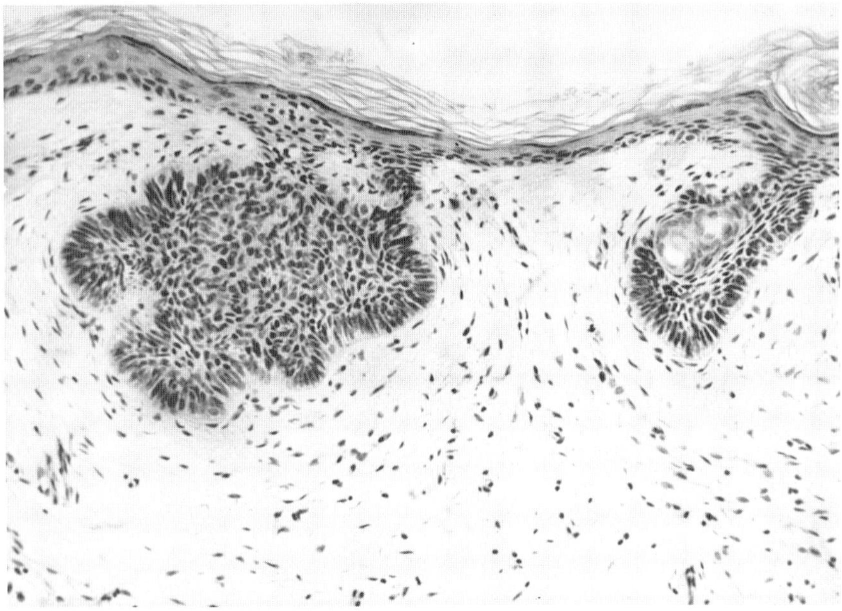

Fig. 3.8. Superficial basal cell carcinoma of the trunk. As well as the characteristic palisading of the tumour margin, the atrophic epidermis is orthokeratotic. A sweat duct is surrounded on the right side. ×175. H & E.

The changes seen in skin subjected to chronic radiodermatitis—for example, on the hands of incautious radiographers and dentists—are essentially similar although the degree of dermal damage, the vascular changes, and some cytological features may be characteristic. The effect of prolonged exposure to fossil-fuel carcinogens is also very similar with both patchy epidermal and more uniform dermal changes. In all these conditions the skin changes are chronic and, in general, progressive even if ultraviolet light and the other agents are avoided. There is, as mentioned above, anecdotal evidence that individual keratoses may disappear spontaneously, as happened with a proportion of the tar warts in animals in the early experiments with chemical carcinogens.

Bowen's disease and its relationship to actinic damage is a puzzling subject, particularly for pathologists who usually lack the opportunity of seeing the clinical manifestations. Considering the range of microscopical changes in the epidermis following each of the different carcinogenic influences, it seems advisable to use the term Bowenoid keratosis for lesions which clinical and other evidence suggest are due to actinic radiation. Bowen's disease (if eponyms continue to be used) can then be reserved for a fairly distinctive clinical entity, the main features of which are the slow, unremitting progression of a red and usually scaly, but sometimes warty, plaque to produce an irregular 'geographical' outline. The appearance can be rather similar to psoriasis but the changes are not modified by the type of treatment which clears psoriatic plaques. The distribution is random over the skin surface, not necessarily associated with actinic changes in the dermis, perhaps tending to favour areas exposed to chronic mild trauma or the lower parts of the legs, especially in women.

There is a distinctive microscopic change seen in some examples of Bowen's disease which is not present in Bowenoid keratosis, and which is more obvious in earlier lesions. In contrast to the sparing of intra-epidermal sweat ducts, the pilosebaceous ducts and possibly part of the sebaceous glands and follicles show precancerous cytological features (Figs. 3.9 and 3.10). On occasion, the change is limited to the pilosebaceous apparatus suggesting that the process begins there and later spreads to the epidermis (Graham *et al.* 1961). The involvement of these structures probably explains the frequency with which multiple punctate recurrence follows superficial treatment of Bowen's disease with cryotherapy or 5-fluorouracil cream, a phenomenon not seen with similarly treated actinic keratoses.

There is evidence to suggest that many more cases of Bowen's disease are due to previous exposure to arsenic than the patients' histories indicate (Graham *et al.* 1961). The hidden sources of arsenic taken perhaps 50 years before were mostly medicinal. Arsenic was previously used very commonly as treatment for a number of common diseases such as psoriasis, eczema and allergic disorders, anaemia, and, in combination with bromide, epilepsy

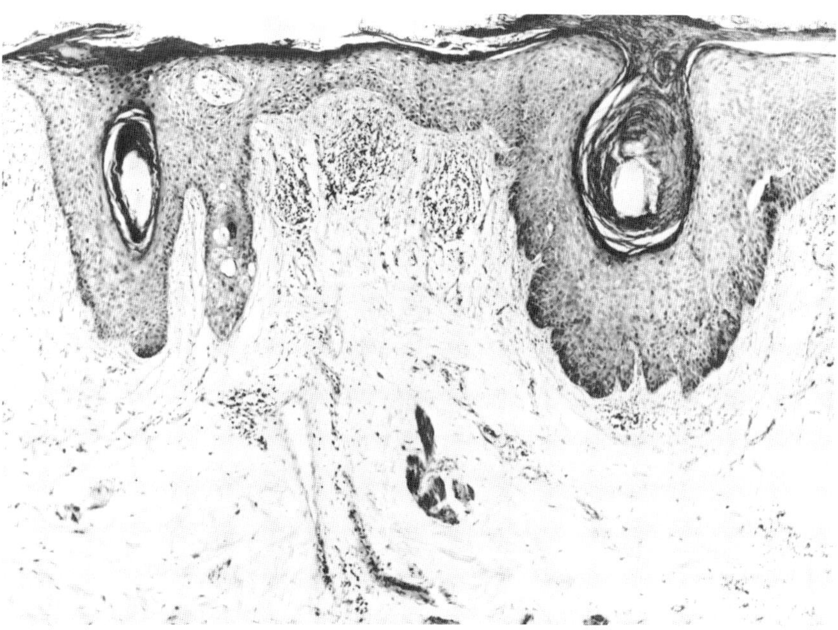

Fig. 3.9. Well-differentiated Bowen's disease involving epidermis and pilosebaceous ducts. ×56. H & E.

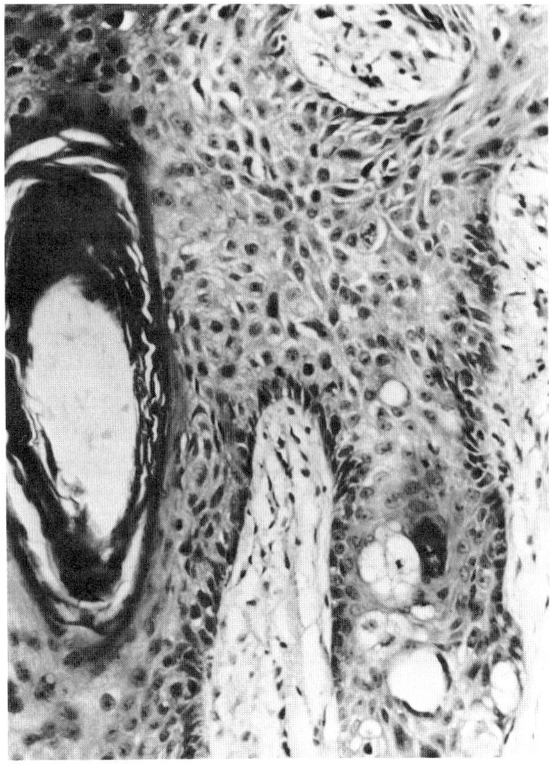

Fig. 3.10. Detail of duct and sebaceous gland. ×195. H & E.

and chorea. It was, and perhaps still is, an ingredient of some proprietary remedies for such disorders. To remember all youthful medication is to ask too much of most patients, but the evidence of raised levels of arsenic in the skin assayed by reliable methods has been found in a sufficient number of patients to make it a likely cause for the majority of such cases. Even in the absence of such assays, repeated careful history taking can get evidence from a patient who intentionally or unintentionally misleads the clinician as the following brief case history shows.

A lady of 64 had multiple red scaly areas on the trunk and limbs for some years which were proved to be Bowen's disease on biopsy. She also had palmoplantar keratoses and had undergone vulvectomy for carcinoma of the vulva. At first she denied exposure to arsenic but later admitted to having dosed herself with Fowler's Solution for acne in her youth. Her father had been a doctor and she had taken advantage of both his textbooks and the medicine cupboard in the surgery, giving herself a substantial dose of arsenic over a period of several years.

In the past, voices have been raised arguing that arsenic is not a proven carcinogen. Occasionally this has been put forward by a committed experimental pathologist unwilling to accept that human patients, too, may be experimental animals at times. Those associated with the manufacture and selling of arsenical products, notably for veterinary use, have a more rational motive for doing so (Frost 1967). There is, however, incontravertible evidence of an epidemiological nature from several areas of the world where the natural water supply is contaminated with arsenic to support the anecdotal evidence of numerous case reports over the last century.

Xeroderma pigmentosum

Xeroderma pigmentosum is a disease in which defects in the enzymic mechanisms for repairing damaged DNA allow the results of ultraviolet radiation on the skin to become manifest in an exaggerated form in childhood or adolescence. Several enzymic processes are involved and variations in the natural history of the disease can be related to different enzyme deficiencies (Cleaver and Bootsma 1975). The disease has an autosomal recessive mode of inheritance and its frequency within a population reflects to some extent the frequency of consanguinous marriages. Heterozygotes do not show symptoms. Cell culture has been the main technique for investigating the biochemical basis of the disease and heterozygous cell lines have levels of excision-repair enzymes that are within the normal range.

In the classical form the skin is normal at birth but the first signs may appear soon afterwards. They consist of erythema or even blistering on exposed areas, provoked by a degree of sun exposure which would not affect normal skin, and after an abnormally long latent period. The later changes resemble in many ways the 'ageing' of exposed skin with atrophy, telangiectasia, variable pigmentation, keratoses, and, later, tumour formation. In advanced cases the scarring may closely resemble an old radiodermatitis with contracture causing ectropion and atresia of mouth and nostrils. Hyperpigmentation is scattered in discrete areas 2-5 mm in diameter resembling freckles or lentigines. It involves not only the exposed skin but also the vermilion of the lips and the bulbar conjunctiva. Other areas show the pallor of scarring with loss of melanocytes. Ocular symptoms include photophobia and conjunctivitis, progressing to precancerous changes or frank conjunctival malignancy. Neurological complications indicate that the disorder is not confined to the skin. These affect only some patients and include microcephaly and mental deficiency, nerve deafness, ataxia, and, in some cases, quadriplegia—the de Sanctis-Cacchione syndrome.

The changes in xeroderma pigmentosum can occur in the coloured races, demonstrating the prime importance of the DNA repair processes. For complete protection from ultraviolet radiation a thick opaque sunscreen for exposed skin and screening sunglasses are required in the most sensitive patients. The prognosis is thus based on several independent factors. The type of enzyme deficiency seems to be the most important determinant of the potential hazard, the intensity of the ultraviolet radiation in the environment and the degree of protection by means of natural skin melanin being of somewhat less significance. The age at diagnosis and thus of the beginning of proper protection is, of course, what determines the actual damage to the DNA. Prenatal diagnosis is thus important.

The example of oculocutaneous albinism makes an interesting contrast as in this disorder the intensity of environmental ultraviolet radiation seems to be the critical factor. Albinos in temperate climates appear to suffer no great increase in skin malignancy but in the tropics or dry sunny places such as South Africa and Central Australia, albino Bantu and aborigines show a high incidence of skin malignancy, including the occasional case of malignant melanoma. Like xeroderma pigmentosum, albinism is an autosomal, recessively inherited disease. The defect is in the melanization of melanosomes, the DNA repair mechanism being normal.

The histological changes of xeroderma pigmentosum in the earlier stages are similar to those of sunburn. Repeated exposure leads to inflammatory changes with pigmentary incontinence, scarring and degenerative changes in the dermis, marked changes in the superficial vasculature with loss of capillary loops, telangiectatic venules, and epidermal atrophy. Similar but less extensive changes may be seen in skin not normally exposed to the sun (Hadida *et al.* 1963). Dysplasia of the epidermis is more extensive, when it appears, than the clinical signs might suggest and tends to cause acanthosis and hyperkeratosis. The tumours that evolve are distinguished mainly by their variability and aggressive behaviour. The microscopist's problem in xeroderma pigmentosum is the recognition of precancerous lesions, particularly pigmented ones, in a generally disturbed population of cells.

For reasons of technical convenience the defects of DNA repair in xeroderma pigmentosum have been studied mainly in fibroblast cultures grown from skin biopsies. The first report (Cleaver 1968) showed that there was a relative failure to carry out excision repair of the damaged DNA. Later work (Cleaver and Trosko 1970) demonstrated that the particular impediment to repair was the presence of cyclobutane pyrimidine dimers induced by the action of ultraviolet light on adjacent pyrimidines in the same strand of DNA. The fibroblasts from xeroderma pigmentosum patients do not differ from those from normal subjects in either their rate of growth or their nutritional needs, and they appear to have a normal karyotype. Many of the cultures are abnormally sensitive to ultraviolet light and to some chemical carcinogens. It has been possible to prove that the common and neurological types of xeroderma pigmentosum are genetically heterogeneous and comprise at least five types, each representing a different defect of excision repair. There is another variant in which the defect is not of excision repair and in which ultraviolet sensitivity is almost normal (Cleaver 1972). In this form of xeroderma pigmentosum the defect is in post-replication repair.

In xeroderma pigmentosum there are precise and measurable biochemical defects which allow a plausible explanation for the excessive sensitivity to ultraviolet light and the inflammation and scarring in the skin which follow. The defects also give clues to some of the events in the early stages of ultraviolet-induced carcinogenesis and of chemical carcinogenesis where the changes in DNA are similar to those from ultraviolet light. The biochemical changes induced by other chemicals, by ionizing radiation, and by viruses are different. The precancerous state can thus arrive through a variety of pathways, and the exploration and charting of these opens up exciting vistas.

References

Cleaver, J.E. (1968). Defective repair replication of DNA in xeroderma pigmentosum. *Nature (London)* **218**, 652.

—— (1972). Xeroderma pigmentosum: Variants with normal DNA repair and normal sensitivity to ultraviolet light. *J. invest. Derm.* **58**, 124.

—— and Trosko, J.E. (1970). Absence of excision of ultra violet-induced cyclobutane dimers in xeroderma pigmentosum. *Photochem. Photobiol.* **11**, 547.

—— and Bootsma, D. (1975). Xeroderma pigmentosum: Biochemical and genetic characteristics. *Ann. Rev. Genet.* **9**, 19.

Deelmann, H.I. (1923). Sur les rapports entré la gènese du cancer du goudron et le traumatisme. *Bull. de l'Assoc. france. p. l'étude du cancer (Paris)* **12**, 715.

Freudenthal, W. (1926). Verruca senilis und keratoma senile. *Arch. Derm. Syph. (Berlin)* **152**, 505.

Frost, D.V. (1967). Arsenicals in biology: retrospect and prospect. *Fed. Proc.* **26**, 194.

Gerstein, W. and Freeman, R.G. (1963). Transplantation of actinically damaged skin. *J. Invest. Derm.* **41**, 445.

Götz, H. (1976). Tar keratosis. In *Cancer of the skin* (eds. R. Andrade, S.L. Gumport, G. L. Popkin, and T.D. Rees), p. 492. W.B. Saunders Company, Philadelphia.

Graham, J.H., Mazzonti, G.R., and Helwig, E.B. (1961). Chemistry of Bowen's disease: relationship to arsenic. *J. invest. Derm.* **37**, 317.

Hadida, E., Marill, F.G. and Sayag, J. (1963). Xeroderma pigmentosum (A propos de 48 observations personelles) *Ann. Derm. Syph. (Paris)* **90**, 467.

Kimura, A., Hera, A., Harada, R., and Nagashima, M. (1978). So-called multicentric pigmented Bowen's disease. Report of a case and a positive etiologic role of human papillomavirus. *Dermatologica* **157**, 229.

Kovi, J., Tillman, R.L. and Lee, S.M. (1974). Malignant transformation of condyloma acuminatum. *Am. J. clin. Path.* **61**, 702.

Lloyd, K.M. (1970). Multicentric pigmented Bowen's disease of the groin. *Archs. Derm. (Chicago)* **101**, 48.

Lutzner, M.A. (1978). Epidermodysplasia verruciformis. An autosomal recessive disease characterized by viral warts and skin cancer. A model for viral oncogenesis. *Bull. Cancer (Paris)* **65**, 169.

McKee, P.H., Wilkinson, J.D., Black, M.M., and Whimster, I.W. (1981). Carcinoma (epithelioma) cuniculatum: a clinico-pathological study of nineteen cases and review of the literature. *Histopathol.* **5**, 425.

Oriel, J.D. and Whimster, I.W. (1971). Carcinoma *in situ* associated with virus-containing anal warts. *Brit. J. Derm.* **84**, 71.

Orr, J.W. (1938). Changes antecedent to tumour formation during treatment of mouse skin with carcinogenic hydrocarbons. *J. Path. Bact.* **46**, 495.

Orth, G., Jablonska, S., Jarzabek-Chorzelska, M., Obalek, S., Rzesa, G., Favre, M., and Croissant, O. (1979). Characteristics of the lesions and risk of malignant conversion associated with the type of human papillomavirus involved in epidermodysplasia verruciformis. *Cancer Res.* **39**, 1074.

Pinkus, H. (1958). Keratosis senilis; a biologic concept of its pathogenesis and diagnosis based on the study of normal epidermis and 1730 seborrheic and senile keratoses. *Amer. J. clin. Path.* **29**, 193.

Ramsay, C.A., Coltart, T.M., Blunt, S., Pawsey, S.A., and Giannelli, F. (1974). Prenatal diagnosis of xeroderma pigmentosum. Report of the first successful case. *Lancet* **2**, 1109.

Tseng, W.P., Chu, H.M., How, S.W., Fong, J.M., Lin, C.S., and Yeh, S. (1968). Prevalence of skin cancer in Taiwan. *J. Nat. Cancer Inst.* **40**, 453.

Wade, T.R., Kopf, A.W., and Ackerman, A.B. (1978). Bowenoid papulosis of the penis. *Cancer* **42**, 1890.

Wyburn-Mason, R. (1957). Malignant changes following herpes simplex. *Brit. med. J.* **2**, 615.

Yeh, S., How, S.W., and Lin, C.S. (1968). Arsenical cancer of the skin. Histologic study with special reference to Bowen's disease. *Cancer* **21**, 312.

4 Precancerous changes in the breast

J.P. Sloane

Breast carcinomas are frequently associated with certain proliferative changes in the adjacent mammary tissues. Such proliferations have a variable appearance and may show a continuous spectrum of changes from normality to malignancy through grades of typical and increasingly atypical hyperplasia. Several interpretations are possible from such a static histological picture. First, carcinogenic agents may induce a variety of benign and malignant changes in a one-stage process. Second, some or all intraductal and intralobular proliferations may represent carcinomas at an early, non-infiltrative stage of their development which would progress inevitably to infiltrating carcinoma given enough time. Third, carcinomas may evolve in a multistage fashion from precursor or *preneoplastic* lesions which are not in themselves neoplastic but have a greater probability of developing into carcinoma than normal tissues. Such considerations are clearly of fundamental interest and also have direct clinical relevance in assessing the possible risks which such lesions may entail.

Although there is much indirect evidence that human breast tumours evolve from precursor lesions, the concept of preneoplasia cannot be investigated adequately in man as it is impossible (or at least unethical) to observe the evolution of malignant tumours in the human breast. In experimental animals, however, morphological changes may be observed at different intervals after administration of carcinogens, but even experiments such as these have their limitations. Ultimately the existence of a preneoplastic state can only be demonstrated satisfactorily if putative precursor lesions are identified, isolated, and transplanted into another site where their subsequent behaviour can be observed. Such experiments have been performed in rodents, and the results of these and other experimental studies are described below. The changes observed in human breast tissues are then considered in the light of this work.

Observations in mice

Mouse mammary tumours may occur spontaneously or in susceptible strains harbouring the mouse mammary tumour virus (MTV) (Bentvelzen and Daams 1969). Tumours may also be induced by chemical carcinogens such as 7,12-dimethyl benz(a)anthracene (DMBA), 20-methylcholanthrene (MCA), dibenzanthracene (DBA), and benzo(a)pyrene (BP) (Biancifiori *et al.* 1961) or by hormonal stimulation with oestrogens or pituitary implants either alone (Muhlbock 1956) or in combination with chemical carcinogens (Faulkin 1966).

Like their human counterparts, mouse mammary carcinomas exhibit a variable histological appearance, not only from tumour to tumour but also within the same lesion (Squartini 1979). Some are well differentiated and composed of uniform cells arranged in acinar structures, and these appear to correspond roughly to the tubular carcinomas of the human. Most tumours exhibit a varied structure with acinar regions, intracystic papillary projections, solid cords, nests, and sheets of cells. Necrosis is not uncommon and squamous metaplasia may occur. The amount of stroma is variable, but in general the extensive dense collagenous and elastotic stroma of the human lesions is not encountered. Another major point of difference is the growth pattern which in mice is expansile; this results in well-circumscribed nodular lesions in contrast to the infiltrative, ill-defined human tumours. Although mouse tumours do metastasize to lymph nodes and the lung parenchyma, they do so later and far less frequently than human breast carcinomas.

Sequential histological studies of 'early' tumours in mice show that they appear to arise either directly from normal tissues or in pre-existing hyperplastic lesions which are of three main types—hyperplastic alveolar nodules (HANs), ductal hyperplasias, and structures known as plaques (Foulds 1956).

Hyperplastic alveolar nodules (Figs. 4.1-4.3)

Hyperplastic alveolar nodules (HANs) were first reported by Apolant (1906) and later described in detail by Haaland (1911) who referred to them as hypertrophic nodules. They exhibit a rather variable appearance but are essentially enlarged lobules with increased numbers of acini which are not usually significantly dilated. The acini may be lined by a single layer of cytologically atypical cells or there may be multilayering and/or atypicality. The size of the nodules varies, and Haaland noted all grades of change from normal lobules to hypertrophic nodules and true tumours. The lesions are usually multifocal and may or may not exhibit secretory changes. They are the main proliferative lesions occurring in mice infected with mammary tumour virus (MTV) or its variants, and they occur less frequently in animals treated with chemical carcinogens where ductal hyperplasias are more common (Medina 1976)—see later.

Using the dissecting microscope, HANs have been identified and removed from the breast of MTV-infected tumour-bearing female mice and transplanted into new hosts either in the subcutis or in mammary fat pads cleared of epithelial tissue (DeOme *et al.* 1959). In these experiments nine out of 19 HANs transplanted into cleared fat pads developed into tumours compared to two out of 19 samples of normal breast tissue. Furthermore, tumours developed from HANs within 13-21 weeks whereas the first

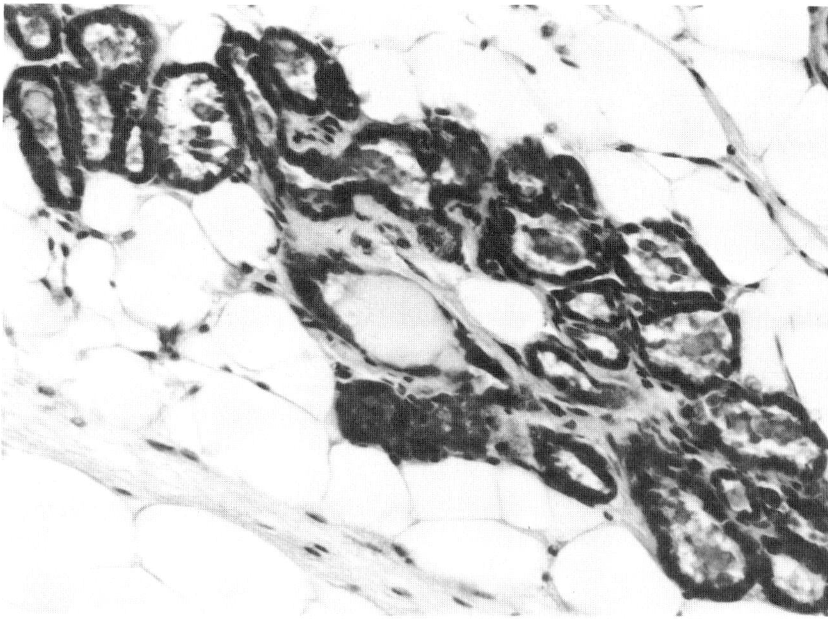

Fig. 4.1. Murine hyperplastic alveolar nodule. There is slight dilatation of the acini which are lined by a single layer of cells with hyperchromatic nuclei. Secretory changes are prominent. ×302. H & E.

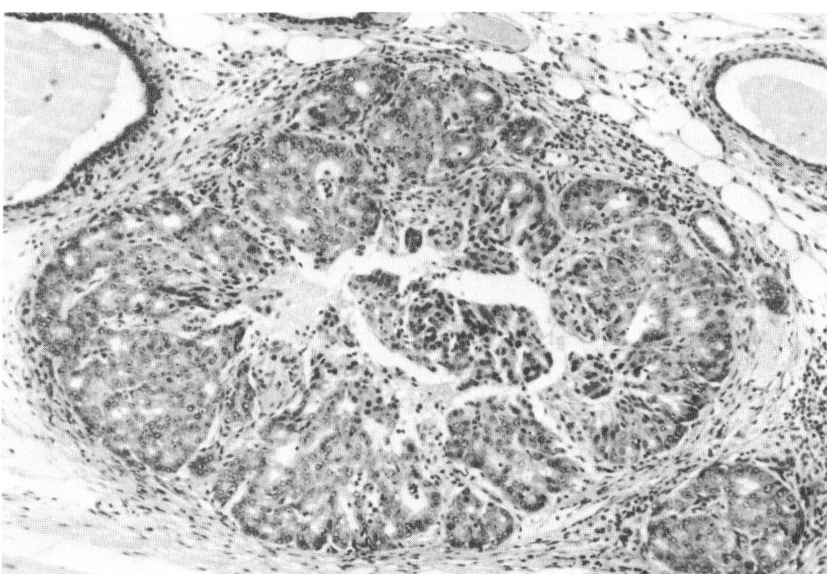

Fig. 4.2. Murine hyperplastic alveolar nodule at a more advanced stage of proliferation than that illustrated in Fig. 4.1. There are numerous acini, many of which are poorly formed. The appearances begin to merge with those of breast carcinoma in this example. ×120. H & E.

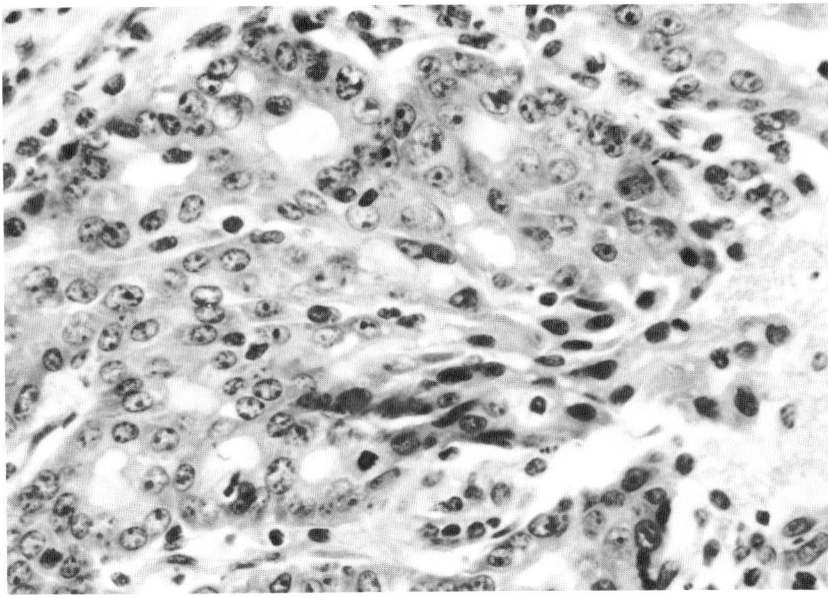

Fig. 4.3. High-power view of the lesion illustrated in Fig. 4.2, showing poorly formed acini mixed with solid areas. There is a mixed cell population of epithelial cells, myoepithelial cells, and lymphocytes. A zone of necrosis can be seen on the right of the picture. ×480. H & E.

tumour from transplanted normal breast tissues appeared at 24 weeks. A further two of the 19 transplants of normal breast tissues developed into HANs. Many of the 80 HANs transplanted into the subcutaneous tissue regressed, and only one gave rise to a tumour. Thus, normal tissues may develop into hyperplastic alveolar nodules which themselves develop into tumour more frequently and more quickly than do normal tissues. Transformation is not, however, inevitable. Normal tissues may also develop into tumours but it is not clear whether this occurs directly or only through intermediate stages. The role of the breast stroma in the proliferation and transformation of normal and preneoplastic cells is clearly an important one.

As a result of experiments such as these, DeOme and Medina (1969) proposed that carcinogenesis in the mouse breast is a two-stage process—from normal to HAN and from HAN to tumour. Statistical studies on human tumours, however, have suggested that as many as six stages may be involved (Armitage and Doll 1954) and this may also be the case in the mouse; the morphological heterogeneity of HANs suggests that they themselves may pass through various stages of development before becoming truly neoplastic.

It has been shown that different HANs vary in their potential for tumour development. Using several HAN out-growth lines derived from individual nodules taken from virus-free hormonally stimulated mice and serially transplanted into new hosts, DeOme and Medina (1969) demonstrated that both the spontaneous incidence of tumours and their latent intervals varied from one cell line to another. Furthermore, the spontaneous incidence could be increased by exposure to MTV, chemical carcinogens, or irradiation, and the susceptibility of each cell line to different agents also varied.

Hyperplastic alveolar nodules have been the subject of many metabolic studies. An isoenzyme of glucose-6-phosphate dehydrogenase (G6PD-1) accounts for about one-third of the total G6PD activity in mammary adenocarcinomas but the enzyme is virtually absent from normal mouse breast. An intermediate value of about 12 per cent is found in HANs (Hilf *et al.* 1973). In some respects HANs are metabolically similar to normal breast tissues, but in others they are more like tumours. Glucose uptake, conversion of glucose to fatty acids, and acetate utilization in HANs are similar to normal breast tissues and greater than in mammary tumours (Bartley *et al.* 1971). The activity of t-RNA methylases is also similar in HANs and normal breast tissues but much lower than in tumours (Abraham and Bartley 1974).

During the change from pregnancy to lactation, however, fatty acid synthesis in the normal breast shifts from predominantly 12-14 carbon fatty acids to those with 10-12 carbon chains, but this qualitative change has not been demonstrated in HANs. Similarly, the fall in DNA and, to a lesser extent, RNA synthesis which occurs in normal breast at the onset of lactation does not occur in HANs or adenocarcinomas (Abraham and Bartley 1974). Banerjee *et al.* (1973) have also shown that HANs may be unresponsive to normal ovarian hormonal control.

On the other hand, Faulkin and DeOme (1960) demonstrated that HANs respond to local growth-controlling influences in a similar fashion to normal mammary epithelium. When HANs are transplanted into cleared mammary fat pads they grow to fill the pad, but they do not overgrow and replace it as do malignant tumours. Furthermore when HANs are transplanted into non-cleared glands, the intact epithelial elements have an inhibitory effect on HAN growth which tumours can override.

HANs have also been examined for their ability to promote angiogenesis, a feature of many malignant tumours. Gimbrone and Gullino (1976) studied the effect of various types of mammary tissue implanted into the irises of rabbits. Ninety per cent of mammary tumours induced significant neovascularization compared to 6 per cent of normal tissues. HANs exhibited intermediate behaviour with about 30 per cent showing a pattern of vessel growth similar to that induced by breast tumours.

In nuclear magnetic resonance studies, spin-lattice relaxation times for hyperplastic alveolar nodules were intermediate between those obtained for normal and neoplastic breast tissues (Beall *et al.* 1980).

It has been shown that cytochalasin B can induce multinucleation in cultured neoplastic mammary epithelial cells whereas normal mammary epithelial cells are much less susceptible to this agent. Medina *et al.* (1980) have used this phenomenon to investigate cultures of preneoplastic cells.

The percentage of multinucleate cells in preneoplastic cultures after treatment with cytochalasin B was similar to that in cultures of normal cells.

Thus, taken as a whole, the functional and metabolic properties of hyperplastic alveolar nodules, like their morphological features, are intermediate between normal and neoplastic breast tissues.

Ductal hyperplasias (Fig. 4.4)

HANs do not occur as frequently in mice treated with chemical carcinogens as in those infected with MTV although they do seem to have the same tumour potential in such animals (Medina 1979). The more usual lesions associated with chemical carcinogens in the breast are ductal hyperplasias and keratinized nodules. The latter consist of a few dilated alveoli filled with keratin-like material and desquamated cells; they exhibit a low growth potential and do not produce tumours on transplantation (Medina). Ductal hyperplasias are of several major types characterized by Medina (1976) as follows.

Simple terminal duct hyperplasia in which there is multilayering of ducts with cytologically typical cells.

Lobular hyperplasia in which acini are completely filled with uniform epithelial cells.

End bud hyperplasia, characterized by proliferation of small or terminal ducts capped by club-like structures composed of uniform epithelial cells.

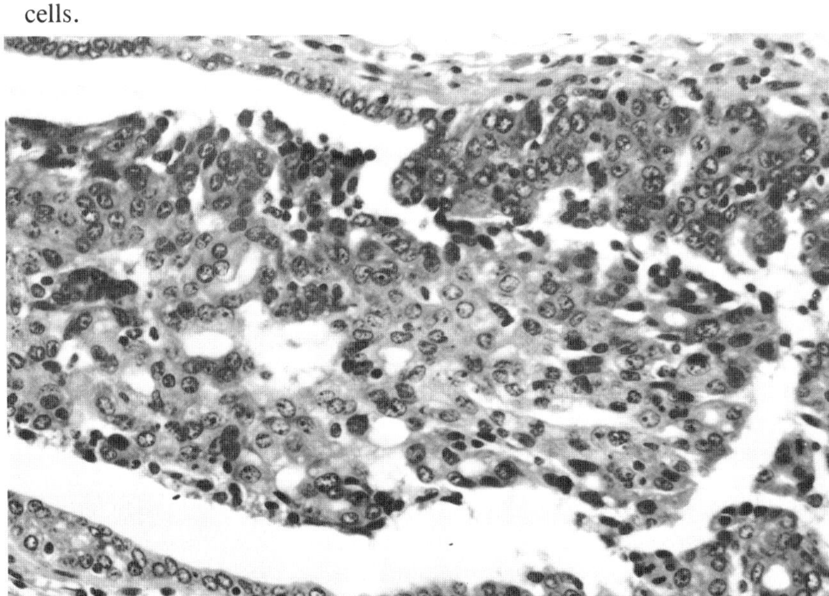

Fig. 4.4. Ductal hyperplasia in the mouse. This is a terminal duct with the beginning of the lobule on the right of the picture. A polypoid mass consisting of epithelial, myoepithelial and lymphoid cells projects into the lumen. ×302. H & E.

Ductal papillary hyperplasia forming intraductal papillary projections ranging from a few simple folds to complex structures resembling papillomas.

The papillae may or may not have connective tissue cores. Cellular atypia may be seen, and in some cases the lesions merge with *in situ* carcinomas.

Outgrowth cell lines have been established from ductal hyperplasias, but unlike those derived from HANs they cannot be serially transplanted indefinitely. Nevertheless they produce tumours on transplantation which demonstrates their preneoplastic nature. Papillary hyperplasias tend to develop into papillary carcinomas, and lobular hyperplasias produce tumours with a multiform appearance. The ductal tissue not producing tumours but serially transplanted tends to exhibit progressively declining growth potential and eventually either reverts to normal or becomes cystic. Thus the cells of these lesions appear to be heterogeneous with regard to their tumour-forming ability, and regression may take place. Some of the cell lines depend on hormones for transformation into tumours.

Ductal hyperplasias have not yet been subjected to extensive functional and metabolic investigations as have HANs.

Plaques

Plaques are disc-like structures usually 0.5-1.0 cm in diameter and 0.1-0.2 cm thick when first recognized clinically (Foulds 1956). They are thus larger than HANs and they are usually single, although two or three plaques may sometimes develop in one breast. They have smooth outlines but are not encapsulated, and they have a symmetrical, organoid structure. There is a central medulla of loose connective tissue in which normal-looking tubules are scattered and a more compact cortex of radially orientated branching tubules lined by pleomorphic cells which may be multilayered. During pregnancy, plaques increase in size by overgrowth of tubules in the cortical zone and regression takes place after parturition. Progression to carcinoma has been observed in these lesions, especially after repeated pregnancies, and the neoplastic change may be either focal (uni- or multifocal) or diffuse. The resulting tumours may or may not be hormone responsive and commonly exhibit a varied growth pattern. Plaques usually occur in MTV-bearing mice (Squartini 1979).

Observations in rats

Mammary tumours may develop spontaneously in all rats but the frequency varies considerably from one strain to another. Tumours may be induced by oestrogens (Geschickter and Byrnes 1942), by chemical carcinogens such as 2-acetylaminofluorene (AF) (Wilson *et al.* 1941), MC (Shay *et al.* 1949), or DMBA (Huggins *et al.* 1961), or by irradiation (Shellabarger *et al.* 1957). At present there is no convincing evidence for a viral aetiology in rat mammary carcinomas. Apart from the strain, the age of the animal also greatly influences the response to tumour-inducing agents (Huggins *et al.* 1961).

Although there is a considerable resemblance between mammary tumours of man and the rat, especially in the range of differentiation exhibited, there are important differences (Young and Hallowes 1973). Like the mouse, the dense stromal fibrosis of human tumours is rarely seen in the rat. Metastases are very uncommon unless the animals are immunosuppressed in various ways (Kim 1979). Fibrocystic disease is a rare accompaniment of rat tumours except in those induced by oestrogens.

It has been suggested that rat mammary tumours may arise from HANs, ductal hyperplasias, or direct from normal mammary epithelium. Middleton (1965) induced tumours in female Wistar rats using AF, MC, and DMBA, and histological examination of the resulting 'early' lesions showed that most arose in ducts, ductules, or end-buds and a minority in acini. Middleton concluded that no lesions were encountered which could be regarded as morphological precursors of neoplastic transformation although his observation that the early end-bud carcinomas closely resembled normal end-buds in growing breasts underlines the major problem of subjectivity in characterizing lesions as preneoplastic or neoplastic by histology alone.

Hyperplastic alveolar nodules (HANs)

The evidence for the preneoplastic status of HANs in rats is conflicting. Beuving *et al.* (1967*a*) induced carcinomas in 50-day-old female Sprague-Dawley rats with a single intragastric dose of 20 mg DMBA. The tumours were accompanied by HANs which accounted for 75 per cent of the lesions observed, the remainder being distended alveolar nodules, 'area nodules', and fibrous nodules; ductal hyperplasias were not mentioned. The authors concluded that HANs were likely to be preneoplastic as they did not occur in untreated control animals, were present at the first appearance of tumours, and (like the tumours themselves) increased in number with increasing time after carcinogen treatment. Transplantation experiments were later undertaken with 50-60-day-old Fischer rats given a single intragastric dose of 20, 15, or 10 mg DMBA (Beuving *et al.* 1967*b*). Tumours and HANs were found only in the treated animals together with distended alveolar nodules, fibrous nodules, and ductal hyperplasias, but transplantation of HANs into cleared fat pads of 3-week-old rats resulted in hyperplastic outgrowths but no tumour formation. It was concluded that the low tumour-forming capabilities of HANs from Fischer rats may be related to the known relative lack of sensitivity of this strain to breast tumour induction. The experiments were therefore repeated using Lewis rats in which the incidence of hyperplastic lesions is approximately five times that of other rat strains (Beuving 1968). This time, about 20 per cent of the HAN outgrowths produced tumours within 11-52 weeks after transplantation.

Russo *et al.* (1977) administered 20 mg DMBA to 55-day-old Sprague-Dawley rats by gastric instillation and observed the evolution of tumours at intervals over the ensuing weeks. Although HANs were observed they did not appear to give rise to tumours which were all intraductal in origin—see below. Sinha and Dao (1974) also treated 55-day-old Sprague-Dawley rats with single doses of DMBA both intravenously (5 mg) and by direct application to the breast (300μg, 100μg, or 25μg). With intravenous administration, the animals developed both HANs and mammary tumours but the inguinal glands developed more HANs than the others, whereas tumour incidence was highest in the axillary glands. This lack of correlation between the number of HANs and the number of tumours led to the conclusion that HANs were not preneoplastic. Furthermore, local application of DMBA to the gland resulted in the appearance of carcinomas without the formation of HANs. These findings prompted the suggestion that normal cells transform directly to neoplastic ones and require no intermediate steps. The neoplastic outgrowth developing from some HANs may simply indicate that HANs contain a neoplastic cell population.

HANs in rats have been studied biochemically but not as extensively as those of the mouse. Dao *et al.* (1975) found that both the rate of DNA synthesis and the oestrogen-binding protein concentration in HANs were lower than in both normal mammary epithelium and in mammary tumours—an observation which would be against their preneoplastic status. DNA synthesis was, however, determined on breast tissue from normal animals 60-66 days old at a time when extensive lobular-alveolar development is taking place (Russo *et al.* 1977) whereas HANs were taken from animals about 45 days older when the normal labelling index would be expected to be lower; but the differences in oestrogen binding protein concentrations cannot easily be explained away. Both HANs and normal tissues can increase casein synthesis in response to hormonal stimulation whereas mammary tumours fail to respond.

The situation relating to the preneoplastic status of rat hyperplastic alveolar nodules is thus a complicated one although there are certain consistent threads running through the experimental data. In mice, transplanted HANs exhibit varying neoplastic potentials which can be increased by further exposure to carcinogenic agents. HAN formation in this species is strongly related to the presence of MTV, and the tumour potential of HANs from MTV-infected mice is greater than from those from MTV-free animals on transplantation (Blair and DeOme 1961)—possibly due to the continued presence of the oncogenic agent. Presumably there are inherent (possibly genetic) factors operating in high-tumour strain animals which favour malignant transformation of normal or preneoplastic breast tissues and this might explain why, in rats, the preneoplastic status of HANs is only revealed in high-tumour strains. It thus seems that rat HANs are potentially preneoplastic but (at least in most strains) are part of a relatively unimportant route in neoplastic transformation, and that this major difference from mouse neoplasia is at least partly related to the different aetiologies of breast tumours in the two species.

Ductal hyperplasias

The evolution of carcinomas from mammary ducts has been observed by sequential observations on DMBA- and MCA-treated rats rather than by transplantation experiments (Russo *et al.* 1977; Sinha and Dao 1975; Fisher *et al*, 1975*a*, *b*). The carcinogens have usually been administered intragastrically to 50-60-day-old rats in which breast development is incomplete and lobules not yet formed. Although some lobular development takes place during the course of the experiments, the distinction between ductal and lobular origin may not be relevant. Nevertheless, the changes are most marked in the peripheral parts of the duct system while the larger ducts are less frequently involved. The earliest changes occur in the terminal end-buds which become larger due to hyperplasia and hypertrophy of the lining cells, producing several layers of relatively incohesive cells. These intraductal proliferations (IDP) later develop secondary lumina giving rise to cribriform and papillary patterns. The periductal tissues become fibrotic and infiltrated with lymphocytes. Individual IDP tend to coalesce to form lobules of a single tumour, and eventually the histological features are unequivocally those of carcinoma. The weight of evidence suggests that most carcinomas developing in rats treated with chemical carcinogens arise from the ductal system in this way rather than from HANs, a conclusion that is consistent with the findings in carcinogen-treated mice (Medina 1979).

Fisher *et al.* (1976*a*, *b*) classified the proliferative lesions into three main grades of severity: mild hyperplasia, advanced hyperplasia, and cancer. Ultrastructurally, the cells comprising advanced hyperplasia and cancer were indistinguishable. Both showed a disrupted or deficient basal lamina around cell aggregates, pseudopodial extensions of the cell cytoplasm, and an absence of myoepithelial differentiation. These abnormalities were not present in mild hyperplasias. Some ultrastructual abnormalities such as accumulation of cytoplasmic lipid, polyribosomal aggregates, secretory vacuoles, Golgi structures and condensation of nuclear chromatin were noted in mild hyperplasias but were not as pronounced in advanced hyperplasia or cancer.

In their system, mild hyperplasia could also be induced by the administration of oestradiol or progesterone but, although the changes were morphologically indistinguishable from those induced by carcinogens, they did not progress to advanced hyperplasia or to cancer. This led Fisher and his colleagues to use chromosome analysis in an attempt to distinguish between the various forms of ductal hyperplasia. In normal mammary glands, 95 per cent of the cells had the normal diploid number with 2 per cent polyploid and 3 per cent aneuploid forms. Seven per cent of cells from early hyperplasias induced by MCA exhibited aneuploidy and 4 per cent contained major aberrations such as chromosome breaks, fragments, and marker chromosomes. Twenty-seven per cent of cells from advanced ductal hyperplasias were aneuploid and 7 per cent exhibited major aberrations. Cancers contained 32 per cent aneuploid cells and 12 per cent showed major aberrations. Ductal hyperplasias induced by hormones were cytogenetically normal.

Ductal lesions induced by chemical carcinogens and by hormones could also be distinguished by transplantation experiments. When 3-mm cubes of biopsy material were transplanted into the subcutaneous tissues of syngeneic recipients, growth occurred only with advanced hyperplasias and cancers produced by MCA. Histologically, the transplants faithfully reproduced the appearance of the donor lesions and the hyperplasias did not undergo malignant transformation. Most lesions began to regress after about 15 days.

Observations in dogs

Cameron and Faulkin (1971) described hyperplastic lesions in the mammary glands of female beagle dogs. All were alveolar in origin and no primary extralobular duct lesions were seen. Lesions were of two main types: lobules which were merely enlarged with all constituents present in normal proportions, and atypical lobules with focal or diffuse overgrowth or epithelial and/or myoepithelial cells. Some of the lobular lesions were regarded as neoplastic. Atypical nodules, as well as normal and neoplastic tissues, were later transplanted into the cheek pouches of immunosuppressed hamsters (Richmond and Faulkin 1975). All tissues survived but none exhibited growth or transformation, the histological appearances remaining the same over the 45-day test period. Thus, although fundamental transplantation evidence is still lacking, the evidence seems to point to a lobular origin for mammary tumours in the beagle and to the existence of preneoplastic lesions not dissimilar to the HANs of rodents. It should, however, be noted that established mammary tumours in the beagle bitch are extremely diverse in their histology, many of them having no obvious counterpart in the human.

Observations in humans

The normal human breast

The human breast consists of about 15-20 segments which converge on the nipple to form lactiferous sinuses and collecting ducts. The lactiferous sinuses communicate distally with a branching system of interlobular ducts which eventually end in numerous terminal ducts, each of which supplies a lobule. The lobules consist of acini (or ductules) surrounded by stroma which is looser than that in the interlobular zones (Fig. 4.5 (a)). The terminal ducts and lobules are collectively known as 'terminal duct-lobular units' (TDLU). The epithelial lining of the whole duct system consists of a double epithelial layer comprising an inner luminal layer of cuboidal epithelial cells and an outer layer of myoepithelial cells. The latter may assume a number of different forms. Sometimes, especially in atrophic breasts, the myoepithelial cells are obviously myoid in appearance and are spindle-

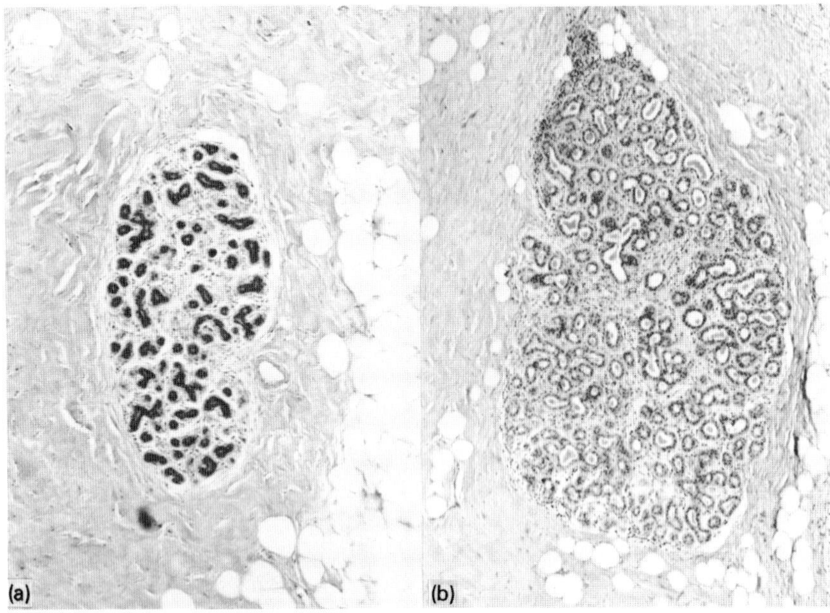

Fig. 4.5. (a) Normal lobule of human breast. (b) Lobule showing adenosis for comparison. ×50. H. & E.

shaped with abundant cytoplasm. Myofibrils may be demonstrated with conventional muscle stains such as phosphotungstic acid-haematoxylin (PTAH). In pregnancy and lactation, by contrast, they form a thin, barely recognizable layer around the acini. In the normal resting state, they are cuboidal in outline and difficult to distinguish morphologically from the epithelial cells; enzyme histochemical and immunocytochemical techniques may be required (Fig. 4.6).

'Benign breast disease'

This term, along with many others including fibrocystic disease, cystic mastopathy, and fibroadenosis, has been used to describe a number of morphological lesions of a largely cystic and proliferative nature which frequently but not invariably coexist. The various terms have a number of disadvantages. Different patients exhibit different types of lesions either alone or in combination, and there is no proof that these changes share a common aetiology; certainly, recent studies have shown that they do not have the same precancerous potential. The use of the word 'disease' is also questionable in view of the frequency with which some of the lesions occur in the general population. When reporting non-malignant breast biopsies, it is our policy merely to describe the changes present without attempting to group them into a single disease entity or even necessarily to give them a pathological significance.

Cysts (Figs. 4.7 and 4.8) are formed by dilatation of acini and for this reason usually appear in clusters. They vary greatly from microscopic

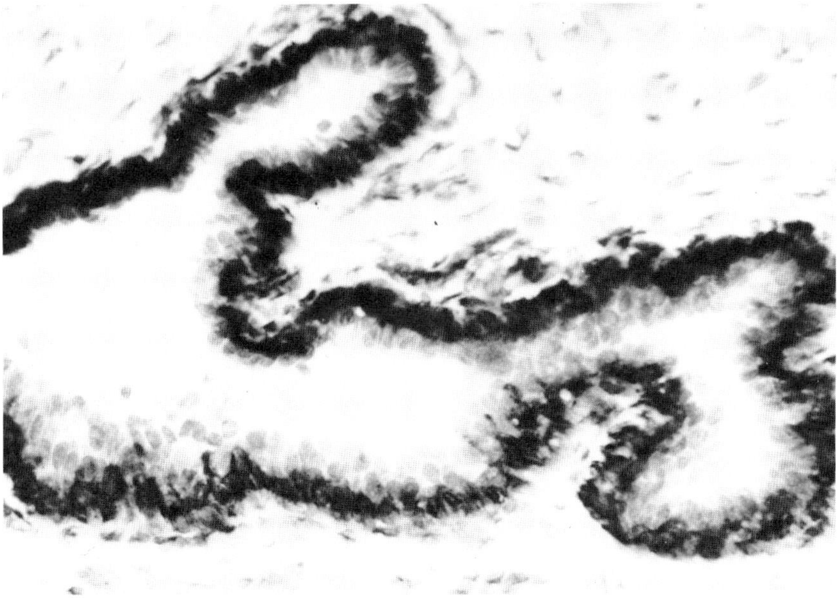

Fig. 4.6. Frozen section of normal interlobular human breast duct stained for alkaline phosphatase. The dark reaction product is present in the cytoplasm of the outer myoepithelial cells. ×302.

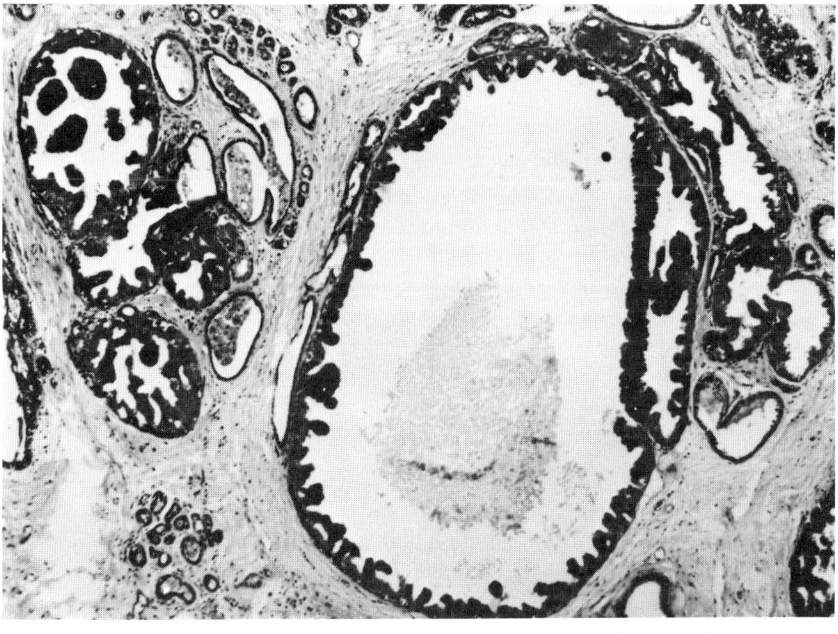

Fig. 4.7. Cluster of apocrine cysts in which lobular architecture is still discernible. There are residual normal lobular elements on the left of the picture. Intraluminal papillary proliferation is prominent. ×48. H & E.

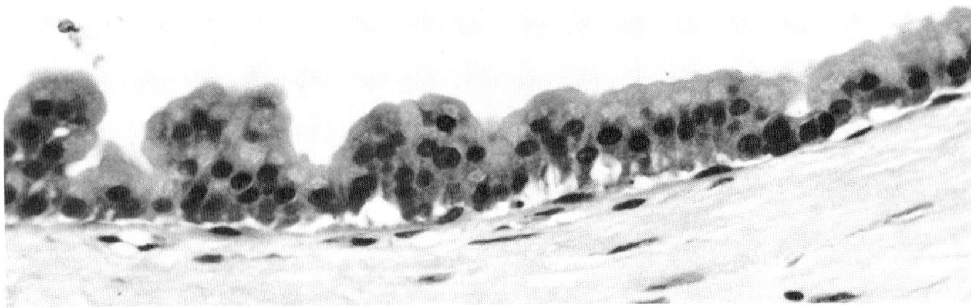

Fig. 4.8. High-power view of cyst wall showing large apocrine cells with copious, deeply eosinophilic cytoplasm exhibiting foci of intraluminal papillary tufting. ×302. H & E.

lesions to spaces measuring several centimetres in diameter. The lining epithelium is usually flattened or exhibits metaplasia toward large apocrine-like cells with copious, deeply eosinophilic cytoplasm which exhibits luminal budding. The normal two-cell layer may be retained and intra-luminal papillary proliferations may be observed.

Duct ectasia (Fig. 4.9). Dilatation of ducts may also vary considerably in degree. The double-cell layer is usually preserved and apocrine metaplasia is exceptional. The dilated ducts appear as sausage-shaped structures and frequently contain large numbers of foamy macrophages. Duct ectasia is commonly associated with cyst formation. There is also another form of duct ectasia which appears to form a separate entity, also referred to as plasma cell mastitis. Here, there is involvement of the collecting ducts and

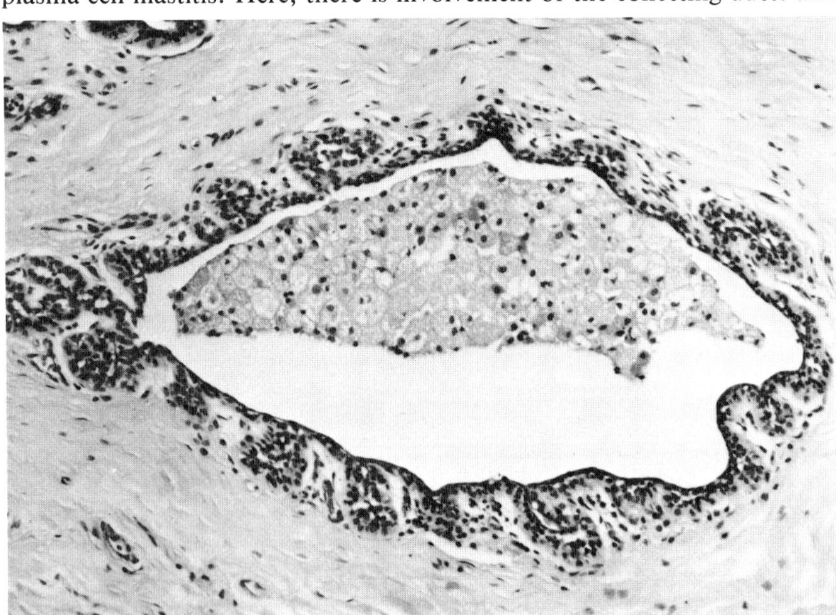

Fig. 4.9. Ectatic duct containing foamy macrophages. ×120. H & E.

lactiferous sinuses which show dilatation and marked periductal chronic inflammation which progresses to fibrosis. The fibrous tissue may subsequently retract, giving rise to indrawing of the nipple which can be misinterpreted as clinical evidence of carcinoma.

Autopsy studies indicate that more than 70 per cent of allegedly normal breasts may exhibit some degree of cyst formation or duct ectasia by the time of the menopause (Frantz *et al.* 1951; Sandison 1962).

Adenosis (Fig. 4.5(b)). Used on its own, this term refers to enlargement of lobules due to increased numbers of normal appearing acini; but it should be noted that normal lobules may show a considerable variation in size even in the same patient. Wellings *et al.* (1975) noted that lobules were best developed in the central and lateral parts of the breast.

Sclerosing adenosis (Figs. 4.10 and 4.11). Although it appears to have no significant precancerous potential, this lesion is of considerable practical importance to diagnostic histopathologists as it may be confused both macroscopically and microscopically with infiltrating carcinoma. At low power, the lobular architecture is preserved, and this is usually the main clue to the correct diagnosis. The individual lesions are composed of narrow tubules and solid cords with characteristically spiky and distorted outlines. In the early stages, the stroma is delicate but fibrosis ensues with compression of epithelial elements. These lesions are undoubtedly infiltrative and may even exhibit local vascular and perineural invasion (Taylor and Norris

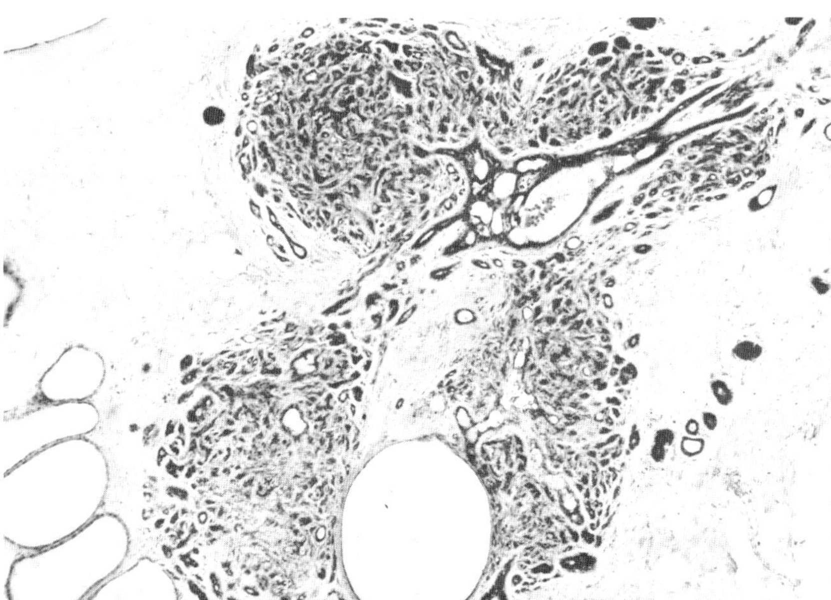

Fig. 4.10. Sclerosing adenosis. Despite the infiltrative appearance, the lobular architecture is retained. ×48. H & E.

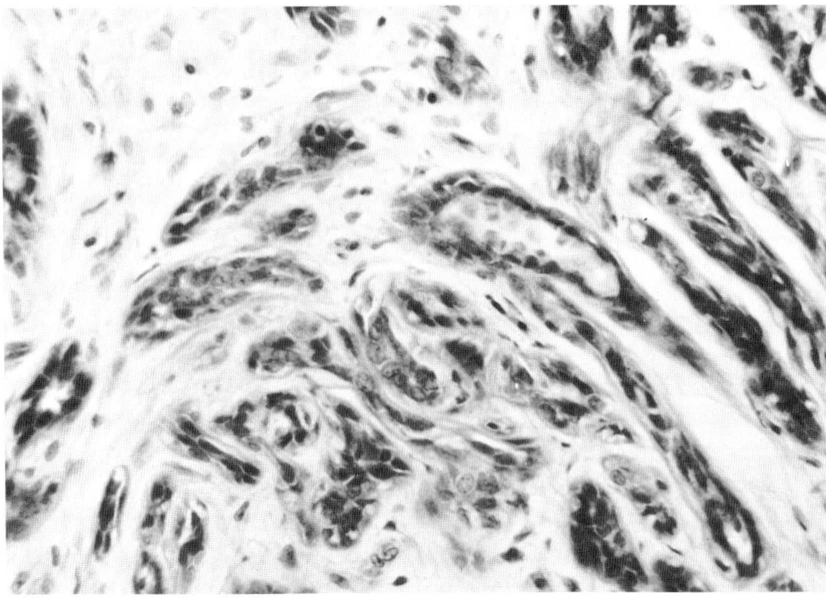

Fig. 4.11. Sclerosing adenosis. High-power view of lesion illustrated in Fig. 4.10. Note the infiltrative appearance of the acini which have very poorly formed lumina. The cells do not exhibit cytological features of malignancy and there is a prominent myoepithelial layer. ×302. H & E.

1967; Eusebi and Azzopardi 1976). In Sandison's (1962) autopsy series, about 10 per cent of subjects over the age of 50 exhibited sclerosing adenosis.

Lactational foci (Fig. 4.12). About 3-4 per cent of normal breasts examined at autopsy contain occasional lobules which show changes virtually indistinguishable from those of normal pregnancy or lactation (Frantz *et al.* 1951; Sandison 1962). These lesions sometimes occur in the absence of a previous pregnancy but, even in these circumstances, they have been shown by immunohistochemical methods to secrete milk protein (Bailey *et al.* 1982).

Intraductal hyperplasia (epitheliosis) and carcinoma

Sandison (1962) found some degree of intraductal proliferation in over 20 per cent of ostensibly normal breasts from autopsies performed on women over the age of 40. In 68 per cent of these cases it was graded as mild, in 25 per cent as moderate, and only in the remaining 7 per cent as severe.

There is considerable variation both in the extent of proliferation and degree of cytological change. Ducts may be normal in calibre or considerably distended. In obviously benign examples (Fig. 4.13), the cells exhibit no nuclear hyperchromatism or significant pleomorphism and mitotic figures are scarce or absent; abnormal mitoses are not seen. The nucleo-cytoplasmic ratio is normal and cytoplasmic outlines are indistinct. Two cell

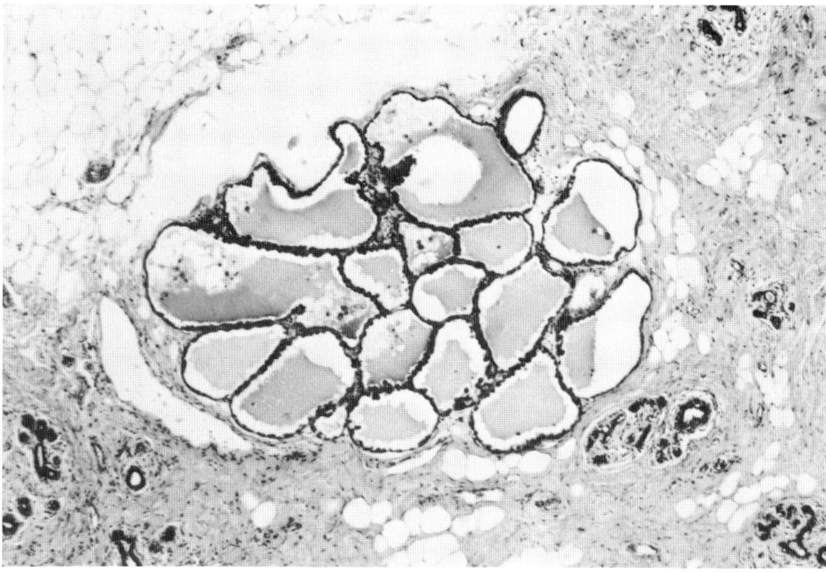

Fig. 4.12. Lactational focus in nonpregnant breast. The acini are dilated, contain abundant secretion, and are lined by hypertrophic cells. ×48. H & E.

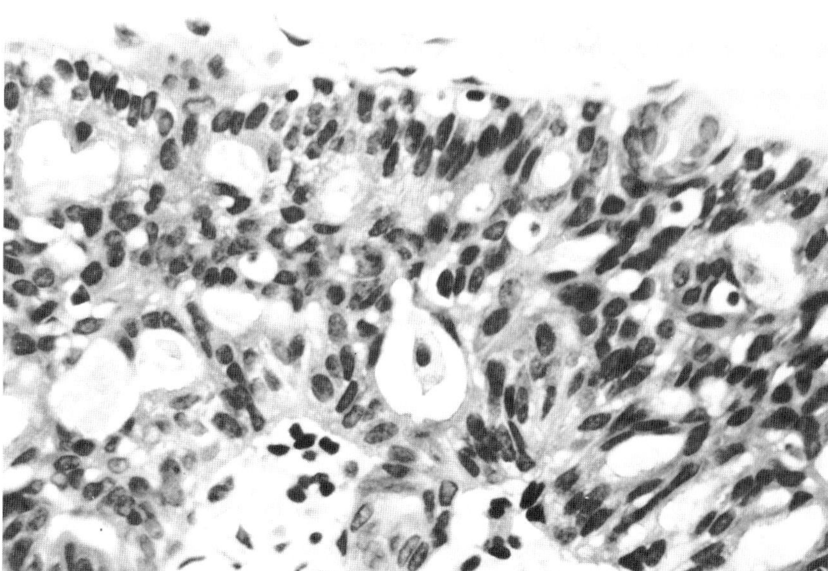

Fig. 4.13. Epitheliosis in an interlobular duct. The cells are polymorphic and lack cytological features of malignancy. The lumina have irregular ill-defined outlines. ×302. H & E.

types are often present—rounded cells resembling normal epithelial cells and more ovoid cells with smaller, darker nuclei which may be myoepithelial elements. Apocrine metaplasia is very uncommon in the solid examples but somewhat more frequent in the papillary types. Necrosis and haemorrhage are rare in the absence of obvious trauma. The growth pattern may be solid, cribriform, or papillary. In the cribriform type, the spaces are irregular in outline and usually exhibit a shaggy appearance due to the presence of protruding cytoplasmic blebs from the lining cells. Foamy macrophages, similar to those seen in duct ectasia, may be seen in the lumina. In the truly papillary examples, vascular connective tissue cores are present within the papillary processes. If the papillary changes are localized to produce a well circumscribed mass, the lesion is designated as an *intraduct papilloma* (Figs. 4.14 and 4.15).

In atypical ductal hyperplasia (atypical epitheliosis) the proliferative changes tend to be intermediate in character between those described above and carcinoma *in situ*. The cells are of one type and may exhibit pleomorphism, nuclear enlargement, and hyperchromatism. Mitotic figures may be seen but are not abnormal. Necrosis and haemorrhage are still rare but organized connective tissue cores are frequently lacking from the papillary types.

In intraduct carcinomas, there is cytological atypicality with nuclear pleomorphism, hyperchromatism, and generally increased cell size. Despite the pleomorphism of the cells, the appearance is generally more uniform

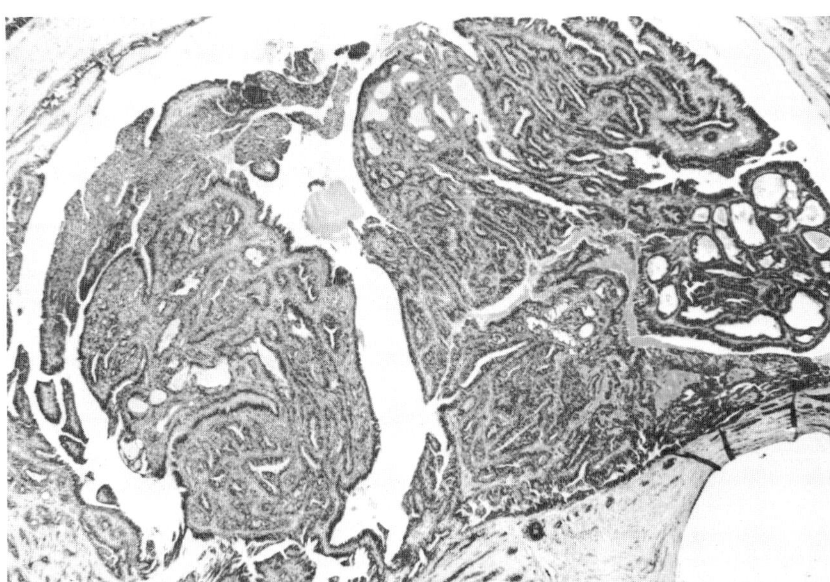

Fig. 4.14. Intraduct papilloma. Note the well-developed arborizing connective tissue cores of the papillae. ×34. H & E.

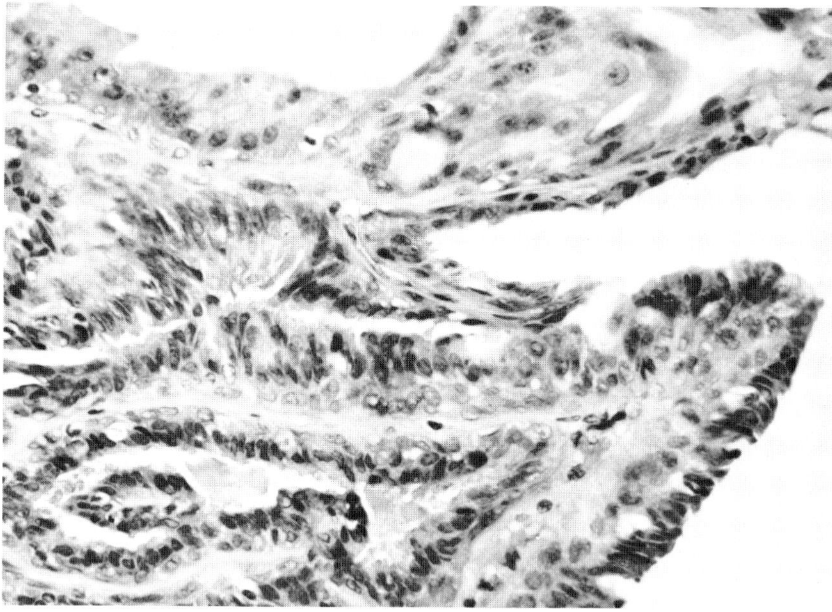

Fig. 4.15. High-power view of lesion illustrated in Fig. 4.14. The papillae have connective tissue cores and are covered by a double layer of cells which lack atypical features. There is a zone of apocrine metaplasia at the top of the picture. ×302. H & E.

than epitheliosis because there is only one cell type. Mitoses are usually frequent and abnormal forms may be present. Focal necrosis and haemorrhage are common, but apocrine metaplasia is hardly ever seen. The growth pattern may be solid, comedo, papillary, cribriform, or clinging (Azzopardi 1979). The comedo variety is essentially solid but with a central zone of necrosis (Fig. 4.16). The papillary types differ from papillomatosis not only in their cytological features but also in the lack of connective tissue cores within papillary processes (Fig. 4.17). In the cribriform types the lumina are rounded and show clean truncated margins. Azzopardi uses the term clinging to describe those *in situ* cancers in which the dilated ducts are lined by just a few layers of cells around a large empty lumen (Fig. 4.18). The proliferations described above have been traditionally classified as ductal in origin presumably because of the size of the structures involved. But the clustering of the lesions in conventional sections and the general lobular configuration seen in dissecting microscope studies (Wellings *et al.* 1975) suggests that they usually arise in terminal ducts and lobules which become markedly distended and distorted as proliferation progresses (Fig. 4.19). Thus, the major differences between them and the lobular lesions described below seem to be cytological rather than anatomical.

Intralobular hyperplasia and carcinoma

These proliferations are much more easily recognized as being of terminal-duct and lobular origin as they produce less ductular distension and

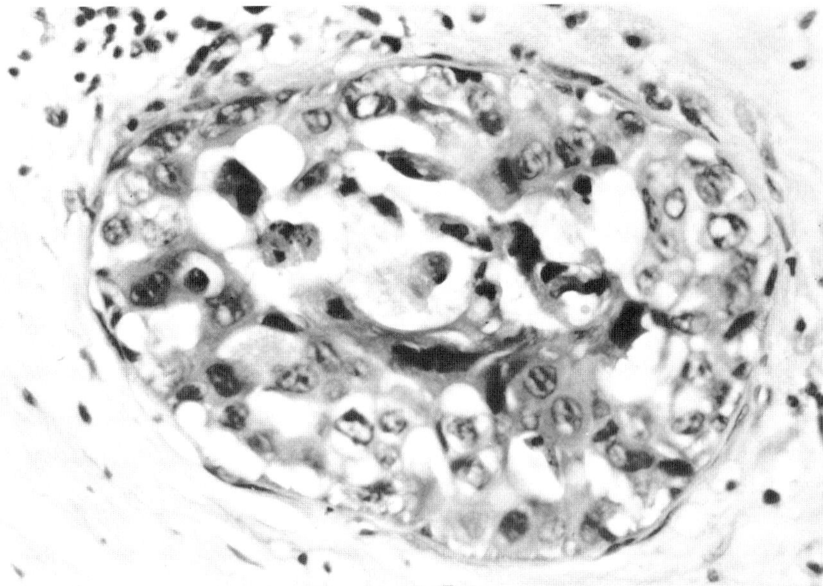

Fig. 4.16. Solid intraduct carcinoma of comedo type. The cells are large and pleomorphic and there is a central zone of necrosis. ×302. H & E.

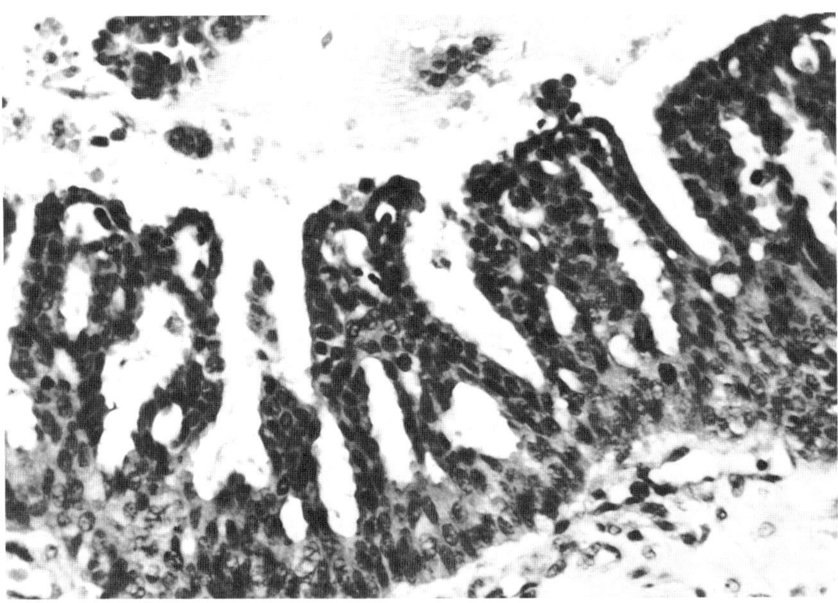

Fig. 4.17. Papillary intraduct carcinoma. There is a densely cellular papillary proliferation of atypical cells without connective tissue cores. ×302. H & E.

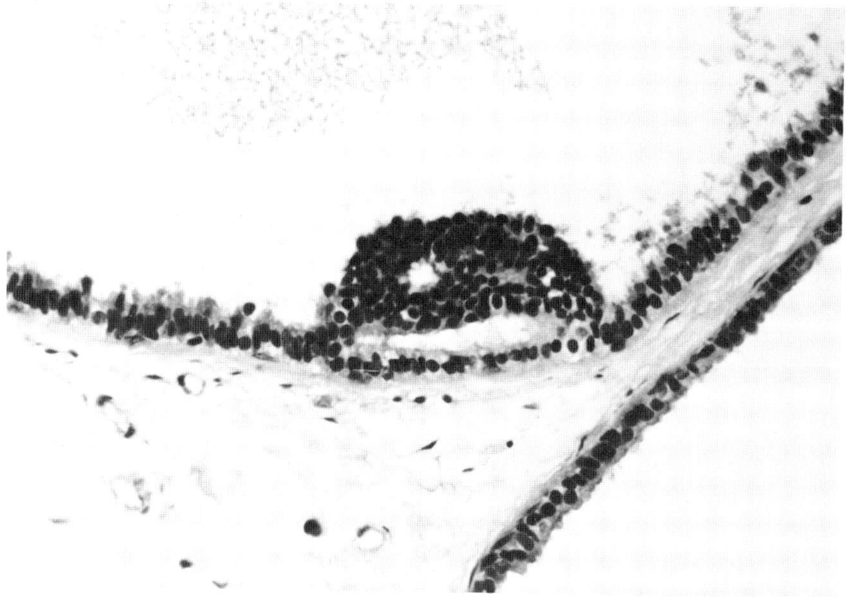

Fig. 4.18. Clinging carcinoma. The malignant cells are mostly one cell thick with only occasional zones of multilayering. ×302. H & E.

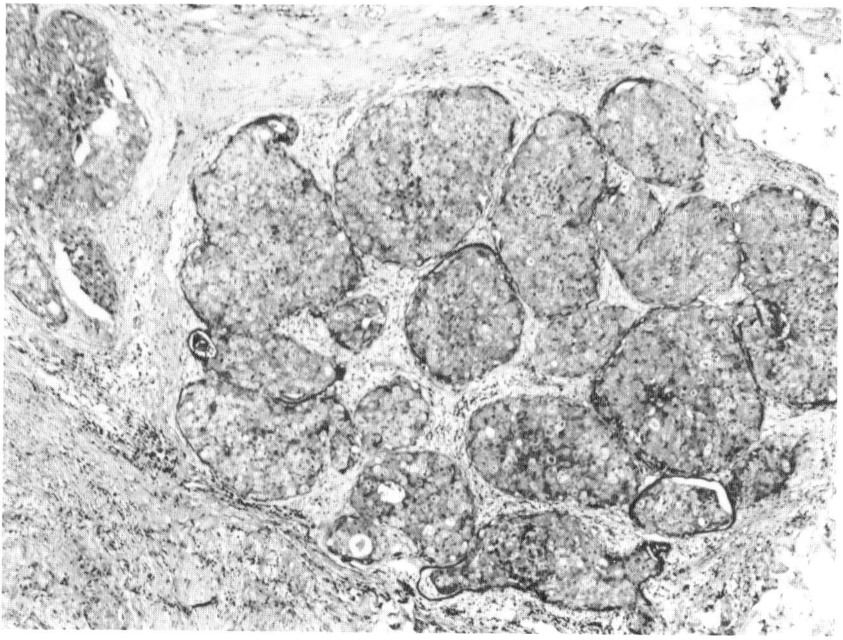

Fig. 4.19. Small solid intraduct carcinoma. Despite the size of the distended ducts the lesion exhibits a lobular architecture with a terminal duct at the top left. ×48. H & E.

disturbance in lobular architecture. A complete spectrum of changes exists between normal lobules on the one hand and lobular carcinoma *in situ* on the other.

In lobular carcinoma *in situ* (Figs. 4.20 and 4.21), lobules are usually clearly distended with uniform, rounded, loosely-cohesive cells which have a rather bland and monotonous appearance. The lumina are completely obliterated and, although the cells are larger than normal breast epithelial cells, they are smaller than the cells of ductal carcinomas—hence the occasional use of the term small-cell carcinoma. Histochemically the cells are frequently found to contain intracytoplasmic inclusions which stain with Alcian blue-periodic acid Schiff (PAS) stains for epithelial mucin. The periphery of the inclusions stain as acid mucin with the Alcian blue and the centre stains as neutral mucin with PAS (Gad and Azzopardi 1975). The lumina also stain with antisera against cell surface components such as epithelial membrane antigen (Sloane and Ormerod 1981).

Atypical lobular hyperplasia (Fig. 4.22) merges with lobular carcinoma *in situ* and the two conditions are frequently difficult to tell apart. The acini are less distended and less crowded in atypical lobular hyperplasia, and a central lumen is usually visible. The cells are somewhat smaller, more cohesive and less uniform in appearance and vary in size, shape and staining intensity. Microcalcification may occur in lobular hyperplasia, but this feature is hardly ever seen in intralobular carcinoma.

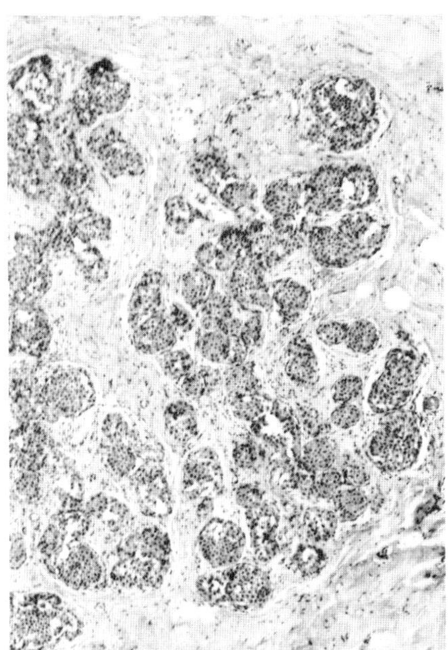

Fig. 4.20. *In situ* lobular carcinoma, showing lobular enlargement but clear retention of lobular architecture. Compare with Fig. 4.5(a). ×48. H & E.

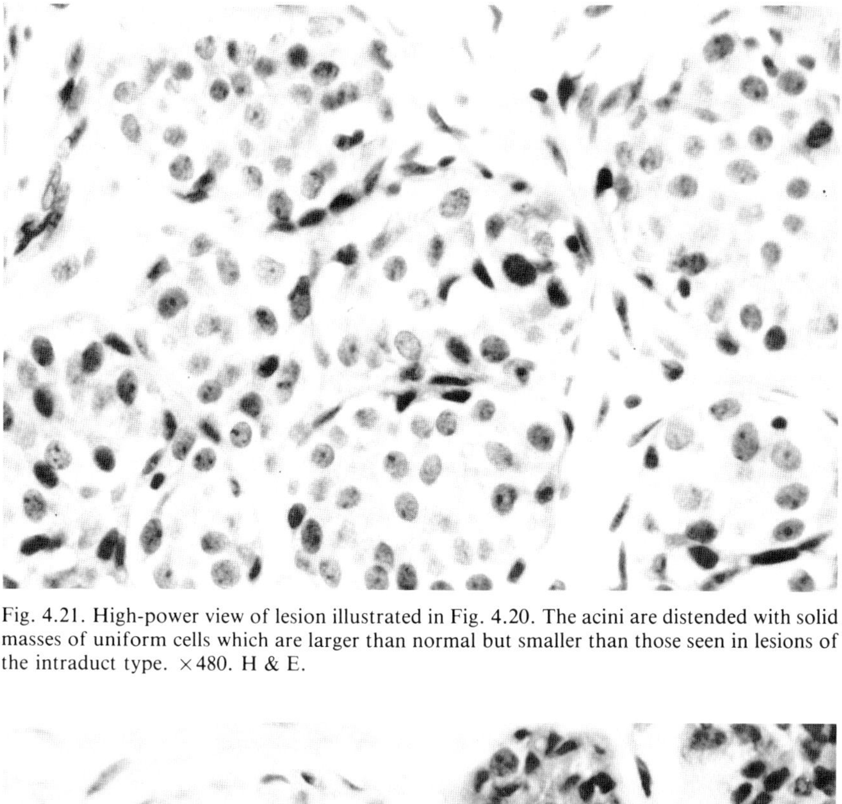

Fig. 4.21. High-power view of lesion illustrated in Fig. 4.20. The acini are distended with solid masses of uniform cells which are larger than normal but smaller than those seen in lesions of the intraduct type. ×480. H & E.

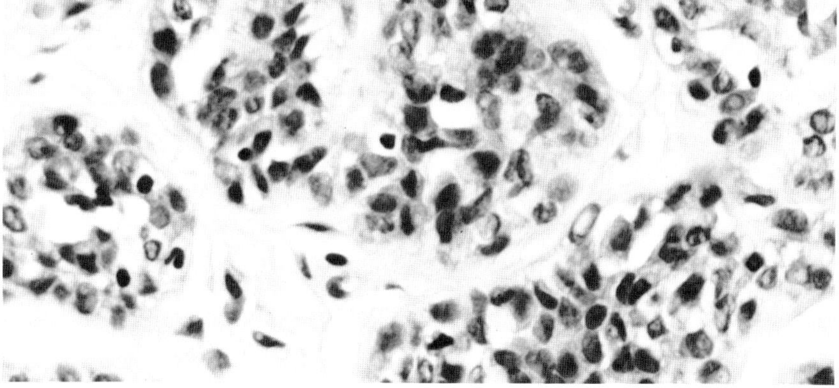

Fig. 4.22. Atypical lobular hyperplasia. The acini are less distended and there are many residual lumina. The cells are polymorphic and smaller than those seen in lobular carcinoma *in situ*. ×480. H & E.

Breast lesions which may coexist with carcinoma

A number of studies have been performed in which the histological changes occurring in breasts harbouring carcinomas have been compared to those in noncancerous breasts. Foote and Stewart (1945*b*) looked for the presence of eleven lesions often collectively and loosely referred to as chronic cystic mastitis in 300 cancerous and 200 noncancerous breasts. The lesions examined were as follows: cysts, duct papillomatosis, blunt duct adenosis, apocrine change, stasis in and distension of ducts, periductal mastitis, fat necrosis, hyperplasia of duct epithelium, fibroadenoma, and fibroadenomatoid hyperplasia. If any one of these was necessary to make the diagnosis of chronic cystic mastitis, then the condition was present in 83 per cent of cancer-bearing breasts and 90 per cent of the controls. If the criteria for diagnosis were restricted to any one of the first five changes, then the incidence dropped in both groups but still remained slightly higher in the noncancer cases. If the diagnostic criteria were made even more rigid by insisting on at least three out of the first five lesions, then the overall figures were lowered even further but were still somewhat higher in the non-malignant group even when corrected for age. Thus, there did not appear to be an assocation between chronic cystic mastitis and carcinoma although the results have to be interpreted with some caution in view of the nature of the control group: this consisted of surgical biopsy specimens in which the frequency of the various lesions would be expected to be higher than in the general population. Furthermore, the small size of most surgical biopsies can lead to sampling problems. Despite such reservations, Foote and Stewart (1945*a*) found that although orderly papillary hyperplasia occurred with similar frequency in cancerous and noncancerous breasts, papillary hyperplasia with cytological atypia was about five times more frequent in the malignant group.

Later studies of this type employed autopsy material for controls, thus overcoming both the problems of selection and sampling. Ryan and Coady (1962) examined the changes in 100 cancer-bearing breasts and compared them to those occurring in 100 pairs of breasts taken from routine autopsies. Serial 1-cm slices were made through the breast tissue and blocks taken from any macroscopically suspicious areas and routinely from the axillary tail, the subareolar region and all four quadrants of the breast itself. The study focused on one pathological change—proliferation of ductal epithelium. The proliferative changes were graded from I to IV with Grade-I changes being merely the multilayering of well-differentiated epithelial cells and Grade IV as carcinoma *in situ*. Proliferative changes were four times more common in the malignant series but this increase rose by a factor of seven if only Grade-III and -IV changes were considered.

Karpas *et al.* (1965) examined 645 consecutive benign and malignant surgical specimens of breast. As in the study of Foote and Stewart (1945*a, b*), the control group consisted of breast tissue which would be reasonably expected to contain an increased number of benign lesions. Although the incidence of all proliferative changes was similar in each group, atypical proliferations were 14 times more common in the malignant series. Thus atypical hyperplasias form a greater proportion of the total number of proliferative lesions in breasts containing cancer than in benign breast diseases.

In the study of Gallager and Martin (1969), sixty radical mastectomy specimens were examined in immense detail taking 200 to 300 5 × 7 inch slides from each specimen. Ductal epithelial hyperplasia of considerable extent was present in every specimen, ranging from simple hyperplasia to *in situ* carcinoma. There was no sharp demarcation between the various degrees of change which merged into one another suggesting the possibility of progression. Changes in mammary lobules varying from simple hyperplasia to lobular carcinoma *in situ* were present in 40 per cent of the breasts. Those breasts without lobular lesions were generally removed from patients older than 65.

A numerical grading system was developed by Black and Chabon (1969) to describe epithelial proliferation in the breast. Letters were used to describe the site of the proliferation and numbers to indicate the degree of atypicality. Thus the letter A was used for primary ducts and major interlobular ducts, B for terminal interlobular ducts, C for preterminal intralobular ducts, D for acini, and AP for areas of apocrine metaplasia. Grading was based on the most severe change in a specimen and was recorded as 1 for normal, 2 for hyperplasia, 3 and 4 for atypical hyperplasia of varying severity, and 5 for carcinoma *in situ*. An *in situ* carcinoma of a major duct would thus be designated as A5. This system has one important limitation in that it is often difficult to determine the exact site of the duct system involved, especially with the more florid proliferations which result in marked expansion and distortion of the duct system (see below). Of 97 samples of breast tissue removed for nodularity, suspicious mammographic changes or local tenderness, only 12 per cent showed changes in excess of Grade 3 and one in excess of Grade 4. In 55 breasts containing invasive carcinoma 77 per cent had changes in excess of Grade 3.

Perhaps the most detailed study of this type is that of Wellings *et al.* (1975) who adapted the subgross sampling technique used in rodents to human breasts. The whole breast was cut into 50 to 150 2-mm slices which were stained with haematoxylin and examined under the dissecting microscope. Lesions were thus selected for conventional histology and the procedure considerably reduced sampling problems. Another advantage was that the low-power, three-dimensional view afforded by the dissecting microscope gave a clearer appreciation of the micro-anatomy of the lesions under study. The morphological evidence gained from this study supported the idea that most lesions grouped as fibrocystic disease including apocrine cysts, sclerosing adenosis, fibroadenomas, ductal carcinoma *in situ*, and lobular carcinoma *in situ* arise either in terminal duct lobular units or within the lobules themselves. The evidence that ductal carcinoma *in situ* develops from the terminal duct lobular units was that the tumours had a lobular configuration, were connected to terminal interlobular ducts, and occasionally contained residual normal acini. Furthermore, the subgross technique allowed the recognition of the most minute ductal carcinoma *in situ* (DCIS) in which the lobular architecture is even more readily recognized.

The study concentrated on atypical lobules which were divided up into type A (ALA) and type B (ALB). Each was graded from I to V. In ALA, the changes were similar to those described above under ductal hyperplasia. (The authors argued that these lesions, although conventionally regarded as of ductal origin, are, like duct carcinoma *in situ*, usually derived from terminal-duct lobular units.) Grade-I and -II lesions exhibited proliferation and apocrine metaplasia without atypia; cellular atypia appeared at Grade III and increased in severity at Grade IV. Grade V corresponded to DCIS. In ALB the changes corresponded to those described under lobular hyperplasia above. Grade-I and -II lesions exhibit intralobular proliferation of uniform cells without increase in lobular size. Lumina are preserved in Grade-I but not Grade-II lesions. Grades III and IV exhibit varying degrees of lobular enlargement due to masses of cohesive uniform cells. Grade V is lobular carcinoma *in situ* (LCIS) which consists of larger and less cohesive cells than Grade IV.

In breasts taken from routine autopsies, AL grades I and II were common at all ages but grades in excess of III were rare. In contrast, in breasts containing clinically evident carcinoma, ALs of Grade III or more were frequent. Grade-I and -II ALs were also more frequent than in autopsy breasts in patients past the fourth decade. ALA were more frequent than ALB and duct carcinoma *in situ* occurred in 40 per cent of the cancerous breasts whereas LCIS occur in only 20 per cent. Four per cent of the autopsy glands contained DCIS and none contained LCIS. Atypical lobules as a whole occurred almost four times more frequently in cancer-containing breasts than in autopsy glands (Jensen *et al.* 1976).

Prospective studies

There have been many studies which have attempted to assess the risk of developing breast carcinoma in patients from whom various non-malignant breast lesions have been excised. Most of them are prospective observational studies reported in retrospect. In some of these investigations the benign lesions have not been characterized histologically whereas in others general terms such as chronic cystic mastitis, cystic disease, or benign breast disease have been employed. Clearly it is difficult to identify a lesion as preneoplastic in studies of this type simply because of the immense variety of changes which may be present.

Further problems in defining lesions result from the subjectivity of histopathological interpretation. An atypical intraductal hyperplasia described by one pathologist may be classified as an *in situ* carcinoma by another, so it is necessary to use high-quality illustrations and to define terminology as precisely as possible.

Another obvious difficulty is that the lesions identified have themselves been removed and the assumption has to be made that similar lesions of no greater severity, such as an occult carcinoma, remain in the breast.

Sampling problems also exist in the control groups. Proliferative lesions often do not produce symptoms and are often discovered simply because of the presence of clinically overt associated lesions such as cysts or zones of fibrosis. Control groups would thus contain a proportion of undiscovered hyperplasias and this would tend to minimize the significance of putative preneoplastic lesions.

The evolution of mammary carcinoma in the human appears to be a slow process and patients have to be followed for a very long time; this often proves to be difficult. Furthermore there is a clear geographical variation in the incidence of breast carcinoma, and the incidence of cancer in patients with various benign lesions has to be seen in the context of the natural incidence in the area from which the patients are drawn.

Davis *et al.* (1964) followed 284 patients who had had local excisions for cystic breast disease for an average of 13 years. The term cystic disease covered a variety of lesions as diverse as cysts and papillary hyperplasia. Carcinoma developed in 2.4 per cent of these patients which was about 1.7 times the expected incidence. Individuals with ductal hyperplasia developed carcinoma at 2.5 times the expected frequency compared to 1.2 in those without hyperplastic changes. These authors also reviewed 20 previous studies performed between 1892 and 1960. The results were very variable and the proportion of patients with cystic disease who developed carcinoma varied from 0 to 10.3 per cent. Only four of the studies included a calculated risk factor, and this varied from 3 to 4.5 times the expected frequency. Much of the variation in the results of these studies can be explained by the problems outlined above.

In their follow-up study of chronic mastopathy, Kodlin *et al.* (1977) used the Black and Chabon (1969) grading system described earlier. The letter prefixes were not, however, employed so that the part of the duct system harbouring the proliferative changes was not recorded. The 2092 patients with scores of 1 or 2 had an increased risk of cancer development of 2.3 which rose to 2.4 for the 262 patients with Grade-3 changes, 6.0 for 49 patients with Grade 4, and 16.7 for the 8 subjects with Grade 5 (carcinoma *in situ*). Thus the cancer risk increased with degree of atypia in the proliferative lesions. The overall incidence rate for cancer in this series was similar to that which the authors obtained by pooling data from previous studies.

In a critical and detailed study, Page *et al.* (1978) followed 925 patients in Nashville, Tennessee for 15-24 years after biopsy for a benign lesion with a 94 per cent follow-up rate. The histological lesions under study were carefully defined and included cysts, duct ectasia, sclerosing adenosis, fibroadenoma, apocrine change, papillary apocrine change, ductal hyperplasia with and without apocrine-like changes, ductal hyperplasia with atypia, and atypical lobular hyperplasia. The cancer incidence for each subgroup was compared to that obtained for their group as a whole, to those quoted in the Third National Cancer Survey of the USA, and to that obtained from a previous study of white women in Atlanta, Georgia. The risk of developing lobular carcinoma was increased sixfold in patients with atypical lobular hyperplasia who were aged under 45 at the time of biopsy. This fell to threefold in patients aged over 45. The increased risk in patients with ductal lesions was different in magnitude and age pattern, being associated with a threefold increase in risk of invasive cancer over the age of 45 but with no increased risk below this age. Surprisingly, atypical ductal lesions did not exhibit a greater risk than ductal proliferations without atypia. Apocrine change with papillary tufting had an elevated cancer risk with a similar age pattern to that of ductal hyperplasia.

The natural history of ductal carcinoma *in situ* has been difficult to assess from prospective studies as patients are usually treated with mastectomy and/or radiotherapy. In two recent laborious, but ingeniously designed studies, cases of intraduct carcinoma treated by biopsy alone were identified as diagnostic errors in a very large number of breast biopsies reported as benign. In the series of Betshill *et al.* (1978) and later updated by Rosen *et al.* (1980), more than 8000 breast biopsies were reviewed and 30 found to contain ductal carcinoma in situ. Follow-up data were available in 15 of these 30, and 10 subsequently developed ipsilateral clinical cancer an average of 9.7 years later. This gives an incidence of 67 per cent if only the patients followed-up are included in the denominator or 33 per cent if the patients lost to follow-up are assumed not to have suffered from recurrent disease. Page *et al.* (1982) reviewed 11 760 biopsies reported as benign and identified 28 cases of intraduct carcinoma. All 28 patients were followed-up; 3 for less than 3 years and the remaining 25 for 8-27 years (mean 16.25 years). Seven of the 25 patients with adequate follow-up (28 per cent) subsequently developed invasive carcinoma 3-10 years later, all in the same breast. The authors quoted a previous study in which residual carcinoma was found in 60 per cent of mastectomy specimens removed following a biopsy diagnosis of intraduct carcinoma; this indicates that the whole lesion is likely to be removed by biopsy alone in almost half the cases. Page *et al.* thus felt that their best estimate of the chance of a residual intraduct carcinoma developing into invasive carcinoma was about 50 per cent.

Lobular carcinoma *in situ*, on the other hand, is not infrequently treated by local excision. In one group of 99 patients with lobular carcinoma *in situ* followed for an average of 24 years, breast carcinoma developed in about one-third of patients either in the same, opposite, or both breasts (Rosen *et al.* 1978). This was nine times the expected frequency. Toker (1974) used a rather unconventional classification in his study of small-cell dysplasia and *in situ* carcinoma of mammary ducts and lobules. Lesions composed of small cells of the type seen in lobular carcinoma *in situ* and atypical lobular hyperplasia were studied, but some cases exhibited a cribriform growth pattern with marked ductal and lobular distension. These would have been classified as ductal carcinoma by some workers but they formed only a small minority of cases in the study. Dysplastic changes were graded from I to III, with type III being equivalent to carcinoma *in situ* and types I and II to varying degrees of atypical lobular hyperplasia. Five per cent of patients with type-III lesions had developed infiltrating carcinoma at 5 years. This figure rose to 21 per cent at 10 years and 45 per cent at 15 years. This compared to 25 per cent at 15 years for type II and 12 per cent at 15 years for patients with type-I lesions.

Retrospective studies

Black *et al.* (1972) took a group of breast cancer patients attending clinics in Saskatchewan who had previously had a benign breast biopsy. For each of these 'reference' cases, three controls were chosen who had not subsequently developed carcinoma and who were matched for age and date of biopsy. The Black and Chabon system was used to grade epithelial proliferation. On reviewing the histological sections some breasts were re-classified as carcinoma *in situ* (Grade 5) and this change was found five times more frequently in the reference group. Duct grades 3 or 4 were found in 30 per cent of the reference group and in 8 per cent of the controls. The risks of developing cancer within the test period was five times greater for patients exhibiting grade 3 and 4 changes compared to those exhibiting grades 1 and 2. Diffuse apocrine metaplasia, intraductal papilloma, fibroadenoma, blunt duct adenosis, and sclerosing adenosis were found not to be associated with an increased risk.

Ultrastructural studies

Ultrastructural observations tend to confirm the light-microscopic impression that breast epithelial hyperplasias are morphologically intermediate between carcinomas and normal mammary tissue (Ozzello 1974). In hyperplasias, as in carcinomas, there is a general tendency for organelles to become more prominent. Golgi complexes, rough endoplasmic reticulum, fine filaments, and microtubules are conspicuous. Mitochondria are increased in number and may exhibit abnormal forms. Intracytoplasmic lumina (structures lined by membranes with microvilli which may or may not communicate with the surface of the cell) are rarely if ever found in normal mammary cells but are not infrequently seen in mammary carcinomas. They are occasionally observed in mammary hyperplasias. In general the cytoplasmic changes tend to parallel the degree of epithelial proliferation.

Normal mammary epithelial cells are surrounded by an intact basal lamina unlike nests of infiltrating carcinoma cells. *In situ* carcinomas may exhibit attenuated or incomplete basal laminae and epithelial cells may protrude through the gaps but without losing contact with cells inside the ducts. In hyperplasias, the basal lamina may show thinning or even thickening and multilayering.

Scanning electromicroscope (SEM) studies have shown that breast carcinoma cells have poorly developed or absent microvilli and that normal appearing or hyperplastic cells from breasts harbouring carcinomas also have abnormal microvilli. They may be thickened and irregular or exhibit clumping at their tips, and contacts may even form between the microvilli or adjacent cells (Spring-Mills and Elias 1976).

General biological properties of human proliferative lesions

If a lesion is preneoplastic, then it should occur at an earlier average age than the corresponding neoplasm. In Black and Chabon's 1969 series, the average age of patients with 'benign lumps' was 44 compared to 53 for carcinoma. A similar age difference was found by Kodlin *et al.* (1977) with an average of seven years between the benign and malignant diagnoses.

Some insight into the behaviour of lobular carcinoma *in situ* is given by its age distribution. In Rosen's 1978 series the average age was 45 and only one patient was older than 59. The average age of patients with infiltrating carcinoma associated with an *in situ* lobular component was 47 in Black and Chabon's 1969 study and this contrasted with an average age of 53 overall and 58 for cases of breast cancer without *in situ* lobular carcinoma. In the 1978 study of Page *et al.* the risk of developing carcinoma in patients under 45 with atypical lobular hyperplasia was double that for patients who were older than 45. These data suggest that both atypical lobular hyperplasia and lobular carcinoma *in situ* may regress after the menopause and that a continued stimulus (presumably hormonal) is often necessary not only for their maintenance but also for their progression to infiltrating neoplasia.

As nearly all human breast carcinomas are known to be aneuploid, there have been several studies aimed at detecting karyotypic abnormalities in non-neoplastic lesions. Two main techniques have been used. The first is Feulgen microspectrophotometry in which sections are stained by the Feulgen method for DNA and the light absorption by nuclei measured with a microspectrophotometer; normal cells such as lymphocytes are used as controls. This technique has the advantage of identifying precisely the cytological features and anatomical location of the cells under test, but its major disadvantage is insensitivity. In one study (Zippel and Kunze 1977) twelve cases of lobular carcinoma in situ and three cases of invasive lobular carcinoma were studied. All infiltrative and one-third of the *in situ* lesions gave DNA values in the diploid-to-tetraploid range. The remaining two-thirds of the *in situ* carcinomas were diploid. The authors concluded that the diploid-to-tetraploid cases of lobular carcinomas *in situ* represented a more advanced stage in neoplastic evolution than the diploid examples.

Fisher and Paulson (1978) used the alternative technique of chromosomal analysis which is more sensitive and has the added advantage of enabling recognition of morphological chromosomal abnormalities. However, it is impossible to know from what part of a potentially heterogenous piece of tissue the test cells are derived. Six fibroadenomas were studied and the proportion of aneuploid cells varied from 0 to 11 per cent in five and was 30 per cent in the sixth. No morphologically abnormal chromosomes were seen. Aneuploidy was seen in 0-12 per cent of cells from non-proliferative tissues which included lesions such as sclerosing adenosis, blunt duct adenosis, apocrine metaplasia, and simple cysts. The chromosomes again appeared normal. Six samples showing notable intraductal hyperplasia and varying cellular atypia, but no histological evidence of cancer, exhibited 7-40 per cent of aneuploid cells. Three of these samples showed morphologically aberrant chromosomes. All cells from invasive carcinomas exhibited aneuploidy and morphologically abnormal chromosomes.

Lymphocytes are regularly seen within normal breast epithelium as indeed they are in epithelium from other sites such as the skin and the intestine; the phenomenon has been termed emperipolesis. Black and Chabon (1969) noted that these intra-epithelial lymphoid accumulations persist in hyperplastic epithelium but decrease or disappear in atypical hyperplasia and *in situ* and infiltrating carcinoma.

Transplantation studies

Using the subgross sampling technique, Jensen and Wellings (1976) were able to identify individual lobules in breast biopsies and mastectomy specimens. The structures were bisected with half the tissues retained for histological examination and the other half transplanted into the cleared fat pad of athymic nude mice and observed for up to 27 weeks. In some transplants, the epithelium did not survive and apparently only the stroma remained. In others, the epithelium remained unchanged but in some it 'dedifferentiated'. The dedifferentiation process was defined as hyperplasia of epithelium with variable degrees of disorganization and immaturity within enlarged ductular units. This phenomenon was seen in 20 out of 61 normal lobules removed from breasts containing cancer, and in 11 out of 48 removed from breasts without cancer. The data obtained from transplantation of atypical lobules were too scanty for analysis. None of the transplants filled the fat pads as do HANs from mice, and none underwent malignant change. It was suggested that the denser stroma of the human lobule and the residual immunocompetence of the B-lymphocyte system in the recipient animals may have contributed to the failure of the tissue to grow.

Although transplantation techniques of this kind could be useful in assessing the malignant potential of human lesions there are major drawbacks. Even if a malignant change could be induced, the process may be too slow to have clinical value. Either some way of accelerating the process is needed or some reliable end-point short of actual malignancy. Furthermore, factors operating in the host may be necessary for progression and these would not be taken into account.

Conclusions

Given that current methods of treating breast carcinoma have little influence on prognosis there is a strong case for concentrating more effort on methods of prevention; better understanding of preneoplastic processes would clearly form an important part of such endeavours.

Animal studies have an essential role to play in view of the insurmountable problems of adequately studying the evolution of human breast carcinomas. Although such investigations do not rule out the possibility that direct origin from normal tissues may sometimes take place, they do establish preneoplasia as a valid concept in the development of breast cancer.

The relevance of such models to the human disease has, however, been questioned as the tumours produced by viruses and high doses of carcinogens are circumscribed and metastasize infrequently. Furthermore they have short latent intervals and are often highly immunogenic. This is often related to their inability to metastasize and, in Fisher's chromosome studies, splenectomy was performed in order to encourage metastatic growth. It has been shown that in animals treated with low concentrations of carcinogens, the latent period of tumours is increased and immunogenicity reduced (Prehn 1975). Such tumours would seem to be better models for human disease and studies on precancerous lesions in such animals would be of great value.

The relevance of rodent studies has been further questioned because of the lack of any lesion in the human which closely resembles the hyperplastic alveolar nodule of the mouse. Indeed, these lesions do not seem to have the same significance in the rat. The explanation may lie in their relationship to the mouse mammary tumour virus as there is no convincing evidence of a viral aetiology in either the rat or man. The lesions produced by chemical carcinogens are, however, similar in both species of rodent and these in turn are not dissimilar to those seen in humans; thus, they form a more acceptable model for human disease.

Apart from establishing the general concept of preneoplasia, animal experiments demonstrate several fundamental points. First, not all lesions which are morphologically similar have the same aetiology or the same malignant potential. In Fisher's experiments, certain exogenous hormones produced proliferative lesions which were indistinguishable from the less severe forms induced by methylcholanthrene, but they did not undergo malignant change. Many of the observations in humans also suggest that there are functional subgroups of morphologically homogeneous lesions which have differing capacities for malignant change. Chromosome analysis may prove to be an effective tool for analysing such lesions and should be investigated further.

Factors in the host may also be important. This is evidenced by the higher rate of malignant transformation of HANs when transplanted into virally infected mice and the influence of strain on malignant transformation of preneoplastic lesions in rats. The failure of HANs to transform when transplanted subcutaneously underlines the importance of local factors within the breast itself.

If patients with preneoplastic lesions are merely closely observed, then they may well develop carcinoma, by which time it will be too late for radical treatment to be effective. If they are treated by mastectomy, then many patients will have needless radical surgery. The clinical dilemma is that conservative treatment is likely to be ineffective and that effective treatment may be inappropriate. Further work is required to establish what factors in the lesions and in the patients themselves determine the likelihood of malignant change. Such investigations might generate new data on the behaviour of the lesions and suggest alternative modes of therapy. The rarity of lobular carcinoma *in situ* developing after the menopause, for example, suggests hormonal dependence which in turn might suggest a role for hormone receptor blocking agents.

Effective screening is perhaps the major problem as several clinicopathological studies suggest that the lesions with the greatest potential for neoplastic change usually produce no premonitory symptoms and are discovered only incidentally. It is impossible to biopsy repeatedly the whole population and even so the sampling problems would be great. Developments in imaging techniques such as xeroradiography and ultrasonography may be helpful, but the lesions are frequently too small for visualization. Cytological techniques may be important but these are also not without considerable problems. Fluid containing cells can be aspirated from the non-lactating breast but it is usually very small in quantity. Furthermore, animal and human studies now seem to be in agreement that carcinomas generally arise from the most distal parts of the ductal system. Some method of stimulating breast secretion would be necessary.

Nevertheless, research along these lines would be justified as it would generate new fundamental information which could be applied to the problem of preventing human breast carcinoma.

References

Abraham, S. and Bartley, J.C. (1974). Comparison among the metabolic characteristics of normal, preneoplastic, and neoplastic mammary tissues. In *Hormones and cancer* (ed. K.W. McKerns), p. 29. Academic Press, New York, London.

Apolant, H. (1906). Die epithelialen Geschwulste der Maus. *Arb. Inst. Exp. Ther. Frankfurt* **1**, 7.

Armitage, P. and Doll, R. (1954). The age distribution of cancer and a multi-stage theory of carcinogenesis. *Brit. J. Cancer* **VIII**, 1.

Azzopardi, J.G. (1979). *Problems in breast pathology*. W.B. Saunders Co. Ltd.

Bailey, A.G., Sloane, J.P., Trickey, B.S., and Ormerod, M.G. (1982). An immunocytochemical study of α-lactalbumin in human breast tissue. *J. Pathol.* **137**, 13-23.

Banerjee, M.R., Mehta, R.C., and Wagner, J.E. (1973). DNA polymerase and DNA synthesis in preneoplastic nodule outgrowths of BALB/C and C3H mouse mammary gland. *J. Nat. Cancer Inst.* **50**, 339.

Bartley, J.C., McGrath, H., and Abraham, S. (1971). Glucose and acetate utilization by hyperplastic alveolar nodule outgrowths and adenocarcinomas of mouse mammary gland. *Cancer Res.* **31**, 527.

Beall, P.T., Asch, B.B., Chang, D.C., Medina, D., and Hazlewood, C.F. (1980). Distinction of normal, preneoplastic, and neoplastic mouse mammary primary cell cultures by water nuclear magnetic resonance relaxation times. *J. Nat. Cancer Inst.* **64**, 335.

Bentvelzen, P. and Daams, J.H. (1969). Hereditary infections with mammary tumor viruses in mice. *J. Nat. Cancer Inst.* **43**, 1025.

Betshill, W.L., Rosen, P.P., Lieberman, P.H., and Robbins, G.F. (1978). Intraduct carcinoma. Long-term follow-up after treatment by biopsy alone. *J. Am. med. Assn.* **239**, 1863.

Beuving, L.J. (1968). Mammary tumor formation within outgrowths of transplanted hyperplastic nodules from carcinogen-treated rats. *J. Nat. Cancer Inst.* **40**, 1287.

——, Faulkin, L.J. Jr., DeOme, K.B., and Bergs, V.V. (1967*a*). Hyperplastic lesions in the mammary glands of Sprague-Dawley rats after 7,12-Dimethyl-benz(a)-anthracene treatment. *J. Nat. Cancer Inst.* **39**, 423.

——, Bern, H.A., and DeOme, K.B. (1967*b*). Occurrence and transplantation of carcinogen-induced hyperplastic nodules in Fischer rats. *J. Nat. Cancer Inst.* **39**, 431.

Biancifiori, A., Bonser, G.M., and Caschera, F. (1961). Ovarian and mammary tumours in intact C3Hb virgin mice following a limited dose of four carcinogenic chemicals. *Brit. J. Cancer* **15**, 270.

Black, M.M. and Chabon, A.B. (1969). In situ carcinoma of the breast. *Pathol. Ann.* **4**, 185.

——, Barclay, T.H.C., Cutler, S.J., Hankey, B.F., and Asire, A.J. (1972). Association of atypical characteristics of benign breast lesions with subsequent risk of breast cancer. *Cancer* **29**, 338.

Blair, P.B. and DeOme, K.B. (1961). Mammary tumor development in transplanted hyperplastic alveolar nodules of the mouse. *Proc. Soc. exp. Biol. Med.* **108**, 289.

Cameron, A.M. and Faulkin, L.J. (1971). Hyperplastic and inflammatory nodules in the canine mammary gland. *J. Nat. Cancer Inst.* **47**, 1277.

Dao, T.L., Sinha, D., Christakos, S., and Varela, R. (1975). Biochemical characterization of carcinogen-induced mammary hyperplastic alveolar nodule and tumor in the rat. *Cancer Res.* **35**, 1128.

Davis, H.H., Simons, M., and Davis, J.B. (1964). Cystic disease of the breast: relationship to carcinoma. *Cancer* **17**, 957.

DeOme, K.B., Faulkin, L.J. Jr., Bern, H.A., and Blair, P.B. (1959). Development of mammary tumors from hyperplastic alveolar nodules transplanted into gland-free mammary fat pads of female C3H mice. *Cancer Res.* **19**, 515.

—— and Medina, D. (1969). A new approach to mammary tumorigenesis in rodents. *Cancer* **24**, 1255.

Eusebi, V. and Azzopardi, J.G. (1976). Vascular infiltration in benign breast disease. *J. Pathol.* **118**, 9.

Faulkin, L.J. Jr. (1966). Hyperplastic lesions of mouse mammary glands after treatment with 3-methylcholanthrene. *J. Nat. Cancer Inst.* **36**, 289.

—— and DeOme, K.B. (1960). Regulation of growth and spacing of gland elements in the mammary fat pad of the C3H mouse. *J. Nat. Cancer Inst.* **24**, 953.

Fisher, E.R., Shoemaker, R.H., and Sabnis, A. (1975*a*). Relationship of hyperplasia to cancer in 3-methylcholanthrene-induced mammary tumorigenesis. *Lab. Invest.* **33**, 33.

—— ——, and Palekar, A.S. (1975*b*). Identification of premalignant hyperplasia in methylcholanthrene-induced mammary tumorigenesis. *Lab. Invest.* **33**, 446.

—— and Paulson, J.D. (1978). Karyotypic abnormalities in precursor lesions of human cancer of the breast. *Amer. J. clin. Pathol.* **69**, 284.

Foote, F.W. and Stewart, F.W. (1945*a*). Comparative studies of cancerous versus noncancerous breasts. *Ann. Surg.* **121**, 6.

—— —— (1945*b*). Comparative studies of cancerous versus noncancerous breasts. *Ann. Surg.* **121**, 197.

Foulds, L. (1956). The histologic analysis of mammary tumors of mice. II. The histology of responsiveness and progression. The origins of tumors. *J. Nat. Cancer Inst.* **17**, 713.

Frantz, V.K., Pickren, J.W., Melcher, G.W., and Auchincloss, H. Jr. (1951). Incidence of chronic cystic disease in so called "normal breasts". *Cancer* **4**, 762. **4**, 762.

Gad, A. and Azzopardi, J.G. (1975). Lobular carcinoma of the breast: a special variant of mucin-secreting carcinoma. *J. clin. Path.* **28**, 711.

Gallager, H.S. and Martin, J.E. (1969). Early phases in the development of breast cancer. *Cancer* **24**, 1170.

Geschickter, C.F. and Byrnes, E.W. (1942). Factors influencing the development and time of appearance of mammary cancer in the rat in response to oestrogen. *Arch. Pathol.* **33**, 334.

Gimbrone, M.A. Jr. and Gullino, P.M. (1976). Neovascularization induced by intraocular xenografts of normal, preneoplastic and neoplastic mouse mammary tissues. *J. Nat. Cancer Inst.* **56**, 305.

Haaland, M. (1911). *Spontaneous tumours in mice.* Fourth scientific report of the Imperial Cancer Research Fund.

Hilf, R., Rector, W., and Abraham, S. (1973). A Glucose-6-phosphate dehydrogenase isoenzyme characteristic of preneoplastic and neoplastic mouse mammary tissue. *J. Nat. Cancer Inst.* **50**, 1395.

Huggins, C., Grand, L.C., and Brillantes, F.P. (1961). Mammary cancer induced by a single feeding of polynuclear hydrocarbons, and its suppression. *Nature* **189**, 204.

Jensen, H.M. and Wellings, S.R. (1976). Preneoplastic lesions of the human mammary gland transplanted into the nude athymic mouse. *Cancer Res.* **36**, 2605.

——, Rice, J.R., and Wellings, S.R. (1976). Preneoplastic lesions in the human breast. *Science* **191**, 295.

Karpas, C.M., Leis, H.P., Oppenheim, A., and Merscheiner, W.L. (1965). Relationship of fibrocystic disease to carcinoma of the breast. *Ann. Surg.* **162**, 1.

Kim, U. (1979). Factors influencing metastasis of breast cancer. In *Breast cancer* (ed. W.L. McGuire) Vol. 3, p. 1. Plenum Medical Book Company.

Kodlin, D., Winger, E.E., Morgenstern, N.L., and Chen, U. (1977). Chronic mastopathy and breast cancer. *Cancer* **39**, 2603.

Medina, D. (1976). Preneoplastic lesions in murine mammary cancer. *Cancer Res.* **36**, 2589.

—— (1979). Serial transplantation of chemical carcinogen-induced mouse mammary ductal dysplasias. *J. Nat. Cancer Inst.* **62**, 397.

—— Oborn, C.J., and Asch, B.B. (1980). Distinction between preneoplastic and neoplastic mammary cell populations *in vitro* by cytochalasin B-induced multinucleation. *Cancer Res.* **40**, 329.

Middleton, P.J. (1965). The histogenesis of mammary tumours induced in the rat by chemical carcinogens. *Brit. J. Cancer* **19**, 830.

Muhlbock, O. (1956). The hormonal genesis of mammary cancer. In *Advances in cancer research* (ed. J.P. Greenstein and A. Haddow), p. 371. Academic Press, New York.

Ozzello, L. (1974). Electron microscopic study of functional and dysfunctional human mammary glands. *J. invest. Dermatol.* **63**, 19.

Page, D.L., Van de Zwagg, R., Rogers, L.W., Williams, L.T., Walker, W.E., and Hartmann, W.H. (1978). Relation between component parts of fibrocystic disease complex and breast cancer. *J. Nat. Cancer Inst.* **61**, 1055.

——, Dupont, W.D., Rogers, L.W., and Landenberger, M. (1982). Intraduct carcinoma of the breast; follow-up after biopsy only. *Cancer* **49**, 751.

Prehn, R.T. (1975). Relationship of tumor immunogenicity to concentration of the oncogen. *J. Nat. Cancer Inst.* **55**, 189.

Richmond, R.E. and Faulkin, L.J. Jr. (1975). Survival and differentiation of canine mammary tissues in the hamster cheek pouch. *Cancer Res.* **35**, 791.

Rosen, P.P., Lieberman, P.H., Braun, D.W. Jr., Kosloff, C., and Adair, F. (1978). Lobular carcinoma *in situ* of the breast. *Amer. J. Surg. Pathol.* **2**, 225.

Rosen, P.P., Braun, D.W., and Kinne, D.E. (1980). The clinical significance of pre-invasive breast carcinoma. *Cancer* **46**, 919.

Russo, J., Saby, J., Isenberg, W.M., and Russo, I.H. (1977). Pathogenesis of mammary carcinomas induced in rats by 7, 12-Dimethylbenz(a)anthracene. *J. Nat. Cancer Inst.* **59**, 435.

Ryan, J.A. and Coady, C.J. (1962). Intraductal epithelial proliferation in the human breast—a comparative study. *Can. J. Surg.* **5**, 12.

Sandison, A.T. (1962). An autopsy study of the adult human breast. *Nat. Cancer Inst. Monogr. No. 8.*

Shay, H., Aegerter, E.A., Gruenstein, M., and Komarov, S.A. (1949). Development of adenocarcinoma of the breast in the Wistar rat following the gastric instillation of methylcholanthrene. *J. Nat. Cancer Inst.* **10**, 255.

Shellabarger, C.J., Cronkite, E.P., Bond, V.P., and Lippincott, S.W. (1957). The occurrence of mammary tumors in the rat after sublethal whole-body irradiation. *Rad. Res.* **6**, 501.

Sinha, D. and Dao, T.L. (1974). A direct mechanism of mammary carcinogenesis induced by 7, 12-Dimethylbenz(a)anthracene. *J. Nat. Cancer Inst.* **53**, 841.

—— —— (1975). Site of origin of mammary tumors induced by 7, 12-Dimethylbenz(a)anthracene in the rat. *J. Nat. Cancer Inst.* **54**, 1007.

Sloane, J.P. and Ormerod, M.G. (1981). Distribution of epithelial membrane antigen in normal and neoplastic tissues and its value in diagnostic tumor pathology. *Cancer* **47**, 48.

Spring-Mills, E. and Elias, J.J. (1976). Cell surface changes associated with human breast cancer. *Scanning electron microscopy*, Part V. p. 1. Proceedings of the Workshop on Advances in Biomedical Applications of the SEM.

Squartini, F. (1979). Tumours of the mammary gland. In *Pathology of tumours in laboratory animals* (ed. V.S. Turusov), p. 53. IARC Scientific Publications No. 23.

Taylor, H.B. and Norris, H.J. (1967). Epithelial invasion of nerves in benign diseases of the breast. *Cancer* **20**, 2245.

Toker, C. (1974). Small cell dysplasia and in situ carcinoma of the mammary ducts and lobules. *J. Pathol.* **114**, 47.

Wellings, S.R., Jensen, H.M., and Marcum, R.G. (1975). An atlas of subgross pathology of the human breast with special reference to possible precancerous lesions. *J. Nat. Cancer Inst.* **55**, 231.

Wilson, R.H., DeEds, F., and Cox, A.J. Jr. (1941). The toxicity and carcinogenic activity of 2-acetaminofluorene. *Cancer Res.* **1**, 595.

Young, S. and Hallowes, R.C. (1973). Tumours of the mammary gland. In *Pathology of tumours in laboratory animals* (ed. V.S. Turusov), p. 31. IARC Scientific Publications No. 5.

Zippel, H.H. and Kunze, W.P. (1977). The nuclear DNA content of lobular neoplasia of the mammary gland. *Arch. Gynak.* **22**, 265.

5 Precancerous states in the head and neck

L. Michaels

Cancers of the head and neck are as diverse as the organs and tissues which occur in this region. Most of these cancers are rare and little or nothing is known of their precursor states. The commoner malignancies are the epidermoid carcinomas of the oral cavity and larynx, and some knowledge of the morphological changes leading up to these malignancies is available. A third tumour—nasopharyngeal carcinoma—is rare in the West but common in certain Chinese populations. Its morphological antecedents are not known, but information from epidemiology, genetics, and virology can logically be regarded as important contributions to characterizing the precancerous states for this particular tumour. The three sites discussed in this chapter—oral cavity, larynx, nasopharynx—serve to illustrate the diversity of approaches to precancerous states.

Oral cavity

Leukoplakia, erythroplakia, and submucous fibrosis

From the time of the development of cytological-smear techniques for recognizing malignancy of the uterine cervix, there has been intense activity directed at gaining knowledge of this form of malignant disease by pathologists and gynaecologists (see Chapter 12). This work has led to a greater degree of understanding of precancerous conditions of the cervix than in any other organ. It is natural, therefore, to compare progress in the oral cavity with that in the cervix. In the uterine cervix, workers in the field of precancerous states have abandoned the use for classification of macroscopic descriptions such as leukoplakia, even though such appearances are common features of precancerous states of the cervix. Gross changes are useful in identifying regions which require biopsy, but a histological assessment of such lesions is essential for full evaluation. In the classification of premalignant states of the oral mucosa, by contrast, importance is still given to leukoplakia and erythroplakia. Pindborg (1980*a*) defines *leukoplakia* as a white patch which cannot be removed by scraping and cannot be attributed to any other diagnosable disease (Fig. 5.1). It is subdivided into homogeneous and nodular (or speckled) forms, and it is the nodular form

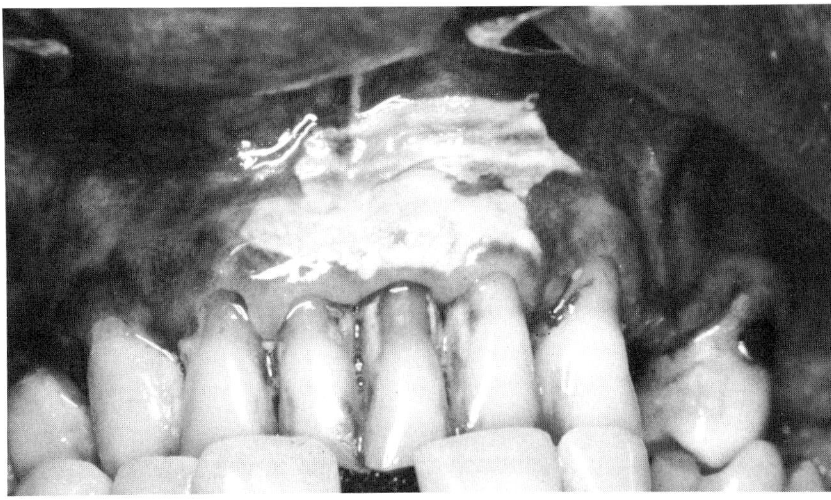

Fig. 5.1. Leukoplakia of the gum. (Courtesy of Dr F.F. Nally, Eastman Dental Hospital, London.)

that is considered to carry the higher risk for the development of subsequent malignancy. Leukoplakia of the floor of the mouth is the most dangerous form of the condition: histological examination of leukoplakic zones from this region shows some 43 per cent of leukoplakias to represent dysplasia, carcinoma *in situ*, or invasive carcinoma as compared with 12-24 per cent of leukoplakia showing such changes in other parts of the oral cavity (Waldron and Shafer 1975). Such a variety of different histological entities clearly indicates that leukoplakia is an inaccurate designation for any classification. Even histologically 'innocent' leukoplakia in the floor of the mouth carries a greater risk of malignant change than histologically innocent lesions in other sites (Kramer *et al.* 1978).

Erythroplakia is a well-defined patch with a fiery red velvety surface (Pindborg 1980*a*). There is growing interest in these lesions, since it has been shown that 80 per cent of them are premalignant or malignant. Two distinct types are recognized (Mashberg 1980). The first is a granular, red, velvety lesion with stippled or patchy white areas of keratin at the centre and the edges (Fig. 5.2). The second is a smooth, non-granular, red patch with minimal or no white areas. The erythematous character of the lesion appears to be related to vascular congestion associated with inflammation beneath abnormal epithelium. Unlike leukoplakia, all areas of the oral mucosa showing erythroplakia are very likely to be malignant.

Submucous fibrosis of the oral cavity has recently been associated with an increased tendency for local cancer development (Pindborg 1980*a*). This is a chronic lesion affecting any part of the mucosa of the oral cavity and occasionally extending into the pharynx and oesophagus. The squamous epithelium is atrophic, and fibroelastic tissue is deposited in the lamina

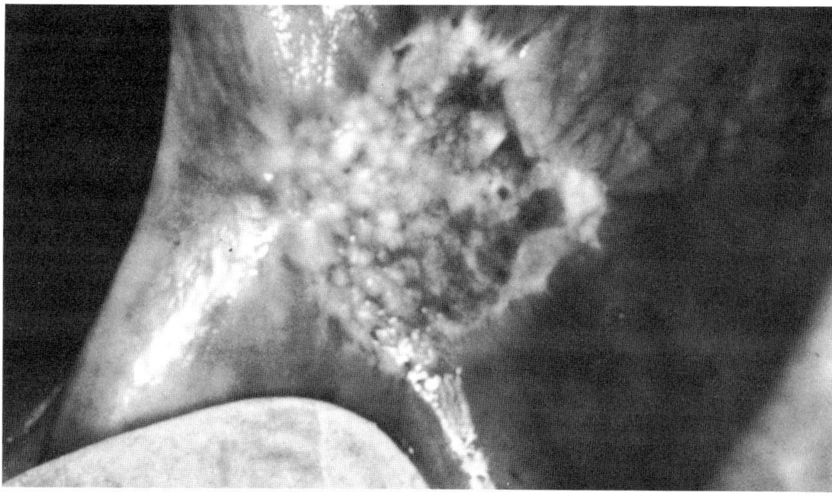

Fig. 5.2. Erythroplakia of the inner surface of the cheek. Note the granular red appearance of the lesion with a whitish circumference and numerous white patches. (Courtesy of Dr F.F. Nally, Eastman Dental Hospital, London.)

propria. The condition is always accompanied by an inflammatory reaction (Figs. 5.3 and 5.4). The disease occurs mainly among Indians, but sporadic cases have been observed in other countries in East Asia.

It has been calculated that about 250 0G0 cases of submucous fibrosis are present in India. Evidence from India for the predisposition of cases with submucous fibrosis to develop local squamous-cell carcinomas may be summarized as follows:

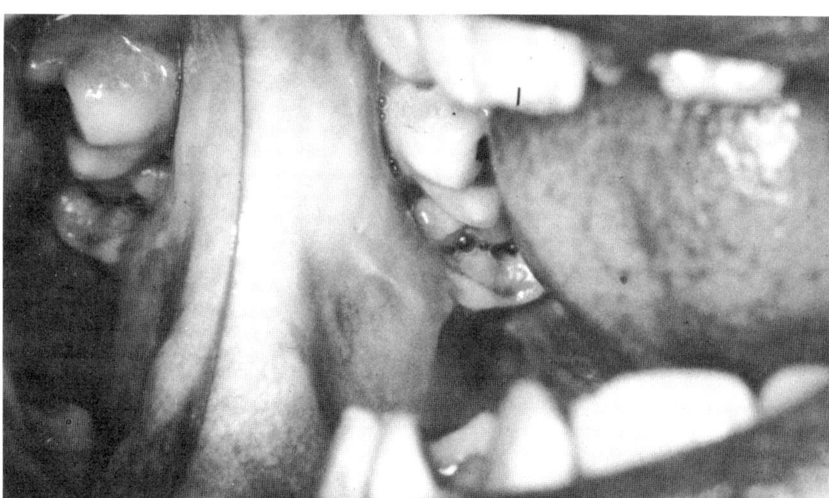

Fig. 5.3. Submucous fibrosis of the inner surface of the cheek. (Courtesy of Dr F.F. Nally, Eastman Dental Hospital, London.)

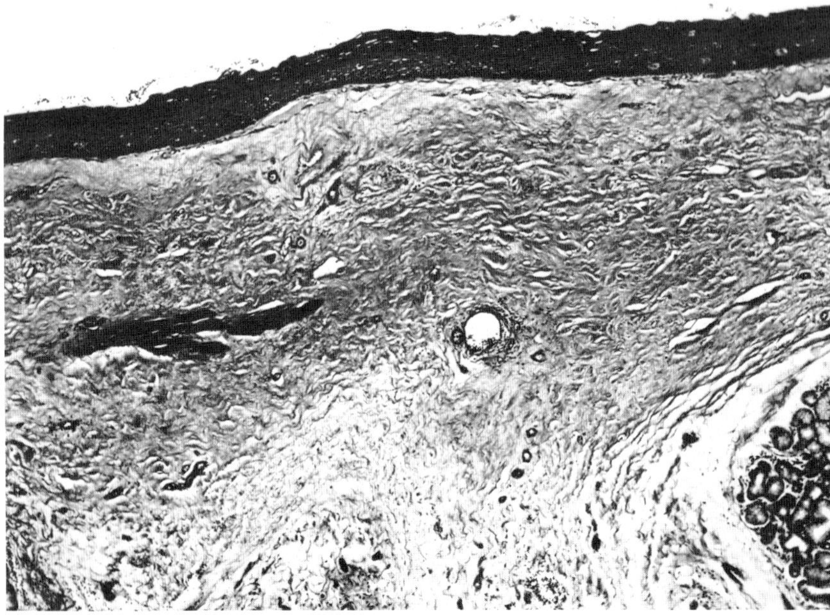

Fig. 5.4. Submucous fibrosis of cheek. The squamous epithelium is flat and somewhat atrophic. There is a marked increase of poorly cellular fibrous and elastic tissue in the lamina propria which has engulfed some skeletal muscle fibres, the remnants of which are seen as a band running horizontally on the left. A venule, surrounded by lymphocytes, is seen in the middle of the field. ×38. H & E. (Specimen submitted by Dr K. Lee, Institute of Dental Surgery, London.)

1. There is a higher incidence of leukoplakia in patients with submucous fibrosis (13-27 per cent).
2. There is a higher incidence of epithelial atypia in submucous fibrosis (about 14 per cent).
3. 40-49 per cent of patients with oral cancer in India show submucous fibrosis.
4. 3-6 per cent of cases of submucous fibrosis also have coexisting microscopic squamous cancers.
5. Follow-up studies of cases with submucous fibrosis seen at the Tata Memorial Hospital in Bombay indicate that one-third of the patients subsequently develop squamous-cell carcinoma. An hypothesis for the relationship of submucous fibrosis to carcinoma has been put forward by Pindborg and Sirsat (1966) who propose that the lesion starts in the connective tissues as an inflammatory reaction which is followed by fibroelastic deposition. These changes may be due to hypersensitivity to chili, betel nut, or tobacco, or may perhaps be related to vitamin deficiencies. As a result of the connective tissue changes there is atrophy of the overlying epithelium which becomes more vulnerable to the carcinogenic

affects of chewed tobacco. Thereafter the epithelium becomes increasingly hyperplastic and dysplastic, and squamous carcinomas develop.

Histopathology of precancerous lesions of squamous epithelium

The stage of precancerous histological change which immediately precedes invasive squamous carcinoma is carcinoma *in situ*. This is generally accepted as a lesion consisting of neoplastic cells extending through the full thickness of the epithelium, but with an intact basement membrane. Lesser degrees of involvement of the epithelium by dedifferentiated cells is by general agreement known as dysplasia in cervical epithelium (Stafl and Matlingly 1973), and this term has become widely accepted for similar changes in all squamous mucosal surfaces including the oral epithelium.

The detailed cellular changes of dysplasia are similar in all squamous cell epithelia. Kramer (1969) has used the computer to reduce the subjective element in the analysis of histopathological changes of premalignant lesions of the oral epithelium. Detailed microscopic findings of many cases were submitted to the computer which was programmed in such a way as to analyse this information and place it into groups that seemed to correspond to conventional diagnostic categories such as lichen planus or squamous carcinoma. Computer analysis of an 'unknown' case was felt to represent a more objective approach to the diagnosis than the usual assessment by the pathologist. The method is very time-consuming, and there has been no rush of pathologists to use computer methods in day-to-day diagnosis of premalignant lesions; but the method promises objectivity and further development may lead to its wider adoption in histopathological practice. In the process of reviewing histological material for these computer-based studies, Kramer (1980) has made a detailed analysis of the cellular appearances of dysplastic oral epithelium; his findings are applicable to dysplastic changes affecting squamous epithelium in the head and neck in general and are summarized in Table 5.1 and Figs. 5.5-5.7.

Table 5.1. *Dysplastic changes in squamous epithelium*

1. 'Drop-shaped rete processes'.
Rete processes normally taper progressively or else form structures with almost parallel sides and blunt ends. Rete processes which are wider at their deeper part than superficially are described as 'drop-shaped' and occur frequently in dysplastic epithelia.

2. Disturbed cellular polarity
This feature applies mainly to the polarity of the basal cells which normally lie in the long axis, parallel to the mucosal surface.

3. Nuclear hyperchromatism, prominent nucleoli, increase in nuclear-cytoplasmic ratio

4. Basal-cell hyperplasia with the related features of disturbed maturational sequence; cell crowding; and increased numbers of mitoses, mitoses in upper epidermal layers and abnormal mitoses.

Aetiological agents in the genesis of cancer of the oral epithelium

Tobacco and betel nut. It is generally accepted that tobacco usage, whether smoked or chewed, is an important aetiological factor in the development of cancer of the oral epithelium. Intra-oral carcinomas are more common among smokers but the association, at least in the West, is not straightforward. Any such association has to explain the declining incidence of oral cancers in the last 30 years in the face of increased smoking and a spectacular rise in incidence of tobacco-associated carcinomas of the bronchus. On the other hand, a high incidence of smoking runs parallel with a high incidence of oral cancers, and of leukoplakia, in India and South-east Asia.

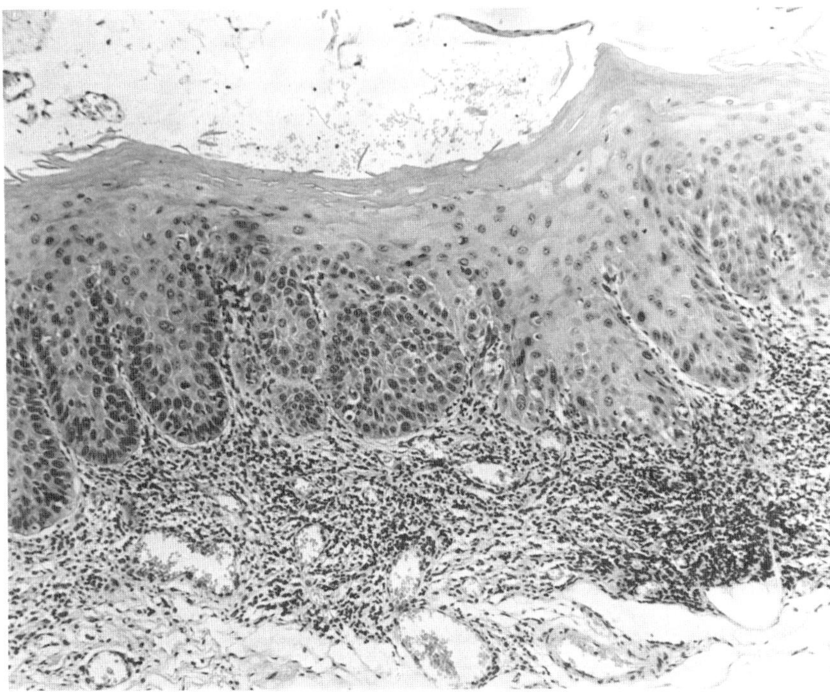

Fig. 5.5. Moderate dysplasia of oral epithelium. The rete processes are 'drop-shaped' and there is a dense inflammatory infiltrate under the epithelium. ×95. H & E. (Specimen submitted by Professor I.R.H. Kramer, Institute of Dental Surgery, London.)

Cancer of the buccal mucosa is commoner in these regions than in any other part of the world. The situation is, however, complicated by the additional prevalent factor of chewing betel nut (Fig. 5.8 (a), (b)). The betel nut, alone, apparently does not induce tumours and it seems to be the *combined* usage of betel nut and tobacco which provides the carcinogenic stimulus. The betel nut quid is placed in the lower buccal sulcus, and the majority of cancers in betel nut chewers starts in that location. Snuff

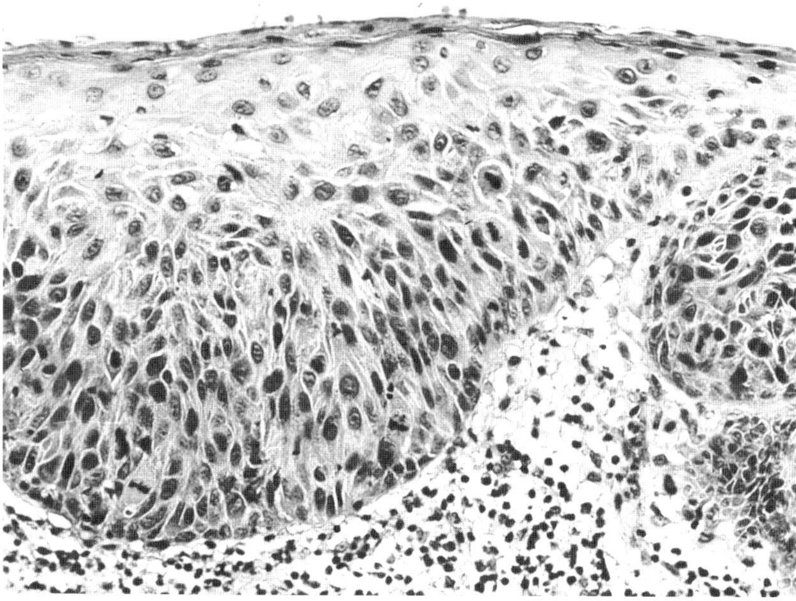

Fig. 5.6. Dysplasia of oral epithelium. There is disordered polarity of the basal layer and disturbed maturation. ×18. H & E. (Specimen submitted by Professor I.R.H. Kramer, Institute of Dental Surgery, London.)

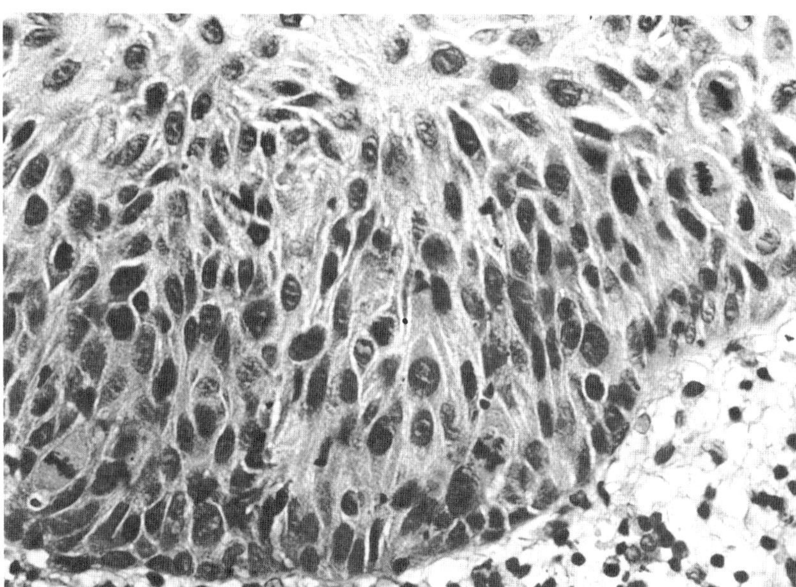

Fig. 5.7. Higher-power view of part of previous illustration showing numerous mitotic figures, prominent nucleoli, and increased nuclear-cytoplasmic ratios. ×360. H & E. (Specimen submitted by Professor I.R.H. Kramer, Institute of Dental Surgery, London.)

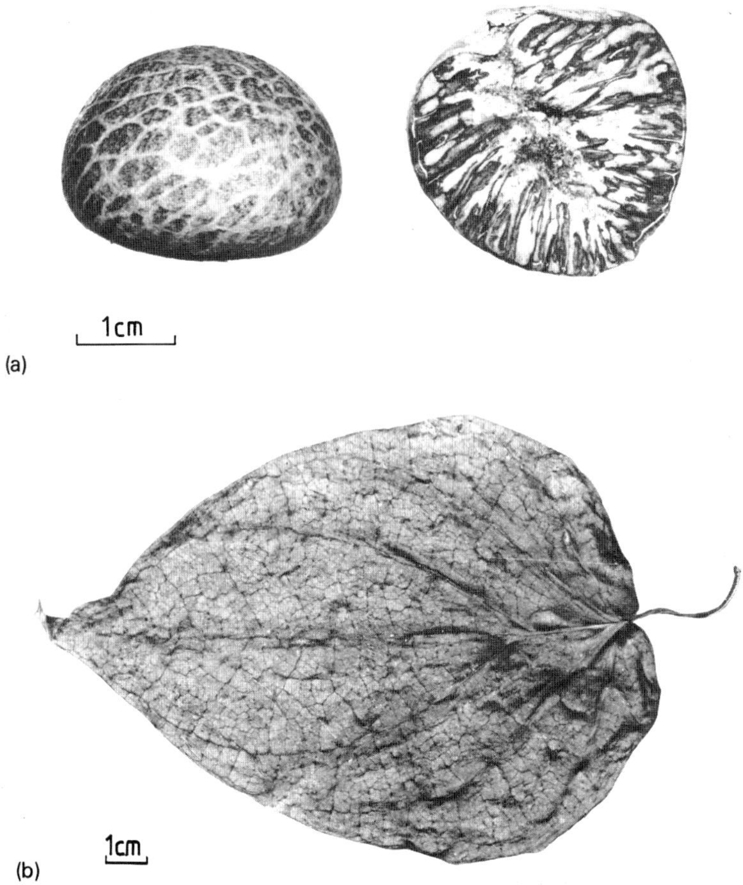

Fig. 5.8. (a) Betel nut: surface and cut surface. The dark areas are reddish brown in colour. (b) Betel leaf, a different species of plant altogether from the nut. The nut is eaten by first crushing it, adding spices, and then wrapping the mixture within the leaf to form a quid.

dipping, a habit which consists of the placement and retention of finely ground or powdered tobacco in the oral vestibule between the gum and cheek, has been related to a high incidence of oral cancer among women (to whom the habit is largely confined) in the southern United States (Winn *et al.* 1981).

In some parts of India the bizarre practice of smoking by placing the lighted end of the cigarette in the mouth is carried out. The carcinogenic effects, which may be a combination of heat and carcinogens contained in the smoke, are seen as squamous carcinomas mainly on the hard palate and to a lesser extent on the dorsum of the tongue (Reddy *et al.* 1974).

Candida infection. Lesions associated with *Candida albicans* infection are under some suspicion as a possible premalignant factor (Bánóczy 1977; Cawson and Binnie 1980). Such lesions take the form of white patches with adjacent reddening of the mucosa. Histologically the reddened areas correspond to atrophy of the epithelium and the white areas to mucosal hyperplasia with intraepithelial microabscesses. Keratinization is common and dysplastic changes are frequently present in the mucosa; it is believed that the process may, under certain circumstances, go on to invasive carcinoma. It should, however, be emphasized that the particular circumstances in which *Candida* infections may contribute to the development of oral cancers are unclear: such infections are, of course, quite common and may coexist with a local tumour.

Syphilis. Syphilitic infection has long been considered as a predisposing factor in the development of oral leukoplakia and oral (particularly lingual) cancer. A recent study from Hungary showed a 2.5 per cent frequency of syphilis in patients with leukoplakia; syphilis was present in 10 per cent of cases of oral carcinoma (Bánóczy 1977). The endarteritis associated with syphilitic infections of the tongue leads to an atrophy of the overlying lingual mucosa which may be rendered more vulnerable to the action of exogenous carcinogens.

Sideropenic dysphagia. The Paterson-Kelly syndrome or sideropenic dysphagia has been associated with an increased frequency of oral as well as hypopharyngeal carcinoma. This observation would explain the higher frequency of oral cancer in females than in males noted in northern Sweden by Larsson *et al.* (1975). Iron-deficiency states induce atrophy of the epithelium of the upper respiratory and digestive tracts.

Relationship of virus infection to oral cancer. It has not been possible to relate viral infections of any kind to the development of oral cancer. It is of interest in this connection that an oral epithelial abnormality which resembles carcinoma *in situ* microscopically has been suggested as being of viral aetiology and not to have a premalignant connotation (see Fejerskow *et al.* 1977).

Experimental oral carcinogenesis

The hamster cheek pouch. Many experimental studies on the effects of carcinogens on oral squamous epithelium have made use of the hamster cheek pouch and thrown some light on precancerous states of the oral mucosa. The Syrian hamster possesses two cheek pouches which communicate with the mouth on either side. They arise from immediately inside the commissures of the lips and extend back almost as far as the clavicles passing under the skin so that the muscle layer of the face lies medial to the pouch; they can easily be everted for gross examination. The pouches are lined by a layer of stratified squamous epithelium 4-6 cells thick which does not possess rete ridges and does not give origin to minor salivary glands.

The experiments most relevant to precancerous changes have been carried out with 7,12-dimethylbenz(a)anthracene (DMBA), and the early studies by Salley (1954) and Morris (1961) established the main features. Initially there is an inflammatory reaction to the application of DMBA which soon subsides. The treated pouches subsequently develop papillomatous growths which enlarge to more than 1 cm in diameter. Microscopic examination shows that from the time of six applications of DMBA, the squamous epithelium lining the pouch becomes hyperplastic, thickening to six to eight layers. There is also evidence of increased surface keratinization. Dysplastic changes are first seen among hyperplastic cells. The underlying connective tissue also proliferates. At fifteen applications of DMBA and thereafter, papillomatous lesions are present, covered by somewhat dysplastic squamous mucosa. These dysplastic and hyperplastic changes become more severe and, by nine weeks, there is marked invasion of the underlying epithelium by nests and sheets of malignant epithelial cells. The entire mass of malignant epithelium rests on a network of loosely arranged connective tissues. Metastases in cervical lymph nodes have occasionally been observed. These early observations have been widely confirmed in the more recent studies which are reviewed by Smith (1980).

The invasive tumours that develop following DMBA applications to the hamster cheek pouch differ from human oral carcinoma in their gross appearance. Most human oral cancers, and indeed squamous-cell carcinomas of the mucosae of the head and neck in general, arise from a wide flat field of malignant squamous epithelium; and although there may sometimes be some heaping up of malignant epithelium into exophytic papillary processes there is nearly always at the same time an infiltrative nonpapillary element which may extend widely on either side of the papillary component. Microscopically, however, the features of the squamous carcinomas are identical in man and in the hamster cheek pouch, and it is of interest that the stages of hyperplasia, dysplasia, and carcinoma *in situ* confirm the stages of precancerous development that have been inferred from the individual 'still pictures' observed in biopsies from human lesions. Additional studies of hamster cheek pouch carcinomas by histochemical and electron microscopical methods have not shown significant differences from human oral carcinomas (Smith 1980).

The application of DMBA to the hamster cheek pouch epithelium thus provides a reliable and quick source of oral epithelial changes comprising stages of hyperplasia and dysplasia leading on to carcinoma. Franklin and Smith (1980) have taken advantage of this system to quantitate the microscopic appearances. Changes of malignant potential produced by DMBA were compared with non-malignant hyperplastic changes induced by a solution of 50 per cent oil of turpentine in liquid paraffin. Franklin and Smith used the light microscope and a variety of stereological parameters to analyse the alterations in the epithelium of the cheek pouch tumours in sections, paying close attention to the adequacy of sampling. Three parameters gave results that were promising in respect of their relationship to the stage of the malignant process.

1. *Nuclear-cytoplasmic ratio.* This showed a progressive increase with the development of increasing malignant change in the DMBA lesions. In the turpentine-painted lesions the hyperplastic cells had a value lower even than the control cheek pouch epithelium, indicating a very marked difference between precancerous and hyperplastic changes.
2. *Nuclear numerical density* (numbers of nuclei per unit volume of epithelium). In stereological analyses for this feature it was found that there were more nuclei per unit volume in turpentine-painted cheek pouches than in normal controls. In DMBA-induced hyperplasia, however, there were even more nuclei than in the turpentine-painted pouches and the density of nuclei increased progressively with dysplasia and invasive carcinoma. These results appear to differ from those obtained in similar quantitative studies with the human cervix where, after rising to a maximum in terms of cell crowding for a unit area, the degree of crowding falls off in microinvasive and in invasive carcinoma (Hillemanns *et al.* 1968).
3. *Volume/surface area ratios of epithelium.* This investigation was similar to that carried out on small-intestine epithelium by Dunnill and Whitehead (1972) in patients with the malabsorption syndrome. The turpentine-painted pouch epithelium showed a reduction in volume/surface area ratio as compared with controls, and in dysplasia the ratio was still lower. Changes in this parameter have not been studied in human oral precancerous lesions. It is possible that they are relevant only to the malignant process in the special environment provided by the hamster cheek pouch.

Larynx

Squamous-cell carcinomas in the oral cavity develop from the normal covering squamous epithelium, and considerations of the relevant precancerous states are concerned only with changes in squamous epithelium. In the larynx, similar considerations apply only to squamous-cell carcinomas arising strictly from the vocal cord which is normally covered by squamous epithelium; squamous cancers developing at other sites within the larynx arise from areas which are normally lined by respiratory epithelium. Personal observations indicate that invasive squamous carcinomas of the larynx arising from regions lined by respiratory epithelium may originate in the following ways.

Directly from respiratory epithelium;
From squamous epithelium derived by metaplasia from respiratory epithelium;
From dysplastic or intraepithelial carcinomatous change of squamous epithelium derived by metaplasia from respiratory epithelium.

It follows that hyperplastic conditions of respiratory epithelium and squamous metaplasia of respiratory epithelium should be included in a consideration of precancerous states as well as dysplasia and carcinoma *in situ* of squamous epithelium.

Histogenesis of epidermoid metaplasia

It is likely, in view of its frequency, that the transformation of respiratory epithelium to epidermoid epithelium is carried out by a direct mechanism. The traditional view (Moore 1945) is that basal cells of the respiratory epithelium regenerate to produce epidermoid cells instead of ciliated or mucous columnar epithelial cells, the previously differentiated epithelial cells being shed to give way to the new type. Clear histological evidence for the stages of this process has not, however, been adduced and the work of Elizabeth McDowell and her colleagues at the University of Maryland School of Medicine strongly suggests that epidermoid metaplastic epithelium may frequently result from the direct transformation of mucous cells without multiplication of undifferentiated basal cells (Trump *et al.* 1978; see also Chapter 6). These studies have been carried out on the respiratory epithelium of the trachea, bronchus, and bronchioles in man and animals, but it is likely that the results apply to respiratory epithelium in general. In a study of many areas of epidermoid metaplasia with and without keratinization and also in prolonged culture of human bronchial epithelium deprived of vitamin A, the metaplastic epithelium was often seen to undergo an abrupt transition from epithelium showing mucous goblet cell hyperplasia. Areas of 'stratification' were also frequent in proximity to epidermoid metaplasia, i.e. a multilayering of mucus-secreting cells. Histochemical study of the epidermoid metaplastic cells themselves, particularly using Alcian blue-periodic acid-Schiff (PAS) stains, showed cytoplasmic mucosubstances in the cells of the metaplastic epithelium. A glycocalyx, a thin rim of heavily stained mucosubstance, was usually seen on the luminal aspect of the flattened surface cells of the metaplastic epidermoid epithelium. Basal cells did not contain mucosubstances. Electron microscopy confirmed the mucus content of many superficial keratinizing cells. Differentiated mucous cells of the tracheobronchial epithelium have been shown to incorporate tritiated (^{3}H) thymidine and to undergo cell division. These cells share with basal cells the responsibility for the primary repair process after injury of respiratory epithelium. It seems probable that they are a direct source of the epidermoid cells in epidermoid metaplasia, wherever this change may be found.

Epidermoid metaplasia in the larynx

Personal observations made on the appearances of metaplastic squamous-cell epithelium in the human larynx lend support to the ideas on the histogenesis of epidermoid metaplasia put forward by McDowell and her co-workers. Variable degrees of epidermoid metaplasia are regularly seen in the adult larynx. In the subglottis, small islands of squamous metaplasia are found in as many as 40 per cent of the non-smoking, non-bronchitic urban population (Stell *et al.* 1980). In the supraglottis, areas of non-dysplastic squamous epithelium are common in cases of laryngeal carcinoma whether or not they have been previously irradiated.

Metaplastic squamous epithelium in the supraglottis was studied in 15 laryngectomy specimens containing squamous-cell carcinomas. For controls, the epithelial lining of the pyriform fossa was examined in 15 larynges in which portions of that mucosa had been removed together with the larynx.

In the supraglottic tissues, areas of mucous secretory epithelium adjacent to epithelium showing squamous metaplasia were heaped in a manner resembling the 'stratification zones' described by Trump *et al.* (1978) in bronchial epithelium. These areas showed a gradual transition to epithelium showing definite epidermoid metaplasia (Fig. 5.9) and, in a few places, dysplasia or carcinoma *in situ.* In the epidermoid areas many zones were seen in which the cells were vacuolated. Such groups of cells were situated in an intermediate position between the basal layer of the epithelium and the surface of the keratinized layer. The vacuoles range in size from multiple small vesicles in the same cell to empty spaces covered by a thin rim of cytoplasm (Fig. 5.10). With the Alcian blue method, they stained faintly in some cases and in other cases not at all. Vacuolated cells were also seen in some larynges in which the vacuoles stained in a basophilic fashion with haematoxylin and eosin and were strongly positive with Alcian blue. An occasional rim of Alcian blue-staining material was seen on the surface of metaplastic squamous epithelium similar to the glycocalyx described by Trump *et al.* (1978). No areas provided any evidence for the origin of squamous cells from the basal layer or of any process indicating a pushing aside of respiratory epithelium from below by newly formed squamous epithelium. Vacuolated cells were not present in squamous epithelium from the pyriform fossae in any of the 15 cases that were examined. These observations are in keeping with the origin of squamous cells in squamous metaplasia from among the mucous secretory cells of the respiratory epithelium. Cells actually containing stainable mucus are seen in the midst of the epidermoid cells. More commonly, various degrees of vacuolation are present which may represent degenerative changes in the mucous secretory

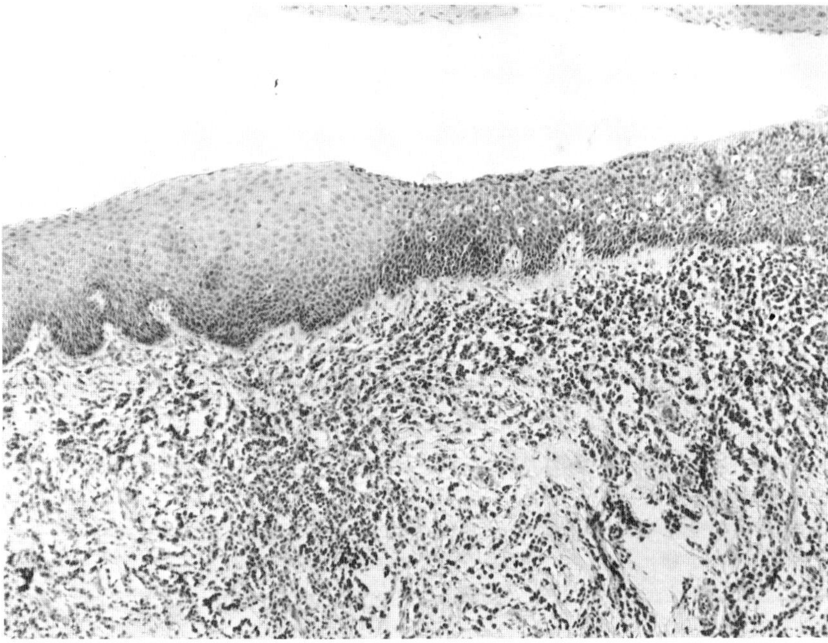

Fig. 5.9. Laryngeal epithelium from supraglottic region showing metaplastic squamous epithelium on the left which is sharply separated from a 'stratification zone' comprising multilayered secretory cells on the right. ×95. H & E.

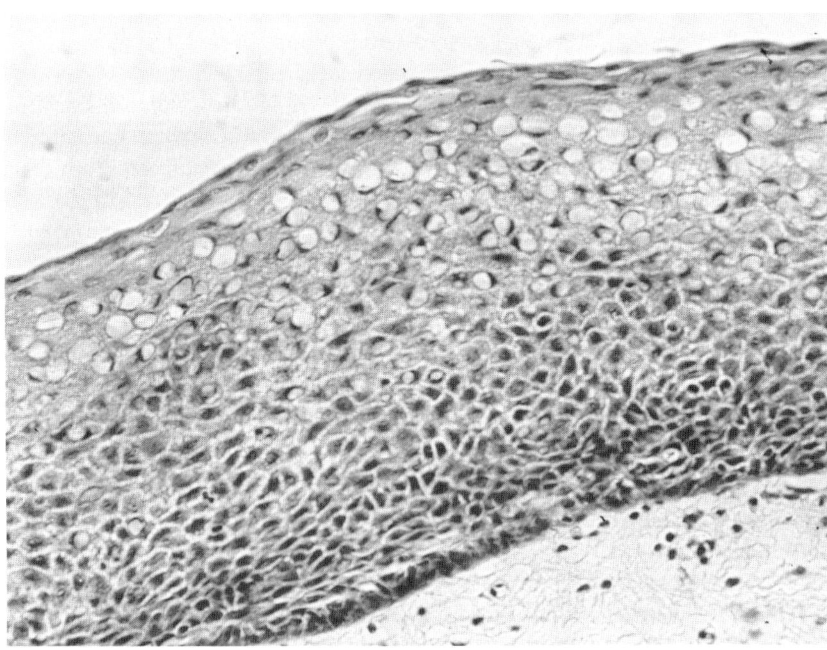

Fig. 5.10. Vacuolated cells in metaplastic squamous epithelium of larynx. ×240. H & E.

cells. This interpretation is strengthened by the deterioration in Alcian blue positivity which accompanies progressive vacuolation.

Classification of precancerous states of the larynx

As in the oral cavity, the classification of precancerous states of the larynx was at one time closely associated with the degree of keratinization of the epithelium. Insufficient attention was paid in a number of studies relating keratosis and malignancy to the degree of atypical mucosal changes seen histologically (Putney and O'Keefe 1953); once again 'leukoplakia', defined as a clinically observed white plaque on the epithelium produced by keratosis, was felt to be a premalignant lesion. This impression was widely accepted in spite of Kleinsasser's early (1963) insistence on a classification of squamous-cell lesions of the vocal cord based on dysplastic changes. He proposed three categories:

Simple hyperplasia;
Hyperplasia with foci of atypical cells;
Precancerous epithelium (carcinoma *in situ*).

It was not until the 1974 Centennial Conference of Laryngeal Cancer, held in Toronto, that there was general agreement that the term 'leukoplakia' should not be used for laryngeal lesions. At this conference the injunction was repeated throughout the relevant discussions that the assessment of malignant potential in laryngeal squamous lesions should be based on the degree of epithelial dysplasia (Fechner 1974). Several assessments of the negative role of keratosis as a precancerous lesion in the larynx had been published before the 1974 Conference. Norris and Peale (1963), for example, followed 30 patients with keratosis but without dysplasia and only one developed cancer, but, of 86 patients showing keratosis of the larynx accompanied by dysplasia, 11 developed cancer. McGavran *et al.* (1960) studied 84 patients with laryngeal keratosis for periods of 5 to 15 years and only three developed invasive carcinoma. These authors concluded that the most important prognostic feature was the presence or absence of cellular atypia (Fig. 5.11). Hellquist *et al.* (1982) have recently studied biopsies from 193 patients which they classified into three categories:

Group 1, slight dysplastic changes often accompanied either by superficial keratosis or by hyperplasia;
Group 2, intermediate between Group 1 and Group 3;
Group 3, severe dysplasia (squamous differentiation identified on the epithelial surface (Fig. 5.12(a), (b)) or carcinoma *in situ* (little if any squamous differentiation on the surface).

The biopsies in these patients were obtained from all areas of the larynx, the majority from the vocal cord region.

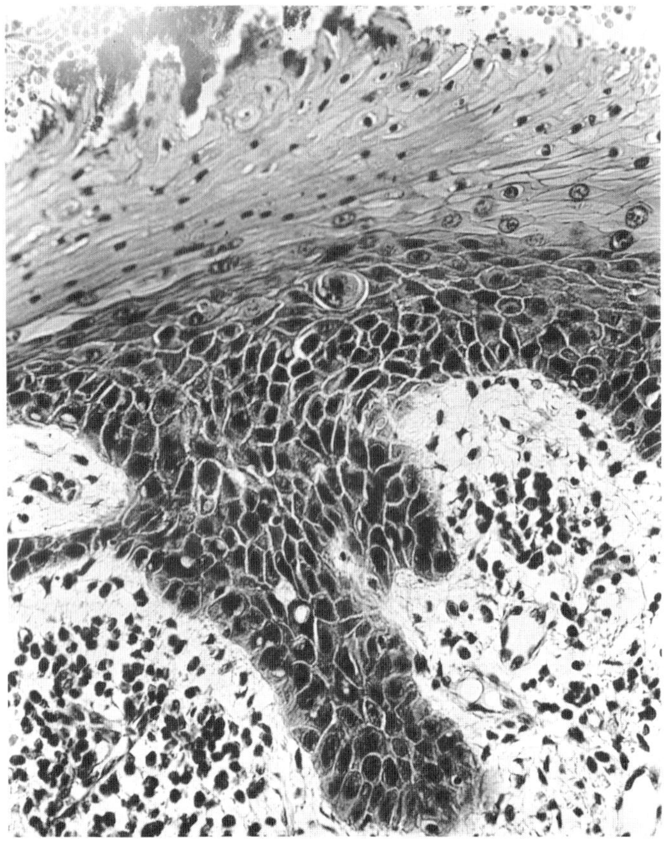

Fig. 5.11. Severe dysplasia of laryngeal squamous epithelium with marked overlying keratosis. The latter (seen grossly as a 'leukoplakic' patch) bears no relation to the assessment of the degree of precancerous change, but the presence of dysplasia is critical. ×240. H & E.

In Group 1 out of 98 patients available for follow-up, two developed severe dysplasia and two invasive carcinoma. In Group 2 out of 24 patients available for follow-up, severe dysplasia developed in three patients and invasive carcinoma in three patients. In Group 3 out of 39 patients 16 were given radiotherapy as the primary form of treatment. 23 cases were treated primarily by excision or stripping of the vocal cords. Five of these cases developed invasive carcinoma.

The work of Hellquist's group thus confirms that in precancerous states of the larynx, the degree of mucosal atypia—the basis of the classification into three groups—is the most important histological criterion since it is closely correlated with the subsequent incidence of invasive carcinoma. These results not only indicate the importance of placing cases of severe dysplasia in the 'most severe' category with carcinoma *in situ*, but also show that severe dysplasia with keratosis has a worse prognosis than severe dys-

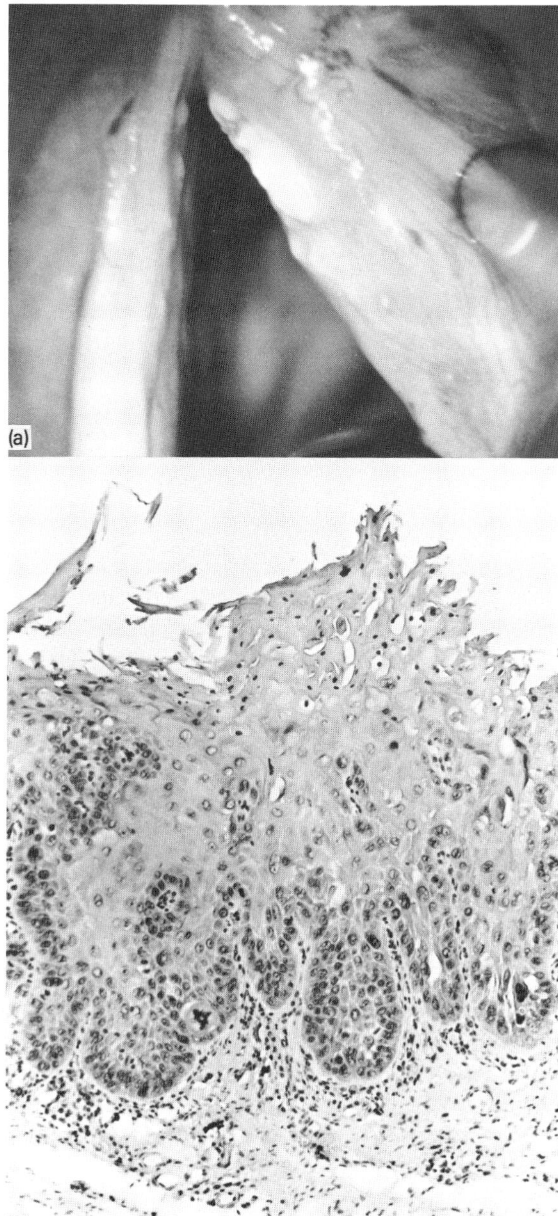

Fig. 5.12. (a) Vocal cords seen at microlaryngoscopy. There is a greyish-white focus at the anterior end of a somewhat oedematous right vocal cord. The free margin of the right vocal cord has been turned upwards by the suction tube, the free end of which is visible on the right. (b) Biopsy of right vocal cord showing a severe degree of dysplasia with keratosis (well-differentiated type). (From Hellquist *et al.* (1982).)

plasia and carcinoma *in situ* of the classic type without keratosis. Seven out of nine cases of invasive carcinoma developed from severe dysplasia with keratosis but no invasive carcinoma developed from carcinoma *in situ* of classic type and only two from severe dysplasia without keratosis. This work reverts in a sense to a serious interpretation of keratotic changes in the larynx—but with the important proviso that the keratosis must be accompanied by severe dysplasia.

Hellquist has refined these histological observations by computerized microspectrophotometry in Feulgen-stained 9μm thick plastic-embedded sections. In Groups 1 and 2 the nuclear DNA content and nuclear size were not different from normal; it was particularly noteworthy that the cases in Group 2 which later developed severe dysplasia showed no spectrophotometric difference from normal. The photometric values for severe dysplasia and carcinoma *in situ* differed markedly from those with lesser degrees of dysplasia and were comparable to those of invasive carcinoma. A more reliable assessment than by histological inspection could be made by photometry of the nuclear atypia in cases of severe dysplasia which were well differentiated, emphasizing the particularly serious nature of this lesion. Reference was made earlier in this chapter to the use of a computer in grouping epithelial changes in oral mucosa into disease categories and later to the use of microscopic measurements in assessing precancerous states more precisely. Microspectrophotometry of laryngeal biopsies illustrates a third mode of quantitation that offers refinement to the pathologist's qualitative visual assessment. Whether these methods will come into routine use in the future is unclear, but there has been much justifiable criticism of the subjective nature of many of the conclusions of histopathologists in precancerous lesions of squamous epithelium. It seems reasonable, therefore, that any methods which give greater objectivity to these judgements should in the course of time be adopted.

Technical problems in the diagnosis of precancerous states of the larynx

The diagnosis of precancerous states of the larynx is usually made after examination of small punch biopsies removed at endoscopy. The first requisite for an accurate histological assessment is the correct selection of tissue for biopsy by the surgeon. Failure to remove a representative area for biopsy or the removal of insufficient tissue may result in a mistaken histological interpretation of the lesion which may not be realized until the patient returns with more advanced disease. Some regions are difficult or impossible to inspect with the laryngoscope—the subglottis, for example, because of the overhanging vocal cords, or the deep and narrow saccule. Marked inflammatory change and oedema may make it impossible to obtain an adequate biopsy, although it must be admitted that such severe changes are usually to be found in the presence of invasive carcinoma rather than carcinoma *in situ* alone. There is an impression among clinicians that precancerous changes of the larynx will always provide some gross surface appearances which, at most sites, will be detected by careful microlaryngoscopy. The point has not been adequately tested, but it seems likely that some areas of carcinoma *in situ* or severe dysplasia are associated with an unremarkable surface appearance and might not be seen at laryngoscopy and biopsied. The clinician may hinder the pathological assessment by tearing the biopsy fragments in the course of removal so that severe artefacts are seen in the final histological preparation.

In the laboratory correct handling by technologists is vital. Endoscopic punch biopsies are small and considerable experience in their correct embedding is required to avoid the production of tangential sections of epithelium; with such sections the diagnosis of carcinoma *in situ* is impossible since a decision about the presence or absence of invasion requires observation of the relationship of surface epithelium to lamina propria (Fig. 5.13).

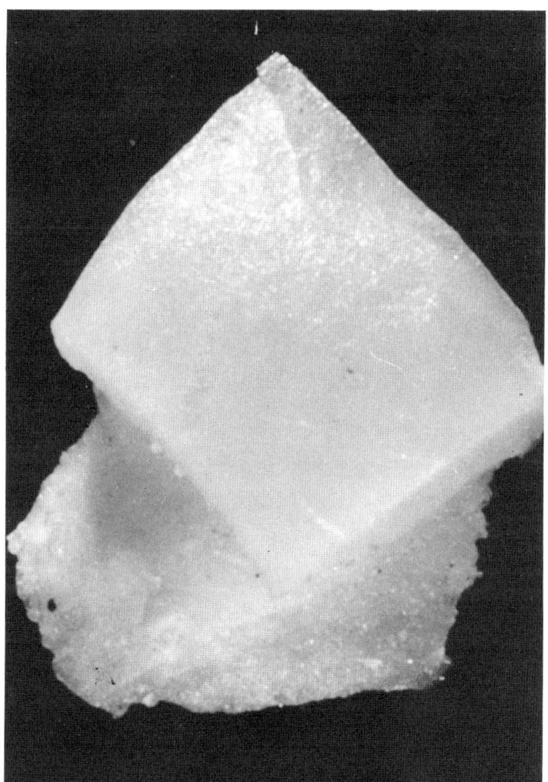

Fig. 5.13. Biopsy-sized fragment of laryngeal mucosa seen under dissecting microscope. The mucosal surface is uppermost and is smooth and shiny. It is important that this is recognized during embedding so that sections are cut at right angles to the mucosal surface.

Differential diagnosis of precancerous states of the larynx

The overdiagnosis of severe dysplasia in the larynx as carcinoma *in situ* is of no serious consequence, since both are probably equally proven to be associated with invasive carcinoma (Hellquist *et al.* 1982). Particular concern should be given to detecting the well-differentiated form of severe dysplasia in view of the possibility of its even worse outlook.

Inflammatory and other non-malignant lesions may be associated with hyperplasia and dysplasia of the overlying squamous epithelium—the so-called 'pseudoepitheliomatous hyperplasia'. Such changes are well known in relation to tuberculosis and granular cell myoblastoma and careful examination of the lamina propria is necessary in any biopsy showing atypical epithelial changes. The specific histological features of tuberculosis may, in particular, be slight and the amount of material available is often very small. The site of a previous biopsy and the surface of a laryngeal nodule may show dysplasia that falsely suggests the possibility of a precancerous lesion. One of the commonest causes of dysplastic change in laryngeal biopsies which is often severe in degree, is previous irradiation (Fig. 5.14). The pathologist should always know the clinical history, particularly with regard to previous lesions of the larynx and their treatment.

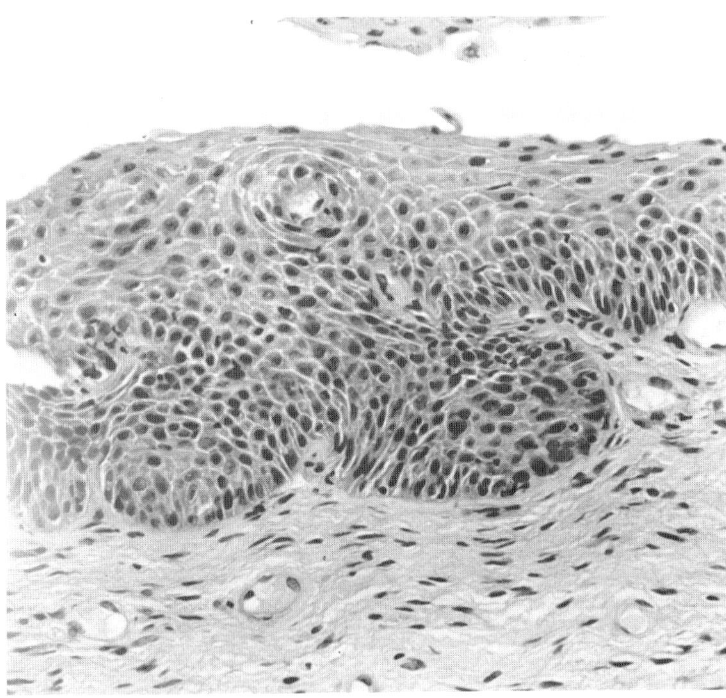

Fig. 5.14. Dysplastic change in vocal cord epithelium following irradiation. The patient had received 6800 rads 9 months previously for squamous-cell carcinoma. The appearances do not indicate precancerous change. ×400. H & E.

Carcinomatous tissue identified below the surface of the covering epithelium does not always mean that *invasive* carcinoma is present. Carcinoma *in situ* may grow along clefts of the surface, and it is particularly prone to develop in relation to the columnar cells of the ducts of seromucinous glands of the larynx (Figs. 5.15 and 5.16). The columnar cells often degenerate and disappear and the appearances may be misinterpreted as a focus of invasive cell carcinoma.

Carcinoma in situ *of the larynx*

There is information from an extensive study by Auerbach *et al.* (1970) about the incidence, site, detailed morphology, and relationship to smoking of carcinoma *in situ* of the larynx. Nine hundred seventy-one larynges from autopsies performed on male veterans were examined microscopically in

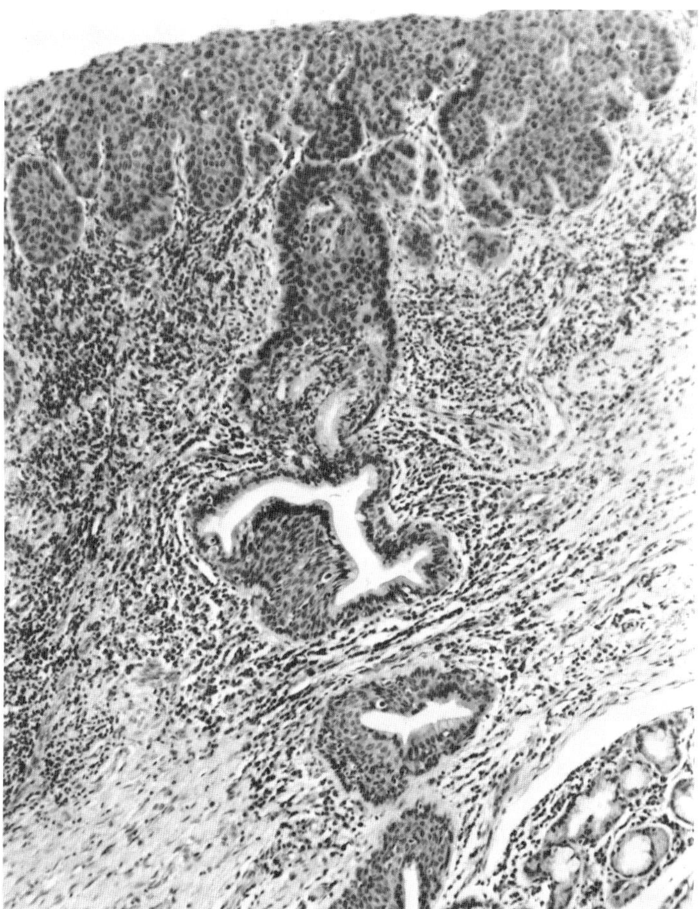

Fig. 5.15. Carcinoma *in situ* of surface epithelium of the larynx, with extension along the duct of a seromucinous gland. ×100. H & E.

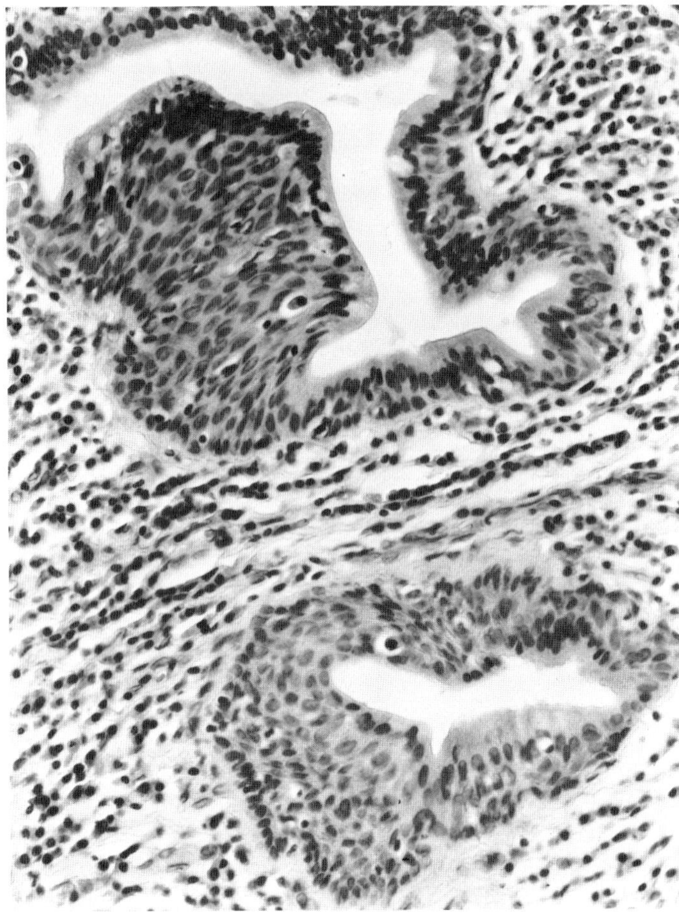

Fig. 5.16. Higher power of part of previous illustration showing cells of carcinoma *in situ* closely opposed to epithelial lining cells of duct of seromucinous gland. ×250. H & E.

four vertical slices on each side, each comprising part of the false vocal cord, the true vocal cord, and the areas above and below the cords. Thus in each of the eight sections from the larynx there were four epithelial areas the changes of which were recorded, a total of 32 areas being available for study from each case.

Carcinoma *in situ* was found in the true vocal cord in 11.4 per cent of the larynges and in the false cord in 4.9 per cent. The other two areas showed a very low incidence of carcinoma *in situ.* Carcinoma *in situ* is depicted by the authors as arising directly from respiratory epithelium in the areas other than the true vocal cords by a process of hyperplasia and atypical change of basal cells.

The degree of atypical change of the epithelium of the true vocal cord was strongly related to smoking habits. The atypical changes were much more marked in cigarette-smokers than in people who had never smoked; they increased in proportion to the number of cigarettes smoked per day before death and were seen to a greater degree in cigarette-smokers than in cigar- and pipe-smokers. Ex-cigarette-smokers had fewer such changes than men who continued to smoke cigarettes up to the time of death.

Carcinoma *in situ* of the larynx shows similar microscopic features to carcinoma *in situ* of the oral cavity (Figs. 5.17 and 5.18).

Carcinoma in situ *associated with invasive carcinoma*

If it is accepted that carcinoma *in situ* is a frequent lesion in the larynx, the question arises: is there a particular area in which diagnostic and therapeutic activity can be concentrated so as to prevent the development of invasive carcinoma? The brief answer is that, unfortunately, carcinoma *in situ* may arise anywhere in this complex organ. A particular problem is that the lesion frequently coexists with invasive carcinoma. Bauer (1974) studied 354 laryngeal cancers by making serial longitudinal blocks of the entire laryngeal mucosa after removing the laryngeal cartilages from the specimen. In this paper three pairs of illustrations are given for three cases showing on the one hand the gross surface appearances of the mucosa and on the other a

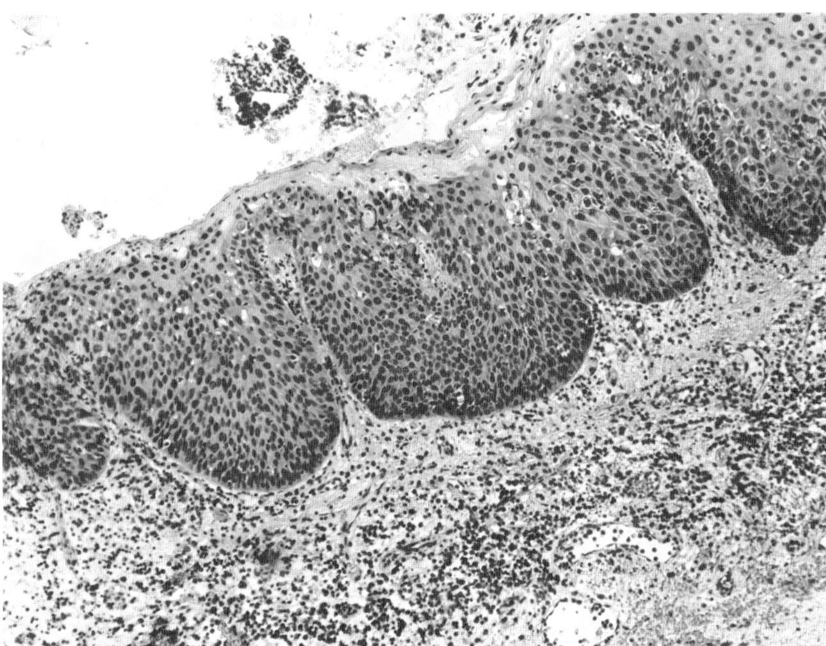

Fig. 5.17. Carcinoma *in situ* of vocal cord. The rete processes are drop-shaped, there is a disturbance of polarity of the basal layer and maturation is defective throughout the epithelium. The component cells of the epithelium show cytologic features of malignancy. ×100. H & E.

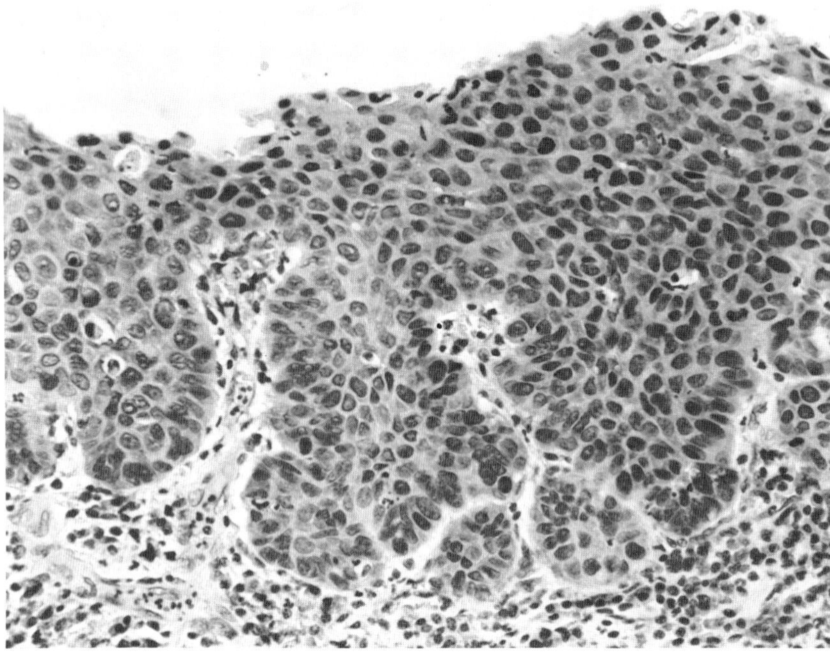

Fig. 5.18. *In situ* carcinoma of laryngeal epithelium. Note 'drop-shaped' rete processes, disturbed polarity of basal cells, disturbed maturational sequence, cell crowding, and a high nucleo-cytoplasmic ratio. ×240. H & E.

diagram of the surface outline of invasive, superficially invasive, and carcinoma *in situ* areas. The area of carcinoma *in situ* was of variable width and followed round the edge of the invasive carcinoma as a tortuous convoluted zone. In the photographs some mucosal areas of carcinoma *in situ* are clearly without gross features. Of the 374 invasive carcinomas 172 (49 per cent) showed carcinoma *in situ*. Seventy-three per cent of the supraglottic cancers were accompanied by carcinoma *in situ*, but lesser numbers of the other anatomical forms of cancer. When squamous carcinoma of the larynx is separated into non-keratinizing and keratinizing forms, Bauer found that significantly greater numbers of cases of non-keratinizing carcinoma (76 per cent) were accompanied by carcinoma *in situ* than keratinizing carcinoma (29 per cent).

I have studied the same problem in a much smaller series of 37 consecutive cases of invasive squamous-cell carcinoma of the larynx or hypopharynx that presented at the Royal National Throat, Nose, and Ear Hospital in London. In each case transverse slices of the larynx and hypopharynx were made on a motorized slicing machine by the method of Michaels and Gregor (1980) and representative blocks of tumour and surrounding tissue were taken for histological examination. The area of each block was marked on 'Polaroid' photographs so that the site of the *in situ* carcinoma could be ascertained whenever found. Sixteen of the 36 cases of laryngeal or hypopharyngeal carcinoma contained areas of carcinoma *in situ*, the sites of which are listed in Table 5.2. The invasive components in these cases were usually adjacent, though more extensive. Exceptions were provided by two cases of carcinoma *in situ* affecting the saccule in which the invasive squamous carcinoma arose not from the saccule but from the adjacent aryepiglottic fold. The distance of the further edge of a zone of carcinoma *in situ* from the adjacent invasive carcinoma was measured and found to vary from 1 to 9 mm. In contrast to Bauer's findings, 9 of the 16 cancers in which carcinoma *in situ* as well as invasive carcinoma was present were moderately or well differentiated with ample keratin production. Table 5.2 also illustrates—and again in contrast to Bauer's findings—that carcinoma *in situ* may accompany any position of origin of squamous-cell carcinoma in the larynx or hypopharynx.

Table 5.2. *Sites of carcinoma* in situ *in cases of invasive carcinoma of larynx and hypopharynx*

	Number of cases
Epiglottis and false cord	2
Saccule (invasive carcinoma was present on nearby aryepiglottic fold in both cases)	2
Ventricle	3
True cord	4
Subglottis	3
Pyriform fossa	3

Epidemiological factors and experimental studies in laryngeal carcinoma

Cigarette-smoking. There is strong epidemiological evidence of a correlation between heavy cigarette-smoking and the incidence of carcinoma of the larynx (Stell 1973). In histological studies on autopsy larynges, the relationship of dysplasia and carcinoma *in situ* to smoking history was found to be close (Auerbach *et al.* 1970). In a more recent autopsy study of 148 vocal cord specimens (Mueller and Krohn 1980) dysplasia and carcinoma *in situ* were found in only 4.2 per cent of non-smokers, rising to 12.5 per cent in light to 22.5 per cent in moderate and to 47.2 per cent in heavy smokers. In ex-smokers these precancerous changes were present in only 12.5 per cent, the level of light smokers.

Experimental studies have recently achieved a striking specificity in studying the relationship of cigarette smoke to laryngeal cancers. Progressive refinement of experimental techniques has led to a method in which a high incidence (about 50 per cent) of precancerous changes and carcinoma of the larynx was induced in animals exposed to cigarette smoke: the system is described by Bernfeld *et al.* (1979). Important factors in obtaining this particularly high yield of precancerous and cancerous lesions of the larynx included the use of males of an inbred strain of Syrian golden hamster which appeared to be particularly susceptible to laryngeal carcinogens, and the design of a positive-pressure cigarette-burning machine with intermittent as opposed to continuous exposure of the animals to smoke. As many as 496 hamsters were studied histologically which had been exposed to smoke for 59 weeks or more—a sufficient period of time for neoplastic and preneoplastic changes to be detectable histologically. 36.8 per cent of larynges from the exposed group of animals showed invasive carcinoma and an additional 9.4 per cent contained lesions of early carcinoma or carcinoma *in situ*, making a total of 47.4 per cent of larynges with malignant change. Some larynges showed epithelial hyperplasia or squamous papilloma with or without malignant changes of the epithelium. The malignant changes in the larynx appeared to be dose-dependent. By the use of 100 per cent tobacco, the figure given above of 47.4 per cent of larynges showing malignant change was obtained, but the incidence fell to 21.7 per cent malignant change with 50 per cent tobacco. With exposure to Cytrel, a special tobacco supplement, no neoplastic changes were identified. The pathological features of squamous papillomatosis, squamous metaplasia of respiratory epithelium, dysplasia of squamous epithelium, and squamous carcinoma (well or poorly differentiated) in these experiments were strikingly similar to the lesions found in the human larynx (Homburger *et al.* 1979).

Alcohol consumption. There is also less strong, but reliable, evidence of an association between alcohol consumption and carcinoma of the larynx (Hinds *et al.* 1979). It is possible that the effect of alcohol consumption on laryngeal carcinoma may be through alcohol-related nutritional deficiencies particularly those of zinc and vitamin A (McCoy *et al.* 1980). On the other hand a direct synergistic effect of 10 per cent alcohol intake on the carcinogenic effect of benzo(a)pyrene in the larynx in hamsters has been observed by Stevens (1979) although the numbers were small: seven out of twenty alcoholic hamsters developed carcinoma as compared with two out of twenty non-alcoholic benzo(a)pyrene-treated hamsters.

Asbestos. There is a proven relationship between asbestos exposure and carcinoma of the lung. It might be imagined that a similar relationship would exist between asbestos and carcinoma of the larynx and retrospective studies to support this view have been published by Stell and McGill (1973). Asbestos bodies have been recovered from laryngeal tissues at autopsy in two of five patients with occupational asbestos exposure, but no dysplastic epithelial changes were observed in the mucosa (Roggli *et al.* 1980). Recent prospective studies of possible asbestos exposure in cases of laryngeal carcinoma have, however, shown no definite relationship (Hinds *et al.* 1979; Newhouse *et al.* 1980) and the question remains open.

Morphologically recognizable precancerous states in oral cavity and larynx: their aetiology, diagnosis, and treatment

A tacit assumption in work on precancerous states of the oral cavity and larynx has been that dysplasia may progress to carcinoma *in situ* which itself may go on to invasive carcinoma. This assumption is difficult to substantiate in any single clinical or even experimental study. But the cumulative weight of the large numbers of observations of both types that have been made confirms that the assumption is a valid one. Tobacco is the most important aetiological agent; even where other factors may play a part in the development of a precancerous state, such as betel-nut chewing in the mouth or alcohol consumption in the larynx, these factors may act together with tobacco. In the diagnosis of the cancerous states emphasis is being increasingly placed on sites where precancerous changes may be particularly found. This approach is important because, unlike the cervix uteri, the potential cancer-bearing areas of the oral cavity and larynx are extensive and impossible to remove in their entirety without a highly disfiguring surgical operation. In order to reduce the subjective element in the histological diagnosis of these conditions, mensuration of microscopic features has been introduced and also computerized analysis of the various microscopic features that enable a diagnosis of the various precancerous entities to be made. The value of these additional laboratory studies has yet to be proved on a large scale. The therapy of precancerous states in these anatomical regions is still largely surgical, but the lesions are often too widespread for adequate excision and, as progression of the condition is not certain, the necessity for surgery frequently cannot be adequately assessed in any particular case. The value of radiotherapy remains controversial.

Nasopharynx

In a classification proposed by the World Health Organization (Shanmugaratnam 1978), three histological types of nasopharyngeal carcinoma (NPC) were proposed.

1. Squamous-cell carcinoma (keratinizing squamous-cell carcinoma);
2. Non-keratinizing squamous-cell carcinoma;
3. Undifferentiated carcinoma.

Nasopharyngeal carcinoma is rare in Europe and North America but much more frequent among Mongoloid populations living in or derived from Southern China; groups with an intermediate incidence of NPC occur in the North African littoral and in East Africa. The undifferentiated carcinomas, in which there are often numerous accompanying lymphocytes, predominate in Chinese populations, but there is evidence from light and electron microscopical studies of surgical biopsies (Michaels and Hyams 1977) and from autopsy material in a Chinese population (Teoh 1957) that these three forms do not represent sharp categories; they appear to merge into each other, each being related to epidermoid carcinoma with greater or lesser degrees of squamous differentiation.

The morphological aspects of precancerous states in relation to NPC have received little attention. A recent investigation of nasopharyngeal biopsies from 15 Chinese cases of NPC and 15 controls showed similar (mild) mucosal dysplasia in both groups (Gusterson *et al.* 1983). Immunohistochemical studies with epithelial membrane antigen and carcinoembryonic antigen (EMA,CEA) showed positive staining of mucosal cells near regions of inflammation in both groups; no distinctive staining was seen in the dysplastic zones. These findings are similar to those previously described in immunohistological studies of squamous epithelium from other sites in the head and neck and elsewhere (Sloane *et al.* 1982). Certain *non-morphological* features such as genetic constitution and exposure to Epstein-Barr (EB) virus are, however, important factors in the development of NPC and merit brief discussion.

The wide variation in incidence rates of NPC has already been noted, ranging from $<1/10^5$ to $10\text{-}20/10^5$ in different parts of the world (Hirayama 1978). Convincing evidence has emerged from studies mainly carried out in Hong Kong and Singapore that high-risk people in those areas—that is, individuals of Southern Chinese origin—have a distinctive HLA profile (Simons *et al.* 1974, 1975, 1978; Chan *et al.* 1981). NPC in the Southern Chinese is associated with an increased incidence of HLA-A2 and B sin 2, an association which holds for both initial susceptibility to NPC and for survival after diagnosis. Increased risk also seems to be associated with BW17, and a decreased risk with A11. A comparable pattern has not yet been found in the intermediate-risk group of NPC cases from North Africa (Betuel *et al.* 1975), but investigations in these regions have not been extensive. The significance of altered HLA patterns in the aetiology of NPC among high-risk populations is unclear. The question of hypothetical disease susceptibility genes has been postulated which may be linked with other genes that influence antibody responses—see later. Preliminary results have also been recorded on the distribution of certain genetically controlled erythrocyte enzymes and serum protein systems in Chinese cases of NPC—for instance, glucose 6-phosphate dehydrogenase, red-cell acid phosphatase and transferrin (Kirk *et al.* 1978). This is an interesting line of enquiry, but more information is needed from other ethnic groups in high, intermediate, and low-risk regions in other parts of the world.

A close relationship between NPC and EB virus is now extensively documented. Data based mainly on seroepidemiological studies indicate an association that appears to operate in all groups investigated broadly irrespective of ethnic origin or degree of risk (De Thé *et al.* 1978; Henle and Henle 1981). Certain aspects of the antibody response to EB virus in patients with NPC are unusual. Work with high-risk Chinese groups has shown a particular tendency for such patients to produce IgA antibodies to EB virus-related antigens (Henle *et al.* 1978). The high frequency and (often) high titres of EB virus-related serum IgA antibodies appear to be a characteristic feature of NPC. Still more interesting is the observation that a similar pattern of IgA antibody formation against EB virus antigens is seen in apparently unaffected family members of NPC patients (Ng *et al.* 1978). No specific preneoplastic lesions have yet been identified in biopsy material from such individuals (De Thé *et al.* 1981). The possibility of links between these distinctive IgA antibody responses and genetic constitution has been raised (Levine *et al.* 1981), but more information is necessary to strengthen such a proposal. Detailed studies of the structure of the EB virus genome are now available, but restriction endonuclease maps of 8 EBV DNAs have so far failed to reveal any characteristics which could be linked with pathological origin—from NPC, or Burkitt's lymphoma or infectious mononucleosis (Kieff *et al.* 1981).

Despite the obvious importance of genetic predisposition and exposure to EB virus, several other aetiological features remain to be identified in NPC. Exogeneous chemicals are likely to be involved and the role of putative ingested carcinogens, in the form of salted fish, has attracted much attention (Huang 1978).

References

Auerbach, O., Hammond, E.C., and Garfinkel, L. (1970). Histologic changes in the larynx in relation to smoking habits. *Cancer* **25**, 92.

Bánóczy, J. (1977). Follow-up studies in oral leukoplakia. *J. Maxillofac. Surg.* **5**, 69.

Bauer, W. (1974). Concomitant carcinoma in situ and invasive carcinoma of the larynx. Centennial conference in laryngeal cancer. Workshop No. 2, p. 127. Appleton Century Crofts, New York.

Bernfeld, P., Homburger, F., Soto, E., and Pai, K.J. (1979). Cigarette smoke inhalation studies in inbred Syrian golden hamsters. *J. Nat. Cancer. Inst.* **63**, 675.

Betuel, H., Camoun, M., Colombani, J., Day, N.E., Ellouz, R., and De-Thé, G. (1975). The relationship between nasopharyngeal carcinoma and the HL-A system among Tunisians. *Int. J. Cancer* **16**, 249.

Cawson, R.A. and Binnie, W.H. (1980). Candida leukoplakia and carcinoma: a possible relationship. In *Oral premalignancy. Proceedings of the First Dows Symposium* (ed. I.C. Mackenzie, E. Dabelsteen, and C.A. Squire), pp. 23-4. University of Iowa Press.

Chan, S.H., Day, N.E., Khor, T.H., Kunaratnam, N., and Chia, K.B. (1981). HLA markers in the development and prognosis of NPC in Chinese. In *Nasopharyngeal carcinoma* (ed. E. Grundmann, G.R.F. Krueger, and D.V. Ablashi), p. 205. Cancer Campaign Volume 5. Gustav Fischer, Stuttgart, New York.

De Thé, G., Lavoue, M.F., and Muenz, L. (1978). Differences in EBV antibody titres of patients with nasopharyngeal carcinoma originating from high, intermediate and low incidence areas. In *Nasopharyngeal carcinoma: etiology and control* (ed. G. de Thé and Y. Ito), pp. 471-81. IARC Scientific Publications No. 20. International Agency for Research on Cancer, Lyon.

——, Desgranges, C., Zeng, Y., Wang, P.C., Bornkamm, G.W., Zhu, J.S., and Shang, M. (1981). Search for precancerous lesions and EBV markers in the nasopharynx of IgA-positive individuals. In *Nasopharyngeal carcinoma* (ed. E. Grundmann, G.R.F. Krueger, and D.V. Ablashi), p. 111. Cancer Campaign Volume 5. Gustav Fischer, Stuttgart, New York.

Dunnill, M.S. and Whitehead, R. (1972). A method for the quantitation of small intestinal biopsies. *J. clin. Path.* **25**, 243.

Fechner, R.E. (1974). *Workshop No. 2. Centennial conference on laryngeal cancer*, p. 110. Appleton Century Crofts, New York.

Fejerskow, O., Roed-Peteren, B., and Pindborg, J.J. (1977). Clinical, histological and ultrastructural features of a possible virus induced oral leukoplakia. *Acta Pathol. Microbiol. Scand.* **A25**, 897.

Franklin, C.D. and Smith, C.J. (1980). Stereological analysis of histological parameters in experimental premalignant hamster cheek pouch epithelium. *J. Pathol.* **130**, 201.

Gusterson, B.A., Mitchell, D.P., Warburton, M.J., and Carter, R.L. Epithelial markers in the diagnosis of nasopharyngeal carcinoma: an immunocytochemical study. *J. Clin. Path.* **36**, 628.

Hellquist, H., Lundgren, J., and Olofsson, J. (1982). Hyperplasia, keratosis, dysplasia and carcinoma *in situ* of the vocal cords—a follow-up study. *Clin. Otolaryngol.* **7**, 11.

Henle, W. and Henle, G. (1981). The association of Epstein-Barr virus with nasopharyngeal carcinoma. In *Nasopharyngeal carcinoma* (ed. E. Grundmann, G.R.F. Krueger, and D.V. Ablashi), p. 1. Cancer Campaign Volume 5. Gustav Fischer, Stuttgart, New York.

—— ——, and Ho, J.H.C. (1978). Epstein-Barr virus-related serology in nasopharyngeal carcinoma and controls. In *Nasopharyngeal carcinoma: etiology and control* (ed. G. de Thé and Y. Ito), pp. 427-37. IARC Scientific Publications No. 20. International Agency for Research on Cancer, Lyon.

Hillemanns, H.G., Sixtus-Klug, B., and Prestel, E. (1968). Cytoplasma-Kern relationen der Malignitätsstufen des Cervixepithels gemessen mit dem Integrationsocular. I. Zum Carcinoma in Situ und Microcarcinom der Cervix. *Arch. Gynaek* **206**, 82.

Hinds, M.W., Thomas, D.B., and O'Reilly, H.P. (1979). Asbestos, dental X-rays, tobacco and alcohol in the epidemiology of laryngeal cancer. *Cancer* **44**, 1114.

Hirayama, T. (1978). Descriptive and analytical epidemiology of nasopharyngeal cancer. In *Nasopharyngeal carcinoma: etiology and control* (ed. G. de-Thé and Y. Ito). pp. 167-89. IARC Scientific Publications No. 20. International Agency for Research on Cancer, Lyon.

Homburger, F., Soto, H., Althoff, J., Dalquen, P., and Heitz, P. (1979). Carcinoma of the larynx in hamsters exposed to cigarette smoke. *Amer. J. Pathol.* **95**, 845.

Huang, D.P., Ho, J.H.C., Saw, D., and Teoh, T.B. (1978). Carcinoma of the nasal and paranasal regions in rats fed Cantonese salted marine fish. In *Nasopharyngeal carcinoma: etiology and control* (ed. G. de-Thé and Y. Ito), pp. 315-28. IARC Scientific Publications No. 20. International Agency for Research on Cancer, Lyon.

Kieff, E., Dambaugh, T., Heller, M., King, W., Van Santen, V., and Cheung, A. (1981). Structure and function of the Epstein-Barr virus genome: a brief overview. In *Nasopharyngeal carcinoma* (ed. E. Grundmann, G.R.F. Krueger, and D.V. Ablashi), p. 87. Cancer Campaign Volume 5, Gustav Fischer, Stuttgart, New York.

Kirk, R.L., Blake, N.M., and Serjeantson, S. (1978). Genetic components in susceptibility to nasopharyngeal carcinoma. In *Nasopharyngeal carcinoma: etiology and control* (ed. G. de Thé and Y. Ito), p. 283. IARC Scientific Publications No. 20. International Agency for Research on Cancer, Lyon.

Kleinsasser, O. (1963). Die Klassification und Differentialdiagnose der Epithelialhyperplasien der Kehlkopfschleimhaut auf Grund histomorphologischer Merkmale. II. Mitteilung. *Z. Laryngol. Rhinol. Otol.* **42**, 339.

Kramer, I.R.H. (1969). Precancerous conditions of the oral mucosa. A computer aided study. *Ann. R. Coll. Surg. Eng.* **45**, 340.

—— (1980). Basic histopathological features of oral premalignant lesions. In *Oral premalignancy. Proceedings of the 1st Dows Symposium* (ed. I.C. MacKenzie, E. Dabelsteen, and C.A. Squire), pp. 23-4. University of Iowa Press.

——, El-Labban, N.G., and Lee, K.W. (1978). The clinical features and risk of malignant transformation in sublingual keratosis. *Brit. Dent. J.* **144**, 171.

Larsson, L.G., Sandstrom, A., and Westling, P. (1975). Relationship of Plummer-Vinson disease to cancer of the upper alimentary tract in Sweden. *Cancer Res.* **35**, 3308.

Levine, P.H., Chan, S.H., Terasaki, P., and Hewetson, J. (1981). Studies on HLA antigens and EBV antibodies: implications for the prevention of nasopharyngeal carcinoma. In *Nasopharyngeal carcinoma* (ed. E. Grundmann, G.R.F. Krueger, and D.V. Ablashi), p. 247. Cancer Campaign Volume 5. Gustav Fischer, Stuttgart, New York.

Mashberg, A. (1980). Clinical features of oral malignancy in relation to prognosis. In *Oral premalignancy. Proceedings of the 1st Dows Symposium* (ed. I.C. Mackenzie, E. Dabelsteen, and C.A. Squire), p. 292. University of Iowa Press.

McCoy, G.D., Hecht, S.S., and Wynder, E.L. (1980). The roles of tobacco, alcohol and diet in the etiology of upper alimentary and respiratory tract cancers. *Preven. Med.* **9**, 622.

McGavran, M.H., Bauer, W.C., and Ogura, J.H. (1960). Isolated laryngeal keratosis. Its relation to carcinoma of the larynx based on a clinicopathologic study of 87 consecutive cases with long term follow up. *Laryngoscope* **70**, 932.

Michaels, L. and Hyams, V.J. (1977). Undifferentiated carcinoma of the nasopharynx. A light and electron microscopical study. *Clin. Otolaryngol.* **2**, 105.

—— and Gregor, R.J. (1980). Examination of the larynx in the histopathology laboratory. *J. clin. Pathol.* **33**, 705.

Moore, R.A. (1945). *A textbook of pathology*, p. 113. W.B. Saunders Company, Philadelphia and London.

Morris, A.L. (1961). Factors influencing experimental carcinogenesis in the hamster cheek pouch. *J. dent. Res.* **40**, 3.

Mueller, K.-M. and Krohn, B.R. (1980). Smoking habits and their relationship to precancerous lesions of the larynx. *J. Cancer Res. clin. Oncol.* **96**, 211.

Newhouse, M.L., Gregory, M.M., and Shannon, H. (1980). Etiology of carcinoma of the larynx. In *Biological effects of mineral fibres*, Vol. 2, p. 687 (ed. J.C. Wagner). IARC Scientific Publications No. 30, Lyon.

Ng, M.H., Ho, H.C., and Kwan, H.C. (1978). The genetic and antigenic basis for the IgA antibody response to Epstein-Barr viral capsid antigen. In *Nasopharyngeal carcinoma: etiology and control* (ed. G. de Thé and Y. Ito), pp. 449-58. IARC Scientific Publications No. 20. International Agency for Research on Cancer, Lyon.

Norris, C.M. and Peale, A.R. (1963). Keratosis of the larynx. *J. Laryngol.* **77**, 635.

Pindborg, J.J. (1980*a*). Lesions of the oral mucosa to be considered premalignant and their epidemiology. In *Oral premalignancy. Proceedings of the First Dows Symposium* (ed. I.C. Mackenzie, E. Dabelsteen, and C.A. Squire), pp. 2-14. University of Iowa Press.

—— (1980*b*). *Oral cancer and precancer.* John Wright and Sons, Bristol.

—— and Sirsat, S.M. (1966). Oral submucous fibrosis. *Oral Surg.* **22**, 764.

Putney, F.J. and O'Keefe, J.J. (1953). Clinical significance of keratosis of the larynx as a premalignant lesion. *Ann. Otol. Rhinol. Laryngol.* **62**, 348.

Reddy, C.R.R.M., Kameswari, V.R., and Raju, M.V.S. (1974). Palatal epithelial changes in reverse smokers having carcinoma of the hard palate. *Indian J. med. Res.* **62**, 195.

Roggli, V.L., Greenberg, S.D., McLarty, J.L., Hurst, G.A., Spivey, C.G., and Heiger, L.R. (1980). Asbestos body content of the larynx in asbestos workers. A study of five cases. *Arch. Otolaryngol.* **106**, 533.

Salley, J.J. (1954). Experimental carcinogenesis in the cheek pouch of the Syrian hamster. *J. dent. res.* **33**, 253.

Shanmugaratnam, K. (1978). *Histological typing of upper respiratory tract tumours.* International histological classification of tumours, no. 19. World Health Organization, Geneva.

Simons, M.J., Wee, G.B., Day, N.E., Morris, P.J., Shanmugaratnam, K., and de-Thé, G. (1974). Immunogenetic aspects of nasopharyngeal carcinoma. I. Differences in HL-A antigen profiles between patients and comparison groups. *Int. J. Cancer* **13**, 122.

—— —— ——, Chan, S.H., Shanmugaratnam, K., and de-Thé, G.B. (1975). Probable identification of an HL-A second-locus antigen associated with a high risk of nasopharyngeal carcinoma. *Lancet* **1**, 142.

——, Chan, S.H., Darmalingam, S., Wee, G.B., Shanmugaratnam, K., Prasad, U., Goh, E.H., Betuel, H., Ho, J.H.C., Chau, J.C.W., Day, N.E., and de-Thé, G. (1978). Nasopharyngeal carcinoma and histocompatibility antigens. In *Nasopharyngeal carcinoma: etiology and control* (ed. G. de-Thé and Y. Ito), pp. 271-82. IARC Scientific Publications No. 20. International Agency for Research on Cancer, Lyon.

Sloane, J.P., Ormerod, M.G., Carter, R.L., Gusterson, B.A., and Foster, C.S. (1982). An immunocytochemical study of the distribution of epithelial membrane antigen in normal and disordered squamous epithelium. *Diagnost. Histopathol.* **5**, 11.

Smith, C.H. (1980). Experimental animal models for oral premalignancy. In *Oral premalignancy. Proceedings of the First Dows Symposium* (ed. I.C. MacKenzie, E. Dabelsteen, and C. Squire), p. 78. University of Iowa Press.

Stafl, A. and Matlingly, R.F. (1973). Colposcopic diagnosis of cervical neoplasia. *Obstet. Gynecol.* **41**, 168.

Stell, P.M. (1973). Smoking and laryngeal cancer. *Lancet* **1**, 617.

—— and McGill, T. (1973). Asbestos and laryngeal cancer. *Lancet* **2**, 416.

——, Gregory, I., and Watt, J. (1980). Morphology of the human larynx. II. The subglottis. *Clin. Otolaryngol.* **5**, 389.

Stevens, M.H. (1979). Synergistic effect of alcohol on epidermoid carcinogenesis in the larynx. *Otolaryngol. Head Neck Surg.* **87**, 751.

Teoh, T.B. (1957). Epidermoid carcinoma among Chinese: a study of 31 necropsies. *J. Path. Bact.* **73**, 451.

Trump, B., McDowell, E.M., Glavin, F., Barrett, L.A., Becci, P.J., Schuerch, W., Kaiser, H.E., and Harris, C.C. (1978). The respiratory epithelium. III. Histogenesis of epidermoid metaplasia and carcinoma *in situ* in the human. *J. Nat. Cancer Inst.* **61**, 563.

Waldron, C.A. and Shafer, W.G. (1975). Leukoplakia revisited. A clinicopathologic study of 3,256 oral leukoplakias. *Cancer* **36**, 1386.

Winn, D.M., Blot, W.J., Shy, C.M., Pickle, L.W., Toledo, A., and Fraumeni, J.F. Jr. (1981). Snuff dipping and oral cancer among women in the Southern United States. *New Engl. J. Med.* **304**, 745.

6 Preneoplasia in the lungs and the potential of cells to have modulated phenotypes

B.A. Gusterson

> ... it must be emphasized that there is only one entity, *carcinoma of the lung.*
> (Willis, R.A. (1948). *Pathology of tumours.* Butterworth, London.)

The variety of cell phenotypes often seen in different regions of a single bronchial tumour raises considerable difficulties in the classification and histogenesis of this group of neoplasms. Such apparent diversity may be explained by the retention in a tumour population of cells which can still undergo functional adaptation to the local microenvironment (McDowell *et al.* 1978*b*). Thus the goblet-cell hyperplasia and squamous metaplasia seen in bronchial mucosa following exposure to carcinogens and to non-specific irritants may find their counterparts in areas of glandular and squamous differentiation within a predominantly anaplastic tumour. Alternatively, the tumours may arise from pluripotential stem cells, or most of them may be polyclonal. The recent detailed studies of normal and neoplastic bronchi in hamsters (Becci *et al.* 1978*a,b*) and in man (McDowell *et al.* 1978*a,b*) suggest that the morphological heterogeneity of lung tumours is reflected by the lability of the phenotype of some of the normal cells in the bronchial wall. Recent developments in the identification and interrelationships of the cells composing the normal lung are considered here with particular emphasis on their relevance to various preneoplastic changes and to tumours arising in the bronchial tree, bronchial glands, and alveoli.

The normal lung

The cell types present in the normal lung that are potential targets for carcinogens are those elements (a) which are exposed to the active forms of carcinogenic agents, and (b) which can still proliferate—that is, they are not terminally differentiated. It is generally accepted that most lung carcinogens enter through the airways (US Department of Health, Education, and Welfare 1968; Mohr *et al.* 1975) so that the bronchial tree is directly exposed to relatively high concentrations of both carcinogens and non-carcinogenic, but otherwise toxic, substances. *In vivo* labelling experiments using tritiated [^{3}H]-thymidine have shown that both basal and mucous cells in the hamster bronchial tree can proliferate (Barrett *et al.* 1976); so, too, do the small mucous granule-containing cells in the bronchus of the rat (Bindreiter *et al.* 1968). Similar cell types have been shown to incorporate tritiated thymidine in long-term cultures of human bronchial epithelium (Barrett *et al.* 1976) as have the mucous cells in the submucosal bronchial glands of the hamster (McDowell *et al.* 1980). The ciliated cells in the bronchi are generally considered to be terminally differentiated and incapable of division, but recent results suggest that these cells can also incorporate [^{3}H]-thymidine (Ayers and Jeffery 1982). The peripheral endocrine cells of the bronchial tree and bronchial glands have not been shown to be capable of proliferation in man, but the structural and functional relationship between these cells and carcinoid tumours and oat-cell tumours (Bensch *et al.* 1968) makes them the obvious candidates for the origin of at least some of these neoplasms. In the bronchioles, basal cells are absent and mucous cells form a minority population; but the Clara cells in this region (in the rat) have been shown to have proliferative capacity (Evans *et al.* 1978). In the alveoli, Type II pneumocytes can undergo hyperplastic changes and in the rat they incorporate tritiated thymidine (Kauffman *et al.* 1974), but their role as the possible cell of origin of bronchio-alveolar carcinoma is still debated (Kuhn 1972; McDowell *et al.* 1978*b*). Thus on the grounds of carcinogenic access and proliferative capacity there are many cells in the lung which are potential sites of origin for bronchial carcinomas. It might be expected that by comparing the ultrastructural characteristics of these normal cells with those of the tumours some indication might be obtained about the histogenesis of the major categories of lung tumours. Recent studies, however, suggest that individual cells are more phenotypically heterogeneous than might be suspected at the light microscope level (McDowell *et al.* 1978*a*).

Much confusion in lung pathology stems from two observations:

1. that bronchial mucosa is capable of undergoing a metaplastic change to a keratinizing or non-keratinizing squamous type of epithelium;
2. the widely held belief that small-cell anaplastic carcinomas take their origin from a derivative of the neural crest and hence from a cell type *dissimilar* from the other endodermally derived cells lining the respiratory tract and the bronchial glands.

The subject of squamous metaplasia will be referred to later, but for the future discussion of preneoplasia in relation to small-cell carcinoma it is necessary to consider further the relationship of the peripheral neuroendocrine cells to other cells in the bronchial tree.

With the establishment of the APUD concept (Pearse 1969)—APUD being a synonym for amine precursor uptake and decarboxylation—it was postulated that cells having the property of concentrating and decarboxylating amine precursors shared a common embryological origin from the neural crest. This view has been perpetuated by other common characteristics such as membrane electrical excitability and the production of peptide hormones (Tischler 1978). In the lung both calcitonin (Becker *et al.* 1980) and bombesin (Wharton *et al.* 1978) have been proposed as the hormones normally produced by bronchial Kultschitzky cells. Bombesin has also been demonstrated in small-cell anaplastic carcinomas (Cutz *et al.* 1982; Erisman *et al.* 1982) and in the plasma of some patients with this tumour (Moody *et al.* 1981; Wood *et al.* 1982). The neurone-specific enzyme enolase is another molecular marker for both peripheral and central neuro-endocrine cells (Schmechel *et al.* 1978) which has been reported to be present in five out of five oat-cell carcinomas (Tapia *et al.* 1981). More recently a unique cell-surface protein has been demonstrated for human small cell lung carcinomas which is shared with neuroblastomas but is not present on non-small cell lung carcinomas (Baylin *et al.* 1982). This supports the neural features of this group of tumours but, as the authors state, this finding emphasizes that embryologically diverse cells with similar function may be expected to share common cell-surface proteins. The evidence is thus in favour of the conclusion that these shared features with neural tissue are better explained as an expression of functional requirement rather than of common embryological origin. Among the cells encompassed by the APUD concept are the islet cells of the pancreas and the Kultschitzky cells of the gut (Pearse and Takor 1976)—two tissues that are now proven to be of endodermal rather than of neuro-ectodermal origin (Cheng and Leblond 1974; Sidhu 1979). Kultschitzky cells in the lung are normally too few to carry out embryological studies, but the presence of surface microvilli on human lung endocrine cells (Cutz *et al.* 1975; McDowell *et al.* 1978*a*) and the demonstration of tonofilament bundles in similar cells in many species of fetal lungs (Hage 1974; Cutz *et al.* 1974, 1975) support an origin from endoderm rather than neural ectoderm. Microvilli and tonofilaments are found in gut endocrine cells (Sidhu 1979) but neither microvilli nor tonofilaments have been demonstrated in APUD cells of proven neural crest derivation. Tonofilament bundles have also been reported in a human bronchial carcinoid tumour (An 1978) and in a similar tumour after prolonged culture *in vitro* (Bensch *et al.* 1976). These observations, combined with the recognition of typical neurosecretory granules in goblet cells of the human segmental bronchi (Terzakis *et al.* 1972), indicate that the endocrine cells of the lungs and the tumours that arise from them cannot be considered in isolation: they represent part of the general ability of both normal and malignant bronchial epithelium to undergo phenotypic change. Recent reports suggest that similar lability of phenotype is present in other tissues—for example, the gastrointestinal tract in the rat in which all the elements comprising the normal colonic mucosa including endocrine cells appear to be derived from a common undifferentiated cell (Shamsuddin and Trump 1981).

Advances in the identification of squamous and glandular differentiation at the ultrastructural and immunocytochemical level have demonstrated that single normal cells can express both phenotypes simultaneously. Tonofilaments can be reasonably construed as ultrastructural markers of squamous differentiation—but recent reports indicate that keratin-like polypeptides are present in basal cells and intermediate cells of the normal bronchus (Schlegel *et al.* 1980) and we have demonstrated similar materials in the ducts of normal bronchial glands, the mucus-secreting cells of the bronchial mucosa, and in the serous elements of the bronchial glands (Gusterson *et al.* 1982). This ability of a cell to express more than one differentiated function poses obvious difficulties in nomenclature. The problem of using keratin-like peptides as markers of squamous differentiation is compounded further by the observation that these materials form part of the normal cytoskeleton of many epithelial cells (Schlegel *et al.* 1980).

Recent studies on regenerating tracheal epithelium in hamsters (McDowell *et al.* 1979) and on normal human bronchial epithelium *in vitro* (Barrett *et al.* 1976) illustrate the potential modulation of the normal phenotype and some of the problems involved. Following mechanical trauma, the hamster tracheal mucosa is completely repaired within 96 hours (McDowell *et al.* 1979). Basal-like cells and mucous granule-containing cells migrate first and close the defect. They proliferate and, after 48 hours, a non-keratinizing multilayered structure is formed of cells containing both tonofilaments and mucous granules. At this time the cells of the basal layer become depleted of mucous granules. After a further 24 hours the surface cells are totally undifferentiated and must (presumably) have arisen from dividing basal and/or mucous cells. These undifferentiated cells gradually develop cilia and mucous granules, some cells containing both, and the epithelium is completely reconstituted. Similar phenotypic changes can be seen in human bronchial mucosa in organ culture where there is a decrease in the number of goblet cells, a loss of ciliated cells, and the maintenance of cells with both mucous granules and ultrastructural features of squamous differentiation (Barrett *et al.* 1976). This ability of non-malignant bronchial epithelium to demonstrate combined squamous and glandular differentiation has been interpreted by some workers as evidence for origin of mixed tumours from the bronchial mucosa (McDowell *et al.* 1980)—a topic which is discussed later.

It thus appears that there is considerable evidence to support the view that cell populations in the normal bronchial mucosa can undergo various phenotypic changes. Such changes are not absolute and they reflect quantitative differences in the expression of various differentiation pathways: the end result is that typical mucous cells may contain tonofilaments and cells showing squamous metaplasia can contain mucous granules (McDowell *et al.* 1979). With this degree of normal lability it is hardly surprising that pulmonary tumours may show a similar spectrum of phenotypic expression. Having discussed modulated phenotypes among cells in the normal bronchus, it is now appropriate to consider phenotypic heterogeneity in various animals models and in human tissues that are potentially preneoplastic.

Preneoplastic lesions of the lungs in animals and man

The identification of preneoplasia is important both to determine the histogenesis of specific tumour types and to recognize changes which may be of prognostic significance as markers of malignant potential. There is very little evidence in human studies relating potential preneoplastic states to tumour type and, in particular, the pathogenesis and histogenesis of small-cell carcinoma is not understood—see later.

The main criticism of the experimental models that are available is that the histological types and behaviour of the tumours induced in animals do not have close counterparts in man. Of the systems used to date, the Syrian golden hamster has produced the most useful data, although experiments in dogs and rodents have supported the view that squamous metaplasia is probably an essential part of the progression from a normal bronchial cell to squamous carcinoma. Sequential studies in animals have helped to clarify the evolution of preneoplastic and neoplastic lesions, but in man the evidence for preneoplastic lesions is more difficult to assess.

Animal models

Many attempts have been made to establish relatively simple systems whereby animals are exposed to controlled concentrations of pure carcinogens. A recent review by Stenbäck (1977) on the application of the Syrian golden hamster to study respiratory-tract tumours covers many of the problems of experimental models, and the author points out that the hamster, unlike other laboratory animals, develops a spectrum of lung tumours with a similar morphology to some of those seen in man. Much of the earlier work on carcinogen-induced lesions was carried out at the light-microscope level and was concerned with acute changes in the hamster tracheo-bronchial epithelium (Port *et al.* 1973). Saffiotti *et al.* (1968), for example, instilled benzo(a)pyrene into the trachea of hamsters and induced squamous metaplasia and squamous carcinomas, adenocarcinomas, and large-cell anaplastic carcinomas.

Detailed ultrastructural studies comparing preneoplastic lesions in the bronchial tree of hamsters and man have demonstrated very close correlations between the preneoplastic lesions and the tumours produced in both species (Becci *et al.* 1978*c*; Trump *et al.* 1978). When a mixture of benzo(a)pyrene and ferric oxide is instilled into the trachea of Syrian hamsters a sequence of changes takes place starting with an acute reaction within 24 hours to produce goblet-cell hyperplasia (Becci *et al.* 1978*c*). There is extrusion of ciliated cells and mitotic activity is seen in mucous cells. The extrusion of ciliated cells continues until, one week after the initial instillation, the mucosa consists of a basal layer with a homogeneous surface layer of cuboidal cells which are recognizable ultrastructurally as mucous cells. These cells are found in the normal bronchial mucosa of man (McDowell *et al.* 1978*a*) and the hamster (Becci *et al.* 1978*a*) and are referred to as small mucous granule cells (SMGC). They are considered to represent mucous cells at the early stage of the secretory cycle and they are capable of replication. With continued application of the carcinogen the epithelium becomes hyperplastic, forming five- to ten-cell layers. At this stage the mucosa takes on the light-microscopic features of squamous metaplasia. Ultrastructurally, however, these cells are still recognizable as mucous cells containing both mucous granules and a few tonofilaments. Eventually there is an increase in the number of cytoplasmic tonofilament bundles and the epithelium becomes cornified with abundant desmosomes and the typical features of keratinizing epithelium. It is important to note that even in these well-keratinized cells neutral mucins are still detectable histochemically, indicating that the metaplastic cells retain the expression of both glandular and squamous differentiation pathways (Becci *et al.* 1978*c*). Thus a single cell type can apparently show a range of phenotypic expression from a predominantly mucous cell with a few tonofilaments to a keratinizing cell which nevertheless retains markers of its original mucin production. It is not possible to prove that individual cells *in vivo* undergo these transitional changes, but evidence is strongly compatible with this view. These areas of squamous metaplasia eventually progress to carcinoma *in situ* in which the cells become pleomorphic with full-thickness atypia characteristic of *in situ* lesions at other sites. Ultrastructurally, the *in situ* carcinomas contain cells exhibiting both squamous and mucoid elements. The *in situ* lesions progress and develop into adenocarcinomas, squamous carcinomas, and large-cell anaplastic carcinomas similar at both the light and ultrastructural level to those seen in man (Becci *et al.* 1978*b*). In control animals, given the carrier (0.9 per cent sterile sodium chloride solution) alone, the metaplastic lesions were indistinguishable from those in the carcinogen-treated group but, unlike the latter, they were reversible and did not progress to *in situ* or invasive carcinoma.

The importance of these observations lies in two main fields. In relation to the role of squamous metaplasia as a premalignant state it is clear that, as in other animal models including the dog (Kobayashi *et al.* 1978), squamous metaplasia is a concomitant and a precursor of later *in situ* and invasive bronchial carcinoma. It is, however, equally clear that similar metaplastic lesions are found in animals exposed to other, non-carcinogenic, toxic materials. Although no differences have been detected between one type of squamous metaplasia and another at either light or ultrastructural level, markers may eventually be developed to identify those cells that have malignant potential. From a biological standpoint, the confirmation of Stenbäck's earlier observations that in squamous metaplasia the individual cells (even in keratin whorls) contain mucins (Stenbäck 1973) is of fundamental importance. An obvious explanation is provided for the observation that some bronchial squamous carcinomas, adenocarcinomas, and large-cell anaplastic carcinomas with both mucous and squamous elements develop in the hamster (Becci *et al.* 1978*b*) and in man (McDowell *et al.* 1978*b*). More recently it has been demonstrated that cloned lines from an adeno-squamous carcinoma arising in the rat trachea will produce adeno-squamous carcinomas *in vivo* further demonstrating the instability of differentiation (Steele and Nettesheim 1981). Multiple phenotypes appear to be expressed not only in normal but also in the preneoplastic bronchial epithelium.

It is often difficult to assess the relevance of animals models, but members of Auerbach's group (Schreiber *et al.* 1974) who have carried out the most exhaustive epidemiological and histological studies of lung cancer in man were unable to distinguish between the cytological changes induced by the benzo(a)pyrene-ferric oxide mixture in hamsters and those described in cigarette smokers with lung cancer (Saccomanno *et al.* 1974). It appears that the hamster is a satisfactory model for studying preneoplasia in relation to the development of squamous carcinoma, adenocarcinoma, and large-cell anaplastic carcinoma; but the major drawback of the system is the very low incidence of small-cell anaplastic carcinomas. Their rarity suggests that if these tumours can in fact be induced in hamsters, either they develop from a different cell type or a different carcinogenic agent is involved in the evolution of this tumour which produces cells with a different transformed phenotype.

Small-cell anaplastic tumours are very rare in all laboratory animals and in 126 hamsters treated with benzo(a)pyrene (Becci *et al.* 1978*b*) there was one solitary, carcinoid-like lesion. Recent studies with nitrosamines, however, in the same animal model would indicate that this carcinogen may be more appropriate. The incidence of small-cell anaplastic carcinoma is related to smoking and it is thus of interest that nitrosamines are formed from nicotine both *in vitro* and during tobacco curing (Hecht *et al.* 1978).† Female Syrian hamsters given subcutaneous injections of *N*-diethylnitrosamine, *N*-dibutylnitrosamine, or *N*-nitrosomorpholine developed hyperplasia of small groups of bronchial APUD-cells containing neurosecretory granules (Reznik-Schüller 1977*a, b*). Nodules formed in the peripheral bronchioles and, after 5-9 weeks, tonofilaments appeared within the APUD-like cells, sometimes arranged in perinuclear whorls typical of squamous cells. With time the granules became less prominent and the concentration of tonofilaments increased until the cells were no longer

† *N*-nitrosamines are also bound and metabolized by cultured human bronchial mucosa (Harris *et al.* 1977).

identifiable as having originated from neurosecretory elements. The fact that benzo(a)pyrene does not produce similar lesions suggests that such nodules cannot be regarded as non-specific reactions, but further studies are required to demonstrate their malignant potential and their possible relationship to small-cell carcinomas in man. Endocrine-cell hyperplasia has also been induced recently in the rat lung using asbestos (Cole *et al.* 1981). The demonstration of squamous metaplasia by neurosecretory cells supports their common embryological origin with the other cells lining the bronchial mucosa, and it is a further example of phenotypic lability which can also be seen within squamous elements of some small-cell anaplastic carcinomas (MacKay *et al.* 1977).

Animal models of bronchiolo-alveolar cell carcinomas have been reported in the dog (Auerbach *et al.* 1970) but the tumours illustrated are histologically different from bronchiolo-alveolar carcinomas of man. Some interesting observations have, however, been made in the hamster after subcutaneous injections of *N*-nitrosomorpholine (Reznik-Schüller 1977*b*). It has been claimed that, after three weeks of treatment, lamellar bodies, similar to those normally seen in Type II pneumocytes, develop in the non-ciliated Clara cells of the terminal bronchioles. These cells become hyperplastic and eventually develop into invasive tumours resembling human alveolar carcinomas. Some of the cells in these tumours contained tonofilaments and/or dense core granules. The question of bronchiolo-alveolar cell carcinoma as a specific histopathological entity will be mentioned later, but this observation again suggests that lung cells can adopt phenotypic patterns seen in cells of common embryological derivation when irritated or when undergoing neoplastic change. A cautionary note should also be added that the ultrastructural features of a tumour may be more indicative of functional phenotype than of histogenesis.

Human studies

In animal models it is possible to demonstrate a sequence of histological events progressing to invasive carcinoma. Investigations in man are mainly limited to epidemiologically-related autopsy studies, and although the changes described in the bronchial epithelium are similar to those seen in animals a direct relationship between carcinoma *in situ* and a prediction of future invasive potential cannot be established. Current data would suggest that the majority of lung carcinomas, including the peptide hormone-producing tumours, develop from cells lining the bronchial mucosa and that the histological variability seen in the lung tumours may develop after the preneoplastic and early invasive phases.

From the classical studies of Auerbach's group on the detailed histology of the bronchial tree in smokers and uranium miners (Auerbach *et al.* 1961, 1978, 1979), it can be concluded that certain morphological changes in the bronchial tree are potentially preneoplastic. Loss of cilia, epithelial hyperplasia, and non-keratinizing squamous metaplasia, all with varying degrees of cytological atypia (Figs. 6.1 and 6.2), can be found in both smokers and non-smokers. Marked atypia in former smokers appears to be reversible (Auerbach *et al.* 1979). It is thus essential to specify the context in which such changes are occurring because they are certainly not specific. As in the animal studies, the question arises of distinguishing between the toxic regenerative responses of the bronchial mucosa and the potentially malignant manifestations of a carcinogenic insult. Metaplastic changes, for example, are clearly not necessarily a manifestation of early neoplasia (Nettesheim 1976); they are commonly found in non-smoking city-dwellers (Spain *et al.* 1970) and in other circumstances including the bronchi of patients who have required prolonged intubation (Trump *et al.* 1978).

Is it possible to distinguish between metaplastic lesions that will progress to infiltrative carcinoma and those that will not? From the animal and human studies so far carried out at both the light- and the electron-microscope level there are no detectable differences between areas of squamous metaplasia induced by local noncarcinogenic irritation and those found in association with overt carcinoma—although the lack of cornification in the former was suggested as a possible point of distinction (Trump *et al.* 1978). Cellular atypia can be seen both in response to nonspecific irritation and in smokers with lung cancer; but the combination of loss of cilia and marked mucosal atypia progressing to complete full thickness epithelial dysplasia

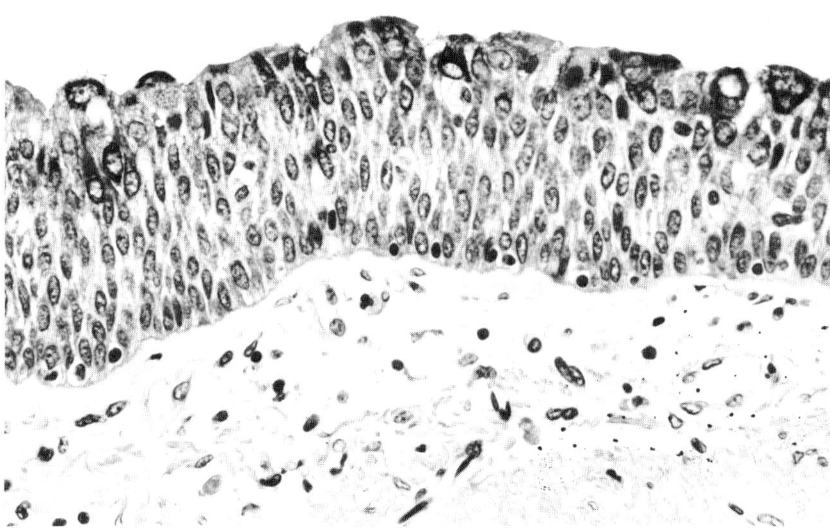

Fig. 6.1. Photomicrograph of bronchial wall stained immunocytochemically for keratin with a haemalum counterstain. There is loss of cilia and stratification. Early squamous metaplasia is indicated by positive keratin-like immunoreactive material in the cytoplasm of the more superficial cells. ×320.

(carcinoma *in situ*)—Fig. 6.3—is only observed in smokers. The degree of atypia produced by tobacco smoke is dose-dependent (Auerbach *et al.* 1961), and it is tempting to suggest a progression from squamous metaplasia through degrees of atypia to carcinoma *in situ* and eventually to invasive carcinoma. Unfortunately this scheme ignores the potential toxic but noncarcinogenic effects of other constituents of tobacco smoke. Despite such reservations it must be said that in some cases the cytological similarity between the *in situ* carcinoma and the invasive tumour (Figs. 6.3 and 6.4) strongly suggests that carcinoma *in situ* is the antecedent lesion.

Ultrastructural studies have demonstrated that in hyperplasia and in carcinoma *in situ* of the human bronchus, the proliferating cells are probably both basal cells and mucous cells; also that these potentially neoplastic lesions consist of cells which vary from squamous to mucous with many cells demonstrating elements of both glandular and squamous differentiation (Trump *et al.* 1978). A technique recently developed clearly demonstrates the presence of keratin and mucin in the same cells at the light microscope level (Mitchell and Gusterson 1982). Analogies between man and the hamster (see earlier) are close. It would thus appear likely that the hyperplastic and *in situ* lesions described by Auerbach's group are produced by proliferation of both basal and mucous cells. Tumours arising from

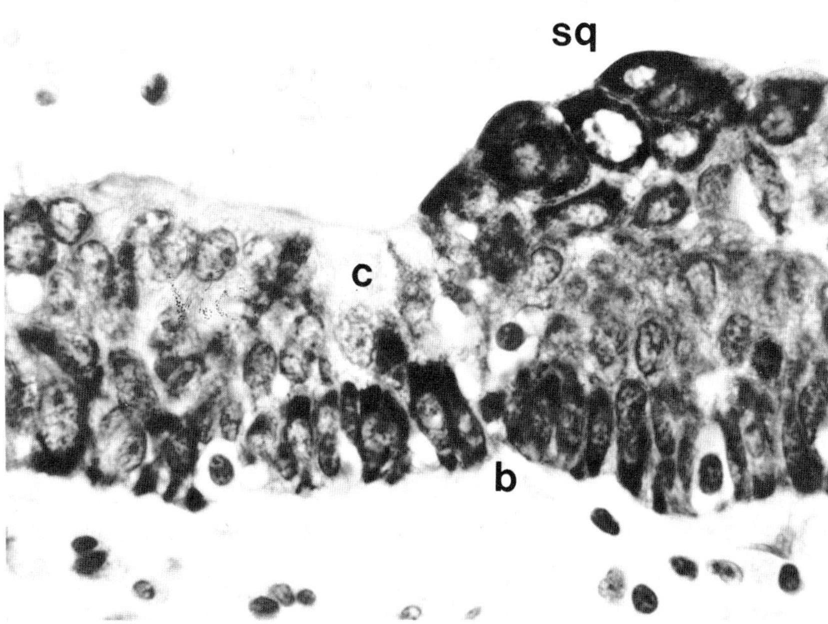

Fig. 6.2. Photomicrograph of a section of bronchial wall stained immunocytochemically for keratin—an area of squamous metaplasia (sq) is strongly positive with absence of staining in the adjacent ciliated cells (c). Staining of basal cells (b) is also marked in this area. ×600. (Reproduced with permission of *Virchows Archives* (*Pathol. Anat.*) (1982) **394**, 271.)

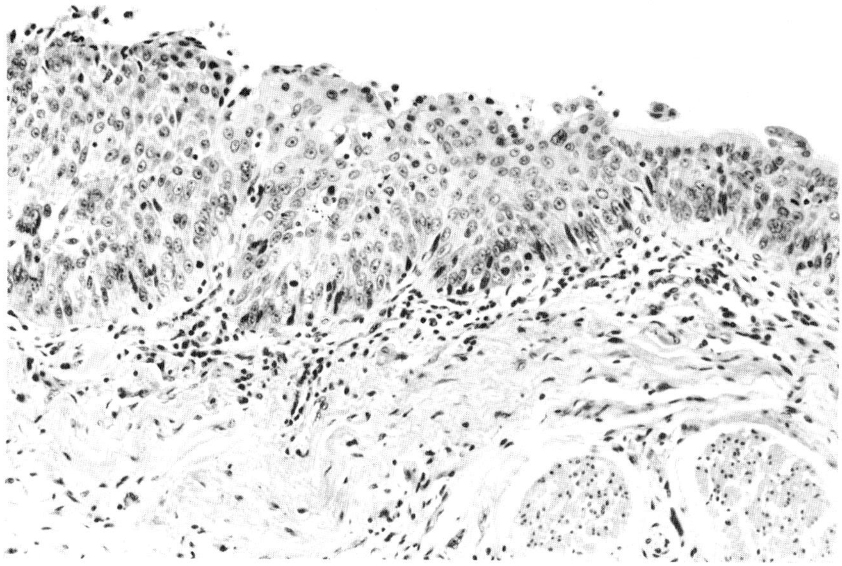

Fig. 6.3. Photomicrograph of bronchial wall showing carcinoma *in situ*. The degree of atypia and pleomorphism is not marked, but is identical to the infiltrative tumour shown in Fig. 6.4. ×157. H & E.

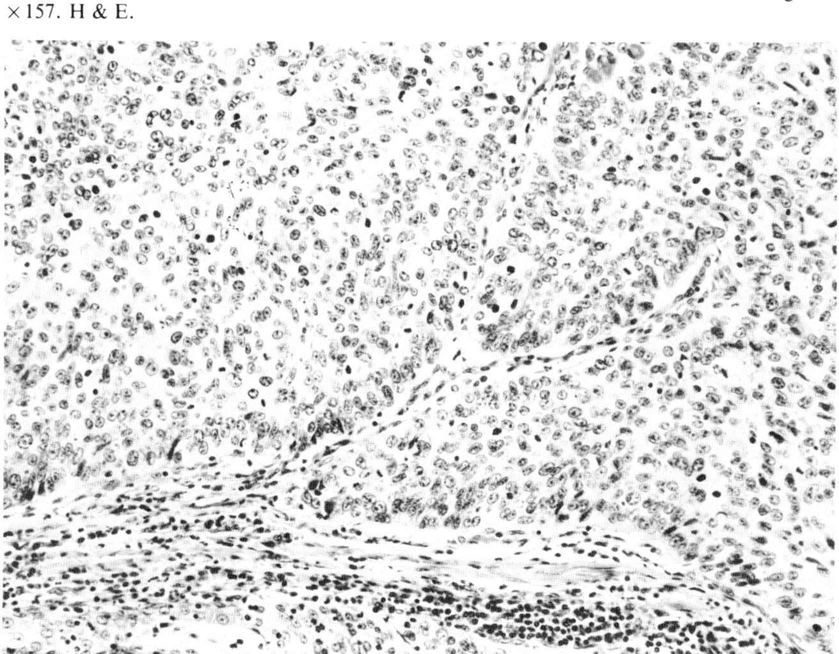

Fig. 6.4. Photomicrograph of infiltrating carcinoma with similar cytological features to the *in situ* component seen in Fig. 6.3. Some of the tumour showed well-differentiated squamous areas with keratin pearls and the tumour was classified as an epidermoid (squamous) carcinoma. ×157. H & E.

these sites might therefore be expected to be squamous carcinomas, adenocarcinomas, and tumours with mixed glandular and squamous elements according to the dominant phenotype expressed (McDowell *et al.* 1978*b*, 1980). Current evidence supports the thesis that many lung carcinomas at the ultrastructural level contain both mucous and squamous features and, if classified histogenetically, some of the tumours placed in the small-cell anaplastic, large-cell anaplastic, poorly differentiated squamous, and poorly differentiated adenocarcinoma groups have mixed phenotypic patterns (McDowell *et al.* 1978*b*). Examples are illustrated in Figs. 6.5 and 6.6.

The cellular origin of small-cell anaplastic carcinoma remains much more controversial, and it must be stated that there is no clinical or histological justification for the subclassification of these tumours as proposed in the World Health Organization Classification of 1967: Hattori *et al.* (1972) have described all histological subtypes within the same tumour. Clinical studies have failed to ascribe any prognostic significance to the different cell types (Cohen and Matthews 1978) and recent work by Hansen (1980) has shown no correlation between peptide hormone production and the histological subtypes.

The relation of small-cell anaplastic carcinomas to the normal Kultschitsky cells found in the bronchi, peripheral bronchioles, and the bronchial glands is of fundamental importance. The observation that many small-cell carcinomas contain cytoplasmic neurosecretory granules similar to those seen in carcinoid tumours and normal-lung Kultschitzky cells (Bensch *et al.* 1968) suggested a common histogenesis for these tumours. This view was supported by the subsequent demonstration of peptide hormone production by both carcinoid tumours and small-cell anaplastic carcinomas *in vivo* (Rees 1976; Yesner 1978) and *in vitro* (Ellison *et al.* 1976). Certain observations have, however, complicated the issue. Large-cell anaplastic, squamous cell, and adenocarcinomas may all contain neurosecretory granules (Yesner 1978; Gould and Chejfec 1978; McDowell *et al.* 1981) and be associated with hormone production (Yesner, 1978; McDowell *et al.* 1980). Furthermore, some small-cell anaplastic carcinomas contain bundles of tonofilaments (Sidhu and Fresko 1978) and have definite squamous regions detectable with the light microscope (Walter and Pryce 1960; Churg *et al.* 1980). Thus within the broad classification of lung carcinoma there is considerable overlap in the phenotypic pattern both in endocrine and non-endocrine tumours supporting Willis's contention that 'there is only one entity, *carcinoma of the lung*,' (Willis 1948). This commonality of phenotypic expression is most easily understood if it is accepted that all the cells in the bronchial tree that are a potential source of lung carcinomas have a common embryological origin from the endoderm of the gut.

If small-cell anaplastic carcinomas are histogenetically related to normal-lung Kultschitzky cells, it might be expected that lesions analogous to the hyperplastic nodules described in hamster lungs (Reznik-Schüller, 1977*a*)

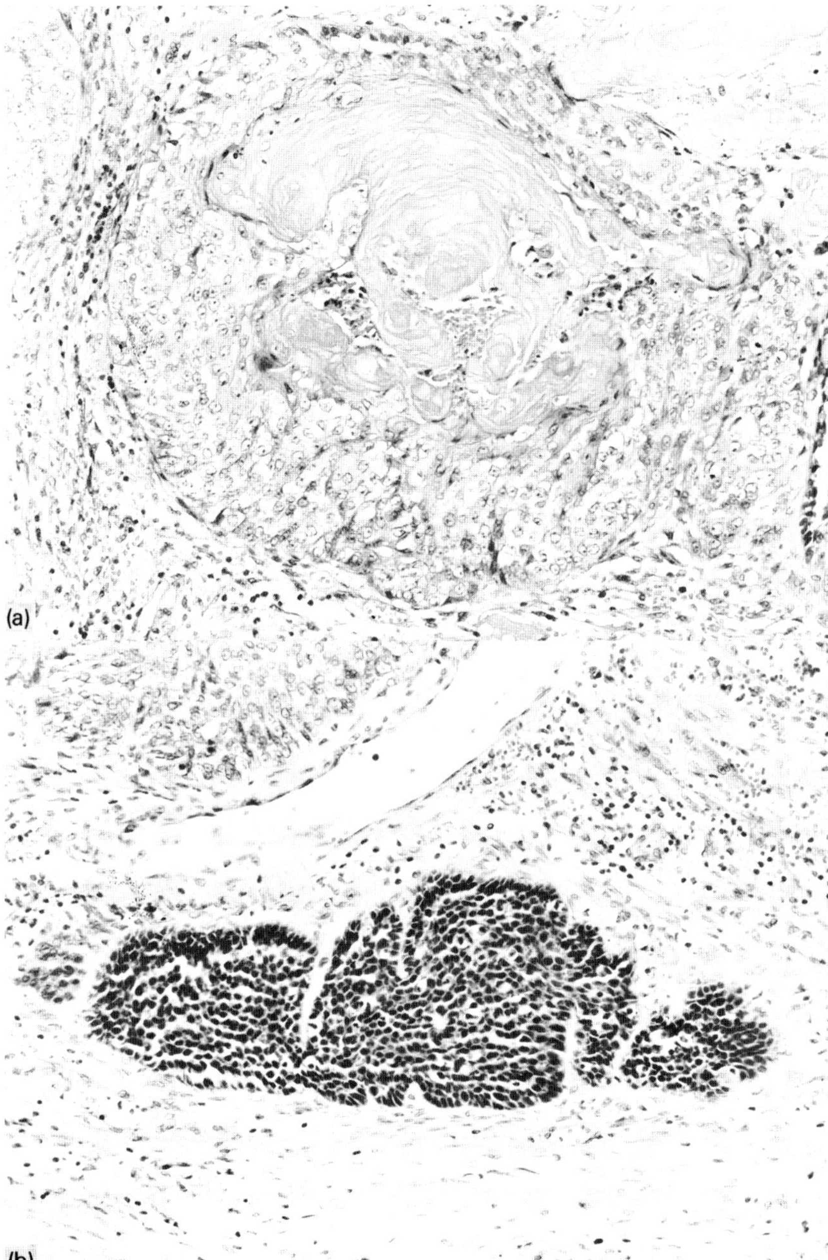

Fig. 6.5. This tumour consisted predominantly of intermediate-sized anaplastic cells arranged in a trabecular pattern with areas of keratin formation (a). Within this tumour there was a carcinoid-like focus with smaller cells arranged in definite trabeculae (b). On levelling this region merged through cytologically intermediate areas to form a morphological continuum with the larger anaplastic cells seen in the top left hand corner. ×150. H & E.

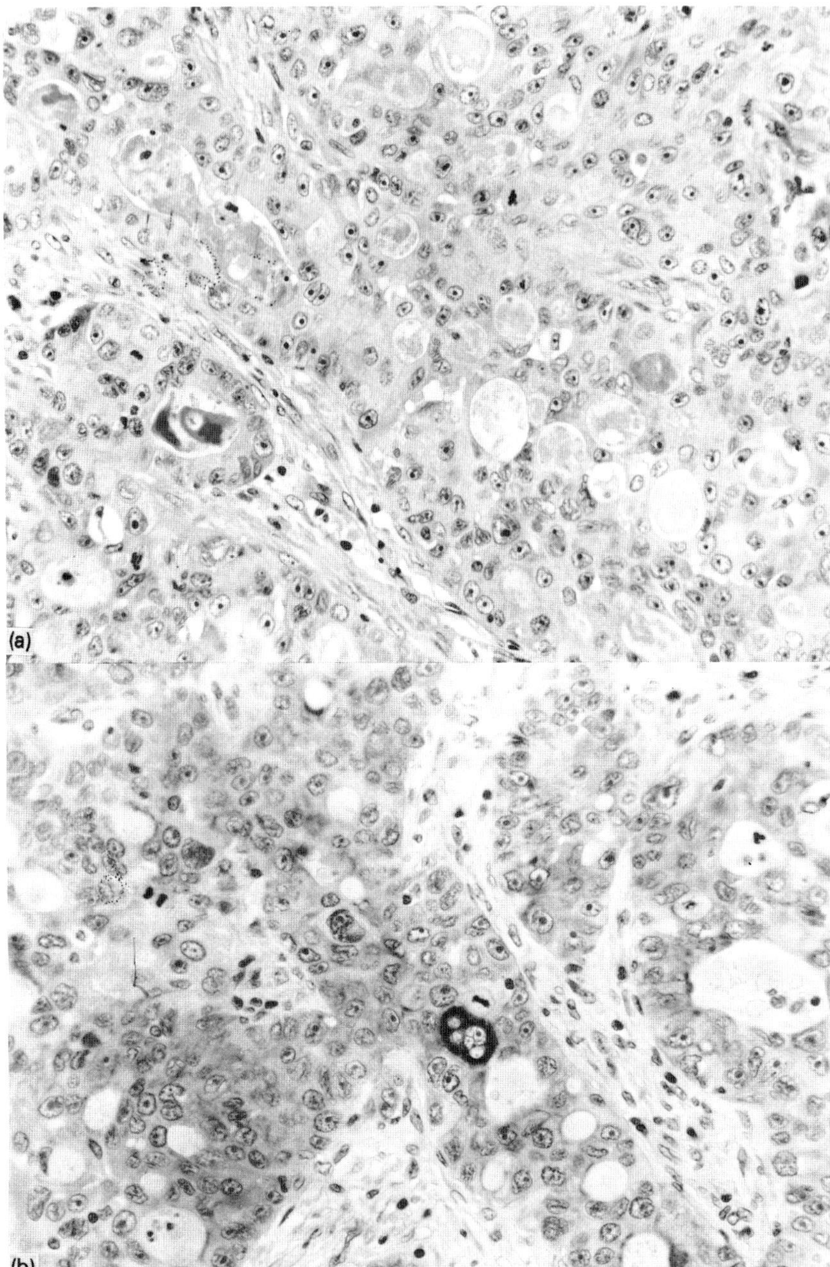

Fig. 6.6. Photomicrographs of a large-celled anaplastic carcinoma with mucin production. The majority of the mucin was cytoplasmic or in pools as shown by the PAS staining after diastase digestion (a). No clear ductal structures or acini were formed. (b) The same tumour stained immunocytochemically for keratin. The majority of cells contained keratin-like immunoreactive material and occasional mononuclear and multinucleate cells were strongly positive. $\times 250$.

would be found in autopsies at a reasonable frequency. Tumourlets have been described in association with small-cell anaplastic carcinoma (Ranchod 1977) but these hyperplastic nodules, composed of Kultschitzky-type cells containing neurosecretory granules, are more commonly found in the lung periphery as rare incidental post-mortem findings. Such nodules have been reported in patients with Cushing's syndrome but there is no evidence that they develop into small-cell anaplastic carcinomas. The other obvious group of patients to examine for preneoplastic changes associated with small-cell carcinomas are uranium miners who have a 41 per cent incidence of small-cell anaplastic carcinoma as compared with 11 per cent in a control group (Auerbach *et al.* 1978). Although detailed histological studies were made by these authors, they presented no evidence identifying any histologically specific *in situ* lesion in association with any particular tumour type. There is no mention of Kultschitzky-cell hyperplasia in the bronchial glands although *in situ* lesions with similar histology to those in the bronchi were identified. There have been isolated reports in the literature identifying *in situ* carcinoma, composed of small uniform cells indistinguishable from those in the primary small-cell carcinoma (Walter and Pryce 1955; Williams and Howard 1958), but the dearth of information available suggests that the preneoplastic lesions in most small-cell carcinomas are similar to those described for other lung tumours. If this is the case, then there is further support for considering these tumours as part of the general spectrum of lung carcinomas rather than as a separate pathological entity.

Recent data suggest that although there is no clinical correlation with the histological subtypes of small-cell carcinoma defined according to the 1967 WHO criteria, this group of tumours is heterogeneous in terms of phenotypic expression and response to therapy (Greco *et al.* 1978). Given more precise methods of classification, it might be possible to select those tumour phenotypes that are associated with an improved prognosis and more suitable for intensive therapy. McDowell *et al.* (1978*b*, 1980) have suggested that within the group of small-cell anaplastic carcinomas there are tumours that ultrastructurally should be considered as squamous, adeno, or mixed adeno/squamous carcinomas (in addition to those tumours with characteristics of endocrine cells). These findings are consistent with the fact that not all small-cell carcinomas are associated with peptide hormone production (Tischler 1978). With this degree of overlapping phenotype in all the common lung tumours, the future challenge is to identify prospectively the phenotypic pattern that correlates with potential curability. A number of biochemical parameters can be measured as potential treatment markers, but none of them has been correlated with any specific histological type (Richardson *et al.* 1978). Recent investigations with a small number of lung tumours (Table 6.1) have demonstrated the variable distribution of keratin-like materials, and it will be interesting to see whether this marker proves to be any more useful than others (Gusterson *et al.* 1982). On the

Table 6.1. *Bronchial carcinoma and immunoreactive keratin-containing cells*[a]

Classification (WHO 1967)	No. of tumours	No. containing positive cells
Epidermoid	8	8
Large cell—without mucin	12	6
Large cell—giant cell	1	0
Adenocarcinoma—bronchogenic		
Acinar	5	1
Papillary	1	1
Small cell		
Polygonal	5	0
Fusiform	10	2
Muco-epidermoid	1	1

[a] Sections of formol-saline fixed and paraffin-embedded material were stained with a human anti-keratin antiserum at a dilution of 1/100. The cells containing keratin-like immunoreactive materials were visualized using an anti-rabbit alkaline phosphatase conjugated second antibody.

basis of past experience it is likely that any single reagent will be of little value when used alone, but may be more useful when combined with other cellular markers. It is worth noting that two small-cell anaplastic carcinomas containing positive cells (Fig. 6.7) were identified in metastatic sites after intensive therapy, suggesting a possible selection by treatment of a clone of cells with a different phenotype and with (potentially) a different response to therapy. Such examples of a labile phenotype in small-cell carcinoma are well documented *in vivo* (Abeloff *et al.* 1979; Sidhu and Fresko 1978; Ewing *et al.* 1980), and *in vitro* (Gazdar *et al.* 1980).

Another potential marker of early neoplastic change is the production of pro-hormones. This line of investigation arises from the fact that peptide hormone-producing tumours at any site also tend to produce the larger precursor polypeptide molecules which are usually undetectable in the circulation. 'Big-ACTH', for example, can be extracted from human-lung tumours and has been detected in extracts of dysplastic bronchi from smoking dogs (Gewirtz and Yalow 1974). This observation prompted the ultrastructural examination of neuroendocrine cells in human bronchi by Gould *et al.* (1978) who concluded that neuroendocrine cells in dysplastic bronchi contained fewer secretory granules than the controls and showed other features of structural abnormalities of the secretory apparatus. Such results suggest that it might be possible to detect early dysplasias of these cells by the demonstration of pro-hormones either in tissue sections or in peripheral blood.

It is generally accepted that mucoepidermoid tumours and adenoid cystic carcinomas, with a similar histology to salivary gland tumours, arise from the bronchial glands and the associated ducts; but the origin of bronchiolo-alveolar carcinoma is much more controversial (Kuhn 1972). On the basis of

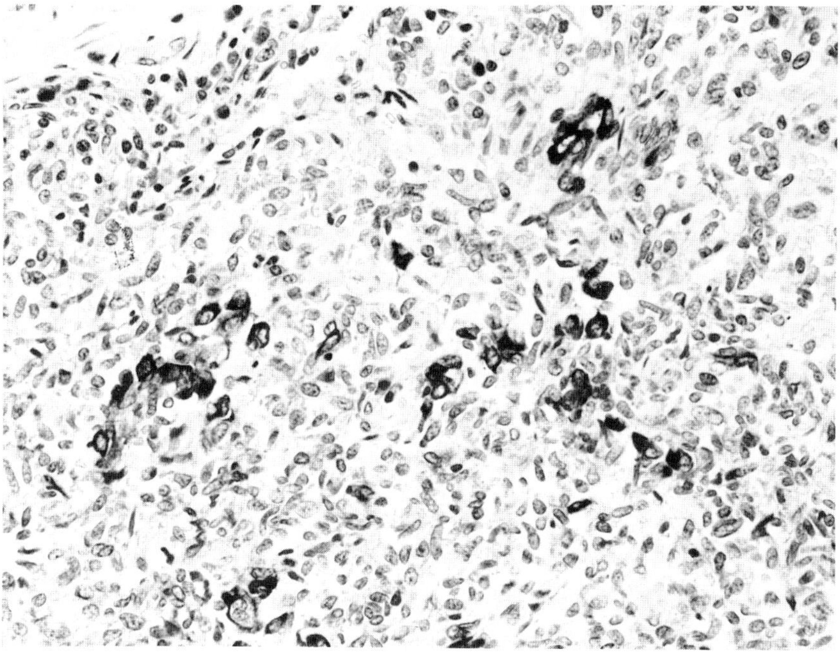

Fig. 6.7. Photomicrograph of an adrenal metastasis from a small-cell anaplastic carcinoma of the lung. Keratin-like immunoreactive material is demonstrated immunocytochemically in the cytoplasm of a proportion of the cells. These cells could not be identified as a separate population using standard staining techniqнes. ×250.

animal studies mentioned earlier, it is suggested that Clara cells can give rise to tumours with this growth pattern. The subject has been recently reviewed (McDowell *et al.* 1980) in relation to the histogenetic classification of lung tumours based on ultrastructural features. McDowell and her colleagues concluded that tumours morphologically fulfilling the diagnostic criteria of bronchiolo-alveolar-cell carcinomas were a heterogeneous group ultrastructurally and that there was no justification for regarding them as a separate entity. At the present time, however, it is still not clear whether the cases in this study would fulfil the criteria of other workers in the field for the designation of bronchiolo-alveolar-cell carcinoma.

General comments

Advances in the understanding of the heterogeneity of lung tumours have been restrained by the dogma that changes in phenotype within a given population can only occur by the proliferation of a pluripotential cell capable of initiating new populations with a different differentiated function. An alternative explanation that is supported by the detailed ultrastructural studies referred to earlier (McDowell *et al.* 1980), is that a cell with one identifiable phenotype can express some other part of its genome in response either to intrinsic or extrinsic factors. Data presented also suggest that individual cells can express more than one pattern of differentiation, and that the resultant phenotype seen at the light-microscope level merely represents quantitative differences. The early detection of phenotypic change may aid the identification of preneoplastic lesions.

From the material discussed here it is apparent that the heterogeneity of phenotypic expression within bronchial carcinomas is reflected by the lability of the differentiated function of cells in the normal and preneoplastic bronchial epithelium, a feature common to both animals and man. It may be reasonable to conclude that histogenesis can usually be inferred from a direct comparison of the differentiated pattern in the primary tumour and the cells which normally express this function, but, while probably correct in most circumstances, this approach ignores certain obvious exceptions and is in many ways oversimplified. The parameters available at the light-microscope level are limited, and the classification of tumours is usually based purely on the presence or absence of squamous or glandular differentiation with further categorization depending on cell size. Small-cell carcinomas are still referred to as anaplastic even though it is well recognized that some of them have the highly specialized function of synthesizing peptide hormones (Yesner 1978). Future developments may be predicted to demonstrate the limitations of our present reagents for the subclassification of lung carcinomas, and future classifications of more clinical application will only arise by developing markers of biological significance to the neoplastic state. In the case of small-cell carcinomas it has already been suggested that the peptide hormones elaborated by these tumours may act as autostimulatory factors which confer some kind of selective advantage (Ellison 1977). If this interpretation is correct, it might be expected that, in the development of a carcinoma, cells may be identified which produce hormones. There is some support for this view in the work of Gewirtz and Yalow (1974), who reported that the dysplastic bronchial epithelium from smoking dogs contained a higher concentration of the pro-hormone for ACTH than normal bronchial tissues.

From the animal and human studies it can be concluded that most bronchial carcinomas arise from preneoplastic lesions that are indistinguishable at the light-microscope level; an explanation must, therefore, be sought for the heterogeneity seen in the resultant invasive tumours. The presence of squamous metaplasia and goblet-cell hyperplasia in the bronchial tree is well recognized, and it is thus not surprising that bronchial tumours may show regions of squamous and mucous differentiation demonstrating the retention of their ability to express these phenotypes—perhaps in response to local environmental factors. In the case of tumours containing neurosecretory granules and producing peptide hormones, histogenesis is difficult to assess because the normal Kultschitsky cells, the obvious candidates as progenitors, are present in small numbers and are not described as predominant components of human preneoplastic lesions. The observation of human goblet cells containing neurosecretory granules (Terzakis *et al.* 1972) is important, suggesting that other cells in the bronchial wall can express this phenotype and thus the potential cells of origin for peptide-hormone-associated tumours are the same as for all other bronchial tumours. This is supported by the demonstration of hormone production and neurosecretory granules in association with squamous, adeno, and large-cell carcinomas (Yesner 1978; McDowell *et al.* 1980, 1981). Another important result of these observations is that the phenotype of a cell, at the level of the light microscope, is a very poor indicator of functional capacity. Some so-called small-cell anaplastic carcinomas are very well differentiated in terms of their ability to synthesize peptide hormones, while appearing uniform and undifferentiated to the morphologist. The conclusion must be that light microscopy in lung cancer is a poor indicator of biological function, and that all carcinomas arising in the bronchial tree form a continuum expressing quantitatively different proportions of their ability to change their phenotypic pattern.

The question must be asked why peptide hormone production, particularly ACTH and calcitonin, occurs in such a high proportion of lung tumours (Yesner 1978; Hansen *et al.* 1980). Ellison (1977) has suggested that these peptides confer a selective advantage on the cells producing the peptide so that, through a process of natural selection, they survive preferentially in the local environment. If this is true, we can ask whether it is possible to use hormones and their precursors as potential markers of pre-neoplasia. The preneoplastic lesions which may evolve into peptide-hormone-associated tumours are not described, and it is unlikely that more than a few of these tumours arise *de novo* from the neurosecretory cells in the bronchial mucosa; most of them probably develop from *in situ* lesions in which the presence of neurosecretory granules is not a prominent feature.

During the development of a carcinoma it could be envisaged that a number of mutational events occur, some of which would be lethal while others may confer advantage to the cell (Ellison 1977). For example, the ability to invade would be a phenotypic pattern advantageous to a cell. Once an invasive carcinoma with a certain phenotype has developed, it will be constantly exposed to both further mutational events and to local environmental factors that could produce further phenotypic change to select those cells best suited to their local micro-environment. If peptide hormone production is advantageous, it is likely that the proportion of tumours producing these hormones would be greater than predicted on the basis of histogenic information. It might also be expected that such tumours would have a poor prognosis. Recent results indicate that small-cell carcinomas may have a worse prognosis if they are associated with raised plasma calcitonin levels (Sappino *et al.* in press). The ability of small-cell carcinomas to modulate phenotypic expression in response to treatment is suggested in the data presented here (Table 6.1) and by other workers where metastases from small-cell carcinomas have demonstrated squamous differentiation (Abeloff *et al.* 1979)—a feature which may explain the emergence of eventual drug-resistant disease.

At present it is reasonable to conclude that there is one entity, bronchial carcinoma, but that with the development of new markers of biological functions we may be able to subclassify these tumours in relation to their predicted response to therapy. It is hoped that these new markers will be useful in identifying early neoplastic events, which will be of fundamental interest to biologists, pathologists, and clinicians.

References

Abeloff, M.D., Eggleston, J.C., Mendelsohn, G., Ettinger, D.S., and Baylin, S.B. (1979). Changes in morphologic and biochemical characteristics of small cell carcinoma of the lung. *Amer. J. Med.* **66**, 757.

An, T. (1978). Cytoplasmic inclusions in bronchial carcinoid. *Human Pathol.* **9**, 241.

Auerbach, O., Stout, A.P., Hammond, E.C., and Garfinkel, L. (1961). Changes in bronchial epithelium in relation to cigarette smoking and in relation to lung cancer. *New Engl. J. Med.* **265**, 253.

——, Saccomanno, G., Kuschner, M., Brown, R.D., and Garfinkel, L. (1978). Histologic findings in the tracheobronchial tree of uranium miners and non-miners with lung cancer. *Cancer* **42**, 483.

——, Hammond, E.C., Kirkman, D., and Garfinkel, L. (1970). Effects of cigarette smoking on dogs. II Pulmonary neoplasms. *Arch. environ. Hlth (Chicago)* **21**, 754-68.

—— ——, and Garfinkel, L. (1979). Changes in bronchial epithelium in relation to cigarette smoking. *New Engl. J. Med.* **300**, 381.

Ayrers, M.M. and Jeffery, P.K. (1982). Cell division and differentiation in bronchial epithelium. In *Cellular biology of the lung.* Life sciences (eds. G. Cumming and G. Bonsignore), vol. 10, p. 33. Plenum Press, New York.

Barrett, L.A., McDowell, E.M., Frank, A.L., Harris, C.C., and Trump, B.F. (1976). Long-term organ culture of human bronchial epithelium. *Cancer Res.* **36**, 1003.

Baylin, S.B., Gazdar, A.F., Minna, J.D., Bernal, S.D., and Shaper, J.H. (1982). A unique cell-surface protein phenotype distinguishes human small-cell from non-small cell lung cancer. *Proc. Nat. Acad. Sci. USA* **79**, 4650.

Becci, P.H., McDowell, E.M., and Trump, B.F. (1978*a*). The respiratory epithelium. II. Hamster trachea, bronchus, and bronchioles. *J. Natl. Cancer Inst.* **61**, 551.

—— —— —— (1978*b*). The respiratory epithelium. VI. Histogenesis of lung tumors induced by benzo(a)pyrene-ferric oxide in the hamster. *J. Natl. Cancer Inst.* **61**, 607.

—— —— —— (1978*c*). The respiratory epithelium. IV. Histogenesis of epidermoid metaplasia and carcinoma in situ in the hamster. *J. Natl. Cancer Inst.* **61**, 577.

Becker, K.L., Monaghan, K.G., and Silva, O.L. (1980). Immunocytochemical localization of calcitonin in Kulschitsky cells of human lung. *Arch. Pathol. Lab. Med.* **104**, 196.

Bensch, K.G., Corrin, B., Pariente, R., and Spencer, H. (1968). Oat cell carcinoma of lung. *Cancer* **22**, 1163.

——, Bonikos, D.S., and Hockberger, P.E. (1976). Pulmonary carcinoid tumors in tissue and organ culture. *Cancer* **38**, 2006.

Bindreiter, M., Schuppler, J., and Stockinger, L. (1968). Zellproliferation und differenzierung im trachealepithel der ratte. *Exp. Cell Res.* **50**, 377.

Cheng, H. and Leblond, C.P. (1974). Origin, differentiation and renewal of the four main epithelial cell types in the mouse small intestine. V. unitarian theory of the origin of the four epithelial cell types. *Amer. J. Anat.* **141**, 537.

Churg, A., Johnston, W.H., and Stulbarg, M. (1980). Small cell squamous and mixed small cell squamous-small cell anaplastic carcinomas of the lung. *Amer. J. Surg. Pathol.* **4**, 255.

Cohen, M.H. and Matthews, M.J. (1978). Small cell bronchogenic carcinoma: A distinct clinicopathologic entity. *Semin. Oncol.* **5** (3), 234.

Cole, G.A., Polak, J.M., Johnson, N.F., Marangos, P., and Pearse, A.G.E. (1981). Neurone specific enolase as a useful histological marker for the demonstration of asbestos-induced endocrine cell hyperplasia of the rat lung. Pathol. Soc. Abstr. January.

Cutz, E., Chan, W., Wong, V., and Conen, P.E. (1974). Endocrine cells in rat fetal lungs. *Lab. Invest.* **30**, 458.

—— —— —— —— (1975). Ultrastructure and fluorescence histochemistry of endocrine (APUD-type) cells in tracheal mucosa of human and various animal species. *Cell Tissue Res.* **158**, 425.

—— ——, and Track, N.S. (1981). Bombesin, calcitonin and leu-enkephalin immunoreactivity in endocrine cells of human lung. *Experientia* **37**, 765.

—— ——, Kay, J.M., and Chamberlain, D.W. (1982). Immunoperoxidase staining for serotonin, bombesin, calcitonin and leu-enkephalin in pulmonary tumorlets, bronchial carcinoids and oat cell carcinomas. *Lab. Invest.* **46**, 16a.

Ellison, M.L. (1977). Cell differentiation and the biological significance of inappropriate tumour products. *Proc. Roy. Soc. Med.* **70**, 845.

——, Hillyard, C.J. Broomfield, G.A., Rees, L.H., Coombes, R.C., and Neville, A.M. (1976). Ectopic hormone production by bronchial carcinomas in culture. *Clin. Endocrinol.* **5**, Supp. 397, 397s.

Erisman, M.D., Linnoila, R.L., Hernandez, O., Diaugustine, R.P., and Lazarus, L.W. (1982). Human lung small-cell carcinoma contains bombesin. *Proc. Nat. Acad. Sci. USA* **79**, 2379.

Evans, M.J., Cabral-Anderson, L.J., and Freeman, G. (1978). Role of the Clara cell in renewal of the bronchiolar epithelium. *Lab. Invest.* **38**, 648.

Ewing, S.L., Sumner, H.W., Ophoven, J.J., Mayer, J.E. Jr., and Humphrey, E.W. (1980). Small cell anaplastic carcinoma with differentiation: A report of 14 cases. *Lab. Invest.* **42**, 115.

Gazdar, A., Carney, D., Baylin, S., and Guccion, J. (1980). Small cell carcinoma of the lung: Altered morphological, biological and biochemical characteristics in long term cultures and heterotransplanted tumors. *AACR Abst. Biol. Genet.* **21**, 51.

Gewirtz, G. and Yalow, R.S. (1974). Ectopic ACTH production in carcinoma of the lung. *J. clin. Invest.* **53**, 1022.

Gould, V.E. and Chejfec, G. (1978). Ultrastructural and biochemical analysis of "undifferentiated" pulmonary carcinomas. *Human Pathol.* **9**, 377.

——, Yannopoulous, A.D., Sommers, S.C., and Terzakis, J.A. (1978). Neuroendocrine cells in dysplastic bronchi. *Amer. J. Pathol.* **90**, 49.

Greco, F.A., Einhorn, L.H., Richardson, R.L., and Olham, R.K. (1978). Small cell lung cancer: Progress and perspectives. *Semin. Oncol.* **5** (3), 323.

Gusterson, B., Mitchell, D., Warburton, M., and Sloane, J. (1982). Immunohistochemical localisation of keratin in human lung tumours. *Virchows Arch.* [*Pathol. Anat.*] **394**, 269.

Hage, E. (1974). Histochemistry and fine structure of endocrine cells in fetal lungs of the rabbit, mouse and guinea-pig. *Cell Tissue Res.* **149**, 513.

Hansen, M., Hansen, H.H., Hirsch, F.R., Arends, J., Christensen, J.D., Christensen, J.M., Hummer, L., and Kuhl, C. (1980). Hormonal polypeptides and amine metabolites in small cell carcinoma of the lung, with special reference to stage and subtypes. *Cancer* **45**, 1432.

Harris, C.C., Autrup, H., Stoner, G.D., McDowell, E.M., Trump, B.F., and Schafer, P. (1977). Metabolism of acyclic and cyclic N-nitrosamines in cultured human bronchi. *J. Nat. Cancer Inst.* **59**, 1401.

Hattori, S., Matsuda, M., Tateishi, R., Nishihara, H., and Horai, T. (1972). Oat cell carcinoma of the lung. *Cancer* **30**, 1014.

Hecht, S.S., Chen, C.B., Hirota, N., Ornaf, R.M., Tso, T.C., and Hoffman, D. (1978). Tobacco-specific nitrosamines: Formation from nicotine in vitro and during tobacco curing and carcinogenicity in strain A mice. *J. Nat. Cancer Inst.* **60**, 819.

Kauffman, S.L., Burri, P.H., and Weibel, E.R. (1974). The postnatal growth of the rat lung. II. Autoradiography. *Anat. Rec.* **180**, 63.

Kobayashi, N., Okita, M., Yarita, T., Hanzawa, S., Okamoto, T., and Katsuki, H. (1978). A method for experimental induction of bronchogenic carcinoma in subcutaneously implanted bronchial autografts in dogs. *J. Thor. & Cardio. Surg.* **75**, 434.

Kuhn, C. (1972). Fine structure of bronchiolo-alveolar cell carcinoma. *Cancer* **30**, 1107.

Mackay, B., Osborne, B.M., and Wilson, R.A. (1977). Ultrastructure of lung neoplasms in lung cancer. In *Lung cancer: clinical diagnosis and treatment* (ed. M.J. Straus), pp. 71-84. Grune and Stratton, New York.

McDowell, E.M., Barrett, L.A., Glavin, F., Harris, C.C., and Trump, B.F. (1978*a*). The respiratory epithelium. I. Human bronchus. *J. Nat. Cancer Inst.* **61**, 539.

——, McLaughlin, J.S., Merenyi, D.K., Kieffer, R.F., Harris, C.C., and Trump, B.F. (1978*b*). The respiratory epithelium. V. Histogenesis of lung carcinomas in the human. *J. Nat. Cancer Inst.* **61**, 587.

——, Becci, P.J., Schurch, W., and Trump, B.F. (1979). The respiratory epithelium. VII. Epidermoid metaplasia of hamster tracheal epithelium during regeneration following mechanical injury. *J. Nat. Cancer Inst.* **62**, 995.

——, Hess, F.G. Jr., and Trump, B.F. (1980). Epidermoid metaplasia, carcinoma in situ, and carcinomas of the lung. In *Diagnostic electron microscopy* (ed. B.F. Trump and R.T. Jones). John Wiley and Sons.

——, Wilson, T.S., and Trump, B.F. (1981). Atypical endocrine tumors of the lung. *Arch. Pathol. Lab. Med.* **105**, 20.

Mitchell, D.P., and Gusterson, B.A. (1982). Simultaneous demonstration of keratin and mucin. *J. Histochem. Cytochem.* **30**, 707.

Mohr, U., Schmähl, D., and Tomatis, L. (Eds.) (1975). *Air pollution and cancer in man.* IARC Scientific Publications, No. 16.

Moody, T.W., Pert, C.B., Gazdar, A.F., Carney, D.N., and Minna, J.D. (1981). High levels of intracellular bombesin characterise human small cell lung carcinoma. *Science* **214**, 1246.

Nettesheim, P. (1976). Precursor lesions of bronchogenic carcinoma. *Cancer Res.* **36**, 2654.

Pearse, A.G.E. (1969). The cytochemistry and ultrastructure of polypeptide hormone producing cells of the APUD series and the embryological, physiologic and pathologic implications of the concept. *J. Histochem. Cytochem.* **17**, 303.

—— and Takor, T.T. (1976). Neuroendocrine embryology and the APUD concept. *Clin. Endocrinol.* **5**, Supp. 299s.

Port, C.D., Henry, M.C., Kaufman, D.G., Harris, C.C., and Ketels, K.V. (1973). Acute changes in the surface morphology of hamster tracheobronchial epithelium following benzo(a)pyrene and ferric oxide administration. *Cancer Res.* **33**, 2498.

Ranchod, M. (1977). The histogenesis and development of pulmonary tumorlets. *Cancer* **39**, 1135.

Rees, L.H. (1976). Concepts in ectopic hormone production. *Clin. Endocrinol.* **5**, Supp. 363s.

Reznik-Schüller, H. (1977*a*). Ultrastructural alterations of APUD cells during nitrosamine-induced lung carcinogenesis. *J. Pathol.* **121**, 79.

—— (1977*b*). Sequential morphologic alterations in the bronchial epithelium of Syrian golden hamsters during N-nitrosomorpholine-induced pulmonary tumorigenesis. *Amer. J. Pathol.* **89**, 59.

Richardson, R.L., Greco, F.A., Oldham, R.K., and Liddle, G.W. (1978). Tumor products and potential markers in small cell lung cancer. *Semin. Oncol.* **5** (3), 253.

Saccomanno, G., Archer, V.E., Auerbach, O., Saunders, R.P., and Brennan, L.M. (1974). Development of carcinoma of the lung as reflected in exfoliated cells. *Cancer* **33**, 256.

Saffiotti, U., Cefis, F., and Kolb, L.H. (1968). A method for the experimental induction of bronchogenic carcinoma. *Cancer Res.* **28**, 104.

Sappino, A-P., Ellison, M.L., Carter, S.M., and Smith, I.E. (in press). Prognostic value of tumour markers at presentation for treated small cell carcinoma of the lung.

Schlegel, R., Banks-Schlegel, S., and Pinkus, G.S. (1980). Immunohistochemical localization of keratin in normal human tissues. *Lab. Invest.* **42**, 91.

Schmechel, D., Marangos, P.J., and Brightman, M. (1978). Neurone-specific enolase is a molecular marker for peripheral and central neuroendocrine cells. *Nature* **276**, 834.

Schreiber, H., Saccomanno, G., Martin, D.H., and Brennan, L. (1974). Sequential cytological changes during development of respiratory tract tumors induced in hamsters by Benxo(a)pyrene-ferric oxide. *Cancer Res.* 689.

Shamsuddin, A.K.M. and Trump, B.F. (1981). Colon epithelium I. Light microscopic histochemical and ultrastructural features of normal colon epithelium of male Fischer 344 rats. *J. Nat. Cancer Inst.* **66**, 375.

Sidhu, G.S. (1979). The endodermal origin of digestive and respiratory tract APUD cells. *Amer. J. Pathol.* **96**, 5.

—— and Fresko, N.D. (1978). The morphologic spectrum of Clara cell tumors of the lung. *Lab. Invest.* **38**, 365.

Spain, D.M., Bradess, V.A., Tarter, R., and Matero, A. (1970). Metaplasia of bronchial epithelium. Effect of age, sex and smoking. *J. Amer. Med. Assoc.* **211**, 1331.

Steele, V.E. and Nettesheim, P. (1981). Unstable cellular differentiation in adenosquamous cell carcinoma. *J. Nat. Cancer Inst.* **67**, 149.

Stenbäck, F. (1973). Morphologic characteristics of experimentally induced lung tumors and their precursors in hamsters. *Acta Cytolog.* **17**, 476.

—— (1977). Morphology of experimentally induced respiratory tumors in Syrian golden hamsters. *Acta Oto-Laryngol. Suppl.* **347**, 5.

Tapia, F.J., Barbosa, A.J.A., Marangos, P.J., Polak, J.M., Bloom, S.R., and Dermody, C. (1981). Neuron-specific enolase is produced by neuroendocrine tumors. *Lancet* **1**, 808.

Terzakis, J.A., Sommers, S.C., and Andersson, B. (1972). Neurosecretory appearing cells of human segmental bronchi. *Lab. Invest.* **26** (1), 127.

Tischler, A.S. (1978). Small cell carcinoma of the lung: Cellular origin and relationship to other neoplasms. *Semin. Oncol.* **5** (3), 244.

Trump, B.F., McDowell, E.M., Glavin, F., Barrett, L.A., Becci, P.J., Schürch, W., Kaiser, H.E., and Harris, C.C. (1978). The respiratory epithelium. III. Histogenesis of epidermoid metaplasia and carcinoma in situ in the human. *J. Nat. Cancer Inst.* **61** (2), 563.

US Department of Health, Education, and Welfare (1968). *The Health consequences of smoking.* 1968 Supplement to the 1967 Public Health Service Review. Public Health Service Publication No. 1696.

Walter, J.B. and Pryce, D.M. (1955). The site of origin of lung cancer and its relation to histological type. *Thorax* **10**, 117.

—— —— (1960). The frequency of differentiation in oat-cell carcinoma of the lung. *J. Pathol. Bact.* **80**, 121.

Wharton, J., Polak, J.M., Bloom, S.R., Ghatei, M.A., Solcia, E., Brown, M.R., and Pearse, A.G.E. (1978). Bombesin-like immunoreactivity in the lung. *Nature* **273**, 769.

Williams, M.J. and Howard, S.A. (1958). The associations of invasive and in situ anaplastic bronchogenic carcinoma of the oat cell type. *Cancer* **2** (5), 939.

Willis, R.A. (Ed.) (1948). Epithelial tumours of the trachea, bronchi and lung. In *Pathology of tumours.* Butterworth, London.

Wood, S.M., Wood, J.R., Ehatei, M.A., Sorensen, G.D., and Bloom, S.R. (1982). Is bombesin a tumour marker for small-cell carcinoma? *Lancet* **i**, 690.

World Health Organization (WHO) (1967). Histological typing of lung tumours. *Int. Histological Classification Tumours*, no. 1.

Yesner, R. (1978). Spectrum of lung cancer and ectopic hormones. *Pathol. Ann.* **13**, 217.

7 Precancerous states of the oesophagus and stomach

Si-Chun Ming

Many carcinomas of the oesophagus and stomach have a dismal prognosis because they are diagnosed at an advanced stage. Modifications in therapeutic approach have resulted in little significant improvement, and the main hope for increased survival lies in early diagnosis and treatment. In countries where carcinomas of the oesophagus and stomach are common such as China and Japan, mass screening programmes are revealing large numbers of early carcinomas and survival rates have markedly improved (Ackerman *et al.* 1978; Ariga and Takahasi 1976). Such major efforts may not be feasible or justifiable in low-risk countries where it seems more practical to concentrate efforts on patients with recognized precancerous states by frequent follow-up studies. Identification of precancerous states has, therefore, an important role in overall clinical management.

Nagayo (1977) has separated the precursors of gastric cancer into two categories: precancerous *conditions* and precancerous *changes*, an approach which has been adopted by other investigators (Oehlert 1979; Grundmann and Schlake 1979) and applied to other sites. Precancerous conditions are clinical or histological entities in which there is an increased risk of eventually developing cancer. They may be confined to the target organ or they may affect other tissues and organs as well. Precancerous changes occur at the cellular level in the tissues of the target organ. They are diverse in nature but they carry a (variably) increased risk of evolving into a malignant tumour. A rigid distinction between precancerous conditions and precancerous states may be difficult to maintain in all contexts but the two categories provide a useful framework for describing precancerous states in the oesophagus and stomach, and this nomenclature will be used here.

Oesophagus

The oesophagus is lined by squamous epithelium, and the vast majority of oesophageal cancers are squamous-cell carcinomas. Adenocarcinoma is uncommon, arising either from columnar epithelium or from submucosal glands. The latter are rare, but the former have been increasingly recognized in recent years.

The incidence of oesophageal carcinoma varies greatly from country to country and from area to area within the same country. Its relation to the prevalence rates of precancerous states is largely unknown. The most important information comes from investigations in the People's Republic of China where well-organized mass surveys have been in operation for a number of years (Ackerman *et al.* 1978; Coordinating Group for the Research of Esophageal Carcinoma, Chinese Academy of Medical Sciences, and Honan Province 1974). The main tool used in such surveys is cytological examination, and the information obtained deals with precancerous changes. Histopathological surveys have been carried out in North-East Iran (Crespi *et al.*, 1979), and a similar study has recently been reported from another high-risk population in North-West China (Muñoz *et al.*, 1982).

Precancerous conditions

A number of precancerous conditions in the oesophagus have been recognized for many years. Collectively, they account for only a small number of cancers, and knowledge of precancerous conditions for oesophageal cancer in the general population is still scanty.

Oesophagitis. Oesophagoscopy and biopsy studies in North-East Iran, a high-risk region for oesophageal cancer, demonstrated chronic oesophagitis in 80 per cent of the 418 individuals who were examined (Crespi *et al.* 1979). The study also revealed epithelial dysplasia in 16 cases and invasive cancer in 11 patients, all of whom had chronic oesophagitis. There was no evidence of reflux of gastric contents into the oesophagus, and chronic oesophagitis was therefore regarded as a premalignant condition in this particular population. Strikingly similar results have also been reported among 527 individuals from a commune in Northern Linhsien (Linxian), a high-incidence area for oesophageal cancer in the People's Republic of China (Muñoz *et al.* 1982). Chronic oesophagitis was found in 84 per cent of cases, accompanied by epithelial atrophy in 10 per cent and by dysplasia (see later) in 8 per cent. Re-examination of 20 selected subjects one year later showed progression of the oesophagitis to atrophy and dysplasia in 4 individuals and to overt cancer in 4 others. It must be emphasized, however, that some degree of oesophagitis is common in the general population. Thus among 1000 oesophagi examined at autopsy by Postlethwait and Musser (1974) in the US, oesophagitis was present in 766, 'leukoplakia' in 2, invasive carcinoma in 5, and *in situ* carcinoma in 3 cases. These interesting findings indicate that the same rather common condition—chronic oesophagitis—may have different connotations as a potential precancerous condition in different populations with different risks of developing oesophageal cancer.

Stricture. Stricture of the oesophagus due to tissue destruction, inflammation, and fibrosis following ingestion of corrosive chemicals (particularly lye) is associated with an increased incidence of oesophageal cancer. The incidence of such tumours varies between 1 and 4 per cent, and the latent period is between 30 and 40 years (Bigger and Vinson 1950; Bigelow 1953; Hopkins and Postlethwait 1981). All the cancers developed at the site of the stricture and were squamous carcinomas. The effect of strictures on subsequent tumour development has been studied experimentally in hamsters by Dunham and Sheets (1974). Polyethelene cuffs were tied round the lower end of the oesophagus and the hamsters then received five twice-weekly instillations of benzo(a)pyrene to a maximum dose of 50 mg. In the oesophagus of eight animals with such strictures, three contained local lesions: a papillary carcinoma in one, multiple papillomas in one, and mucosal atypia in one. Only one of 18 animals treated with benzo(α)pyrene without stricture developed a papilloma in the oesophagus. Five other control hamsters had mucosal atypia. No carcinomas were found. The hamsters with strictures developed their local lesions at an earlier age than the untreated controls. Tumours of the forestomach were also found more frequently and in larger numbers in animals with strictures than in the controls.

Achalasia. Justa-Vierra and Haight (1969) reviewed 167 cases from the literature of oesophageal carcinomas in patients with achalasia. The reported incidence varied in different series from 0 to 20 per cent. The cancer tended to be located in the dilated and often inflamed segment of the oesophagus rather than at the narrowed cardiac end. Among 101 patients with achalasia including 13 autopsied cases reviewed by Akuamoa (1969), 5 per cent had oesophagitis and 3 patients had carcinoma. Pierce *et al.* (1970) found oesophageal carcinoma in 3 of 110 patients. The average duration of symptoms was 23 years. Intervals of about 28 years between the onset of achalasia and the diagnosis of carcinoma were also noted by Wychulis *et al.* (1971).

Plummer-Vinson (Paterson-Kelly) syndrome. Patients with Plummer-Vinson syndrome have an iron deficiency anaemia, vitamin B deficiency, and dysphagia which is often associated with the presence of a postcricoid web. These patients have a high incidence of carcinoma in the upper gastro-intestinal tract. An early account was given by Simpson (1939). Among 18 of his patients, carcinoma was present in 10 : 4 in the postcricoid region, 1 in the lower third of the oesophagus and 5 at the cardia. Of 69 patients followed by Chrisholm *et al.* (1971), 2 developed postcricoid carcinoma and one died of oesophageal cancer. Wynder *et al.* (1957) studied a group of

Swedish female patients and found a high level of association between the Plummer-Vinson syndrome and hypopharyngeal and oesophageal cancers, particularly the former.

Hiatus hernia, reflux oesophagitis, and Barrett's oesophagus. In 1955, Pattinson *et al.* found 109 cases in the literature with both hiatus hernia and carcinoma in the lower oesophagus or upper stomach, including 4 cases with ectopic gastric epithelium in the oesophagus. Adenocarcinomas outnumbered squamous-cell carcinomas. Adler and Rodriguez (1959) found carcinomas in 21 of 814 patients with hiatus hernia, an incidence of 2.5 per cent. Twelve patients had adenocarcinomas of the stomach and 9 had oesophageal carcinomas, comprising 7 squamous-cell carcinomas and 2 adenocarcinomas.

In 1957 Barrett drew attention to the clinical condition in which the lower oesophagus is lined by columnar epithelium. Since then there have been many studies of this lesion, which is now known as Barrett's oesophagus. It is generally accepted that the columnar epithelium develops as a result of reparative regeneration following the loss of normal squamous epithelium due to reflux oesophagitis. It is not a congenital lesion as Barrett originally thought. There is evidence of a coexisting hiatus hernia or an incompetent lower oesophageal sphincter in most cases. Chronic peptic ulceration and strictures are common. The columnar epithelium is composed of gastric as well as intestinal cells (Ozzello *et al.* 1977). Cardiac glands and a few chief and parietal cells may be present, but the cellular composition varies from one case to another and in different parts of the same lesion. In general, the mucosa resembles that seen in chronic atrophic gastritis; intestinal metaplasia may be present. Compared with the normal squamous epithelium of the oesophagus, the columnar epithelium has greater proliferative activity and a shorter generation time (Herbst *et al.* 1978). These findings correlate with the presence of immature cells seen in the electron microscope (Ozzello *et al.* 1977).

Oesophageal adenocarcinoma, which is rare in the general population, occurs at a high incidence in Barrett's oesophagus. Haggitt *et al.* (1978) identified 12 of 14 primary oesophageal adenocarcinomas as arising from Barrrett's columnar epithelium. In 10 of these patients, additional dysplasia or carcinoma *in situ* were identified near the main cancer. Hiatus hernia with symptomatic reflux oesophagitis was present in all cases. Conversely, Naef *et al.* (1975) found 140 cases of Barrett's oesophagus among 1225 cases of reflux oesophagitis; adenocarcinoma was present in 12 of these 140 cases. This high incidence of cancer in Barrett's oesophagus is reminiscent of the occurrence of gastric cancer in association with chronic atrophic gastritis.

Adenocarcinomas arising in a Barrett's oesophagus contain cells which secrete intestinal-type mucins. Since intestinal metaplasia is common in

Barrett's oesophagus, it is possible that such cancers may originate in the metaplastic epithelium. According to Jass (1981) the carcinoma is most commonly associated with a type of incomplete metaplasia in which columnar cells between the goblet cells secrete sulphomucins, a situation found in nine out of 15 cases studied. We have examined 16 adenocarcinomas, eight of which occurred in association with incomplete metaplasia in the adjacent epithelium. We also found remnants of adenomatous lesions at the periphery of the cancer in five patients. McDonald *et al.* (1977) reported a remarkable case of multiple adenomas with malignant transformation, suggesting that both adenoma and adenocarcinoma may develop in Barrett's oesophagus and that carcinoma may evolve from an adenoma.

Coeliac disease. Adult patients with coeliac disease have a high incidence of lymphomas and gastrointestinal cancers, particularly carcinoma of the oesophagus. Harris *et al.* (1967) reported 6 cases of oesophageal and 3 cases of gastric carcinoma among 29 patients who died with a clinical diagnosis of coeliac disease. The mean duration of coeliac disease in patients with oesophageal cancer was 50 years. A subsequent report from the same institution listed two cases of oesophageal and one case of gastric cancer among 21 patients dying with histologically proven coeliac disease (Holmes *et al.* 1976).

Tylosis: possible familial aggregations. In 1958, Howel-Evans *et al.* reported two families from Liverpool with tylosis in 48 out of 152 total members. Carcinomas of the oesophagus developed in 12 of them. Tylosis was present in 11 of the cancer cases, the twelfth being incompletely documented. By 1969 oesophageal carcinoma had occurred in 6 additional members of one of these families (Harper *et al.* 1970). In addition, Harper *et al.* discovered 2 cases of oesophageal carcinoma among 10 individuals with tylosis from two other families. Apart from these reports, oesophageal carcinoma is not known to show any familial aggregations. Some families in China have been described with oesophageal cancer in several members (Ackerman *et al.* 1978); but since the affected members were not all genetically linked, environmental factors were probably involved.

Precancerous change

Although oesophageal cancer develops more frequently in individuals with certain precancerous conditions, most patients with this disease have no obvious antecedent abnormality. The underlying precancerous lesion has not been clearly identified but there are strong indications that severe dysplasia of the oesophageal epithelium (Figs. 7.1-7.4) may be implicated as such changes are common in the cancerous oesophagus. Of 13 cancerous oesophagi studied by Mandard *et al.* (1978), mild and moderate dysplasia was present in all cases, marked dysplasia in 10 and carcinoma *in situ* in 8 cases. Cells from severely dysplastic oesophageal epithelium have been

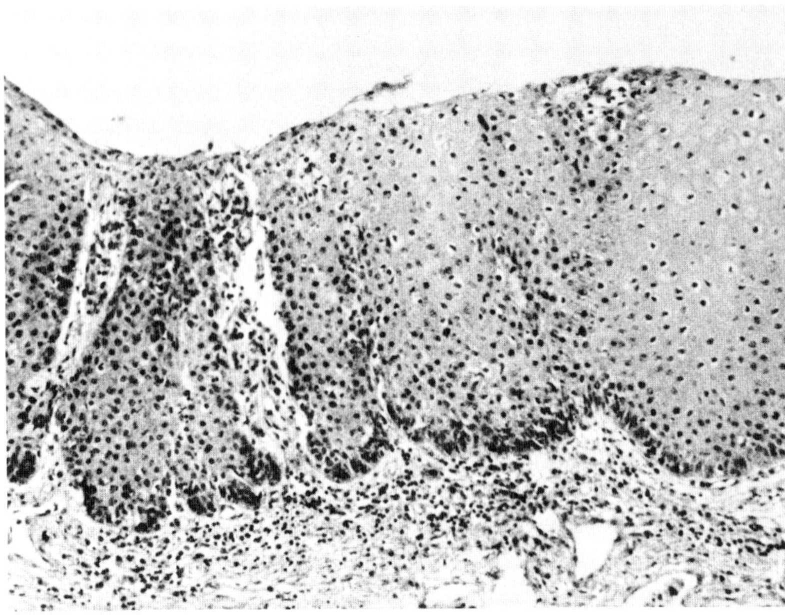

Fig. 7.1. Mild dysplasia of squamous epithelium of the oesophagus showing hyperplasia, focal disorganization, and slight pleomorphism of cells. Maturation toward the surface is normal. ×150. H & E.

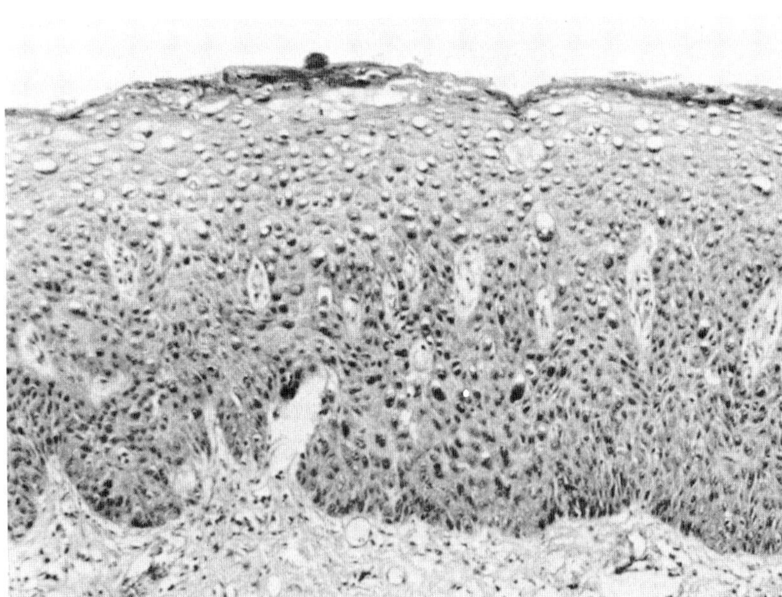

Fig. 7.2. Moderate dysplasia of squamous epithelium of the oesophagus showing hyperplasia, disorganization, and moderate pleomorphism with occasional giant nuclei. Surface cells show parakeratosis. ×150. H & E.

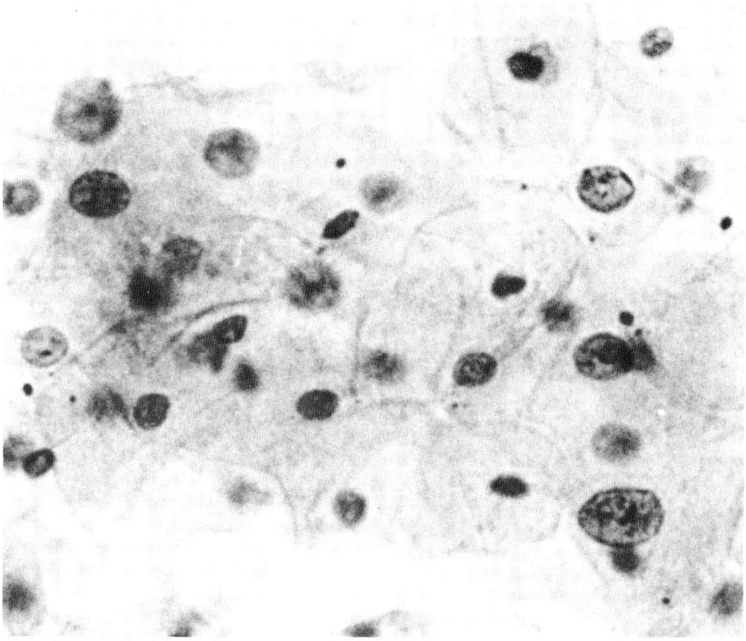

Fig. 7.3. Moderately dysplastic squamous cells in oesophageal washings showing cellular pleomorphism, hyperchromatic nuclei, and reduction of cytoplasm in cells with enlarged nuclei. ×480. H & E.

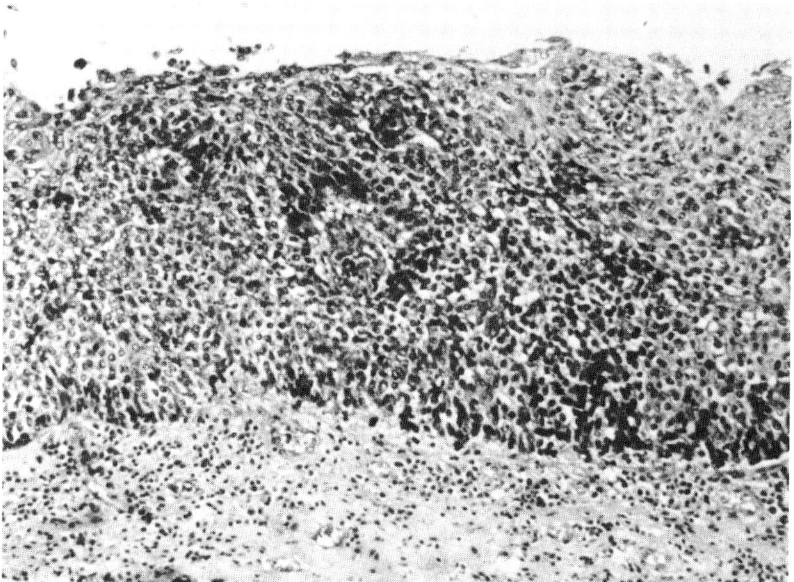

Fig. 7.4. Severe dysplasia of squamous epithelium of the oesophagus showing immature cells throughout the whole thickness of the epithelium. The cell cytoplasm is scanty. ×150. H & E.

shown to be tetraploid or near-tetraploid in karyotype analyses (Mukada *et al.* 1978).

Epidemiologically, oesophageal dysplasia is more frequent among high-risk than low-risk populations. Dysplasia with hyperkeratosis ('leukoplakia') of the oesophagus was present in only 2 of 1000 autopsies in the US (Postlethwait and Musser 1974). In the high-risk population in north-east Iran, it was present in 16 of 418 (3.8 per cent) oesophageal biopsies (Crespi *et al.* 1979). In Japan, mild dysplasia was equally common in high-risk and low-risk areas but severe dysplasia was more frequent in the former (Mukada *et al.* 1976). A cytological screening survey of 62000 Chinese in a high-risk population uncovered marked dysplasia in 2.2 per cent and carcinoma in 1.2 per cent (Li and Shiang 1979). Important follow-up studies in Chinese patients with severe dysplasia revealed oesophageal cancer in 7.9 per cent at 1-2 years, 20.5 per cent at 2-5 years, 34 per cent at 5-9 years, and 53 per cent at 9-12 years (Yang 1980). Valuable information has come from the Coordinating Group for the Research of Esophageal Carcinoma of the Chinese Academy of Medical Science and Honan Province, published in 1974. In Northern Linhsien (Linxian) where the incidence of oesophageal carcinoma is high, mild dysplasia was present in 25 per cent, marked dysplasia in 2.2 per cent, and carcinoma in 1.3 per cent of the 4377 persons from whom cytological material was obtained. By contrast, the incidence of mild dysplasia, marked dysplasia, and carcinoma in the *low* incidence area of Southern Linhsien were 18, 0.7, and 0.7 per cent, respectively. Both dysplasia and cancer rates increased with age. Follow-up studies of these patients over a 2-4-year period provided information on the subsequent evolution of the dysplastic changes: 44.8 per cent of *mildly* dysplastic epithelial changes returned to normal, 40 per cent remained unchanged, and 15.2 per cent progressed to marked dysplasia; *markedly* dysplastic epithelial changes returned to normal in 40.5 per cent, remained unchanged or recurred in 29.9 per cent, and became malignant in 26.6 per cent. Antitumour therapy reduced the incidence of cancer development and increased the regression rate (Cai *et al.* 1980). A more recent survey from a high-incidence area in Northern Linhsien (Linxian) reports a lower incidence of epithelial dysplasia (Muñoz *et al.* 1982) but evolving squamous carcinomas were again documented. These various observations clearly indicate the precancerous nature of severely dysplastic epithelium. On the other hand, it is equally clear that dysplasia is a reversible process and that a significant proportion of dysplastic epithelia may return to normal.

Experimental studies

Squamous-cell carcinoma of the oesophagus has been induced in animals with various *N*-nitroso-compounds—see Table 7.1. Herrold (1966) fed *N*-nitroso-*N*-methylurethane to 16 hamsters. Epithelial hyperplasia and papillomas were induced in all of them and carcinomas developed in 13 animals.

Table 7.1.

N-nitroso-*N*-methylurethane	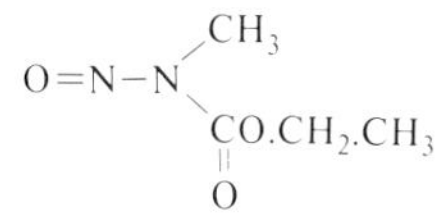
N,*N*-di (2-hydroxypropyl) nitrosamine	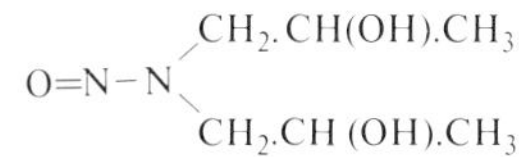
N-methyl-*N*- benzylnitrosamine	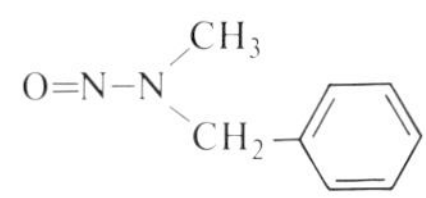
N-methyl-*N*-nitrosoaniline	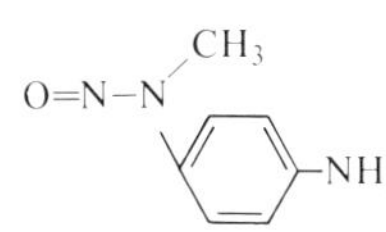
Diethylnitrosamine	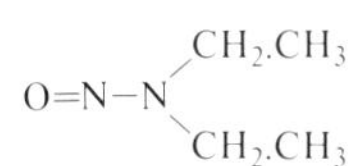
N-nitrososarcosine ethyl ester	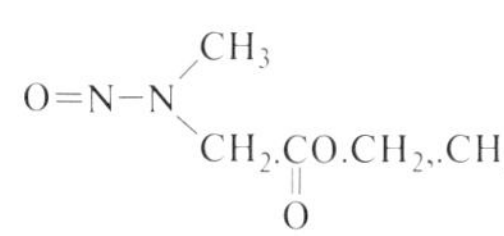
N-ethyl-*N*′-nitro-*N*-nitrosoguanidine	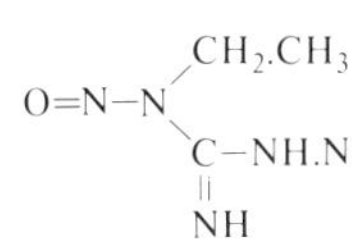

Using rats, Levison *et al.* (1979) induced oesophageal papillomas in one and carcinomas in eight animals treated with di(2-hydroxypropyl)-nitrosamine. Most of the rats with carcinomas also had papillomas and epithelial hyperplasia with cellular atypia. Similar findings were observed by Stinson *et al.* (1978) who gave *N*-methyl-*N*-benzylnitrosamine to 24 rats. Invasive carcinomas were induced in 63 per cent, pedunculated papillary carcinomas in 67 per cent, and papillomas in 100 per cent of the treatment animals. All the oesophagi contained endophytic areas of hyperplasia, often with marked cellular atypia. Local cellular atypia was noted in many of the oesophageal papillomas. Napalkov and Pozharisski (1969) administered *N*-methyl-*N*-nitrosoaniline to 42 rats, 2 of which were killed each month. The earliest changes in the oesophageal epithelium were hyperplasia and dyskeratosis which progressed to form patches of 'leukoplakia'. Continued growth of the epithelium as well as the underlying connective tissue resulted in the formation of papillomas. Increasing dysplasia in the papillomas was followed by the development of overt carcinoma. Dysplasia was thus an integral feature of their malignant transformation. These experiments suggest that the development of experimental oesophageal carcinomas in animals is preceded first by epithelial hyperplasia, then by papillomas which become increasingly dysplastic. True papillomas are, however, exceedingly rare in the oesophagus of man, and human oesophageal carcinomas appear to develop directly from dysplastic epithelium. A comparable animal model was reported by Reuber (1977) in rats treated wth diethylnitrosamine. The initial preneoplastic changes were focal hyperplasia and dysplasia. The hyperplastic epithelium first became nodular and later evolved into carcinoma *in situ* and small early carcinoma. Similar observations have been made by Cai *et al.* (1980*a*) in mice and rats given *N*-nitrososarcosine ethyl ester. Multiple carcinomas and foci of dysplasia and carcinoma *in situ* were induced in three dogs given *N*-ethyl-*N'*-nitro-*N*-nitrosoguanidine by Sasajima *et al.* (1977).

These experimental observations, together with results from clinical material, suggest the following developmental sequence for oesophageal cancers: simple epithelial hyperplasia, mild dysplasia, severe dysplasia, carcinoma *in situ*, and finally invasive carcinoma.

Stomach

Gastric cancers are predominantly adenocarcinomas, other types of carcinoma being rare. Adenocarcinomas of the stomach have complex histological patterns and are conveniently considered in two main histological types. Lauren (1965) observed that most gastric cancers resembled colonic carcinomas, being composed of well-formed acini lined by cells with brush borders; other tumours showed a more diffuse, infiltrative pattern and lacked glandular organization. The former were called *intestinal*-type carcinomas and the latter *diffuse*-type carcinomas (Figs. 7.5 and 7.6). About 14 per cent of tumours could not be classified. This taxonomic scheme has been widely used, particularly in epidemiological studies, but two misconceptions are common. First, the diffuse type of carcinoma has often been equated with undifferentiated carcinoma because of the lack of gland formation. Many cells in such tumours are, however, *well differentiated* in terms of mucin production, the presence of microvilli and enzyme activity. The second misconception is to assume that intestinal-type tumour cells are confined solely to the intestinal type of carcinoma. Such cells occur in both intestinal and diffuse variants of gastric cancer (Lauren 1965), and they have been further documented by histochemical and ultrastructural studies (Goldman and Ming 1968*a, b*; Kobori and Oota 1974; Nevalainen and Jarvi 1977).

Ming (1977*a*) has proposed a classification of gastric carcinomas into expanding and infiltrative types, irrespective of the degree of differentiation

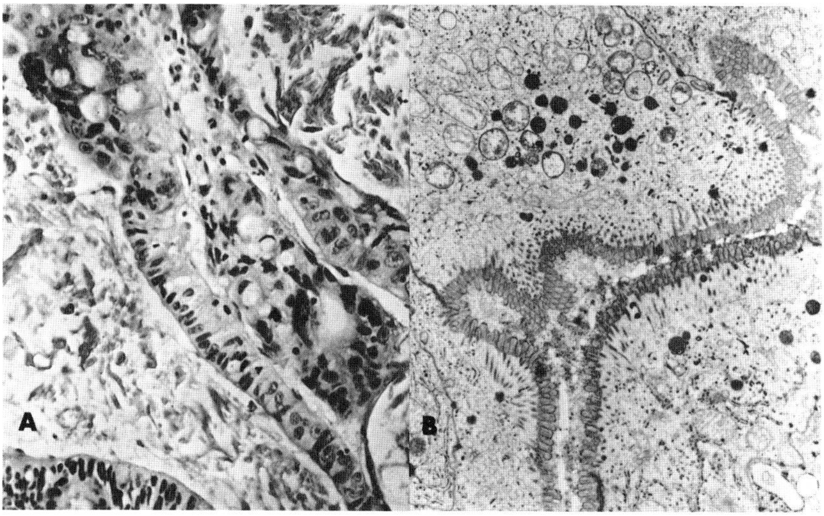

Fig. 7.5. Intestinal (expanding) type of gastric carcinoma. (A) Light-microscopic appearance of the tumour showing well-formed glands, goblet cells, and striated cell borders. ×190. H & E. (B) Electron-microscopic appearance of the tumour showing microvilli and long terminal webs. ×5548.

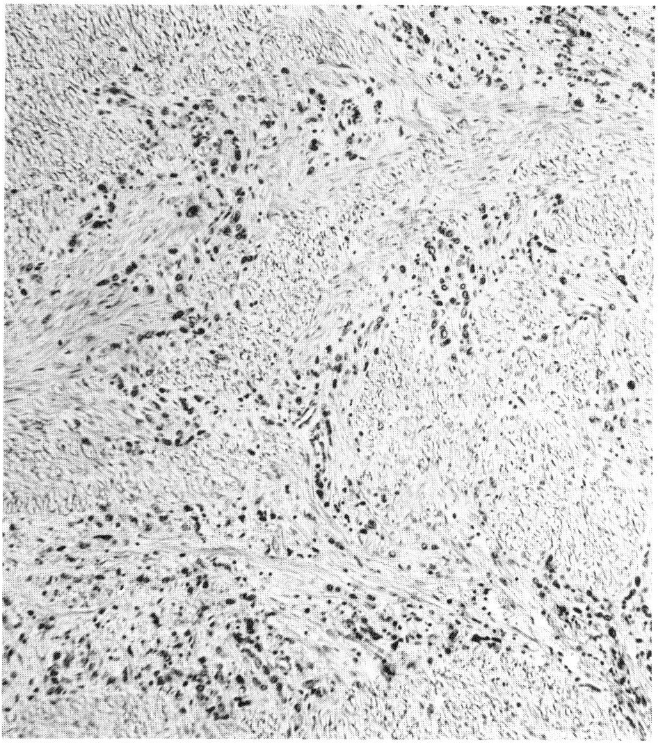

Fig. 7.6. Diffuse (infiltrative) type of gastric carcinoma showing individual cells infiltrating the muscularis propria. ×90. H & E.

and types of cells in the tumour. The critical distinction is based on growth patterns rather than on cytological details. Expanding carcinomas are composed of tumour cells with a relatively cohesive arrangement which form glands or masses and grow into expanding nodules. Infiltrative carcinomas, by contrast, consist of loosely associated or isolated tumour cells which infiltrate individually and often extensively. The expanding carcinoma corresponds to the intestinal type and the infiltrative carcinoma to the diffuse type of cancer described by Lauren. Since this classification is not based on cellular structure the confusion related to the names is avoided, and Lauren's unclassified group can be eliminated. This scheme also allows close correlation between histological pattern and the gross appearance of a tumour. An expanding carcinoma, for example, is likely to form a polypoid tumour and an infiltrative cancer produces a linitis plastica type of lesion. The value of this classification has recently been demonstrated by Ribeiro *et al.* (1981).

Like oesophageal cancer, the geographical distribution of gastric carcinoma shows wide variations between and within countries. Another striking feature is the steady decline in the incidence of gastric cancer in many regions. Some recent epidemiological studies indicate that the different prevalence rates of gastric carcinoma in different countries are related only to the incidence of the intestinal-type cancer which is more common in high-risk than low-risk countries (Muñoz and Matko 1972). Similarly, the decrease in the incidence of gastric cancer among individuals who have moved from a high-risk to a low-risk area is mainly due to a decrease in the incidence of the intestinal type of gastric carcinoma (Correa *et al.* 1973; Haenszel *et al.* 1976). The decline in the incidence of gastric cancer *within* a country may be due to the same reason, a conclusion which emerges from a study in Norway by Muñoz and Asvall (1971). Since the intestinal type of cancer is related to chronic gastritis and intestinal metaplasia, it is not surprising that the incidence of these precancerous conditions is higher in the high-risk countries than in low-risk regions (Imai *et al.* 1971). It should be noted, however, that some investigators have found no difference in the relative incidence of intestinal and diffuse types of gastric cancer either in different locations or at different time periods (Kubo 1974; Oota 1976). Nevertheless, it is quite possible that epidemiological variation in the distribution of gastric cancer is related to the prevalence of the precancerous states which are considered below.

Precancerous conditions

In 1929 Hurst gave the following account of the precursors of gastric carcinoma: 75 per cent of cancers arose from chronic atrophic gastritis, 20 per cent from chronic ulcers, 4.5 per cent from adenomas and 0.5 per cent from polyps. These four diseases are still important precancerous conditions even though their incidence has varied in different reports at different times.

In the last two decades, major efforts in detecting gastric carcinoma have helped to improve survival rates in countries such as Japan where the disease is prevalent. Such efforts have provided many specimens for the study of gastric cancer at early stages of development and for assessing possible antecedent lesions. Early gastric carcinomas have been classified into three major types according to their gross appearance: type I, a protruding tumour; type II, a superficial tumour; and type III, an excavating tumour (Kuru 1967)—see Fig. 7.7. It has been generally inferred that type-I cancers originate in polyps or adenomas, type-II cancers from gastritis or metaplastic mucosa, and type-III cancers from chronic ulcers. Resection of early cancer might have altered the relative importance of various precancerous conditions. Nagayo (1977), for instance, has noted a great reduction in the incidence of type-III early carcinomas in Japan, from 70 per cent in 1934 to about 10 per cent in 1974. The importance of chronic ulcer as a precancerous condition has therefore correspondingly reduced. It is likely that such changes will continue.

Chronic atrophic gastritis and pernicious anaemia. Chronic atrophic gastritis was recognized as a precancerous condition as early as 1913 when Konjetzney reported its presence in 85 per cent of cancerous stomachs; the glands in the atrophic mucosa were hyperplastic and Konjetzney called the condition gastritis hyperplastica atrophicans. Since then the precancerous potential of chronic atrophic gastritis has been hotly debated, but recent studies have generally given confirmatory results. Walker *et al.* (1971) recorded 4 cases of cancer among 40 patients with chronic gastritis. The mean follow-up period was 15 years. Cheli *et al.* (1973) reported that gastric cancer developed in 9 of 65 patients with atrophic gastritis and in none of

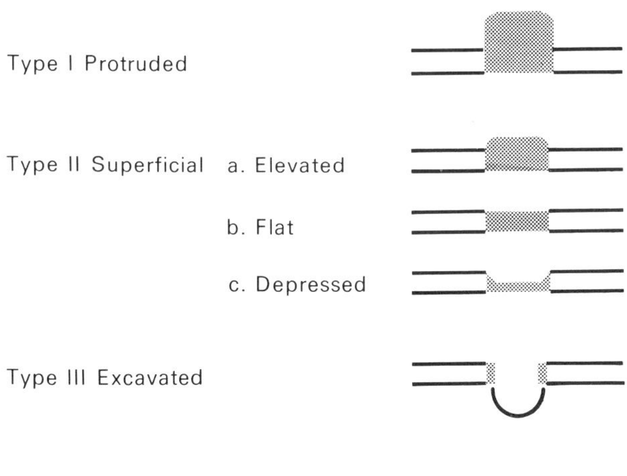

Fig. 7.7. Classification of early gastric carcinoma.

49 patients with other forms of chronic (non-atrophic) gastritis during an observation period of 11-18 years. Among 116 patients with atrophic gastritis followed for 19-23 years by Siurala *et al.* (1974), gastric carcinoma developed in 10 cases and polyps in 8. Furthermore, 13 of 35 biopsies from these patients showed moderate or severe dysplasia of the atrophic mucosa. Studies of early gastric cancer also indicate that chronic atrophic gastritis is a common precancerous condition. In 95 examples of early cancers examined by Majima *et al.* (1965), chronic gastritis was present in 35 patients and shallow ulcers or scars in seven others. All the surface or intramucosal carcinomas investigated by Mason (1974) showed atrophic gastritis in the surrounding mucosa. Epidemiological studies have shown that chronic atrophic gastritis is more prevalent in high-risk than low-risk populations (Imai *et al.* 1971; Correa *et al.* 1976).

The end stage of chronic atrophic gastritis is mucosal atrophy without significant inflammatory reaction. In 1973 Strickland and Mackay proposed that two forms of chronic atrophic gastritis—A and B—should be recognized. Type-A gastritis is associated with the presence of parietal cell antibodies and pernicious anaemia and occurs mainly in the mucosa of the body and fundus. Type-B gastritis primarily involves the mucosa of the antrum and is not associated with parietal cell antibodies and pernicious anaemia. Type-B gastritis is also known as simple atrophic gastritis and occurs commonly in the aged and in postgastrectomy patients. Cancer may occur in either type, but more often in association with Type-B gastritis. The 10 per cent incidence of gastric cancer reported in 40 patients with atrophic gastritis by Walker *et al.* (1971) were all in the Type-B group. Johansen (1978) also emphasized the importance of chronic atrophic gastritis involving the antral mucosa.

An increased incidence of gastric carcinoma in patients with pernicious anaemia has been known for a long time. In a recent report on 877 cases of gastric cancer in Denmark, pernicious anaemia was present in 19, an incidence of 2.2 per cent which represents a threefold increase above the incidence found in the general Danish population (Elsborg and Mosbech 1979). The annual risk of gastric cancer in pernicious anaemia patients was estimated as 0.3 per cent. Most of the carcinomas developed in the body and fundus of the stomach, the sites most frequently affected by mucosal atrophy and gastritis. Creagan and Fraumeni (1973) reported twelve instances of gastric cancer in four generations of an inbred family in which many members had parietal cell antibodies as well as defects in cell-mediated immunity. Gastric polyps are also common in pernicious anaemia. In a report by Elsborg *et al.* (1977) gastric polyps developed in 25 of 68 patients followed for four years. All the polyps were of the regenerative type. Some of them later regressed.

It has been suggested that gastric cancer may develop in patients with pernicious anaemia because of local formation of nitrosamines from nitrites by increased bacterial activity in the achlorhydric, atrophic stomach (Ruddell *et al.* 1978).

As noted above, chronic gastritis is more common in high-risk than low-risk countries (Imai *et al.* 1971). A study in Colombia by Correa *et al.* (1976) also showed that chronic gastritis in high-risk regions occurs in young people much more frequently than in low-risk populations: 50 per cent of the Colombian high-risk population had gastritis by the age of 30 years as compared to 20 per cent in a low-risk population in the same age group. This observation may explain the continued high incidence of gastric cancer among the first-generation immigrants moving from high-risk to low-risk regions.

Intestinal metaplasia. Normal gastric epithelium is composed of a continuous layer of mucus-secreting cells on the surface and in the foveola. Absorptive and goblet cells which occur in the intestine are absent. In intestinal metaplasia, the gastric epithelium is replaced by intestinal cells, and there is partial or complete disappearance of deep oxyntic and pyloric glands (Fig. 7.8). Paneth cells may be present. Ultrastructurally, the absorptive

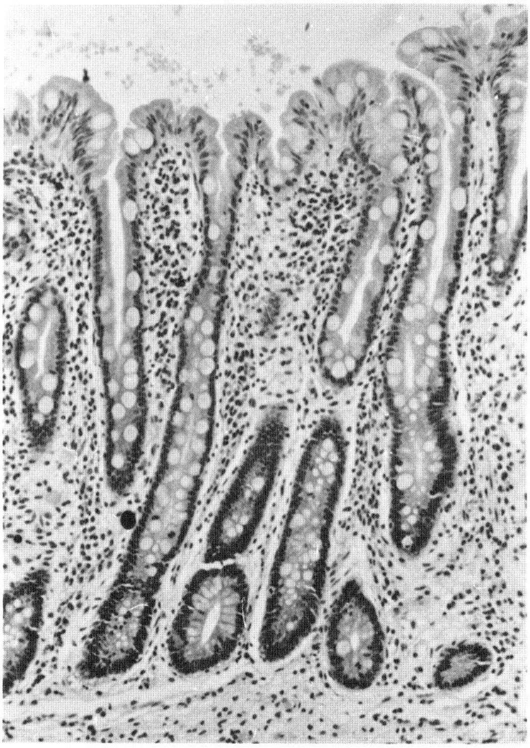

Fig. 7.8. Intestinal metaplasia of the gastric mucosa with complete disappearance of normal gastric glands. ×120. H & E.

and goblet cells in well-developed metaplastic epithelium appear identical with those of the normal small intestine (Goldman and Ming 1968*b*); see Fig. 7.9. The mucus in normal gastric surface epithelium is neutral glycoprotein, but small amounts of sialomucin may be present in the deep foveolar cells. Goblet cells in metaplastic mucosa, on the other hand, contain acidic mucin of small-intestinal or colonic type. The former type of mucin is mainly non-sulphated while the latter is mostly sulphated (Goldman and Ming 1968*a*). Electron-microscopic and histochemical studies have also demonstrated that metaplastic change may be partial or incomplete, with both intestinal and gastric features in the same gland or even in the same cell (Goldman and Ming 1968*a, b*). These observations have been extended in more recent investigations. Kawachi *et al.* (1976) used Tes-Tapes to detect four digestive enzymes, normally present in the intestine, within the metaplastic mucosa of cancerous stomachs; two different patterns emerged. In one form, all four intestinal enzymes were present, and in the other form only two were expressed. Mutsukura *et al.* (1980) have shown that the first pattern is associated with complete metaplasia and the second with incomplete metaplasia. Sulphomucin is also synthesised by gastric mucosa showing incomplete metaplasia and, since this material is secreted by normal

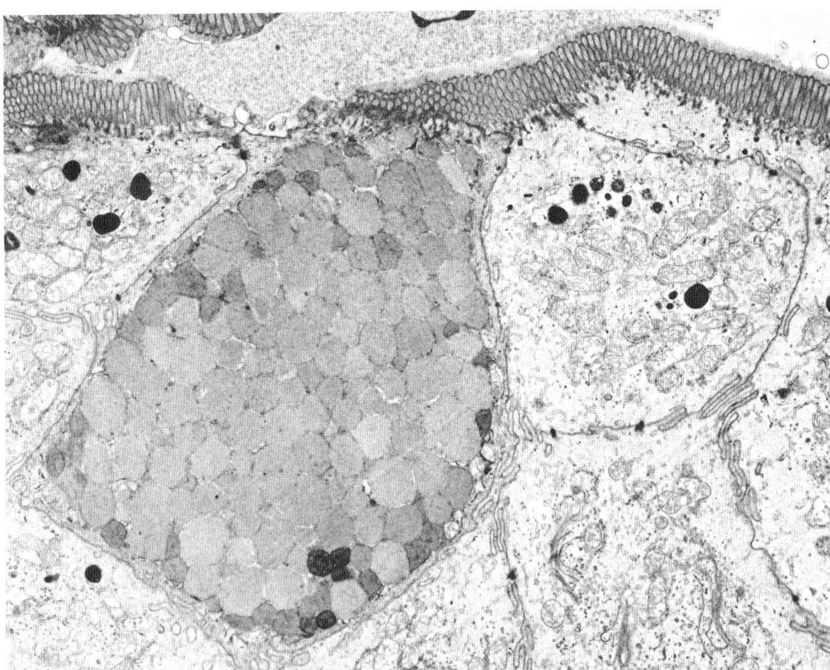

Fig. 7.9. Intestinal metaplasia of the gastric mucosa showing mucin granules in a goblet cell and well-developed microvilli of absorptive cells. ×4800.

colonic mucosa, it has been used to characterize the colonic type metaplasia that is commonly associated with intestinal-type gastric carcinomas (Sipponen 1981; Pagnini and Bozzola 1981). Based on the presence or absence of a colon-specific mucin containing *O*-acylated sialic acid, Teglbjaerg and Nielson (1978) separated metaplastic mucosa from the stomach into small-intestinal and colonic forms. The latter type of mucosa was present in all seven cases of intestinal type cancer examined and in four of sixteen cases with other types of cancer. Jass and Filipe (1979) have found that sulphomucin was present in the metaplastic mucosa in 16 of 21 cancerous stomachs and in only 2 of 13 ulcer cases. These authors have subsequently proposed that intestinal metaplasia in gastric mucosa should be described as complete or incomplete according to the presence or absence of mucus-secreting columnar cells between the goblet cells; the incomplete type is then split into two subtypes, with or without sulphomucin secretion (Jass and Filipe 1981). The association between sulphomucin-secreting incomplete metaplasia and intestinal-type gastric cancer was again established. These studies emphasize the complexity and essentially heterogenous nature of intestinal metaplasia, and our own investigations endorse this view. Based on histological appearances and mucin and enzyme histochemistry, intestinal metaplasia can be divided into five subtypes as listed in Table 7.2.

Although most cases of atrophic gastric mucosa show intestinal metaplasia, some do not. Conversely, intestinal metaplasia may be focal and not associated with generalized atrophy. The extent of intestinal metaplasia varies from case to case and from area to area. The same findings apply to the chronic atrophic gastritis observed in cancerous stomachs (Mason 1974). Chronic atrophic gastritis and intestinal metaplasia are not, therefore, synonymous in terms of their relation to cancer. Since intestinal metaplasia increases with age and is present in nearly all persons above the age of 70 years (Stout 1945), this change was considered by Mason (1974) as only a potentially premalignant (rather than a premalignant) condition. On the other hand, intestinal metaplasia becomes clearly precancerous when it manifests severe dysplastic changes (Ming *et al.* 1967; Ming 1979).

Morson (1955) stressed that gastric cancer may arise from metaplastic mucosa (Fig. 7.10), and the reports cited above confirm this observation. On the other hand, many gastric cancers have been found to originate in non-metaplastic mucosa (Ming *et al.* 1967; Nakamura *et al.* 1968; Johansen 1978). Other studies have shown severe and extensive intestinal metaplasia, particularly in the antrum, in stomachs harbouring the intestinal type of cancer but little or no metaplastic change in stomachs with diffuse-type carcinomas (Lauren 1965; Kawachi *et al.* 1976; Ming 1977*a*; Stemmermann *et al.* 1977). Similar observations have been made in cases of early cancer (Oota 1976; Nagayo 1977; Nakahara 1978; Oohara *et al.* 1982). Furthermore, the incidence of metaplasia runs parallel with the incidence of the

Table 7.2. *Types and main features of intestinal metaplasia*

	Complete		Incomplete		
	Small intestinal	Colonic	Gastric	Small intestinal	Colonic
Cells					
Absorptive cells	+	+	0	0	0
Striated border	+	0	0	0	0
Mucous columnar cells	0	0	+	+	+
Goblet cells	+	+	+	+	+
Paneth cells	+	0	0	0	0
Enzymes					
Alkaline phosphatase	+	0	0	0	0
Trehalase	+	0	−	−	−
Aminopeptidase	+	+	+	+	+
Sucrase	+	+	−	−	−
Mucins in goblet cells					
Neutral glycoprotein	0	0	0	0	0
Sialomucin, *N*-acylated	+	0	+	+	+
Sialomucin, *O*-acylated	±	+	0	±	±
Sulphomucin	0	+	±	+	+
Mucins in mucous columnar cells					
Neutral glycoprotein	N	N	+	±	±
Sialomucin, *N*-acylated	N	N	0	+	±
Sialomucin, *O*-acylated	N	N	0	0	±
Sulphomucin	N	N	0	0	+

+: Present; ±: Variable; 0: Usually absent; −: Unknown; N: Not applicable

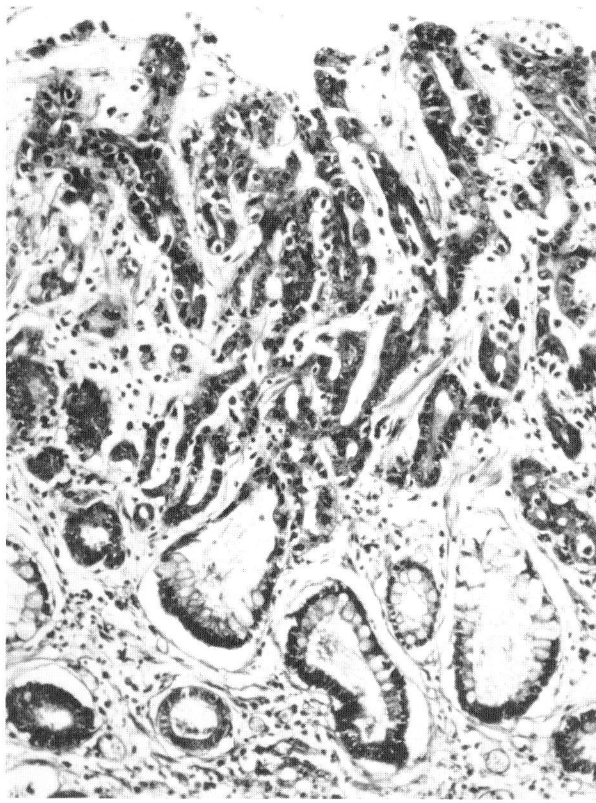

Fig. 7.10. Superficial carcinoma of the stomach arising in metaplastic mucosa. Residual intestinalized glands are present in the deep mucosa. ×150. H & E.

intestinal type of gastric cancer (Muñoz and Matko 1972). All these findings suggest that the intestinal type of gastric carcinomas may arise in metaplastic mucosa. The cell of origin for the diffuse type of cancer has been suspected to be foveolar or neck mucous cells or cells of pyloric glands, as suggested by the demonstration of these cell types in electron-microscopic studies of diffuse carcinomas (Sasano *et al.* 1969; Nevalainen *et al.* 1977; Yamashire *et al.* 1977). On the other hand, intestinal features such as goblet cells, brush borders and stainable acid mucins are present in both cancer types, as discussed above. The presence of intestinal-type cells in a gastric carcinoma does not, therefore, necessarily indicate origin from metaplastic epithelium. In addition to gastric and intestinal cells, argentaffin cells, zymogen cells, and even squamous cells have been identified in some gastric cancers (Sasano *et al.* 1969; Yamashiro *et al.* 1977), and it is possible that gastric cancer may pursue several lines of differentiation irrespective of its cell of origin (Ming *et al.* 1967).

A recent immunohistochemical study of tumour markers in premalignant states of the stomach has been reported by Skinner and Whitehead (1982). Eight markers were examined: pregnancy-specific β-glycoprotein (SP1), human placental lactogen (HPL), carcinoembryonic antigen (CEA), α-fetoprotein (αFP), a tumour-derived colon-specific antigen (t-CSA), ferritin (FE), transferrin (TF) and human β chorionic gonadotrophin (β-HCG). The results are summarised in Table 7.3. Two markers, SP1 and t-CSA, were absent from metaplastic epithelium associated with gastric atrophy but were present both in metaplastic epithelium associated with gastric cancer and in the cancers themselves. CEA was not an effective discriminant in the three groups. More markers were demonstrated in the intestinal metaplasia associated with gastric cancer than in (morphologically identical) metaplasia associated with gastric atrophy and, in terms of the distribution of markers, there were clear similarities between metaplasia associated with

Table 7.3. *Immunohistochemical markers in intestinal metaplasia and gastric carcinoma*

	Overall distribution of markers							
	SP1[a]	HPL	CEA	α-FP	tCSA[b]	FE	TF	β-HCG
Intestinal metaplasia associated with gastric atrophy $n=17$	0	4	14	2	0	6	8	5
Intestinal metaplasia associated with gastric carcinoma $n=13$	4	4	11	6	7	8	8	4
Gastric carcinoma $n=18$	9	9	18	8	10	11	11	10

	Numbers of positive markers/disease category	
	Low	High[c]
	0-3	4-8
Intestinal metaplasia associated with gastric atrophy	13	4
Intestinal metaplasia associated with gastric carcinoma	4	9
Gastric carcinoma	5	13

Compiled from Tables 1 and 2 in Skinner and Whitehead, 1982
See text for abbreviations.
[a] $\chi^2 = 13.41$, $P<0.01$ >0.001; [b] $\chi^2 = 15.12$, $P<0.001$.
[c] $\chi^2 = 10.55$, $P=0.005$

cancer and the cancers themselves. These results again emphasize the heterogenous nature of intestinal metaplasia in gastric mucosa.

Chronic gastric ulcer. The role of chronic gastric ulcer as a precancerous condition has been a controversial topic for many years. Evidence for malignant transformation of a chronic ulcer rests mainly on the development of cancer in a pre-existing ulcer of long duration and the finding of an early focus in the margin of a chronic ulcer. After a careful study of four cases of early carcinoma in an ulcer, Mallory (1940) concluded that carcinoma was the primary disease and that the ulcer developed as a secondary phenomenon. Mallory's view has been generally accepted by pathologists in the US, but later studies from Japan initially pointed to rather different conclusions—despite the observations that the epidemiological distribution of gastric cancer and gastric ulcer were different (Hirohata and Kuratsune 1969). In 1963, Oota found that 85 per cent of gastric cancer cases had pre-existing chronic ulcers. Of 95 cases of early cancer studied by Majima *et al.* (1965), 25 were thought to have developed in an ulcer. According to Kuru (1967), 39 per cent of advanced cancers and 38 per cent of early cancers originated in a deep ulcer. Sano (1971) studied 300 cases of early gastric cancer and found an association with ulcer in 211 cases (70 per cent). More recently, however, the incidence of deeply ulcerating early cancer has decreased markedly (Hirota *et al.* 1980), and the weight of evidence now indicates that chronic ulcer is not an important precursor of gastric cancer in Japan (Oota 1976). Nagayo (1977) reported that the incidence of type-III early cancer and of chronic gastric ulcer had both decreased markedly in Japan, and a current incidence figure of 0.6 per cent for ulcer-cancer among ulcer cases was quoted. A somewhat higher incidence of 2 per cent is reported by other Japanese workers (Yamagata and Hisamichi 1979). In Western countries the incidence of gastric cancer in pre-existing ulcer has been estimated as less than 1 per cent (Mason 1974).

Two further comments on the ulcer-cancer relationship may be made. First, the high incidence of gastric cancer reported in some follow-up studies of medically treated ulcer cases may be due to the inclusion of misdiagnosed patients. Hirohata (1968), for example, found a high incidence of cancer only during the first five years of follow-up and not in cases followed for 8-18 years. The experience of Montgomery and Richardson (1975) was similar. Among 210 ulcer patients followed, the incidence of cancer was 3.9 per cent in the first 18 months but only 0.6 per cent after 5 years. Second, it is well known that gastric cancers themselves may ulcerate, the reported incidence varying from 10 per cent (Mallory 1940) to 25 per cent in advanced tumours (Ming 1977*a*). In 802 early cancers studied by Nagayo (1977), deep ulceration was present in 12 per cent of cases. One commonly cited feature distinguishing malignant from benign ulcers is that the malignant ulcer does not heal. This view has been challenged by Sakita *et al.* (1971) who noted healing in 51 of 72 ulcerated early cancers. Healing was extensive in 18 cases and, in one case, was complete. The authors concluded that malignant ulcers might go through cycles of ulceration and healing and that healing of an ulcer did not exclude malignancy.

Polyps. Gastric polyps may be produced by a variety of conditions. Only epithelial polyps composed of abundant glandular elements are considered here. These lesions have been classified into five major types (Ming 1977*b*). *Inflammatory retention polyps* and *heterotopic polyps* consisting of pancreatic tissue or Brunner's glands are not precancerous. The precancerous status of *hamartomatous polyps* such as those of the Peutz-Jeghers syndrome is uncertain, though a few cases of possible malignant transformation have been reported (Reid 1974). The remaining two types, the *hyperplastic* (*regenerative*) *polyp* and *adenoma*, are subjects of major concern in regard to their relation to cancer.

The premalignant potential of gastric polyps was first recognized by Menetrier in 1888. A long period of confusion ensued in which many conflicting reports were published, and the premalignant potential of gastric polyp became a matter of controversy. When the polyps are evaluated according to their histological features, it becomes evident that they fall into two major categories. Hyperplastic polyps are composed of mature hyperplastic foveolar cells and varying numbers of pyloric-type glands (see Figs. 7.11 and 7.12). Adenomas consist basically of immature or dysplastic glands which often show features of intestinal metaplasia (Ming 1977*b*; Tomasulo 1971; see Figs. 7.13 and 7.14). Although this concept has been

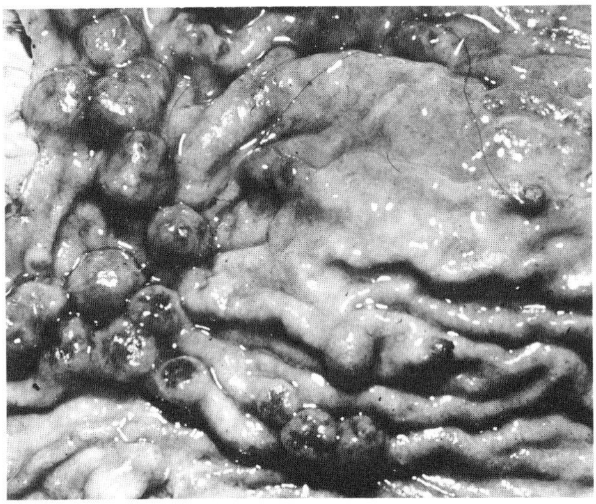

Fig. 7.11. Gross appearance of hyperplastic (regenerative) polyps of the stomach. Surface erosion is present at the tips of several of the polyps.

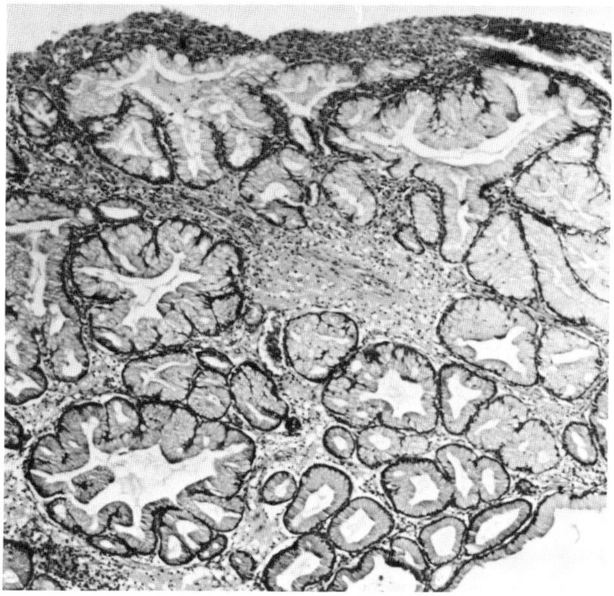

Fig. 7.12. A hyperplastic polyp of the stomach showing hyperplastic and dilated foveolae and stromal inflammation. ×95. H & E.

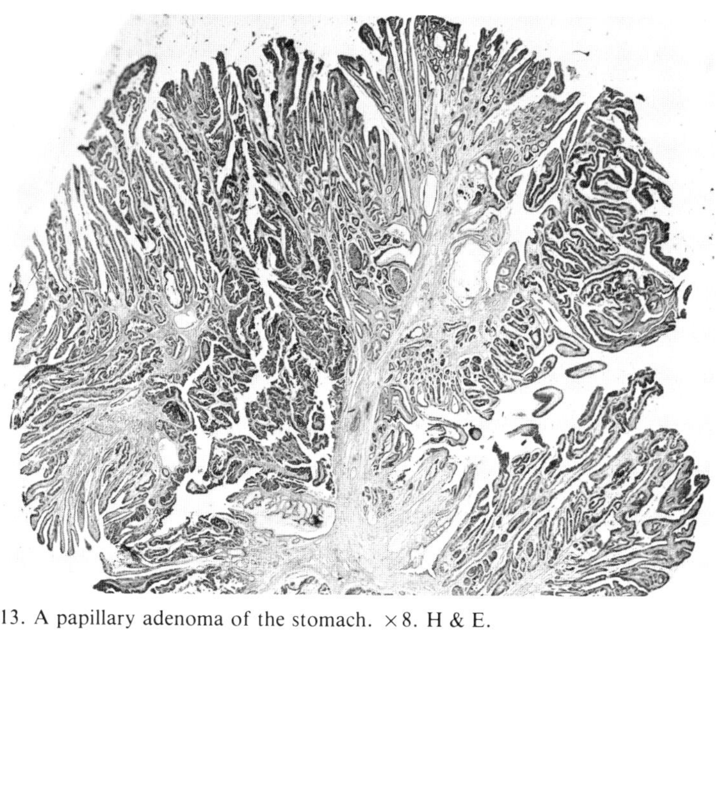

Fig. 7.13. A papillary adenoma of the stomach. ×8. H & E.

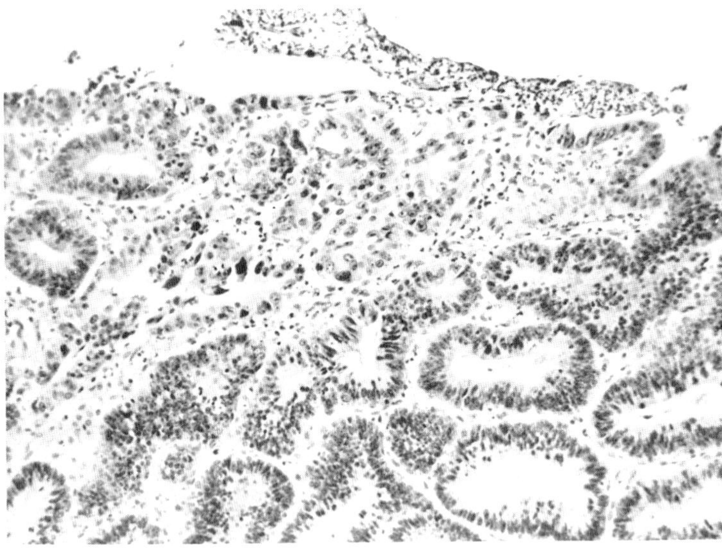

Fig. 7.14. A gastric adenoma showing pseudostratified immature cells in the adenoma together with a focus of carcinoma at the upper centre. ×150. H & E.

widely accepted, nomenclature varies in different accounts. Hyperplastic polyps have also been called hyperplasiogenous polyps (Elster 1976), regenerative polyps (Ming *et al.* 1967), gastric-type polyps (Morson 1955*b*), and type-I polyps (T. Nakamura 1967). Other terms used for gastric adenomas are villous polyps (Koch *et al.* 1979) and intestinal-type polyps (Morson 1955*b*). Hyperplastic polyps were called regenerative polyps by Ming *et al.* (1967) because they were thought to develop as a result of regenerative hyperplasia. The occurrence of such polyps at gastroenterostomy stomata (Janunger and Domelleof 1978; Koga *et al.* 1979; Savage and Jones 1979; Stemmermann and Hayashi 1979) and the spontaneous regression of such polyps noted by Elsborg *et al.* (1977) support this view. Various subtypes of polyps have also been recognized. At the early stage of development, the hyperplastic polyp is sessile. This form of polyp has been called focal foveolar hyperplasia (Elster 1976) and polypoid foveolar hyperplasia (Koch *et al.* 1979). Polyps with erosions and dimple-like depressions at their tips have been called type-II polyps by T. Nakamura (1967). The polyp with abundant, closely-packed, pyloric-type glands has been described as a hyperplastic adenomatous polyp by Koch *et al.* (1979).

Sugano *et al.* (1971) have observed an elevated 'verruca or flowerbed-like' lesion as a clinicopathological entity and called it atypical epithelium. This lesion is a variant of adenoma (Oota 1976) because its histological features are identical with those of a polypoid adenoma (Fig. 7.15). Ming (1977b) described it as a flat adenoma and T. Nakamura (1967) called it a type-III polyp.

The significance of separating gastric polyps into hyperplastic polyp and

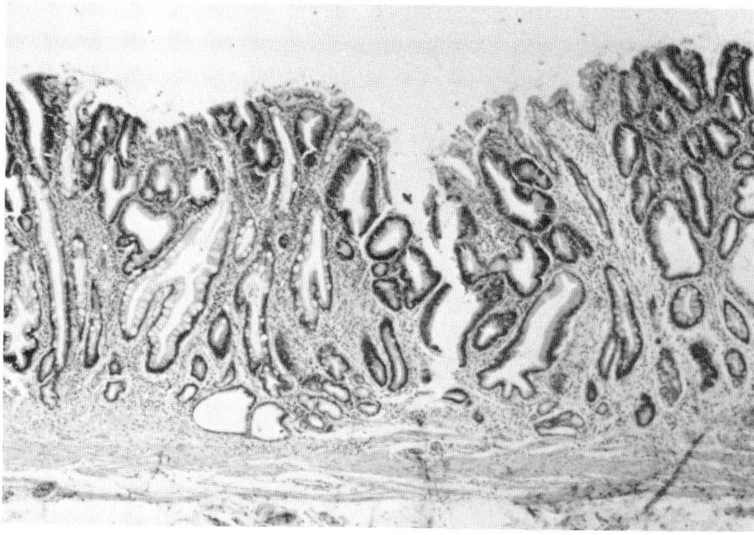

Fig. 7.15. Flat adenoma of the stomach. The adenomatous glands occupy upper one-half of the mucosa. Metaplastic and residual gastric glands are present in the deep mucosa. ×50. H & E.

adenoma lies in their vastly different premalignant potential. Malignant transformation is rarely observed in hyperplastic polyps (despite their wide variety of morphological appearances) though separate, coexisting carcinoma is present in the same stomach in about 22 per cent of cases (Ming 1977*b*). The incidence of cancer increases if metaplastic changes are also present (Kozuka *et al.* 1977). Malignant change in gastric adenomas, on the other hand, is common (see Fig. 7.14) and occurs in an average of 41 per cent of such lesions (Ming 1977*b*). The incidence of carcinoma rises with increasing size of the adenoma (Rieniets and Broders 1946; Walk 1951). Separate but coexisting carcinomas are present in an average of 42 per cent of adenoma cases (Ming 1977*b*). Gastric adenomas are thus clearly precancerous conditions while hyperplastic polyps may be considered precancerous only by virtue of their frequent association with coexisting cancer.

The consequences of partial gastrectomy and gastroenterostomy. There is an increasing awareness in recent years of the precancerous status of gastric remnants following partial gastrectomy for benign conditions. The cancer incidence increases with the length of the postoperative period. Stalsberg and Takdal (1971) reported that gastric cancer developed after partial gastrectomy 3.9 times more frequently than in the intact stomach between 15 and 24 years after the operation. The ratio increased to 5:1 during the next decade and to 8:4, 35 or more years after surgery. Most patients had Billroth II gastrectomies, probably because this is the most common ablative surgical procedure for the treatment of peptic ulcers. The intestinal and diffuse variants of gastric carcinoma occurred with equal frequency in such patients (Hammar 1976). While most authors noted the preoperative diagnosis of duodenal or of gastric ulcer had no effect on the subsequent cancer incidence (Schrumpf *et al.* 1977), some noted a preponderance of gastric ulcer as the original disease (Nicholls 1979).

Other gastric lesions also merit attention. Among 108 gastric stumps examined by endoscopic biopsy, gastritis and intestinal metaplasia were present in 36, dysplasia in 67, and carcinoma in 4 (Schrumpf *et al.* 1977). Dysplasia was severe in 3 cases. Only 1 case had a normal biopsy. The lesions were located at the stoma or in the nearby mucosa. In a series of 42 reoperated patients studied by Janunger and Domelleof (1978), carcinoma was present in 12, adenoma in 3, hyperplastic polyps in 21, and precancerous lesions in 4 cases. Endoscopic biopsy of 63 patients by Savage and Jones (1979) revealed mild-to-moderate dysplasia in about 50 per cent and polyps in 12 per cent of the cases. In occasional cases, the polyp encircled the stoma (Stemmermann and Hayashi 1979; Koga *et al.* 1979). The causc of thc mucosal changes is probably related to the reflux of bile into the stomach (Koga *et al.* 1979; Borchard *et al.* 1979).

Menetrier's disease and hyperplastic gastropathy. In 1888 Menetrier described the occurrence of gastric cancer associated with diffuse mucosal hyperplasia. The hyperplastic mucosa was likened to cerebral convolutions or to ruffled cloth or velvet. Menetrier called it *polyadenome en nappe.* This rare condition is now known eponymously as Menetrier's disease. The cause is unknown. Mild inflammation and oedema are often present but it is not considered to be an inflammatory condition. The main histological feature is hyperplasia of foveolar epithelium with cystic dilatations (Fig. 7.16) and, because of this feature, it may be regarded as a form of hyperplastic gastropathy. In another form, the hyperplasia is an element of the Zollinger-Ellison syndrome but others are clinically asymptomatic. Carcinoma in Menetrier's disease has been reported by Chusid *et al.* (1964), Reese *et al.* (1962), Williams *et al.* (1978), and by Benichou *et al.* (1980). Two types of gastric hyperplasia were called hypertrophic proliferative gastritis and hypertrophic glandular gastritis by Schindler (1965). According to this author 1.7 per cent of gastric carcinoma arose from the former type and 4.2 per cent from the latter type. Gastric carcinoma may be present in asymptomic glandular hyperplasia, but it is not known to occur in Zollinger-Ellison syndrome.

Precancerous change

Chronic atrophic gastritis and intestinal metaplasia are common changes but carcinoma arises in these conditions only infrequently. When carcinoma does develop, the tumour is associated with immature and often abnormal epithelium, particularly in the case of intestinal-type neoplasms (Grundmann

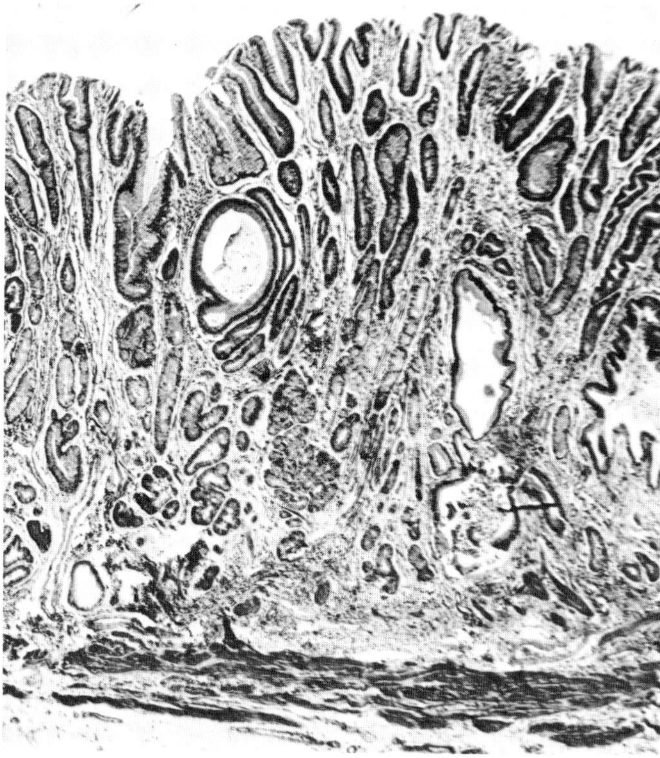

Fig. 7.16. Gastric mucosa in Menetrier's disease showing hyperplastic foveolae, cystic glands and loss of deep glands. ×50. H & E.

1975; Ming *et al.* 1967; Nagayo 1977). Such epithelium is variously called dysplastic, atypical, or anaplastic. Dysplasia is a broad term, implying abnormality of the epithelium at either cellular or tissue level. Any actively proliferating epithelium in normally quiescent regions of gastric mucosa may be considered dysplastic. The terms atypism and anaplasia have more restricted meanings. Atypical epithelium contains malformed cells or glands, and anaplastic epithelium is made up of undifferentiated or very poorly differentiated cells.

The importance of dysplasia as a precancerous change is further illustrated in gastric polyps and in stomachs after partial gastrectomy. Malignant change rarely occurs in hyperplastic polyps composed of mature glands, but it is common in adenomas composed of dysplastic cells (Ming *et al.* 1967). A similar distinction was made by Goldman and Appelman (1972) who divided gastric polyps into two groups depending on the presence or absence of cellular atypism. Carcinoma was present in 9 of 17 polyps with cytological atypia and in none of 105 polyps without atypia. In stomachs operated on more than 15 years earlier, dysplasia may be present at or near the gastroenterostomy stoma which is the favoured location for cancer development in such cases (Hammar 1976; Savage and Jones 1979).

Dysplastic epithelium may show gradations of abnormal proliferation, ranging from regenerative epithelium in an area of inflammation to severely anaplastic epithelium resembling cancer (Nagayo 1971; Ming 1979). These grades are apparent not only morphologically but also from studies of cell kinetics. Proliferation in the normal gastric mucosa occurs at the transition zone between the foveola and the neck of the glands (Oehlert *et al.* 1979). In mature metaplastic epithelium, proliferation occurs at the bottom of the glands (Deschner *et al.* 1972). In the immature or anaplastic epithelium of both metaplastic and nonmetaplastic mucosa, DNA synthesis extends on to the surface epithelium and cell turnover time is much shortened (Deschner *et al.* 1972; Willems and Bleiberg 1978). A detailed kinetic study was made by Oehlert *et al.* (1979) who designated three grades of dysplasia. In grade-1 dysplasia, the nuclear diameter increased from a normal of 6.5-7 μm to 8 μm, the mitotic index from a normal of 0.2-0.5 per cent to 1-1.5 per cent, and the thymidine-labelling index from a normal of 2-5 per cent to 10-15 per cent; the lifespan of cells was reduced to about one-fourth of that in normal glands and the number of proliferating cells doubled. These changes were further enhanced in grade-II and -III dysplasia. In the latter, the lifespan of cells was only about 1 day, compared to 8-20 days in normal gastric mucosa, and the number of proliferative cells per hour increased from 38 in the normal foveola to 170-228 in dysplastic glands. The proliferating zone increased correspondingly.

Several other taxonomic schemes have been proposed in addition to the grading system of Oehlert *et al.* (1979)—see Table 7.4. In 1971 Nagayo classified gastric epithelium into five groups—normal and benign lesions without atypia; benign lesions with slight atypia; borderline lesions; probable carcinoma; and definite carcinoma. In 1975 Grundmann divided dysplasia into low-grade and high-grade types: the latter included carcinoma *in situ* which, in contrast to the focally invasive intraepithelial carcinoma of Schade (1974), was not considered to be truly malignant. Grundmann also advanced evidence to support the view that intestinal-type cancer arose from glandular lesions, signet-ring tumours from the lower part of the tubular neck, and solid anaplastic antral cancers from dysplastic neck cells. Grundmann's classification of dysplasia was subsequently modified and dysplasia was divided into slight, moderate, and severe forms (Grundmann and Schlake 1979). Regenerative changes in inflammatory lesions were excluded. Ming (1979) separated dysplasia into four grades (Figs. 7.17-7.20). Proliferative glands in inflammatory conditions and hyperplastic glands with normal maturation such as those found in hyperplastic polyps and in Menetrier's disease are grouped as grade-1 dysplasia (Fig. 7.17). In grade-2 dysplasia, the glands exhibit excessive active proliferation with immature cells, pseudostratification and reduced secretion of mucus—a prime example

Table 7.4. *Comparison of different grading systems of gastric dysplasia*

Nagayo (1971)	No atypia	Slight atypia	Borderline	Probable cancer	Cancer
Grundmann (1975)	Low grade		High grade		
Grundmann and Schlake (1979)	Inflammatory change	Mild	Moderate	Severe	
Oehlert *et al.* (1979)		Grade I	Grade II	Grade III	
Ming (1979)	Grade 1	Grade 2	Grade 3	Grade 4	
Morson *et al.* (1980)	Inflammatory or regenerative change	Mild	Moderate	Severe	
ISGGC* (1982)	Simple hyperplasia	Severe hyperplasia	—— dysplasia ——	Possible cancer	

* International Study Group on Gastric Cancer

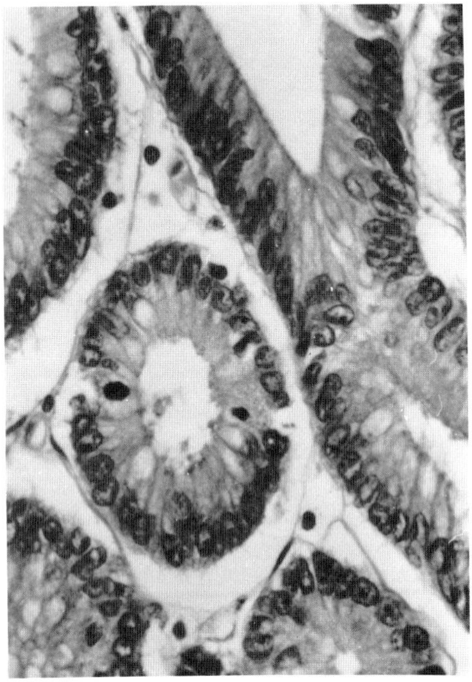

Fig. 7.17. Grade-1 dysplasia of metaplastic gastric glands showing crowded cells, reduced mucus in goblet cells, and mitotic figures. ×426. H & E. An example of simple hyperplasia using ISGGC nomenclature.

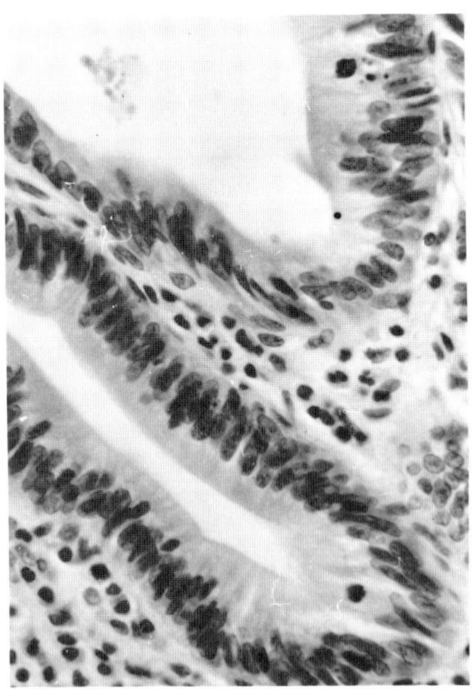

Fig. 7.18. Grade-2 (mild) dysplasia of metaplastic gastric glands showing pseudostratified cells, mitotic figures, and absence of goblet cells. A striated border is present on cells in the lower gland. ×426. H & E. An example of severe hyperplasia by ISGGC nomenclature.

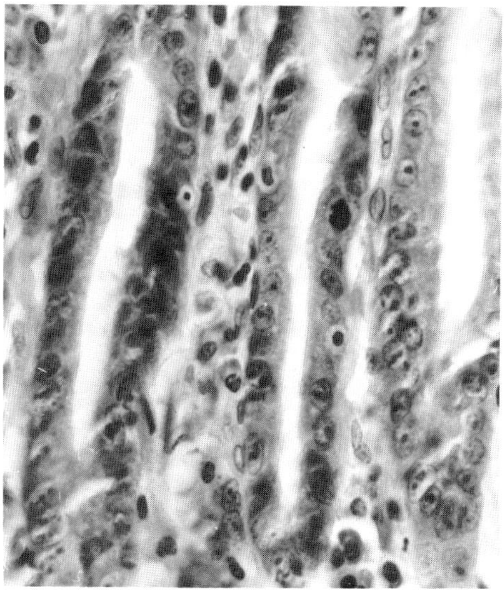

Fig. 7.19. Grade-3 (moderate) dysplasia of nonmetaplastic gastric glands showing immature cells with reduced cell height, loss of mucus secretion, some pleomorphism, and a mitotic figure. ×426. H & E.

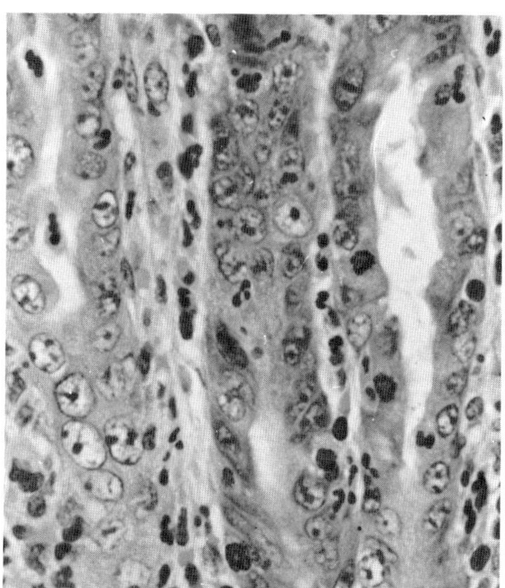

Fig. 7.20. Grade-4 (severe) dysplasia of nonmetaplastic gastric glands showing marked pleomorphism, prominent nucleoli, absence of mucus secretion, and mitotic figures. ×426. H & E.

is the glandular hyperplasia found in chronic gastritis (Fig. 7.18). In grade-3 dysplasia, mitoses and scattered atypical cells are present (Fig. 7.19). This form of dysplasia corresponds to the borderline lesion of Nagayo and is commonly seen in gastric adenomas. In grade-4 dysplasia, the cells are markedly atypical and sometimes anaplastic (Fig. 7.20). This grade corresponds to the severe dysplasia of Grundmann and Schlake and the probable carcinoma of Nagayo. These various classifications have been applied to both metaplastic and nonmetaplastic epithelium. Cuello *et al.*

(1979) have adopted a different approach by separating dysplasias of intestinalized mucosa into two groups: hyperplastic and adenomatous. In the hyperplastic type, the glands are normally spaced while in the adenomatous type the glands are crowded and closely packed. These types were further divided into mild and severe, depending on the degree of cellular disorganization and atypia. Cuello *et al.* also demonstrated that stomachs with mucosal dysplasia contained high concentrations of nitrite and nitrate in the fasting gastric juice. A grading system adopted by a WHO Committee was reported by Morson *et al.* (1980) and subsequently described by Nagayo (1981).

These numerous attempts to classify or grade dysplasia in gastric mucosa illustrate the difficulties of the problem, and the whole issue was recently reviewed by the Pathology Panel of the International Study Group on Gastric Cancer. A workshop meeting in June 1982 recommended that the term dysplasia should be applied only to highly abnormal mucosa. Orderly proliferating epithelium was described as hyperplastic (cf. Fig. 7.17); proliferating epithelium with many immature cells as severely hyperplastic (cf. Fig. 7.18); and moderately to severely abnormal epithelium as dysplastic (cf. Figs. 7.19 and 7.20). When dysplasia is so severe as to resemble cancer repeat biopsies should be undertaken. The more restricted use of the term dysplasia is desirable, but arguments over diagnostic criteria will undoubtedly continue.

Despite the variety of terms and classification systems, the basic concept that dysplasia is a precancerous lesion is generally accepted. It is evident that there are grades of dysplasia and that cancer may develop in severely dysplastic mucosa; but it should again be pointed out that dysplasia may regress and disappear. Among 498 patients with grade-III mucosal dysplasia followed by Oehlert (1979), regression occurred in 74.5 per cent within one year but the regression rate decreased as the duration of persistent dysplasia increased. Of 46 patients who had grade-III dysplasia for more than three years, only 7 showed regression; among the others, gastric carcinomas developed in 4 patients. Oehlert emphasized the importance of additional factors such as genetic composition and immune reactivity of the patient which might influence the natural history of dysplasia.

The association between mucosal dysplasia and carcinoma is clearest for intestinal-type cancers (Grundmann 1975), and malignant change in mucosa showing incomplete metaplasia (see p. 200) is particularly frequent (Onuma *et al.* 1980). On the other hand, some gastric cancers arising in *non-metaplastic* mucosa may also show intestinal features (Ming *et al.* 1967; Nevaillenen *et al.* 1977). Dysplasia is slight or absent in stomachs with diffuse or signet ring cell carcinomas (Grundmann 1975; Nagayo 1977; Ming 1979), and the precancerous lesion for this type of cancer remains to be established.

Experimental studies

Gastric cancers have been induced in animals by various means. The first successful method employed intramural injection of 3-methylcholanthrene; see Stewart (1971). Using this technique, Jarvi and Keyrilainen (1955) produced invasive lesions in the glandular stomach of mice which were composed of three types of cells: tall mucus-secreting cells, nonsecretory cells and small budding cells. The first two cell types had striated borders similar to intestinal cells, while the third category resembled cells from the pyloric region. The possible participation by cells from pyloric glands in the development of gastric cancer was also suggested by Snell *et al.* (1969) who induced gastric cancer in rats by feeding *N,N'*-2,7-fluorenylene-bisacetamide. The precancerous lesions consisted of atrophic glands and foci of hyperplasia and atypia. There was no intestinal metaplasia. The authors advocated a set of strict criteria for the diagnosis of experimental gastric cancer in rodents (see Stewart 1971). Only those tumours which had invaded the whole thickness of the stomach wall were considered as cancerous; histological abnormalities and superficial invasion were regarded as insufficient evidence for malignancy. In 1969 Hirose induced gastric carcinoma in mice by heavy local irradiation. Doses of 10000 rad caused mucosal atrophy in 100 per cent, ulcer in 78 per cent, atypical mucosal hyperplasia in 44 per cent, and adenocarcinoma in 28 per cent of stomachs. Smaller doses of 3000 rad induced intestinal metaplasia in the exceptionally short time of one week, but cancer did not develop during the subsequent observation period of 80 weeks (Watanabe 1978).

N-methyl-*N'*-nitro-*N*-nitrosoguanidine (MNNG) has been found to be a very efficient gastric carcinogen when given in the drinking water to rats and, more recently, to dogs. In most investigations with this compound, the diagnosis of cancer has been based on histological and cytological features rather than the ability of the tumour to invade through the gastric wall or to metastasize (Saito *et al.* 1970; Shimosato *et al.* 1971).

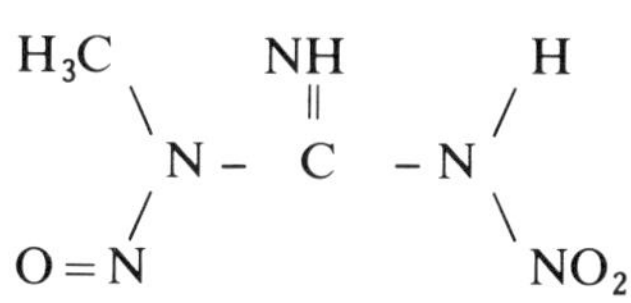

N-methyl-*N'*-nitro-*N*-nitrosoguanidine (MNNG).

Since MNNG regularly produces gastric cancer in susceptible species, the emphasis in experimental work has shifted from the search for an effective model to the identification of precancerous lesions. Cell kinetic studies have indicated that MNNG causes an expansion of the proliferative zone and increased DNA synthesis in gastric glands during the precancerous period (Deschner *et al.* 1979). Morphological investigations by Saito *et al.* (1970) in the rat showed that the initial gastric lesions consisted of mucosal erosion and atrophy followed first by regenerative hyperplasia, then by adenomatous hyperplasia and finally by invasive cancer. Intestinal metaplasia was observed only in stomachs with advanced cancer. Small doses of MNNG induced similar changes over longer time-spans (Fujima *et al.* 1970). Comparable observations have been made by other workers, but the incidence of intestinal metaplasia in the rat varies widely in different accounts (Tabuchi *et al.* 1974; Kobori *et al.* 1976; Matsukura *et al.* 1978). Mice and dogs treated with MNNG show a similar sequence of gastric atrophy, dysplastic hyperplasia and finally cancer, but intestinal metaplasia appears to be rare or absent (Shimosato *et al.* 1971; Saito *et al.* 1978; Sigaran and Con-Wong 1979). On the other hand, the closely related compound *N*-propyl-*N'*-nitro-*N*-nitrosoguanidine causes intestinal metaplasia in rodents *unaccompanied* by any subsequently increased incidence of carcinoma (Furihata *et al.* 1978; Sasajima 1979). These findings cast some doubt on the importance of intestinal metaplasia as a precancerous lesion in experimental animals and merit more detailed investigation.

Gastric polyps and adenomas were sometimes present in MNNG-treated mice (Sigaran and Con-Wong 1979), rats (Fujima *et al.* 1970) and dogs (Sasajima *et al.* 1977; Saito *et al.* 1978) but their relationship to carcinoma is not clear.

The role of chronic ulceration in experimental gastric carcinogenesis has been studied by several investigators. In 1965 Nagayo reported that traumatic gastric ulcers had no effect on cancer formation. Since then chronic ulcers have been induced by implantation of beeswax pellets into the gastric wall (Majima *et al.* 1967), by intramural injections of formalin (Saito *et al.* 1979), and by the administration of iodoacetamide (Takahashi *et al.* 1976): subsequent ingestion of MNNG produced cancers at the ulcer site in these experiments. The role of gastric acidity had also been investigated. Gastric cancer developed less frequently when gastrin was given to MNNG-treated rats (Tatsuta *et al.* 1977), and vagotomy increased the yield of gastric tumours in MNNG-treated dogs (Fujita *et al.* 1979).

Dahm *et al.* (1979) investigated the effects of MNNG on gastric stumps in rats. Carcinoma developed in 25 of 66 gastric remnants remaining after partial gastrectomy. The tumours were preceded by glandular hyperplasia and increasing degrees of dysplasia. The induction period of cancer was reduced by more than ten weeks compared with a group of rats treated with MNNG without gastric surgery. No difference in cancer incidence was seen between rats treated by Billroth I or Billroth II gastrectomies, but the presence of duodenal reflux increased the numbers of tumours.

Most MNNG-induced carcinomas have shown a glandular or intestinal type of histology (Kobori *et al.* 1977; Dahm *et al.* 1979). Diffuse and signet-ring cell carcinomas have occasionally been reported (Saito *et al.* 1970;

Shimosato *et al.* 1971; Sasajima *et al.* 1977; Furihata *et al.* 1978). Electron-microscopic and histochemical studies by Kobori *et al.* (1977) revealed that most tumours were composed predominantly of undifferentiated cells. Highly differentiated gastric and intestinal mucosal cells (and even squamous cells) were also identified, but intestinal metaplasia was absent in the remaining portions of the stomach in this experiment. Such observations are consistent with the view that gastric cancer cells are capable of differentiating into the intestinal type of cells even though they may not have originated from metaplastic epithelium.

General comments

Oesophageal and gastric cancers are deadly diseases. Preventive measures are not yet possible, and early diagnosis and treatment are the best means to reduce their mortality—as documented by reports from China and Japan where mass survey methods are being used most effectively for early detection. Such an approach is justified in these regions because of the exceptionally high incidence of these cancers. In countries with lower incidence rates for oesophageal and gastric cancers, careful and frequent examination of individuals with precancerous states is more feasible. Knowledge of these precancerous states thus not only brings us closer to an understanding of carcinogenic processes in the stomach and oesophagus, but it also enables us to select high-risk populations for close follow-up studies.

Increased risks of oesophageal and gastric carcinomas are known to be prevalent in a number of conditions which have been reviewed in this chapter. They are varied and seemingly unrelated, but the common feature linking them to the malignant process appears to be the increased risk of developing abnormal or dysplastic epithelium.

Precancerous conditions are apparently brought about by factors which are often not inherently carcinogenic. Such factors may be exogenous or endogenous and they are extremely diverse: in the stomach they include the autoimmune gastritis of pernicious anaemia, gastric stumps and gastric polyps and, in the oesophagus, conditions such as lye stricture, achalasia and Barrett's oesophagus. By contrast, precancerous change (i.e. mucosal dysplasia) appears the same irrespective of the wider pathological context in which it develops. Evidence for the precancerous nature of mucosal dysplasia is essentially twofold: dysplasia commonly coexists with cancer in the same organ, and cancer develops frequently in dysplastic epithelium. The first line of evidence has been derived from studies of the cancer-bearing stomach and oesophagus in man (particularly the stomach), and from investigations of the development of gastric and oesophageal cancers in experimental animals. The second line of evidence stems mainly from follow-up studies in man and from experimental work in which animals are examined sequentially at different time periods after administration of a chemical carcinogen. It must, however, be emphasized that dysplastic changes may regress, and that cancer develops only in severely dysplastic epithelium in which the changes have been present for a long time.

Animal experiments have partly clarified our understanding of carcinogenic processes in the stomach and oesophagus, but shortcomings are evident. Experimental induction of oesophageal cancer, for example, commonly produces a large number of benign papillomas which (in man) are rare and do not appear to be precancerous. Experimental studies of gastric carcinogenesis have been much more fruitful. Investigations with MNNG have faithfully reproduced lesions seen in man and they have confirmed the precancerous nature of conditions such as mucosal atrophy, gastric ulcer, and certain postgastrectomy states; but one important question relating to intestinal metaplasia remains unanswered. It was noted earlier that intestinal metaplasia has rarely been observed in MNNG-treated dogs even though most of the MNNG-induced gastric cancers in this species are of intestinal type. It is possible that the metaplastic focus had been replaced by the cancerous tissue, but evidence for this hypothesis is wanting. Thus far, the significance of various lesions found in experimental animals is judged mainly by their coexistence with carcinoma and not by sequential studies of the lesion *in the same animal*. Such investigations are possible in the dog, which is large enough for repeated endoscopic biopsies, and this approach needs to be developed in the future. The precancerous lesion for the diffuse type of gastric carcinoma has so far evaded detection. In man, this form of cancer is often observed developing in otherwise normal gastric epithelium. Signet-ring cells, the prototype of cancer cells in diffuse gastric carcinomas, have been found in experimentally-induced gastric cancers but their relationship to any dysplastic epithelium has not been clarified. This question merits further attention in view of the proposal that intestinal-type and diffuse-type cancers may be tumours with different geographical distributions and perhaps different aetiologies (Muñoz and Matko 1972). It is now well known that the majority of gastric cancer cells (irrespective of their overall histological pattern) have intestinal features, and it has been suggested that they may differentiate into intestinal-type cells even if they arise from nonmetaplastic mucosa (Ming *et al.* 1967). This view is supported by the finding of both gastric and intestinal cells in MNNG-induced tumours, unaccompanied by intestinal metaplasia in the uninvolved mucosa (Kobori *et al.* 1977).

One obvious difference between oesophageal and gastric cancers is that gastric cancers usually occur in an abnormal mucosa while oesophageal cancers are often found in a morphologically normal oesophagus. Several defined precancerous conditions appear to play a significant role in the development of gastric cancers but they are much less apparent in the majority of oesophageal cancers. This situation may simply be due to a previous lack of adequate study as indicated by recent findings of a high incidence of chronic oesophagitis in the high-risk regions of north-east Iran and China (Crespi *et al.* 1979; Muñoz *et al.* 1982). Further confirmation of these observations in other high-risk regions by endoscopic biopsy will help to clarify the importance of chronic oesophagitis as a precancerous condition.

It was noted earlier that the causes of some precancerous conditions are apparently noncarcinogenic. But in certain conditions, notably gastric atrophy and intestinal metaplasia, actual mucosal stimulation by the carcinogen (or carcinogens) may well be an important factor—a conclusion that emerges from several experimental studies. It must, however, be emphasized again that precancerous changes occur in only a minority of patients with precancerous conditions, that such changes are reversible, and that cancer develops in only a small number of patients with severely dysplastic epithelium. The difficulties in quantifying the eventual risk of cancer development are discussed elsewhere in this book, but the present situation with respect to the oesophagus and stomach illustrates some of the basic problems in human carcinogenesis in any target organ. Do the various stages of cancer development described here represent one continuous process or a series of separate processes? And are single or multiple agents involved?

References

Ackerman, L.V., Weinstein, I.B., and Kaplan, H.S. (1978). Cancer of the esophagus. In *Cancer in China* (ed. H.S. Kaplan and P.J. Tsuchitani), p. 111. Alan R. Liss, New York.

Adler, R.H. and Rodriguez, J. (1959). The association of hiatus hernia and gastro-esophageal malignancy. *J. Thoracic Surg.* **37**, 553.

Akuamoa, G. (1969). Achalasia oesophagi and associated diseases. *Acta Chir Scand.* **135**, 421.

Ariga, K. and Takahasi, K. (1976). Gastric mass survey. *Gann Monogr. Cancer Res.* **18**, 99.

Barrett, N.R. (1957). The lower esophagus lined by columnar epithelium. *Surgery* **41**, 881.

Benichou, J., Ohana, S., Testas, P., and Monod-Broca, P. (1980). Menetrier's disease and gastric tumors. *J. Chir.* **117**, 161.

Bigelow, N.H. (1953). Carcinoma of the esophagus developing at the site of lye stricture. *Cancer* **6**, 1159.

Bigger, I.A. and Vinson, P.P. (1950). Carcinoma secondary to burn of the esophagus from ingestion of lye. Report of a case. *Surgery* **28**, 887.

Borchard, F., Mittelstaedt, A., and Kieker, R. (1979). Incidence of epithelial dysplasia after partial gastric resection. *Pathol. Res. Pract.* **164**, 282.

Cai, H.Y., Lin, P.Z., and Guan, X.J. (1980*a*). Studies on experimentally induced cancer and precancerous lesions of the esophagus and forestomach in rats and mice. *Chin. med. J.* **60**, 87.

—— Shu, Y.J., Wang, G.Q., Wu, E.R., Lin, P.Z., Liu, S.F., and Li, M.X. (1980*b*). Treatment of patients with severe dysplasia of esophageal epithelium. I. Observation of the therapeutic effects of antitumor B, antitumor B III and tilorone. *Chin. J. Oncol.* **2**, 92.

Cheli, R., Santi, L., Ciancamerla, G., and Canciani, G. (1973). A clinical and statistical follow-up study of atrophic gastritis. *Amer. J. digest. Dis.* **18**, 1061.

Chisholm, M., Ardran, G.M., Callender, S.T., and Wright, R. (1971). A follow-up study of patients with postcricoid webs. *Quart. J. Med.* **40**, 409.

Chusid, E.L., Hirsch, R.L., and Colcher, H. (1964). Spectrum of hypertrophic gastropathy. Giant rugal folds, polyposis and carcinoma of the stomach—case report and review of the literature. *Arch. intern. Med.* **114**, 621.

Coordinating Group for the Research of Esophageal Carcinoma, Chinese Academy of Medical Sciences and Honan Province (1974). *Studies on the relationship between epithelial dysplasia and carcinoma of the esophagus.* Peking, China.

Correa, P., Sasano, N., Stemmermann, G.N., and Haenszel, W. (1973). Pathology of gastric carcinoma in Japanese populations: comparisons between Miyagi Prefective, Japan, and Hawaii. *J. Nat. Cancer Inst.* **51**, 1449.

—— Cuello, C., Duque, E., Burbano, L.C., Garcia, F.T., Bolanos, O., Brown, C., and Haenszel, W. (1976). Gastric cancer in Colombia. III. Natural history of precursor lesions. *J. Nat. Cancer Inst.* **57**, 1027.

Creagan, R.T. and Fraumeni, J.F., Jr. (1973). Familial gastric cancer and immunologic abnormalities. *Cancer* **32**, 1325.

Crespi, M., Muñoz, N., Grasi, A., Aramesh, B., Amiri, G., Mojtabai, A., and Casale, V. (1979). Oesophageal lesions in northern Iran: a premalignant condition? *Lancet* **2**, 217.

Cuello, C., Correa, P., Zarama, G., Lopez, J., Murray, J., and Cordillo, G. (1979). Histopathology of gastric dysplasias. Correlations with gastric juice chemistry. *Amer. J. Surg. Pathol.* **3**, 491.

Dahm, K., Werner, B., Eichen, R., and Mitschke, H. (1979). Experimental cancer of the gastric stump. In *Gastric cancer* (ed. C.H. Herfarth and P. Schlag), p. 44. Springer-Verlag, Berlin.

Deschner, E.E., Winawer, S.J., and Lipkin, M. (1972). Patterns of nucleic acid and protein synthesis in normal human gastric mucosa and atrophic gastritis. *J. Nat. Cancer Inst.* **48**, 1567.

—— Tamura, K., and Bralow, S.P. (1979). Sequential histopathology and cell kinetic changes in rat pyloric mucosa during gastric carcinogenesis induced by *N*-methyl-*N′*-nitro-*N*-nitrosoguanidine. *J. Nat. Cancer Inst.* **63**, 171.

Dunham, L.J. and Sheets, R.H. (1974). Effects of esophageal constriction on benzo(α)pyrene carcinogenesis in hamster esophagus and forestomach. *J. Nat. Cancer Inst.* **53**, 875.

Elsborg, L., Andersen, D., Myhere-Jensen, O., and Bastrup-Madsen, P. (1977). Gastric mucosal polyps in pernicious anemia. *Scand. J. Gastroenterol.* **12**, 49.

—— Mosbech, J. (1979). Pernicious anaemia as a risk factor in gastric cancer. *Acta med. Scand.* **206**, 315.

Elster, K. (1974). A new approach to the classification of gastric polyps. *Endoscopy* **6**, 44.

Fujima, S., Kogure, K., Sugimura, T., and Takayama, S. (1970). The effect of limited administration of *N*-methyl-*N′*-nitro-*N*-nitrosoguanidine on the induction of stomach cancer in rats. *Cancer Res.* **30**, 842.

Fujita, M., Takami, M., Usugane, M., Nampei, S., and Taguchi, T. (1979). Enhancement of gastric carcinogenesis in dogs given *N*-methyl-*N′*-nitro-*N*-nitrosoguanidine following vagotomy. *Cancer Res.* **39**, 811.

Furihata, C., Kawachi, T., Sasajima, K., Matsukura, N., Sugimura, T., and Matsuda, A. (1978). Experimental stomach carcinogenesis. *Eur. J. Cancer, Suppl.*, p. 31.

Goldman, D.S. and Appelman, H.D. (1972). Gastric mucosal polyps. *Amer. J. clin. Pathol.* **58**, 434.

Goldman, H. and Ming, S.C. (1968*a*). Mucins in normal and neoplastic gastro-intestinal epithelium. Histochemical distribution. *Arch. Pathol.* **85**, 850.

—— —— (1968*b*). Fine structure of intestinal metaplasia and adenocarcinoma of the human stomach. *Lab. Invest.* **18**, 203.

Grundmann, E. (1975). Histologic types and possible initial stages in early gastric carcinoma. *Beitr. Pathol.* **154**, 256.

—— Schlake, W. (1979). Histology of possible precancerous stages in the stomach. In *Gastric cancer* (ed. C.H. Herfarth and P. Schlag), p. 72. Springer-Verlag, Berlin.

Haenszel, W., Kurihara, M., Locke, F.B., Shimuzu, K., and Segi, M. (1976). Stomach cancer in Japan. *J. Nat. Cancer Inst.* **56**, 265.

Haggitt, R.C., Tryzelaar, J., Ellis, F.H., and Colcher, H. (1978). Adenocarcinoma complicating columnar epithelium-lined (Barrett's) esophagus. *Amer. J. clin. Pathol.* **70**, 1.

Hammar, E. (1976). The localization of precancerous changes and carcinoma after previous gastric operation for benign conditions. *Acta Pathol. Microbiol. Scand.* **84A**, 495.

Harper, P.S., Harper, R.M.J., and Howell-Evans, A.W. (1970). Carcinoma of the oesophagus with tylosis. *Quart. J. Med.* **38**, 317.

Harris, O.D., Cooke, W.T., Thompson, H., and Waterhouse, J.A.H. (1967). Malignancy in adult coeliac disease, and idiopathic steatorrhea. *Amer. J. Med.* **42**, 899.

Herbst, J.J., Berenson, M.M., McCloskey, D.W., and Wiser, W.C. (1978). Cell proliferation in esophageal columnar epithelium (Barrett's esophogus). *Gastro-enterol.* **75**, 683.

Herrold, K. McD. (1966). Epidermoid carcinomas of esophagus and forestomach induced in Syrian hamsters by *N*-nitroso-*N*-methylurethan. *J. Nat. Cancer Inst.* **37**, 389.

Hirohata, T. (1968). Mortality from gastric cancer and other causes after medical or surgical treatment for gastric ulcer. *J. Nat. Cancer Inst.* **41**, 895.

—— Kuratsune, M. (1969). The geographical comparison of mortality from cancer of the stomach and ulcer of the stomach in Japan. *Brit. J. Cancer* **23**, 465.

Hirose, F. (1969). Induction of gastric adenocarcinoma in mice by localized X-irradiation. *Gann* **60**, 253.

Hirota, T., Itabashi, M., Kitaoka, H., Oguro, Y., Yamada, T., and Ichikawa, H. (1980). Chronological trend in morphological features of early stomach cancer—recent changes especially of macroscopic findings. *Stomach Intest.* **16**, 13.

Holmes, G.K.T., Stokes, P.L., Sorahan, T.M., Prior, P., Waterhouse, J.A.H., and Cooke, W.T. (1976). Coeliac disease, gluten-free diet and malignancy. *Gut* **17**, 612.

Hopkins, R.A. and Postlethwait, R.W. (1981). Caustic burns and carcinoma of the esophagus. *Ann. Surg.* **194**, 146.

Howel-Evans, W., McConnell, R.B., Clarke, C.A., and Sheppard, P.H. (1958). Carcinoma of oesophagus with keratosis palmaris et plantaris (tylosis). *Quart. J. Med.* (*N.S.*) **27**, 413.

Hurst, A.F. (1929). Precursors of carcinoma of the stomach. *Lancet* **2**, 1023.

Imai, T., Kubo, T., and Watanabe, H. (1971). Chronic gastritis in Japanese with reference to high incidence of gastric carcinoma. *J. Nat. Cancer Inst.* **47**, 179.

Janunger, K.G. and Domelleof, L. (1978). Gastric polyps and precancerous mucosal changes after partial gastrectomy. *Acta Chir. Scand.* **144**, 293.

Jarvi, O. and Keyrilainen, O. (1955). On the cellular structures of the epithelial invasions in the glandular stomach of mice caused by intramural application of 20-methylcholanlrene. *Acta Pathol. Microbiol. Scand. Suppl.* **111**, 72.

Jass, J.R. (1981). Mucin histochemistry of the columnar epithelium of the oesophagus: a retrospective study. *J. clin. Pathol.* **34**, 866.

—— and Filipe, M.I. (1979). A variant of intestinal metaplasia associated with gastric carcinoma: a histochemical study. *Histopathol.* **3**, 191.

—— —— (1981). The mucin profiles of normal gastric mucosa, intestinal metaplasia and its variants and gastric carcinoma. *Histochem. J.* **13**, 931.

Johansen, A. (1978). Atrophic gastritis and intestinal metaplasia as a precancerous stage with special reference to early gastric cancer. *Eur. J. Cancer. Suppl.*, p. 49.

Justa-Vierra, J.O. and Haight, C. (1969). Achalasia and carcinoma of the esophagus. *Surg. Gynec. Obstet.* **128**, 1081.

Kawachi, T., Kurisu, M., Numanyu, N., Sasajima, K., and Sano, T. (1976). Precancerous changes in the stomach. *Cancer Res.* **36**, 2673.

Kobori, O. and Oota, K. (1974). Mucous substances and enzyme histochemistry of non-neoplastic and neoplastic gastric epithelium in man. *Acta Pathol. Jap.* **24**, 119.

——, Gedigk, P., and Totovic, V. (1976). Early changes of glandular stomach in Wistar rats ingesting *N*-methyl-*N'*nitro-*N*-nitrosoguanidine (MNNG); with special reference to light microscopic, electron microscopic and enzyme histochemical study of the regenerating epithelium induced by MNNG. *Z. Krebsforsch.* **7**, 127.

—— —— —— (1977). Adenomatous changes and adenocarcinoma of glandular stomach in Wistar rats induced by *N*-methyl-*N'*-nitro-*N*-nitrosoguanidine. An electron microscopic and histochemical study. *Virchows Arch. Pathol.* (*Pathol. Anat*). **373**, 37.

Koch, H.K., Lesch, R., Cremer, M., and Oehlert, W. (1979). Polyp and polypoid foveolar hyperplasia in gastric biopsy specimens and the precancerous prevalence. *Front. Gastrointest. Res.* **4**, 183.

Koga, S., Watanabe, H., and Enjoji, M. (1979). Stomal polypoid hypertrophic gastritis. A polypoid gastric lesion at gastroenterostomy sites. *Cancer* **43**, 647.

Konjetzny, G.E. (1913). Ueber die Beziehungen des Chronische gastritis mit ihren Folgeerscheinungen und des chronischen Magenulcus zur Entwicklung des Magenkrebses. *Beitr. Z. Klin, Chir.* **85**, 455.

Kozuka, S., Masamoto, K., Suzuki, S., Kubota, K., and Yokoyama, Y. (1977). Histogenic types and size of polypoid lesions in the stomach, with special reference to cancerous change. *Gann* **68**, 267.

Kubo, T. (1974). Geographic pathology of gastric carcinoma. *Acta Pathol. jap.* **24**, 465.

Kuru, M. (1967). *Atlas of early carcinoma of the stomach.* Nakayama-Shoten, Tokyo.

Lauren, P. (1965). The two main histological types of gastric carcinoma: diffuse and so-called intestinal-type carcinoma. *Acta Pathol. Microbiol. Scand.* **64**, 31.

Levison, D.A., Hopwood, D., Morgan, R.G., Coghill, G., Milne, G.A., and Wormsley, K.G. (1979). Oesophageal neoplasia in male Wister rats due to parenteral di(2-hydroxypropyl)-nitrosamine (DHPN): A combined histopathological, histochemical and electron microscopic study. *J. Pathol.* **129**, 31.

Li, F.P. and Shiang, E.L. (1979). Screening for oesophageal cancer in 62000 Chinese. *Lancet* **2**, 804.

McDonald, G.B., Brand, D.L., and Thorning, D.R. (1977). Multiple adenomatous neoplasms arising in columnar-lined (Barrett's) esophagus. *Gastroenterology* **72**, 1317.

Majima, S., Yamaguchi, I., Karube, K., Teshima, T., and Yoshida, K. (1965). A histopathologic study on the origins of early carcinoma of stomach. *Tohoku J. exp. Med.* **86**, 348.

——, Takahashi, T., Yoshida, K., Karube, K., Machida, T., Narisawa, T., Hoshi, H., Hiroki, T., Ito, K., and Kurata, Y. (1967). Atypical epithelial proliferation

in the course of experimental production of ulcer-carcinoma of the stomach. *Tohoku J. exp. Med.* **93**, 363.
Mallory, T.B. (1940). Carcinoma in situ of the stomach and its bearing on the histogenesis of malignant ulcers. *Arch. Pathol.* **30**, 348.
Mandard, A.M., Chasle, J., and Marnay, J. (1978). Cancer of the oesophagus and dysplasia (primary results). *Eur. J. Cancer Suppl.,* p. 15.
Mason, M.K. (1974). Surface carcinoma of the stomach. In *Early gastric cancer: current status of diagnosis* (ed. E. Grundmann, H. Grunze, and S. Witte), p. 39. Springer-Verlag, Berlin.
Matsukura, N., Kawachi, T., Sasajima, K., Sano, T., Sugimura, T., and Hirota, T. (1978). Induction of intestinal metaplasia in the stomachs of rats by *N*-methyl-*N'*-nitro-*N*-nitrosoguanidine. *J. Nat. Cancer Inst.* **61**, 141.
——, N., Suzuki, K., Kawachi, T., Aoyagi, M., Sugima, T., Kifaoka, H., Numajiri, H., Shirota, A., Itabashi, M., and Hirota, T. (1980). Distribution of marker enzymes and mucin in intestinal metaplasia in human stomach and relation of complete and incomplete types of intestinal metaplasia to minute gastric carcinomas. *J. nat. Cancer Inst.* **65**, 231.
Menetrier, P. (1888). Des polyadenomas gastriques et de leurs rapports avec le cancer de l'estomac. *Arch. Physiol. Norm. Path.* **1**, 32.
Ming, S.C. (1977*a*). Gastric carcinoma. A pathobiological classification. *Cancer* **39**, 2475.
—— (1977*b*). The classification and significance of gastric polyps. In *The gastrointestinal tract* (ed. J.H. Yardley and D.M. Morson), p. 149. Williams and Witkins, Baltimore.
—— (1979). Dysplasia of gastric epithelium. *Front. Gastrointes. Res.* **4**, 164.
—— Goldman, H. (1965). Gastric polyps: A histogenetic classification and its relation to carcinoma. *Cancer* **18**, 721.
—— —— Freiman, D.G. (1967). Intestinal metaplasia and histogenesis of carcinoma in human stomach. Light and electron microscopic study. *Cancer* **20**, 1418.
Montgomery, R.D. and Richardson, B.P. (1975). Gastric ulcer and cancer. *Quart. J. Med.* **44**, 591.
Morson, B.C. (1955*a*). Carcinoma arising from areas of intestinal metaplasia in the gastric mucosa. *Brit. J. Cancer* **9**, 377.
—— (1955*b*). Gastric polyps composed of intestinal epithelium. *Brit. J. Cancer* **9**, 550.
——, Sobin, L.H., Grundmann, E., Johansen, A., Nagayo, T., and Serck-Hansen (1980). Precancerous conditions and epithelial dysplasia in the stomach. *J. clin. Pathol.* **33**, 711.
Mukada, T., Sato, E., and Sasano, N. (1976). Comparative studies on dysplasia of esophageal epithelium in four prefectures of Japan (Miyagi, Nara, Wakayama and Aomori) with reference to risk of carcinoma. *Tohoku J. exp. Med.* **119**, 51.
—— Sasano, N., and Sato, E. (1978). Evaluation of esophageal dysplasia by cytofluorometric analysis. *Cancer* **41**, 1399.
Muñoz, N., and Asvall, J. (1971). Time trends of intestinal and diffuse types of gastric cancer in Norway. *Int. J. Cancer* **8**, 144.
—— Matko, I. (1972). Histologic types of gastric cancer and its relationship with intestinal metaplasia. *Recent Results Cancer Res.* **39**, 99.
——, Crespi, M., Grassi, A., Qing, W.G., Quiong, S., and Cai, L.Z. (1982). Precursor lesions of oesophageal cancer in high-risk populations in Iran and China. *Lancet* **i**, 876.
Naef, A.P., Savary, M., and Ozzello, L. (1975). Columnar-lined lower esophagus: an acquired lesion with malignant predisposition. Report on 140 cases of Barrett's esophagus with 12 adenocarcinomas. *J. thorac, cardiovasc. Surg.* **70**, 826.

Nagayo, T. (1965). Effect of oral administration of N,N′2,7-fluorenylene-bisacetamide combined with traumatic ulcers of the glandular stomach of buffalo rats. *J. Nat. Cancer Inst.* **35**, 829.

—— (1971). Histological diagnosis of biopsied gastric mucosae with special reference to that of borderline lesions. *Gann Monogr. Cancer Res.* **11**, 245.

—— (1977). Precursors of human gastric cancer: their frequencies and histological characteristics. In *Pathophysiology of carcinogenesis in digestive organs* (ed. E. Farber), p. 151. Univ. Tokyo Press, Tokyo.

Nakahara, K. (1978). Special features of intestinal metaplasia and its relation to early gastric carcinoma in man: observation by a method in which leucine aminopeptidase activity is used. *J. Nat. Cancer Inst.* **61**, 693.

Nakamura, K., Sugano, H., and Takagi, K. (1968). Carcinoma of the stomach in incipient phase: its histogenesis and histological appearance. *Gann* **56**, 251.

Nakamura, T. (1967). Histopathological classification of gastric polyp and its malignant change. *Recent Advan. Gastroenterol.* **1**, 477.

Napalkov, N. and Pozharisski, K.M. (1969). Morphogenesis of experimental tumors of the esophagus. *J. Nat. Cancer. Inst.* **42**, 927.

Nevalainen, T.J. and Jarvi, O.H. (1977). Ultrastructure of intestinal and diffuse type gastric carcinoma. *J. Pathol.* **122**, 129.

Nicholls, J.C. (1979). Stump cancer following gastric surgery. *World J. Surg.* **3**, 731.

Oehlert, W., (1979). Biological significance of dysplasia of the epithelium and of atrophic gastritis. In *Gastric cancer* (ed. C.H. Herfaith and P. Schlag), p. 91. Springer-Verlag, Berlin.

—— Keller, P., Henke, M., and Strauch, M. (1979). Gastric mucosal dysplasia: What is its clinical significance? *Front. Gastrointest. Res.* **4**, 173.

Onuma, C., Hirota, T., Itabashi, M., Misaka, R., Yoshida, H., Unagami, M., Oguro, Y., Yoshimori, M., Kitaoka, H., Kawachi, T., and Matsukura, N. (1980). Spatial relation between gastric atypical epithelium and subtypes of intestinal metaplasia. *Prog. digest. Endosc.* **17**, 115.

Oohara, T., Tohma, H., Takezoe, K., Ukawa, S., Johjima, Y., Asakura, R., Aono, G., and Kurosaka, H. (1982). Minute gastric cancers less than 5 mm. in diameter. *Cancer* **50**, 801.

Oota, K. (1963). Role of gastric ulcer in the causation of gastric cancer in Japan: a histopathological study of 3000 gastrectomy materials. *Acta Un. Int. Cancer* **19**, 1208.

—— (1976). Early phase of development of human gastric cancer. *Gann Monogr. Cancer Res.* **18**, 77.

Ozzello, L., Savary, M., and Roethlisberger, B. (1977). Columnar mucosa of the distal esophagus in patients with gastroesophageal reflux. *Pathol. Ann.* **12**, 41.

Pagnini, C.A. and Bozzola, L. (1981). Precancerous significance of colonic type intestinal metaplasia. *Tumori* **69**, 113.

Pattinson, J.N., Osborne, G., and Morson, B.C. (1955). Hiatus hernia with adenocarcinoma arising in the region of the cardia. *J. Fac. Radiol.* **7**, 90.

Pierce, W.S., MacVaugh, H., III, and Johnson, J. (1970). Carcinoma of the esophagus arising in patients with achalasia of the cardia. *J. thorac. cardiovasc. Surg.* **59**, 335.

Postlethwait, R.W. and Musser, A.W. (1974). Changes in the esophagus in 1000 autopsy specimens. *J. thorac. cardiovasc. Surg.* **68**, 953.

Reese, D. F., Hodgson, J.R., and Docherty, M.B. (1962). Giant hypertrophy of the gastric mucosa (Menetrier's diseases): a correlation of the roentgenographic, pathologic and clinical findings. *Amer. J. Roentgenol.* **88**, 619.

Reid, J.D. (1974). Intestinal carcinoma in the Peutz-Jeghers syndrome. *J. Amer. med. Assoc.* **229**, 833.

Reuber, M.D. (1977). Histopathology of preneoplastic and neoplastic lesions of the esophagus in BUF rats ingesting diethylnitrosamine. *J. Nat. Cancer Inst.* **58**, 313.

Ribeiro, M.M., Sarmento, J.A. Simoes, M.A.S., and Bastos, J. (1981). Prognostic significance of Lauren and Ming classifications and other pathologic parameters in gastric carcinoma. *Cancer* **47**, 780.

Rieniets, J.H. and Broders, A.C. (1946). Gastric adenomas: a pathologic study. *West. J. Surg. Obstet. Gynecol.* **54**, 21.

Ruddell, W.S., Bone, E.S., Hill, M.J., and Walters, C.L. (1978). Pathogenesis of gastric cancer in pernicious anaemia. *Lancet* **1**, 521.

Saito, T., Inokuchi, K., Takayama, S. and Sugimura, T. (1970). Sequential morphological changes in *N*-methyl-*N′*-nitro-*N*-nitrosoguanidine carcinogenesis in the glandular stomach of rats. *J. Nat. Cancer Inst.* **44**, 769.

——, Sasaki, O., tamada, R., Iwamatsu, and M., Inokuchi, K. (1978). Sequential studies of development of gastric carcinoma in dogs induced by *N*-methyl-*N′*-nitro-*N*-nitrosoguanidine. *Cancer* **42**, 1246.

—— ——, Matsukuchi, T., Iwamatsu, M., and Inokuchi, K. (1979). Experimental gastric cancer: pathogenesis and clinicopathologic correlation. In *Gastric cancer* (ed. C.H. Herfarth and P. Schlag), p. 22. Springer-Verlag, Berlin.

Sakita, T., Oguro, Y., Takasu, S., Fukutomi, H., Miwa, T., and Yoshimori, M., (1971). Observations on the healing of ulcerations in early gastric cancer; the life cycle of the malignant ulcer. *Gastroenterol.* **60**, 835.

Sano, R. (1971). Pathological analysis of 300 cases of early gastric cancer with special reference to cancer associated with ulcers. *Gann Manogr. Cancer Res.* **11**, 81.

Sasajima, K. (1979). Intestinal metaplasia and adenocarcinoma induced in the stomach of rats by *N*-propyl-*N′*-nitro-*N*-nitrosoguanidine. *Nippon Shokakibyo Gakkai Zasshi* **76**, 50.

—— Kawachi, T., Sano, T., Sugimura, T., Simosato, Y., and Shirota, A. (1977). Esophageal and gastric cancers with metastases induced in dogs by *N*-ethyl-*N′*-nitro-*N*-nitrosoguanidine. *J. Nat. Cancer Inst.* **58**, 1789.

Sasano, N., Nakamura, K., Arai, M., and Akazaki, K. (1969). Ultrastructural cell patterns in human gastric carcinoma compared with non-neoplastic gastric mucosa—histogenetic analysis of carcinoma by mucin histochemistry. *J. Nat. Cancer Inst.* **43**, 783.

Savage, A. and Jones, S. (1979). Histological appearances of the gastric mucosa, 15-27 years after partial gastrectomy. *J. clin. Pathol.* **32**, 179.

Schade, R.O.K. (1974). The borderline between benign and malignant lesions in the stomach. In *Early gastric cancer: current status of diagnosis* (ed. E. Grundmann, H. Grunze, and S. Witte), p. 45. Springer-Verlag, Berlin.

Schindler, R. (1965). Gastric carcinoma and gastritis. With reference to coexistence of carcinoma and chronic hypertrophic glandular gastritis. *Amer. J. digest. Dis.* **10**, 607.

Schrumpf, E., Serck-Hanssen, A., Stadaas, J., Aune, S., Myren, J., and Osnes, M. (1977). Mucosal changes in the gastric stump, 20-25 years after partial gastrectomy. *Lancet* **2**, 467.

Shimosato, Y., Tanaka, N., Kogure, K., Fugimura, S., Kawachi, T., and Sugimura, T. (1971). Histopathology of tumors of canine alimentary tract produced by *N*-methyl-*N′*-nitro-*N*-nitrosoguanidine, with particular reference to gastric carcinomas. *J. Nat. Cancer Inst.* **47**, 1053.

Sigaran, M.F. and Con-Wong, R. (1979). Production of proliferative lesions in gastric mucosa of albino mice by oral administration of *N*-methyl-*N'*-nitro-*N*-nitrosoguanidine. *Gann* **70**, 343.

Simpson, R.R. (1939). Anaemia with dysphagia: a precancerous condition? *J. Laryngol. Otol.* **54**, 738.

Sipponen, P. (1981). Intestinal metaplasia and gastric carcinoma. *Ann. clin. Res.* **13**, 139.

Siurala, M., Lehtola, J., and Ihamaki, T. (1974). Atrophic gastritis and its sequelae. *Scand. J. Gastroenterol.* **9**, 441.

Skinner, J.M. and Whitehead, R. (1982). Tumor markers in carcinoma and in premalignant states of the stomach in humans. *Eur. J. Cancer clin. Oncol.* **18**, 227.

Snell, K.C., Stewart, H.L., and Morris, H.P. (1969). The sequential development of atrophy, precancerous lesions and cancer of the glandular stomach and other organs and tissues of rats ingesting *N,N'*-2,7-fluorenylene-bisacetamide. *Gann Monogr.* **8**, 125.

Stalsberg, H. and Takdal, S. (1971). Stomach cancer following gastric surgery for benign conditions. *Lancet* **2**, 1175.

Stemmermann, G., Haenszel, W., and Locke, F. (1977). Epidemiologic pathology of gastric ulcer and gastric carcinoma among Japanese in Hawaii. *J. Nat. Cancer Inst.* **58**, 13.

—— Hayashi, T. (1979). Hyperplastic polyps of the gastric mucosa adjacent to gastroenterostomy stomas. *Amer. J. clin. Pathol.* **71**, 341.

Stewart, H.L. (1971). Experimentally induced gastric adenocarcinomas. Maude Abbott Lecture 1971. *Lab. Invest.* **25**, 672.

Stinson, S.F., Squire, R.A., and Sporn, M.B. (1978). Pathology of esophageal neoplasms and associated proliferative lesions induced in rats by *N*-methyl-*N*-benzylnitrosamine. *J. Nat. Cancer Inst.* **61**, 1471.

Stout, A.P. (1945). Gastric mucosal atrophy and carcinoma of the stomach. *NY State J. Med.* **45**, 973.

Strickland, R.G. and MacKay, I.R. (1973). Reappraisal of nature and significance of chronic atrophic gastritis. *Amer. J. digest. Dis.* **18**, 426.

Sugano, H., Nakamura, K., and Takagi, K. (1971). An atypical epithelium of the stomach. A clinicopathological entity. *Gann Monogr. Cancer Res.* **11**, 257.

Tabuchi, Y., Ogino, T., Mitsuno, T., and Sugimura, T. (1974). Posible role of mucosal damage in stomach carcinogenesis with *N*-methyl-*N'*-nitro-*N*-nitrosoguanidine in the rat. *J. Nat. Cancer Inst.* **52**, 1589.

Takahashi, M., Shirai, T., Fukushima, S., Hahanouchi, M., and Hirose, M. (1976). Effects of fundic ulcers induced by iodoacetamide on development of gastric tumors in rats treated with *N*-methyl-*N'*-nitro-*N*-nitrosoguanidine. *Gann* **67**, 47.

Tatsuta, M., Itoh, M., Okuda, S., Taniguchi, H., and Tamura, H. (1977). Effect of prolonged administration of gastrin on experimental carcinogenesis in rat stomach induced by *N*-methyl-*N'*-nitro-*N*-nitrosoguanidine. *Cancer Res.* **37**, 1808.

Teglbjaerg, P.S. and Nielsen, H.O. (1978). "Small intestinal type" and "colonic type" intestinal metaplasia of the human stomach, and their relationship to the histogenetic types of gastric adenocarcinoma. *Acta Pathol. Microbiol. Scand.* **86A**, 351.

Tomasulo, J. (1971). Gastric polyps. Histologic types and their relationship to gastric carcinoma. *Cancer* **27**, 1346.

Walk, L. (1951). Villous tumor of the stomach. Clinical review and report of 2 cases. *Arch. intern. Med.* **87**, 560.

Walker, I.R., Strickland, R.G., Unger, B., and MacKay, I.R. (1971). Simple atrophic gastritis and gastric carcinoma. *Gut* **12**, 906.

Watanabe, H. (1978). Experimentally induced intestinal metaplasia in Wistar rats by X-ray irradiation. *Gastroenterol.* **75**, 796.

Willems, G. and Bleiberg, H. (1978). Proliferative changes in the gastric mucosa of patients with pernicious anemia. *Eur. J. Cancer. Suppl.,* p. 39.

Williams, S.M., Harned, R.K., and Settles, R.H. (1978). Adenocarcinoma of the stomach in association with Menetrier's disease. *Gastrointest. Radiol.* **3**, 387.

Wychulis, A.R., Woolam, G.L., Anderson, H.A., and Ellis, F.H., Jr. (1971). Achalasia and carcinoma of the esophagus. *J. Amer. med. Assoc.* **215**, 1638.

Wynder, E.L., Hultberg, S., Jacobsson, F., and Bross, I.J. (1957). Environmental factors in cancer of the upper alimentary tract. A Swedish study with special reference to Plummer-Vinson (Paterson-Kelly) syndrome. *Cancer* **10**, 470.

Yamagata, S. and Hisamichi, S. (1979). Precancerous lesions of the stomach. *World J. Surg.* **3**, 671.

Yamashiro, K., Suzuki, H., and Nagayo, T. (1977). Electron microscopic study of signet-ring cells in diffuse carcinoma of the human stomach. *Virchow's Arch. (Pathol. Anat.)* **374**, 275.

Yang, C.S. (1980). Research in esophageal cancer in China: a review. *Cancer Res.* **40**, 2633.

8 Precancerous states of the large intestine

R. Whitehead

It is virtually inevitable that all patients with familial polyposis coli will eventually develop carcinoma of the colon. There is also an increased risk of colon cancer in patients with longstanding ulcerative colitis. The commonest form of colonic cancer is unassociated with these conditions, but evidence has accumulated over the years which points to the fact that this tumour arises in pre-existing adenomatous polyps. Such polyps are relatively common in comparison with cancer, and the polyp→cancer sequence occurs in only a small minority of lesions. It is partly for this reason that the premalignancy of adenomatous polyps has been the subject of heated debate. The indiscriminate use of the term polyp without adequate definition and the use of different terms to refer to the same lesion has clouded the issue. The problem arises out of the practice of removing all polyps so that opportunities for their sequential histological study are rare. Much of the evidence concerning the relationship of polyps to cancer is therefore indirect. Estimates of the polyp→cancer sequence based on improper classification of polypoidal lesions of the colonic mucosa will clearly be erronous. There are certain facts which put the matter into perspective. At autopsy the colon will exhibit one or more polypoidal elevation in 50 per cent of cases (Chapman 1963). The sigmoidoscopic examination of an aged population will reveal similar lesions in 25 per cent of individuals (Gilbertsen *et al.* 1965). Careful histological evaluation can, however, define the problem precisely. Hyperplastic polyps, for example, are about ten times as common as adenomatous polyps (Arthur 1968) and account for most polypoidal lesions of the colon. They are usually distinctive and are regarded as having no malignant potential. There are, however, claims (Goldman *et al.* 1970; Cooper *et al.* 1979; Estrada and Spjut 1980) of a possible relationship between hyperplastic and adenomatous polyps. Especially large hyperplastic polyps may show adenomatous regions, and Skinner and Whitehead (1981) have described two unusually large hyperplastic polyps with a profile of tumour antigens which was similar to that found in adenomatous polyps and adenocarcinomas. A reappraisal of the entrenched universal view of the innocence of these lesions is perhaps indicated. There is little or no evidence that the hamartomatous Peutz-Jegher and juvenile polyps, inflammatory polyps, rarer entities such as the polyps of Cronkhite-Canada syndrome and polyps composed of heterotopic tissues have any significant malignant potential.

Description and classification of adenomatous polyps

The characterization of adenomatous polyps as a separate group has therefore gone a long way towards resolving the inherent difficulty in validating a polyp→cancer sequence. The terms adenomatous polyp, tubular adenoma, villous adenoma, tubulovillous adenoma, papillary adenoma and villous papilloma all describe the same lesion. It is a neoplastic proliferation of colonic glandular epithelium with a variety of growth patterns. The individual cytological changes which go to make up these different growth patterns are identical and, by light microscopy, are usually referred to in terms of increasing dysplasia. Both the size and degree of dysplasia shown by adenomatous polyps may vary in different regions of the large bowel, the larger adenomas with most pronounced dysplasia tending to occur most frequently in the descending colon, sigmoid colon and rectum (Konishi and Morson 1982). Irrespective of size or site, the fundamental change in cell kinetics is a loss of the orderly process of cell division and maturation in the crypt base and migration of the cells to the surface where, after a total life span of three to four days, exfoliation occurs. In adenomatous proliferation the cells retain the power of division whilst losing some or all of their capacity to differentiate and mature. Mitotic activity can be seen in all parts of the irregular glandular structures which have been produced by the disordered cell kinetics.

If enough adenomatous polyps are examined it can be shown that one end of the range comprises polyps with a predominantly tubular structure (Fig. 8.1). The tubules are usually circular in section, they vary in size, and they are frequently and repeatedly branched. Each is surrounded by normal lamina propria. At the other end of the range, polyps are seen with a predominantly villous pattern (Fig. 8.2); in section they appear to be composed of finger-like processes with epithelium covering long thin extensions of the lamina propria. The cells which constitute these patterns of proliferation reflect the capacity for differentiation of the progenitor cells in the abnormal crypt base. They may exhibit a tendency to mature into goblet or absorptive cells but they will show a varying degree of departure from normality and exhibit features usually embodied in the term dysplasia. Thus there is nuclear enlargement, hyperchromasia, pleomorphism, palisading and increased mitotic activity, together with a variety of normal and abnormal cytoplasmic changes (*see* Figs. 8.3-8.7). Electron microscopy will also reveal abnormalities similar to those seen in malignant cells in general. Indeed, like malignant cells, they may also exhibit abnormalities in chromosomal number and configuration (Enterline and Arvan 1967) and, presumably by a process of gene derepression, the cells may acquire a capacity to synthesize a variety

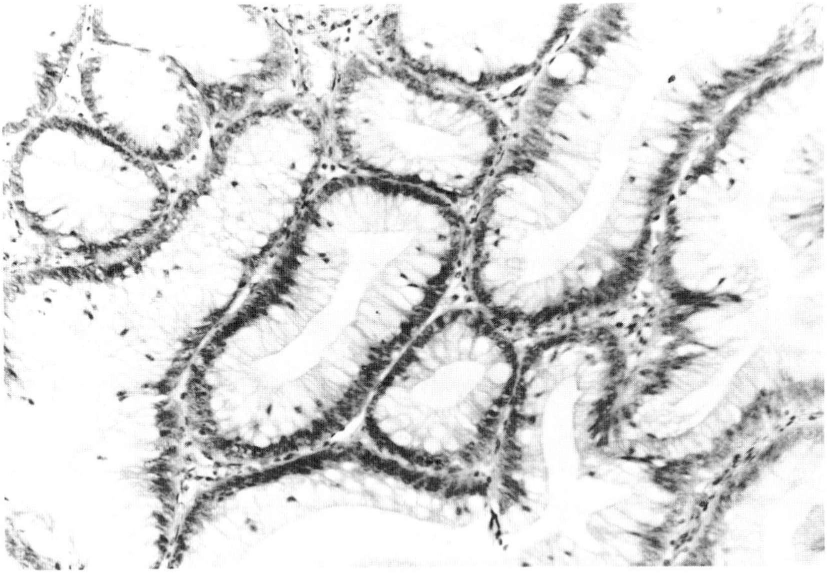

Fig. 8.1. Tubular pattern of glandular epithelial proliferation in an adenomatous polyp. ×280. H & E.

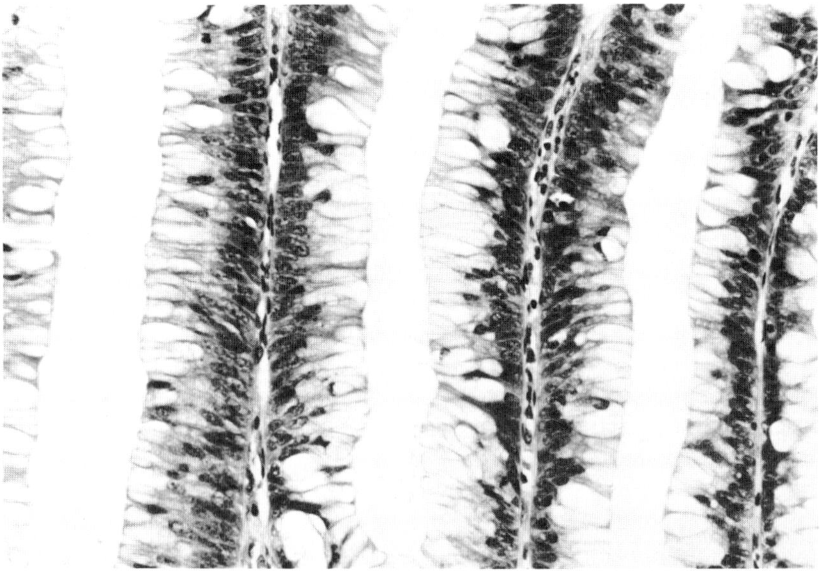

Fig. 8.2. Villous pattern of glandular epithelial proliferation in an adenomatous polyp. ×280. H & E.

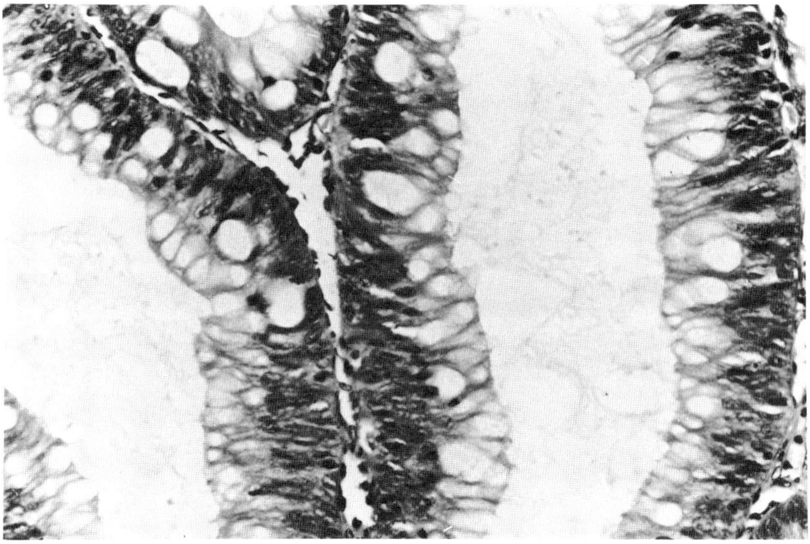

Fig. 8.3. An area of predominantly goblet-cell differentiation in an adenomatous polyp. ×280. H & E.

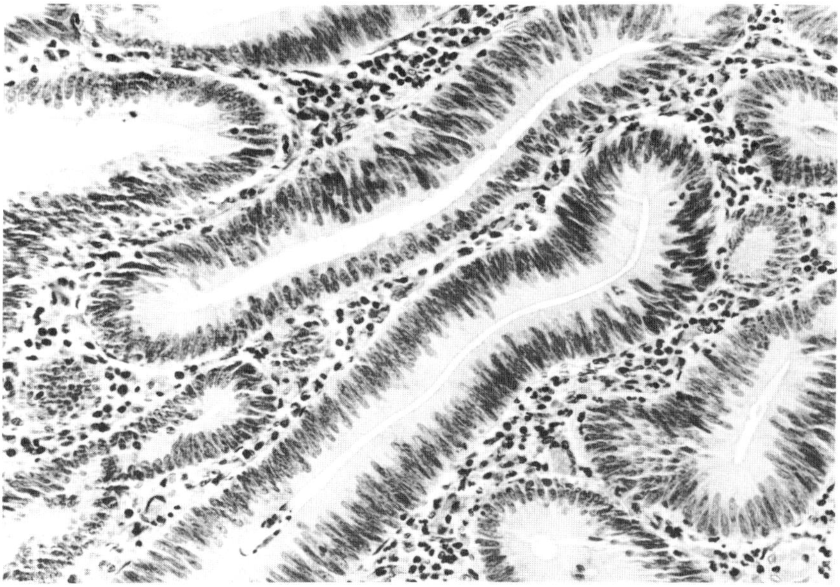

Fig. 8.4. An area of predominantly absorptive-cell differentiation in an adenomatous polyp. ×225. H & E.

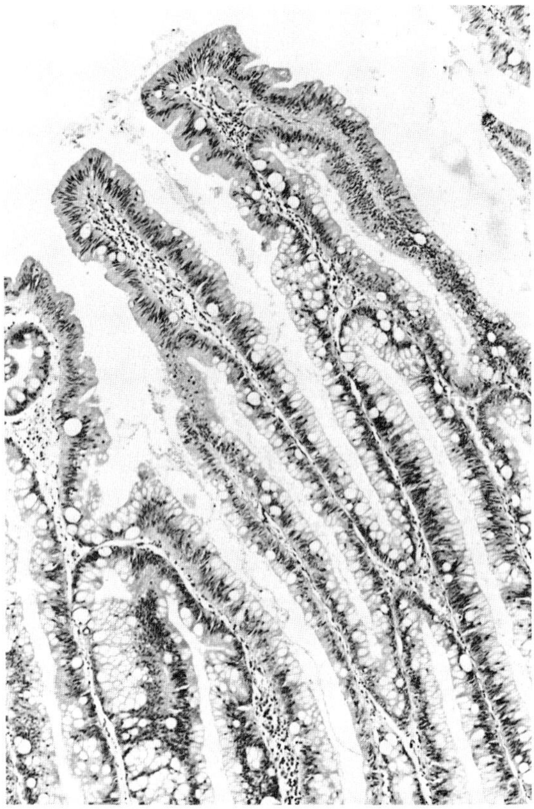

Fig. 8.5. Mixed absorptive- (tips of villous processes) and goblet-cell differentiation (elsewhere) in an adenomatous polyp. ×180. H & E.

of new proteins such as carcinoembryonic antigen or hormones (Isaacson and Le Vann 1976; Skinner and Whitehead 1981).

The latter authors have shown that there is a remarkable similarity between polyps and carcinoma of the colon with respect to their content of the following antigens: carcinoembryonic antigen, human placental lactogen, α-fetoprotein, colon-specific antigen, pregnancy-specific β-lipoprotein 1, human β-chorionic gonadotrophin, placental alkaline phosphatase, iso-ferritins, and transferrin. The progenitor cells of the crypt are also capable of producing cells which undergo metaplasia to Paneth cells, and the presence of these cells in adenomatous polyps is well recognized (Lewin 1968). Endocrine polypeptide cells may also occur in these lesions (Gibbs 1967), but whether they originate from a separate cell line of neural crest origin (Pearse 1966*a*,*b*) or from a common progenitor cell is still disputed (Whitehead and Cosgrove 1979). The polyps which occur in familial polyposis coli are histologically identical to single adenomatous polyps which develop sporadically in ostensibly non-genetically predisposed individuals.

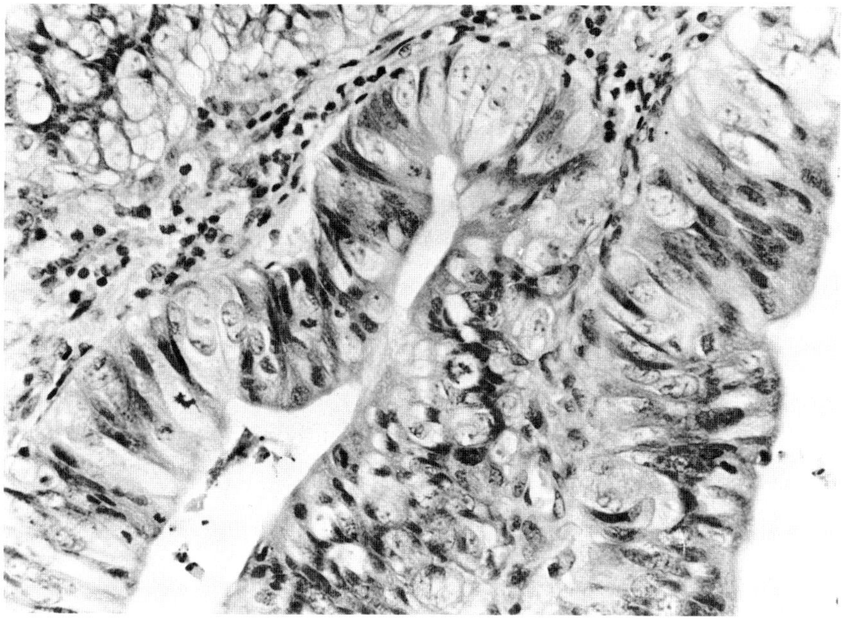

Fig. 8.6. A mixed population of largely undifferentiated cells in an adenomatous polyp. ×360. H & E.

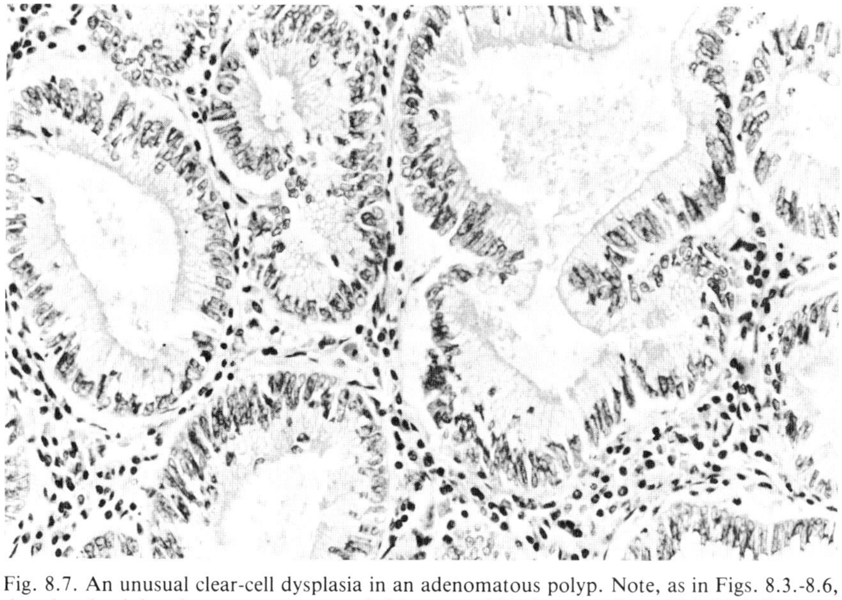

Fig. 8.7. An unusual clear-cell dysplasia in an adenomatous polyp. Note, as in Figs. 8.3.-8.6, that the glandular elements are surrounded by normal lamina propria. ×225. H & E.

Colectomy specimens from patients with familial polyposis have provided the opportunity to study the earliest possible stages of adenoma formation. Deschner and Lipkin (1975), for example, demonstrated ^{3}H-thymidine uptake by cells at or near the surface in crypts which were otherwise histologically normal which suggests a failure of the control mechanisms which normally restrict cell replication to the lower part of the crypt. Indeed unicryptal adenomatous changes recognizable at light-microscope level (Bussey 1975) have also been identified in similar specimens and there are occasional reports (Woda *et al.* 1977) of the same lesions in non-polyposis patients. At this stage in their development all adenomatous polyps are thus histologically identical.

The evolution of a primary tubular or primary villous morphology as the polyps increase in size may well be determined by the nature of the loss of control of crypt kinetics. Of particular importance may be the factor or factors operating in the *normal* gut which are concerned with the production of regular single straight tubular glands orientated at right angles to the muscularis mucosae. There is at least some evidence that part of this mechanism involves an intimate functional interrelationship between the crypt epithelial cells and pericryptal fibroblasts. Pascal *et al.* (1968) and Kaye *et al.* (1968, 1971) have convincingly shown in autoradiographic and electron-microscope studies that fibroblasts in normal epithelium replicate at the same crypt level as the epithelial cells. Their upward migration is also synchronous and, like epithelial cells, the fibroblasts lose their ability to divide when they reach the surface. In adenomatous polyps, however, surface fibroblasts resemble the abnormal epithelial cells in that they retain their capacity for thymidine uptake and cell division. In conventional light-microscope preparations this change is manifested by an obvious thinning of the subepithelial collagen plate at the surface of the polyp, due to diminished collagen synthesis by the immature cells.

Because of their essential pathobiological similarity it would be more satisfactory if all adenomatous polyps were simply referred to as such; but clinical usage and ingrained terminology have determined the final recommendation of the World Health Organization working group on classification of intestinal tumours (World Health Organization 1976). This generally accepted classification recognizes three varieties—a predominantly tubular pattern, a predominantly villous pattern, and a mixed tubulo-villous variety. Predominantly tubular adenomas tend to be smaller, are more frequently pedunculated, and generally exhibit the lesser grades of dysplasia. Predominantly villous adenomas tend to be large and sessile and show severe dysplasia. But these differences are only generalities, and large villous lesions may be composed of partially differentiated goblet cells—a type of polyp which may be associated with hypokalaemia or hypoproteinaemia due to intestinal loss of secretions. On the other hand, quite small predominantly tubular adenomas may exhibit severe dysplastic features.

It needs to be stressed that rigid subdivision of polyps into tubular and villous types is artificial: almost all lesions will contain features of both and only a minority will show a preponderance of one or other pattern. Failure to appreciate this point has contributed significantly to the controversy surrounding the poly→cancer sequence to the extent that some authors have stated that whilst adenomatous polyps (tubular adenomas) have little or no malignant potential, villous papillomas (villous adenomas) frequently undergo malignant change (Spratt *et al.* 1958; Castleman and Krickstein 1962). With increasing size and villous development there is not only a definite trend towards increasing dysplasia, but such lesions may also coexist with invasive adenocarcinoma (Muto *et al.* 1975). On the other hand the larger polyps constitute only ten per cent of all adenomatous polyps, only about ten per cent of colon carcinomas show adenomatous polyps in contiguity (Figs. 8.8 and 8.9), and focal carcinoma will be found in only about one per cent of all adenomatous polyps. The reasons for doubting that *all* adenomatous polyps are precancerous (Horn 1971) are therefore plain.

Further consideration of the likely course of events clarifies the situation. If carcinoma supervenes in the dysplastic epithelium of adenomatous polyps, there is every reason to expect that the change will not take place after a fixed time lapse in each instance. This statement has certainly been confirmed by the study of dysplasia in other sites such as the epithelium of the uterine cervix (see Chapter 12). Indeed, there is evidence for marked variation in the time taken for polyps to become malignant, based on observations from patients who refused to have polyps excised (Muto *et al.* 1975). Furthermore, there are no grounds for believing that all polyps grow at the

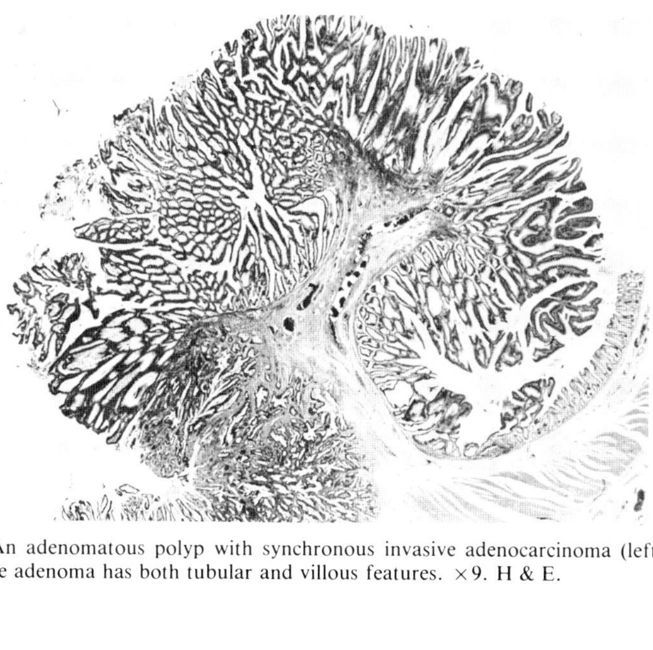

Fig. 8.8. An adenomatous polyp with synchronous invasive adenocarcinoma (left) in continuity. The adenoma has both tubular and villous features. ×9. H & E.

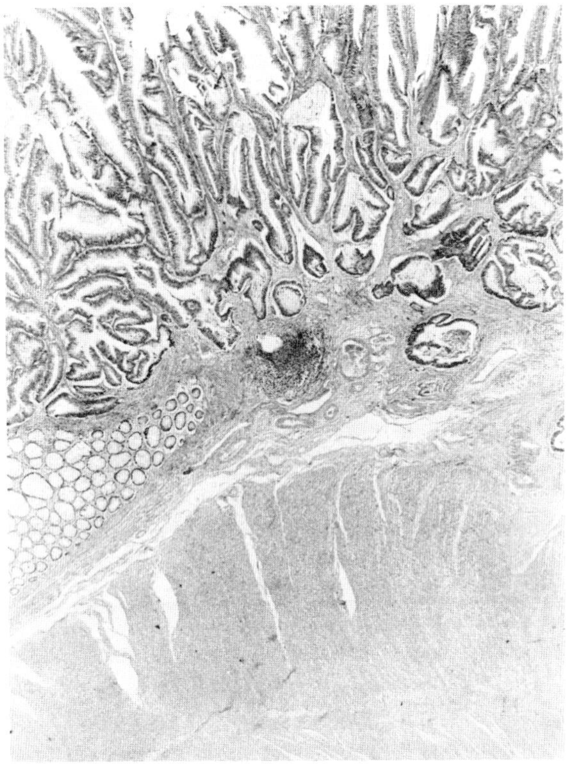

Fig. 8.9. Predominantly villous adenoma with carcinomatous transition and extension beyond the muscularis mucosae. ×18. H & E.

same rate. A large polyp is not necessarily older than a smaller one, and there is radiological evidence that polyps of different sizes may indeed grow at different rates (Welin *et al.* 1963). Carcinoma arising early in the life of a polyp may obviously do so when the polyp is still relatively small—in which case the evidence for any pre-existing lesion would soon be obliterated. The uncommon finding of a pre-existing polyp in most colon carcinomas can therefore be explained quite simply. For purely mechanical reasons very small carcinomas are infrequently diagnosed because they do not usually give rise to symptoms; carcinomas arising in very small adenomatous polyps are thus most unusual though small polyp cancers are described in the literature (Lane *et al.* 1978). In addition, some small carcinomas (3-15 mm in diameter) have been observed in which adenomatous *changes,* as distinct from polyps, were found in the contiguous mucosa (Spjut *et al.* 1979). Such changes are no different from those already referred to as the earliest morphological stages of polyp formation. If carcinoma supervenes late in the life of a polyp, the polyp may well be larger and the pathologist is more likely to observe coexisting cancer and polyps histologically. Larger lesions would clearly precipitate their removal at a time when the coexistent malignant change was still discernible. By this reasoning there are grounds for challenging the frequent statement that large villous tumours have the highest potential for malignant change. There is evidence that at least some of them (Muto *et al.* 1975) may remain unchanged for up to 20 years. Furthermore the cancer which arises in polyposis coli develops from tubular rather than villous adenomas—and the latter are rare lesions in this syndrome. It is thus clear that only a proportion of adenomatous polyps will develop into cancer in their lifetime.

Since most, if not all, carcinomas originate in adenomatous polyps, we are led to examine two lines of evidence: first for the aetiology of adenomatous polyps and second for the possible factors which determine the polyp→cancer sequence.

The aetiology and precancerous potential of adenomatous polyps

There are numerous animal models of carcinoma of the colon (Zedeck 1978) but they are invariably based on the administration of various exogenous chemical carcinogens. Even those systems devised to mimic human colon cancers as closely as possible have several fundamental shortcomings (Pour 1978). A major difficulty lies in the morphological differences between the experimentally induced tumours and colonic cancer in man. The animal tumours, for example, are frequently multiple, a polyp→cancer sequence is unusual, metastatic behaviour is different, synchronous tumours are also induced in a variety of other organs, and there is a quite different time-scale of events. Experimental studies of colon cancer in animals have so far done little to aid understanding of the disease in man, other than to accentuate the importance and interplay of environmental carcinogenic substances and—perhaps—to provide a theoretical means of investigating approaches to treatment. If cancer of the human colon shares similarities with cancer of other organs in man, its aetiology is likely to be multifactorial. Patients with a high susceptibility of genetic determination are clearly those belonging to the familial polyposis group. What role genetic factors play in the acquisition of ordinary carcinoma of the colon is not yet clear, but some evidence for familial susceptibility does exist (Lovett 1976). Studies based on the widely-varying geographic incidences of colon cancer have shown that, coupled with possible individual susceptibility, there is a strong environmental influence (Doll 1969; Stemmerman and Yatani 1976). These environmental factors are primarily related to diet and have been the subject of intensive study (Burkitt 1971; Hill 1974, 1980; Wynder and Reddy 1974; Bone *et al.* 1975). Dietary factors determine gut flora and, in cancer-prone races, the gut bacteria are thought to generate carcinogens from bile acids. In support of this view is the different incidence of colon cancer shown by similar ethnic groups who have different dietary habits (Buell and Dunn 1965; Wynder *et al.* 1969). The importance of dietary factors in the genesis of colon cancer is also shown by the finding that in geographic areas of low cancer incidence adenomatous polyps are also infrequent (Williams and Prince 1975; Stemmerman and Yatani 1976; Haghighi *et al.* 1977; Oluwatope *et al.* 1975). There is some evidence that colonic absorption of deoxycholate, a bacterial metabolite of cholic acid, is increased in patients with adenomatous polyps compared with control subjects (Van der Werf *et al.* 1982), but the precise mechanisms which are involved in the stimulation of adenoma formation and in their subsequent malignant transformation are still to be elucidated. Hill *et al.* (1978) have examined the epidemiological evidence and suggest that there is a recessive gene for adenoma proneness. Environmental factors then determine the development of adenomas in such individuals. Further possibly distinct environmental agents are postulated for continued growth of the adenoma and for the adenoma→carcinoma sequence.

From the practical point of view, cancer of the colon would be prevented if all adenomatous polyps were removed—a view that has been borne out by the results of the 25 year study undertaken by the Minnesota Cancer Detection Centre (Gilbertsen 1974). Mucosal protrusions were systematically removed from 1000 individuals during periodic sigmoidoscopic examinations. The anticipated incidence of rectosigmoid carcinoma was thus effectively reduced by 85 per cent. For preventive medicine, therefore, there is a clear challenge, but a programme which would ensure the easy identification of all asymptomatic adenomatous polyps of the colon and their subsequent removal is fraught with obvious difficulties. This problem aside, the management of polyps which are known to be present can easily be rationalized in the light of present-day knowledge of their now accepted relationship to carcinoma. All adenomatous polyps should be completely removed and examined with great care. An experienced histopathologist will generally be able to offer firm guidelines as to further management. There are, however, certain difficulties in interpretation which are due to a variety of circumstances. First, it is necessary to define accurately when an adenomatous polyp ceases to be a benign lesion and becomes an adenocarcinoma. The subjectivity inherent in such terms as moderate or severe dysplasia and carcinoma *in situ* is obvious, and this has proved to be yet another complicating factor in determining the relationship between adenomatous polyp and colon cancer. In carcinoma of the colon, when the tumour involves only mucosa and submucosa, the cure rate following resection approaches 95 per cent. In all instances of *in situ* (intraepithelial) carcinomas or of carcinomas invading solely into the lamina propria, complete excision results in a 100 per cent cure.

Penetration of the muscularis mucosae by malignant cells appears to be a prerequisite for metastatic spread (Grinnell and Lane 1958), an observation which may well be related to the fact that colonic lymphatics are associated only with the muscularis mucosae and extend no higher than the crypts of Lieberkühn (Fenoglio *et al.* 1973). Theoretically, serial histological study of the entire lesion may be necessary to ensure that invasion beyond the muscularis mucosae has not occurred; more practically, there are inescapable reasons for completely removing all polyps intact with a margin of healthy mucosa. This is becoming increasingly feasible, even for large polyps in the proximal colon, with the growing practice of operative colonoscopy. Even if invasion beyond the muscularis mucosae is demonstrated in polyps removed by this method, further treatment is probably not indicated provided that resection margins are adequate; more surgery may, however, be necessary if the carcinoma is found to be poorly differentiated (Gillespie *et al.* 1979).

A major problem with the larger polyps and some pedunculated tumours is the associated splitting, hyperplasia, and traumatic fibrosis which may be present at the base of the lesion or involving the stalk (Fig. 8.10). Such changes can cause considerable difficulty in deciding for or against invasion through the muscularis mucosae, especially if large lesions are removed piecemeal. Attention has also been drawn to the phenomenon of traumatic pseudoinvasion at the base of polyps (Greene 1974) in which epithelium and sometimes lamina propria are found within or underneath the muscularis mucosae (Fig. 8.11). Such changes represent displacement of tissues and not

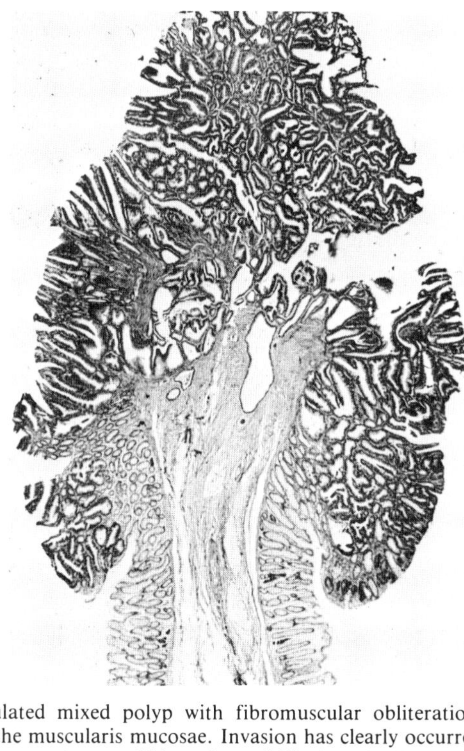

Fig. 8.10. Pedunculated mixed polyp with fibromuscular obliteration of the submucosa tending to obscure the muscularis mucosae. Invasion has clearly occurred but, had the lesion not been intact, interpretation would have been difficult. ×9. H & E.

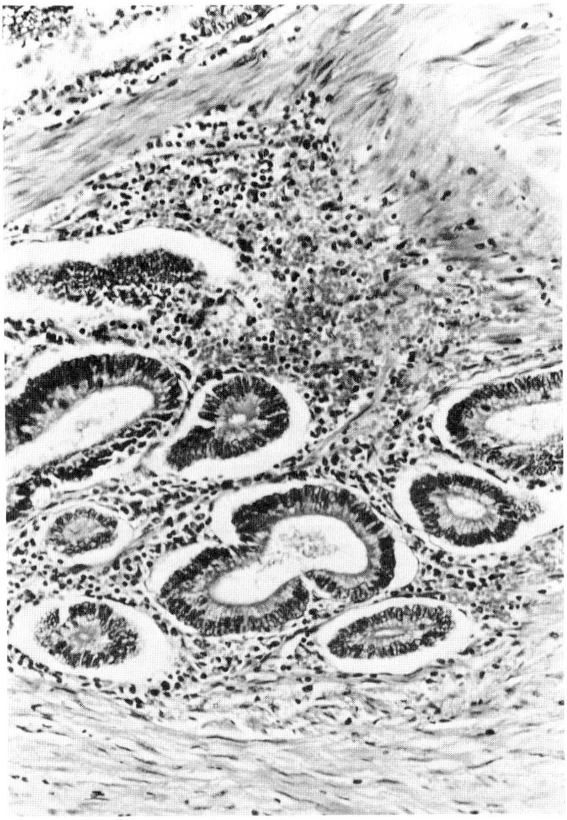

Fig. 8.11. Glandular elements clearly surrounded by the muscularis. This is an example of pseudoinvasion. Note that the glands are surrounded by lamina propria. ×180. H & E.

true invasion. Regions of haemorrhage, fibrosis, and haemosiderin are sometimes found (Fig. 8.12), and cystic dilatation of glands and lakes of escaped mucin occur (Fig. 8.13). These traumatic manifestations are helpful in differential diagnosis and are most frequently seen in pedunculated tumours that are prone to be twisted or pulled along by the colonic movements. On the other hand, trauma can also affect malignant lesions and the pathologist must be able to differentiate innocent displacement from true carcinomatous infiltration. One differentiating feature seen in carcinomatous areas is the absence of any lamina propria around the glandular elements. In its place there is often a conspicuous desmoplastic stromal reaction. But it is prudent to remember that fibrosis can also follow traumatic benign glandular displacement, while haemosiderin may accumulate after trauma to a pedunculated carcinomatous polyp. The only reliable criteria in such instances are the cytological appearances of the epithelial elements themselves: in traumatic pseudoinvasion they will appear no more bizarre than in the overlying polyps. In difficult cases in which only the

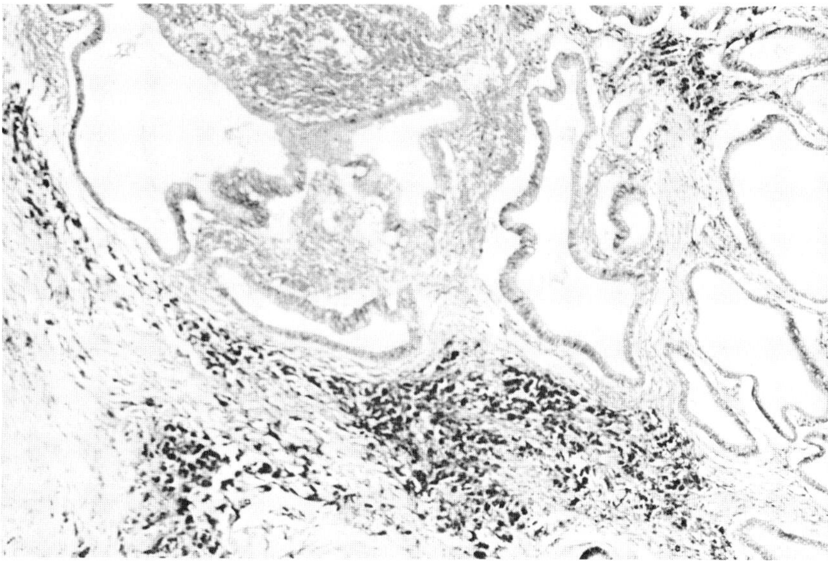

Fig. 8.12. Haemosiderin-laden macrophages adjacent to areas of glandular pseudoinvasion. ×150. Perl's.

muscularis mucosae has been breached, it is more important for the pathologist to ascertain the adequacy of excision of dubious areas.

Familial polyposis coli

This is a disease in which, when fully developed, the large intestine and rectum are the site of hundreds or thousands of adenomatous polyps. Because the number of adenomatous polyps from non-polyposis patients, as well as those from polyposis families, ranges from one to several thousands, Bussey and Morson (1978) have suggested a figure of 100 to separate patients with 'multiple adenomas' and with familial polyposis coli: few if any patients with less than 100 adenomas will give a positive family history. This author has, however, personal experience of a 50-year-old female who died of coronary heart disease and at autopsy was found to have osteomata of the skull, multiple sebaceous cysts, a small caecal adenocarcinoma arising in an adenomatous polyp, and 29 other adenomatous polyps scattered throughout the rest of the colon. This combination of lesions inescapably constitutes Gardner's syndrome and, despite the small number of adenomas, a positive family history was subsequently obtained. Gardner's syndrome is now regarded as the same entity as familial polyposis syndrome but with a greater penetration of the genetic defect and greater expressivity. Various other extracolonic manifestations are sometimes associated with familial polyposis such as osteomas, connective tissue tumours, dental abnormalities, carcinomas of the duodenum and thyroid gland, and gliomas. Patients

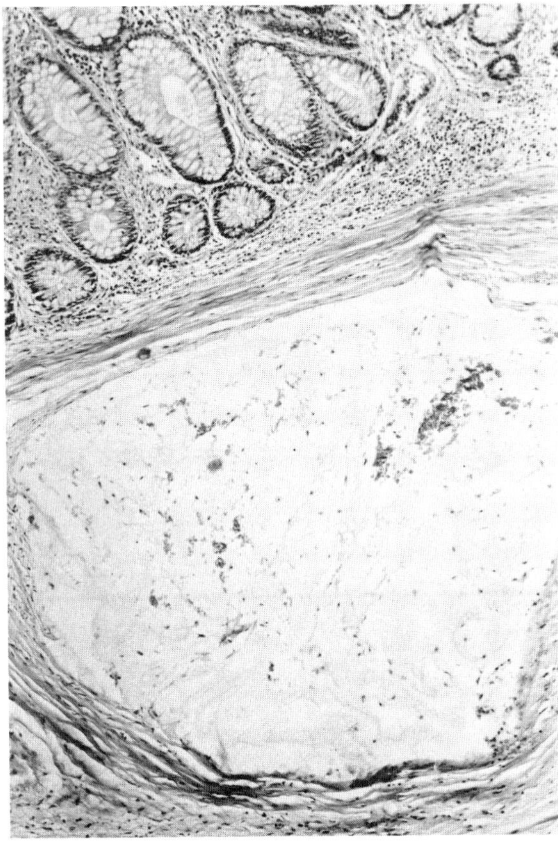

Fig. 8.13. Submucosal lakes of mucin in the stalk of a polyp, another frequent indication of pseudoinvasion. ×180. H & E.

with polyposis coli usually inherit the disease from one or other parent and it is transmitted as a Mendelian dominant character which is not sex-linked.

The adenomas begin to appear in patients in their 20s and 30s but they may only be diagnosed some years later. Microscopically they are essentially similar to single adenomas. The tubular growth pattern predominates, and frankly villous adenomas and adenomas larger than 1 cm are uncommon. The condition acts as the perfect human model in which to study the adenoma→cancer sequence, from the inception of adenoma through to metastatic carcinoma. It is usually stated that carcinoma will inevitably supervene if the condition is left untreated. The carcinomatous change is similar to that which is observed in non-polyposis patients with single or a few polyps and the carcinomas behave in identical fashion, being no less or no more aggressive. The factors which predispose to malignant transformation are unknown but, as in single polyps, they may be partly environmental. When colectomy and ileorectal anastomosis has been performed occasional cases are recorded in which polyps in the rectal stump have *regressed* spontaneously (Hawley 1974). The implications of the observation are of great importance and the phenomenon clearly needs to be substantiated and studied in more detail.

Precancer in ulcerative colitis and Crohn's colitis

It is well established that patients who have ulcerative colitis are prone to develop adenocarcinoma of the colon. The tumours are often multiple and usually run a rapidly progressive course with a correspondingly poor prognosis. Patients particularly at risk are those with disease involving the whole colon for ten or more years.

Onset of colitis in childhood is a frequent and important association. Patients with mild disease appear to be vulnerable, but this may be due to the fact that severe attacks of colitis are more likely to lead to colectomy early in the course of the disease. There is some disagreement whether patients with continuous symptoms (Edwards and Truelove 1964) or with quiescent disease (Svartz and Ernberg 1949) account for the majority who develop carcinoma. Patients who are under continuous medical care are likely to have their carcinomas diagnosed and treated earlier although, paradoxically, the incidence of such tumours tends to be lower than average in special centres where large numbers of colitis patients are regularly seen. The explanation probably lies in the fact that more patients in the high-risk group will have a colectomy before malignancy can supervene.

The view that cancer in ulcerative colitis may be preceded by a histologically distinct, dysplastic mucosal change was put forward by Dawson and Pryse-Davies (1959) who described such changes in sessile polypoidal lesions. Morson and Pang (1967) emphasized that similar dysplasia was more usual in macroscopically flat areas. They found these regions of mucosal dysplasia in rectal biopsies both from patients who had coexistent cancer and dysplastic changes elsewhere and from patients without overt cancer. On the basis of their findings they suggested that regular rectal biopsy in colitics at high risk might identify a group which was entering a precancerous phase and in whom protocolectomy would obviate the development of what is usually an aggressive carcinoma.

Evans and Pollock (1972) and Cook and Goligher (1975) confirmed that rectal dysplastic changes in rectal mucosa could occur in some cases with established colon cancer, but also described cases with carcinoma elsewhere in the bowel without rectal dysplasia. Like Morson and Pang, these authors noted that dysplastic changes may occur in the absence of carcinoma. It is now clear that rectal biopsy alone will fail to reveal dysplastic changes in a proportion of patients with longstanding ulcerative colitis who have already developed dysplastic changes elsewhere or even frank carcinoma. Stepwise biopsy of the entire colon, including macroscopically suspicious areas, is now possible by colonoscopy and dysplastic changes should (in theory) be detected with much greater accuracy than in rectal biopsy alone. But the questions remain as to whether these dysplastic mucosal changes are truly precancerous and, if they are, what proportion of patients with dysplasia develop cancer over what time interval.

Answers to these questions are still not fully available. McGovern (1972) was probably the first to show that mucosal dysplasia in one case of ulcerative colitis preceded invasive cancer by as much as six years. More recently, Lennard-Jones *et al.* (1977) have reported that moderate or severe mucosal dysplasia may revert to normal in up to 50 per cent of patients, but persists in the remainder. On the other hand, if colectomy is carried out in the presence of moderate or severe mucosal dysplasia, a cancer will be found in about 15 per cent of cases. An obvious difficulty in the diagnosis of mucosal dysplasia is that in the presence of active inflammation the differentiation of reactive epithelial features from truly precancerous dysplasia can be notoriously difficult. In childhood especially, the appearances of inflammatory dysplasia may be quite bizarre in one biopsy only to return to a more normal appearance when the attack of colitis has resolved. It has therefore been advocated that precancerous dysplasia should be diagnosed only in the absence of significant inflammation, and there is a clear case for repeat biopsies in such circumstances.

Isaacson (1976), using an immunoperoxidase technique for the demonstration of carcinoembryonic antigen, claims that inflammatory dysplasia which is negative can be differentiated from precancerous dysplasia which is positive. The success of the method is governed by technical skill and by the quality of the antibodies and other reagents used, and the method cannot yet be regarded as having resolved the problem. For the present, therefore, the diagnosis of precancerous dysplasia must be based on criteria such as those proposed by Riddell (1976). The patterns he has described are essentially the same as those seen in adenomatous polyps, but they seem more bizarre in the setting of the abnormal mucosa of chronic ulcerative colitis (Fig. 8.14). Macroscopic features are sometimes present endoscopically, but their recognition will depend on experience and this, except in special centres, will be unusual. The mucosa may, for example, appear similar to velvet which is due to the villous structure of the mucosa that is apparent when it is examined microscopically. Polypoidal lesions may be seen, but these may also be inflammatory as well as truly adenomatous.

Dawson and Pryse-Davies (1959) showed in their original paper that a spectrum of polypoidal lesions may be seen in ulcerative colitis, ranging from the truly inflammatory to the frankly adenomatous. More frequently the areas of dysplastic epithelium in ulcerative colitis have the same macroscopic appearance as the featureless mucosa of uninvolved bowel. If, however, the underlying vessels are difficult to see, biopsy is likely to be rewarding because the mucosa (though flat) may prove to be thickened and dysplastic. The origin of carcinoma in ulcerative colitis from *flat* dysplastic

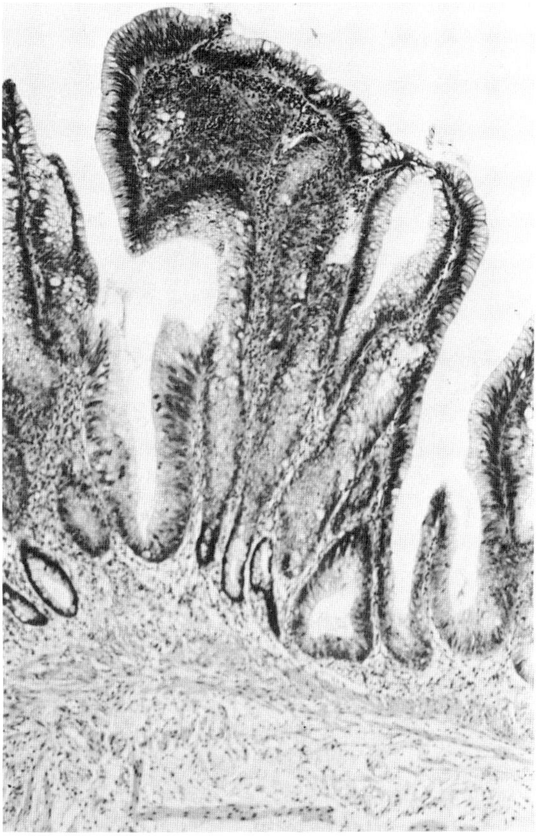

Fig. 8.14. Precancerous dysplasia in ulcerative colitis. Evidence of active inflammatory disease is absent making the abnormality all the more significant. ×150. H & E.

mucosa is strikingly different from the usual polyp→cancer sequence in noncolitics. The development of relatively large non-polypoidal fields of dysplasia may in part be determined by the underlying diffuse inflammatory nature of the disease process and the disturbances of cell kinetics which are induced by it.

Deschner *et al.* (1973) have produced evidence that in colonic mucosa in ulcerative colitis there can be an extension on to the luminal surface of cells still capable of division, even though dysplasia is not present. Riddell (1976) describes two common forms, one identical to the range seen in the usual adenomatous polyps and one referred to as basal-cell dysplasia (Figs. 8.15 and 8.16). The former is found in flat, villous, or polypoid lesions and consists of nuclear atypia, loss or modification of goblet cells, and an increase in mitotic rate in all parts of the epithelium (and not just in the crypt bases). The basal-cell change is seen commonly in flat mucosae and has a strikingly regular appearance. Tubular glands are formed by intensely hyperchromatic

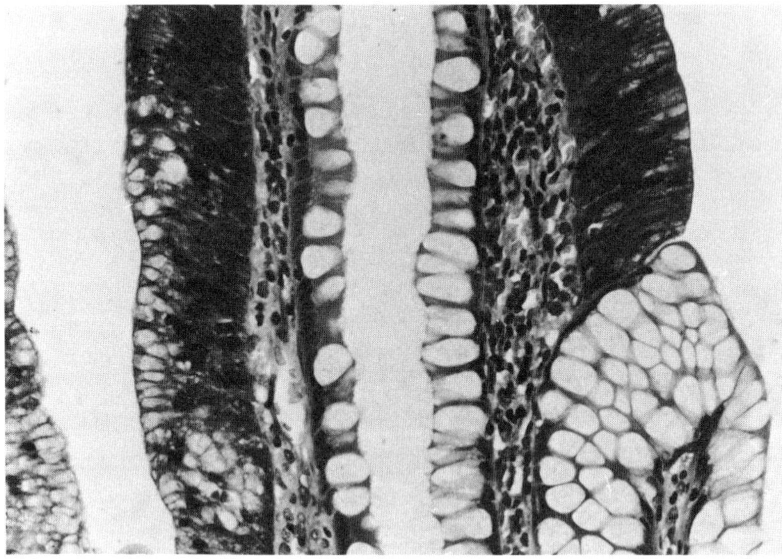

Fig. 8.15. Adenomatous dysplasia in ulcerative colitis. The variation from slight dysplasia with retention of goblet-cell maturation and more obvious atypia in the same or neighbouring tubules is not uncommon. ×280. H & E.

cells arranged in linear fashion parallel to the basement membrane. The nuclei characteristically lie at the basal pole of the cell. Mitoses are frequent but the retained nuclear polarity and uniform appearance is notable, and may be easily overlooked. The cells do, however, have a rather distinct eosinophilic cytoplasm and there is a reduction in the numbers of goblet cells—two features which often assist in the recognition of this change.

Three other, rarer, appearances may be seen—clear cell change, pancellular change, and *in situ* anaplasia. Clear cell change may also seem innocuous but it occurs as a slightly raised lesion macroscopically and has a tubular configuration with an irregular saw-toothed luminal outline in the upper parts of the tubules. The cytoplasm of the cells is clear or ground-glass in appearance and the usual nuclear changes are present although, like basal-cell dysplasia, the nuclei tend to be basally orientated. In pancellular dysplasia the mucosa is flat and composed of enlarged and atypical cells arising from all the usual cell types of the mucosa—goblet cells, absorptive cells, endocrine cells, and even Paneth cells. One or other of these cell types may predominate. *In situ* anaplasia refers to infiltration of malignant cells with or without signet-ring forms in the lamina propria. It usually occurs in association with basal-cell dysplasia in a flat mucosae. The infiltrate is confined to the mucosa, the muscularis mucosae being intact.

Part of the value of categorizing these appearances in such detail lies in attracting the attention of the histopathologist to the possibility that a diagnosis of severe dysplasia in ulcerative colitis should prompt a close sur-

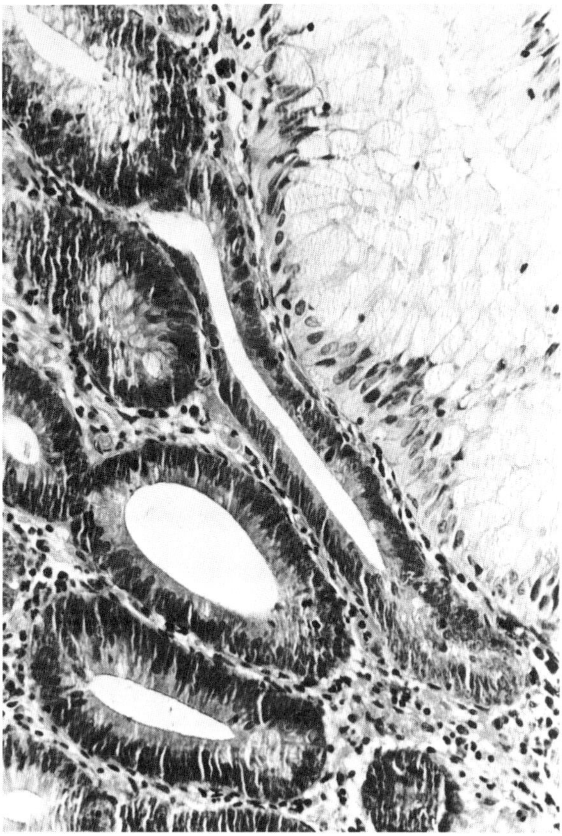

Fig. 8.16. Basal-cell dysplasia in ulcerative colitis. The tubules to the right have a more clear-celled dysplastic appearance and variation of appearances, as in Fig. 8.15, is not unusual. ×280. H & E.

veillance of the patient and help to prevent a cancer death. Because of the nature of the complication the patient will be much younger than the average for colon cancer. If carcinoma in colitis proves always to arise in a dysplastic focus, it seems likely that the precancer period will vary in length. It is in this interim that diagnosis and colectomy will effect a certain cure.

One current approach is to identify the group at high risk and perform sequential colonoscopic biopsies. A decision for proctocolectomy can then be made according to additional clinical data and the severity and persistence of any mucosal dysplasia that is discovered. Whether this policy has advantages over the more empirical approach of elective colectomy in high-risk cases with or without ileorectal anastomosis after ten or more years of disease have elapsed, remains unproven.

Crohn's colitis

There is some evidence that patients with longstanding Crohn's colitis are more prone to develop colonic adenocarcinoma than the normal population (Weedon *et al.*; Gyde *et al.* 1973; Gyde *et al.* 1980). The risk has been assessed as comparable to that in ulcerative colitis. The evidence for the relationship needs to be seen in the light of the more recent definition of Crohn's colitis as a more or less distinct entity, and recognition may have been further delayed due to the greater tendency to resort to surgery in this condition. But given the difficultities in differential diagnosis of inflammatory large-bowel disease, claims for an increased cancer risk in Crohn's disease of the colon need careful evaluation. In some cases the cancer has occurred in an unaffected area, but precancer similar to that which occurs in ulcerative colitis has also been described in the colon (Craft *et al.* 1981). Further studies are clearly needed in order to elucidate the frequency of such lesions. The patchy distribution of the disease in Crohn's disease and the lesser involvement of the mucosa might indicate that factors other than mucosal dysplasia are important. Indeed the cancer in Crohn's colitis may have a greater similarity to the more usual polyp-cancer type.

Schistosomiasis

Infestation with *S. japonicum* and *S. mansoni* is often associated with exuberant inflammatory lesions in the rectum and colon. According to Nebel *et al.* (1974), there is no satisfactory evidence for any consistent relationship between schistosomal polyposis and carcinoma of the colon though the two conditions may sometimes coexist. On the other hand, Ming-Chai *et al.* (1965) described 90 cases of adenocarcinoma of the large intestine complicating schistosomiasis due to *S. japonicum.* The majority had occurred after chronic repeated infection over 10-15 years and the tumours had developed in ulcers, polyps, or areas of abnormal mucosa. According to these authors' description of the lesions the pathogenesis may well be similar to that which is responsible for the malignancy occurring in ulcerative colitis.

Irradiation

Slaughter and Southwick (1957) were probably the first to report the occurrence of radiation-induced colon carcinoma. Since that time Shamsuddin and Elias (1981) refer to seven other cases and describe a patient showing flat mucosal dysplasia similar to that which occurs in ulcerative colitis.

References

Arthur, J.F. (1968). Structure and significance of metaplastic nodules in the rectal mucosa, *J. clin. Pathol.* **21**, 735.

Bone, E., Drasar, B.S., and Hill, M.J. (1975). Gut bacteria and their metabolic activities in familial polyposis. *Lancet* **1**, 1117.

Buell, P. and Dunn, J.E. (1965). Cancer mortality among Japanese Issei and Nisei of California. *Cancer* **18**, 656.

Burkitt, D.P. (1971). Epidemiology of cancer of the colon and rectum. *Cancer* **28**, 3.

Bussey, H.J.R. (1975). Familial polyposis coli, pp. 34-43. Johns Hopkins University Press, Baltimore.
—— and Morson, B.C. (1978). Familial polyposis coli. In *Gastrointestinal tract cancer* (ed. M. Lipkin and R.A. Good), pp. 275-94. Plenum Medical Book Co., New York.
Castleman, B. and Krickstein, H.I. (1962). Do adenomatous polyps of the colon become malignant? *New Engl. J. Med.* **267**, 469.
Chapman, I. (1963). Adenomatous polypi of the large intestine: incidence and distribution. *Ann. Surg.* **157**, 223.
Cook, M.G. and Goligher, J.C. (1975). Carcinoma and epithelial dysplasia complicating ulcerative colitis. *Gastroenterol.* **68**, 1127.
Cooper, H.S., Patchefsky, M.D., and Marks I. (1979) Adenomatous and carcinomatous changes within hyperplastic colonic epithelium. *Dis. Colon Rect.* **22**, 152.
Craft, C.F., Mendelsohn, G., Cooper, H.S., and Yardley, J.H. (1981). *Colonic 'precancer' in Crohn's disease. Gastroenterol.* **80**, 578.
Dawson, I.M.P. and Pryse-Davies, J. (1959). The development of carcinoma of the large intestine in ulcerative colitis. *Brit. J. Surg.* **47**, 113.
Deschner, E.E. and Lipkin, M. (1975). Proliferative patterns in colonic mucosa in familial polyposis. *Cancer* **35**, 413.
Deschner, E.E., Long, F.C., and Katz, S. (1973). Autoradiographic method for an expanded assessment of colonic cytology. *Acta. Cytol.* **17**, 435.
Doll, R. (1969). The geographical distribution of cancer. *Brit. J. Cancer* **23**, 1.
Edwards, F.C. and Truelove, S.C. (1964). The course and prognosis of ulcerative colitis. IV Carcinoma of the colon. *Gut* **5**, 15.
Enterline, R.T. and Arvan, D.A. (1967). Chromosome constitution of adenoma and adenocarcinoma of the colon. *Cancer* **20**, 1746.
Estrada, R.G. and Spjut, H.J. (1980). Hyperplastic polyps of the large bowel. *Amer. J. Surg. Pathol.* **4**, 127.
Evans, D.J. and Pollock, D.J. (1972). *In situ* and invasive carcinoma of the colon in patients with ulcerative colitis. *Gut* **13**, 566.
Fenoglio, C.M., Kaye, G.I., and Lane, N. (1973). Distribution of human colonic lymphatics in normal, hyperplastic and adenomatous tissue. *Gastroenterol.* **64**, 51.
Gibbs, N.M. (1967). The incidence and significance of argentaffin and Paneth cells in some tumours of the large intestine. *J. clin. Pathol.* **20**, 826.
Gilbertsen, V.A. (1974). Proctosigmoidoscopy and polypectomy in reducing the incidence of rectal cancer. *Cancer* **34**, 936.
——, Knatterud, G.L., Lober, P.H., and Wangensteen, O.T. (1965). Invasive carcinoma of the large intestine: a preventative disease? *Surgery* **57**, 363.
Gillespie, P.E., Chambers, T.J., Chan, K.W., Doronzo, F., Morson, B.C., and Williams, C.B. (1979). Colonic adenomas—a colonoscopic survey. *Gut* **20**, 240.
Goldman, H., Ming, S., and Hickok, D.F. (1970). Nature and significance of hyperplastic polyps of the human colon. *Arch. Pathol.* **89**, 349.
Gyde, S.N., Prior, P., Macartney, J.C., Thompson, H., Waterhouse, J.A.H., and Allan, R.N. (1980). Malignancy in Crohn's disease. *Gut* **21**, 1024.
Greene, F.L. (1974). Epithelial misplacement in adenomatous polyps of the colon and rectum. *Cancer* **33**, 206.
Grinnell, R.S. and Lane, N. (1958). Benign and malignant adenomatous polyps and papillary adenomas of the colon and rectum; an analysis of 1,856 tumours in 1,335 patients. *Int. Abst. Surg.* **106**, 519.
Haghighi, P., Nasr, K., Mohallatee, E., Ghassemi, H., Sadri, S., Nabizadeh, I., Sheikholeslami, M., and Mostafavi, N. (1977). Colorectal polyps and carcinoma in southern Iran. *Cancer* **39**, 274.

Hawley, P.R. (1974). Carcinoma of the colon. *Brit. J. hosp. Med.* **11**, 211.
Hill, M.J. (1974). Bacteria and the etiology of colonic cancer. *Cancer* **34**, 815.
—— (1980). Bacterial metabolism and human carcinogenesis. *Brit. Med. Bull.* **36**, 89.
——, Morson, B.C., and Bussey, H.J.R. (1978). Aetiology of adenoma-carcinoma sequence in large bowel. *Lancet* **1**, 245.
Horn, R.C. Jr. (1971). Malignant potential of polypoidal lesions of the colon and rectum. *Cancer* **28**, 146.
Isaacson, P. (1976). Tissue demonstration of carcinoembryonic antigen (CEA) in ulcerative colitis. *Gut* **17**, 561.
—— and Le Vann, H.P. (1976). The demonstration of carcinoembryonic antigen in colorectal carcinoma and colonic polyps using an immunoperoxidase technique. *Cancer* **38**, 1348.
Kaye, G.I., Lane, N., and Pascal, R.R. (1968). Colonic pericryptal fibroblast sheath: replication, migration, and cytodifferentiation of a mesenchymal cell system in adult tissue: II. Fine structural aspects of normal rabbit and human colon. *Gastroenterol.* **54**, 852.
——, Pascal, R.R., and Lane, N. (1971). The colonic pericryptal fibroblast sheath: replication, migration and cytodifferentiation of a mesenchymal cell system in adult tissue. *Gastroenterol.* **60**, 515.
Konishi, F. and Morson, B.C. (1982). Pathology of colorectal adenomas: a colonoscopic survey. *J. clin. Pathol.* **35**, 830.
Lane, N., Fenoglio, C.M., Kaye, G.I., and Pascal, R.R. (1978). Defining the precursor tissue of ordinary large bowel carcinoma: implications for cancer prevention. In *Gastrointestinal tract cancer* (ed. M. Lipkin and R.A. Good), pp. 295-324. Plenum Medical Book Co., New York.
Lennard-Jones, J.E., Morson, B.C., Ritchie, J.K., Shove, D.C., and Williams, C.B. (1977). Cancer in colitis: assessment of the individual risk by clinical and histological criteria. *Gastroenterol.* **73**, 1280.
Lewin, K. (1968). Neoplastic Paneth cells. *J. clin. pathol.* **21**, 476.
Lovett, E. (1976). Family studies in cancer of the colon and rectum. *Brit. J. Surg.* **63**, 13.
McGovern, V.J. (1972). Rectal biopsy in the differential diagnosis of colitis. *Rendiconti di Gastroenterologia,* **4**, 94.
Ming-Chai, C., Jen-Chun, H., P'ei-Yu, C., Ch'i-Juan, C., P'eng-Fei, T., Shen-Hsing, C., Fu-P'an, W., Ts'u-Ling, C., and Shun-Ch'uan, C. (1965). Pathogenesis of carcinoma of the colon and rectum in Schistosomiasis Japonica: a study of 90 cases. *Chinese med. J.* **84**, 513.
Morson, B.C. and Pang, L.S. (1967). Rectal biopsy as an aid to cancer control in ulcertative colitis. *Gut* **8**, 423.
Muto, T., Bussey, H.J.R., and Morson, B.C. (1975). The evolution of cancer of the colon and rectum. *Cancer* **36**, 2251.
Nebel, O.T., Castell, D.O., Fornes, M.F., and Sparks, H.A. (1974). Schistosomal colonic polyposis. Endoscopic and histological characteristics. *Gastroint estinal Endosc.* **20**, 99.
Oluwatope, A., Mabogunje, M.D., Subbuswamy, M.D., and Lawrie, J.H. (1978). Rectal polyps in Zaria, Nigeria. *Dis. Colon Rectum* **21**, 474.
Pascal, R.R., Kaye, G.I., and Lane, N. (1968). Colonic pericryptal fibroblast sheath: replication, migration and cytodifferentiation of a mesenchymal cell system in adult tissue. I. autoradiographic studies of the normal rabbit colon. *Gastroenterol.* **54**, 835.
Pearse, A.G.E. (1966*a*). 5-Hydroxytryptophan uptake by dog thyroid C cells and its possible significance in polypeptide hormone production. *Nature* **211**, 598.
—— (1966*b*). Common cytochemical properties of cells producing polypeptide hor-

mones, with particular reference to calcitonin and the thyroid C cells. *Vet. Res.* **79**, 587.

Pour, P. (1978). A new and advantageous model for colorectal cancer: its comparison with previous models for a common human disease. *Cancer Lett.* **4**, 293.

Riddell, R.H. (1976). The precarcinomatous phase of ulcerative colitis. *Current topics Pathol.* **63**, 179.

Shamsuddin, A.K.M. and Elias, E.G. (1981). Rectal mucosa—malignant and premalignant changes after radiation therapy. *Arch. Pathol. Lab. Med.* **105**, 150.

Skinner, J.M. and Whitehead, R. (1981). Tumor-associated antigens in polyps and carcinoma of the human large bowel. *Cancer* **47**, 1241.

Slaughter, D.P. and Southwick, H.W. (1957). Mucosal carcinomas as a result of irradiation. *Arch. Surg.* **74**, 420.

Spjut, H.J., Frankel, N.B., and Appel, M.F. (1979). The small carcinoma of the large bowel. *Amer. J. surg. Pathol.* **3**, 39.

Spratt, J.S., Ackerman, L.V., and Moyer, C.A. (1958). Relationship of polyps of the colon to colonic cancer. *Ann. Surg.* **148**, 682.

Stemmerman, G.N. and Yatani, R. (1976). Diverticulosis and polyps of the large intestine. *Cancer* **31**, 1260.

Svartz, N. and Ernberg, T. (1949). Cancer coli in cancer of colitis ulcerosa. *Acta Med. Scand.* **135**, 444.

Weedon, D.D., Shorter, R.G., Ilstrup, D.M., Huizenga, K.A., and Taylor, W.F. (1973). Crohn's disease and cancer. *New Engl. J. Med.* **289**, 1099.

Welin, S., Youker, J., and Spratt, J.S. (1963). The rates and patterns of growth of 375 tumours of the large intestine and rectum observed serially by double contrast enema study. (Malmö technique). *Amer. J. Roentogenol., radium ther. Nuclear Med.* **90**, 673.

van der Werf, S.D.J., Nagengast, F.M., van Berge Henegouwen G.P., Huijbregts, A.W.M., and van Tongeren, J.H.M. (1982). Colonic absorption of secondary bile acids in patients with adenomatous polyps and in matched controls. *Lancet* **i**, 759.

Whitehead, R. and Cosgrove, C. (1979). Mucins and carcinoid tumours. *Pathology* **11**, 473.

Williams, A.O. and Prince, D.L. (1975). Intestinal polyps in the Nigerian African. *J. clin. Pathol.* **28**, 367.

Woda, B.A., Forde, K., and Lane, N. (1977). A unicryptal colonic adenoma, the smallest colonic neoplasm yet observed in a non-polyposis individual. *Amer. J. clin. Pathol.* **68**, 631.

World Health Organization (1976). *Histological typing of intestinal tumours.* International histological classification of tumours, no. 15. World Health Organization, Geneva.

Wynder, E.L. and Reddy, B. (1974). Metabolic epidemiology of colorectal cancer. *Cancer* **34**, 801.

——, Kajitani, T., Ischikawa, S., Dodott, P., and Takano, A. (1969). Environmental factors in cancer of the colon and rectum. *Cancer* **23**, 1210.

Zedeck, M.S. (1978). Experimental colon carcinogenesis. In *Gastrointestinal tract cancer* (ed. M. Lipkin and R.A. Good), p. 343. Plenum Medical Book Co., New York.

9 Precancerous states in the liver

K. Weinbren

The identification of pre-neoplastic states in the liver presents several difficulties as the term implies some inevitability of tumour development, a proposition which is usually difficult to sustain. At the same time, there are conditions which are regarded clinically or experimentally as representing a stage in or a background for carcinogenesis on the basis that tumours are found with greater frequency in livers affected by such conditions than in livers which do not show these changes. There is the additional problem of separating other accompanying changes which may be detectable structurally, biochemically, or immunologically from these hepatic lesions which may be regarded as specific stages in the development of a neoplasm. A further complication lies in the fact that substances regarded as carcinogens in some circumstances may also be responsible for other tissue reactions which in themselves may not be part of the process of carcinogenesis, and which should be distinguished from genuine precancerous states.

The main primary neoplasms in the liver arise from hepatocytes, biliary epithelial cells, or littoral (endothelial or peri-sinusoidal) cells. In some species other tumours may be found, but in man the main neoplasms appear to arise from these three categories and the possibility of recognizing separate precancerous states for these lesions is considered here. Reference will be made also to changes observed during the development of tumours in experimental studies.

Hepatocellular carcinoma

This tumour occurs throughout the world, with a particularly high incidence in southern Africa and south-east Asia (Oettlé 1965; Higginson 1970). Several conditions have been considered as possible precancerous states, the most common being cirrhosis. Reports have been published of hepatocellular carcinoma occurring in patients with other liver diseases including viral infections, congenital abnormalities, and metabolic and storage diseases (Roe *et al.* 1979).

Cirrhosis

Results from many studies of patients suffering from cirrhosis and hepatocellular carcinoma (Lee 1966; Anthony 1973; MacSween and Scott 1973; Galambos 1975; Popper 1977; Blenkinsopp and Haffenden 1977) are regarded by most authors as indicating that carcinoma is a complication of cirrhosis and that cirrhosis is reasonably considered to be a precancerous state. While this appears to be a consensus view, it may not apply in all circumstances and evidence of this sequential relationship is not always clear. One of the most recent accounts, from a general hospital in Budapest, describes 181 patients who died with cirrhosis between 1973 and 1976 (Bartók *et al.* 1981). The age incidence for patients who died with carcinoma and cirrhosis was not significantly different from that of patients who died with cirrhosis alone. In addition, although there is in Western countries often clinical evidence of long-standing cirrhosis before carcinoma is recognized (Kew *et al.* 1971), African patients most often present without a clinical history of long-standing cirrhosis and are found at autopsy to have been suffering from carcinoma and cirrhosis (Alpert *et al.* 1969). It may be that the failure to demonstrate in Africans a later average age incidence at autopsy for carcinoma-cirrhosis patients than that for cirrhosis alone rests on a rapid deterioration in patients who develop superimposed carcinoma; but, even if this were so, it might be expected that a prolonged period of cirrhosis would usually precede the development of carcinoma. There may be different relationships between carcinoma and cirrhosis, and it is possible that there is a form of chronic liver disease in which carcinoma and cirrhosis develop together in the same liver. If this form of chronic liver disease is definable, it may be of value to identify early distinguishable characteristics. It is not clear also whether it is possible to identify a form of cirrhosis which is not associated with either superimposed or contemporaneously developing carcinoma.

The type of cirrhosis most frequently associated with carcinoma is macronodular cirrhosis (Lee 1966; Anthony 1973; MacSween 1974). This may imply that neoplasms may be particularly prone to develop in this form of the disease, but it seems that macronodular cirrhosis may develop from micronodular cirrhosis in chronic alcoholic liver disease (Rubin *et al.* 1962). It is conceivable also that the destruction and haemodynamic changes which attend the development of neoplasms within a liver may generate large areas of atrophy and scarring and stimulate further hyperplasia of nodules, thus resulting in an appearance of macronodular cirrhosis. Hepatocellular carcinoma has been described together with cirrhosis thought to be caused by any of the accepted factors including viral infection, metabolic disease, alcoholism, and presumed mycotoxins (Alpert and Davidson 1969; Wogan 1976), and it is likely that the disease state of cirrhosis itself may influence the course of the disease.

The mechanism by which carcinoma develops in these circumstances is not clear; one possibility is that the raised rate of DNA synthesis that inevitably accompanies the formation of hyperplastic nodules in cirrhosis acts as a promoter for cells already initiated by some unknown stimulus, possibly incorporated in the course of the cirrhogenic injury. In this connexion a change in hepatocytes is described which is considered to be a possible stage in the development of the neoplastic process (Anthony *et al.* 1973). This involves groups of hepatocytes containing large irregular nuclei found in parts of the cirrhotic liver and which are distinguishable from tumour. While it is uncertain whether such formations are pre-neoplastic stages of hepatocellular carcinoma or not, these changes are reported to occur, on average, at an earlier age than those associated with fully developed hepatocellular carcinoma. These dysplastic cells are found more frequently in patients with HBsAg positive serum and were particularly common in a series published from Uganda (Vogel *et al.* 1970; Anthony *et al.* 1973).

Hepatic venous lesions

Simson and Middlecote (1973) reported a group of patients presenting with evidence of occlusion or at least obstruction of the outflow from main hepatic veins with the formation of large collaterals and sometimes with evidence of portal hypertension; such patients who live in the north-eastern part of South Africa soon develop the clinical features associated with primary hepatocellular carcinoma. The relationship between the two conditions remains unclear. In most accounts from Europe and the United States, major hepatic venous occlusion results in characteristic morphological changes in the liver (Parker 1959; Gibson 1960) but such patients do not appear to be more liable to develop hepatocellular carcinoma. In reports from Japan of congenital vena caval lesions which result in the clinical features of hepatic venous ostial occlusion, there is a dubious increase in the incidence of primary hepatocellular carcinoma but it is not established whether the increased rate can be related causally to the venous lesion. The survival time after the recognition of the venous lesion is unclear and other factors are usually not excluded (Takeuchi *et al.* 1971).

Veno-occlusive disease (VOD), a lesion involving hepatic venous radicles and sublobular veins (Bras *et al.* 1954), is found particularly in the West Indies after consuming pyrrolizidine alkaloids. The incidence of hepatocellular carcinoma is not epidemiologically associated with chronic Bush tea toxicity and, in general, VOD cannot be regarded as a pre-neoplastic state. Veno-occlusive disease of the liver is reported also in association with the effects of drug therapy, particularly azathioprine, cyclophosphamide, and 6-thioguanine, but such lesions are not known to presage malignant change. Supervoltage radiotherapy (Reed and Cox 1966) is another cause of veno-occlusive disease, and neoplasia has in fact been recorded as a delayed effect (Moore *et al.* 1976). It is difficult to form a balanced view about the neoplastic potential of peliosis in man, as it is not clear whether the peliosis precedes or follows the hepatocyte proliferation. Most observations have been made on necropsy material from patients dying with other chronic diseases such as tuberculosis (Yanoff and Rawson 1964), but more recently Paradinas *et al.* (1977) postulated a mechanical obstruction by hyperplastic hepatic cells of the sinusoidal flow. The patients with periportal sinusoidal dilatation associated with contraceptive steroids have not so far been found to develop hepatic neoplasms (Winkler and Poulson 1975) although benign tumours co-exist with peliosis (Glassburg and Rosenbaum 1976; Paradinas *et al.* 1977) and can undergo malignant change (p. 260-1).

Other vascular conditions

Carcinoma of the liver has been reported in hereditary haemorrhagic telangiectasia (Rendu-Weber-Osler) by Sussman and Sternberg (1975), and benign liver tumours have been associated with cavernous transformation of the portal vein (Klemperer 1928).

With regard to the changes in hereditary haemorrhagic telangiectasia, the fibrous-enmeshed communications between vascular malformations usually show characteristics which are benign, but cirrhosis is sometimes diagnosed (Martini 1959; Feizi 1972). The occasional case of carcinoma appears unlikely to represent a complication of this condition; if any association is warranted, it would be with cirrhosis even though this is a rare change (Daley and Schiller 1976).

The occurrence of four cases of 'adenoma' among 22 patients with cavernomatous transformation of the portal vein described by Klemperer in 1928 suggests *a priori* that this vascular lesion may reasonably be considered a preneoplastic state. While the recorded observation confirms the careful studies made by Klemperer, it is clear that he interpreted the lesions as hyperplastic nodules and subsequent publications indicate that hyperplastic nodules are likely to develop after long-standing portal venous deprivation (Weinbren and Washington 1976; Weinbren 1978; Wanless *et al.* 1980). It is not justifiable on present evidence to consider cavernous transformation of the portal vein as a preneoplastic lesion.

Viral hepatitis

Viral infection of the liver has been recognized for some 40 years and, in most instances, the disease is of limited duration: the patient usually recovers and the liver returns to normal structure and function. Sometimes a more chronic clinical condition develops with the persistence of structural alterations in the liver, and it is recognized that cirrhosis of the liver can sometimes be traced to viral infection.

The relevance of cirrhosis to carcinoma has been referred to and the question that is posed is whether chronic liver disease which is associated with viral infection has a different relationship to hepatocellular carcinoma from chronic liver disease which is associated with cirrhosis which is not primarily virus associated.

From a global point of view, both hepatocellular carcinoma and viral infection by hepatitis B virus are of high incidence and there is a good deal of evidence which indicates that the association between viral infection and hepatocarcinoma is not fortuitous (Peters 1976). The support for this association has been adduced largely from epidemiological studies, in which the incidence of hepatocellular carcinoma has been investigated in relation to various states of viral infection. The criteria on which the diagnosis of hepatocarcinoma is based are generally agreed in such studies, and there appears to be no dispute about the diagnosis. The tumour is associated in about 90 per cent of instances with cirrhosis or some form of chronic liver disease, and only in 10 per cent of cases is the non-tumorous liver reported as normal. For the identification of a state of viral infection, although the clinical and structural changes in the liver are usually recognizable as being associated with viral infection, almost all recent epidemiological investigations have included the serological demonstration of past or present viral infection. It is now clear that the virion of hepatitis B virus is a 42-nm structure, the Dane particle, with a surface coat and an inner core, and that both it and surface antigen (22-nm diam.) are reliably detectable (Dane *et al.* 1970). Antibodies to surface antigen, to core antigen, and to what is probably an inner protein layer in the core (e antibody) are also detectable (Takahashi *et al.* 1979). Thus the designation of viral hepatitis as a precancerous state is related less to the structural changes encountered in this condition than to the persistence of hepatitis B virus in the patient. It is supposed therefore that most patients in whom evidence of virus infection is detected have indeed suffered an episode of viral hepatitis although this is not proven. At the same time, the condition of acute viral hepatitis as defined clinically and morphologically when caused by hepatitis B virus may in fact be an illness from which active chronic hepatitis may develop with persistence of viral infection (Gudat *et al.* 1975). Persistence of infection is not entirely correlated with absence of structural reconstitution as a carrier state may develop after an infection of short duration, and epidemiological studies are based on persistence of infection rather than on structural abnormalities in the liver (Edgington and Chisari 1975). Nonetheless, whatever consensus is reached about the association of hepatitis B infection and hepatocarcinoma these considerations will apply to patients with acute viral hepatitis as, at the present time, it it difficult to identify structural differences between those patients with acute B hepatitis who will have transient infection from those in whom infection will be persistent and detectable.

The evidence linking hepatitis B with hepatocarcinoma has been collated by workers in many parts of the world and is based on a series of correlations. The geographical incidence of hepatocarcinoma is strikingly similar to that of hepatitis B infection (Larouze *et al.* 1977). Moreover the frequency of hepatitis B infection in patients with carcinoma is very high, and the correlation between cancer and hepatitis B infection is striking and similar in countries with a high incidence of hepatocarcinoma and those with a low incidence of hepatocarcinoma (Prince 1980). Recent studies in Iceland with a bank of stored sera have provided interesting information on the natural history of hepatitis B infection and its association with hepatocarcinoma (Heyward *et al.* 1982). The results indicate that hepatitis B infection may occur as little as ten years before hepatocarcinoma is recognized. Seroconversion from HBeAg to anti-HBe occurred as long as six years before the clinical onset of the tumours, and significant increases in serum α-fetoprotein (AFP) were noted two years before hepatocarcinoma was diagnosed. The authors suggest that AFP may be a useful marker for screening high-risk HBsAg carriers after seroconversion from HBeAg to Anti-HBe.

On the structural side, 'ground-glass' hepatocytes containing surface antigen are frequently found in livers from patients with hepatocarcinoma (Deodhar *et al.* 1975) and there is an increased incidence of hepatocarcinoma in patients with chronic liver disease associated with persistent viral infection (Hann *et al.* 1979).

The epidemiological evidence associating B type hepatitis is compelling and it seems justifiable at present to consider that the acute condition may sometimes be a precancerous state. The point must, however, be made that the persistence of infection—which is not necessarily reflected in changes in hepatic morphology—may be the relevant factor in the carcinogenic process.

It may be pertinent then to reflect whether the presence of ground-glass hepatocytes within a liver can reasonably be considered to identify a precancerous state. The evidence suggests that a liver containing such cells is one in which there is persistent viral infection in the form of surface antigen and that the presence of ground-glass Orcein-positive cells, either with active chronic hepatitis or with cirrhosis or in an otherwise normal liver, is indicative of a precancerous state. There is at present no support for the view that the ground-glass cell itself is a pre-neoplastic cell, but this problem does not seem to have been adequately investigated. Comparative studies to confirm the relationship between hepatitis B virus infection and the development of hepatocarcinoma have not been fully developed but a naturally occurring virus infection, similar in some respects to hepatitis B, has been reported in the woodchuck (*Marmota monax*) and this has been closely correlated with the development of hepatocarcinoma in this animal (Summers *et al.* 1978).

Experimental studies on this topic have included studies of base sequences in DNA of patients with hepatocarcinoma (Shafritz and Kew 1981) and in the DNA of cell lines established from human hepatocarcinomas *in vitro* (Knowles *et al.* 1980). Virus DNA base sequences have been found in a very high incidence in liver DNA from patients with hepatocarcinoma in Senegal (Summers *et al.* 1978) and a cell-line has been developed from a patient with hepatocarcinoma in which viral DNA transformations are recoverable (MacNab *et al.* 1976).

The pathogenic mechanism which underlies the malignant transformation of hepatocytes in the presence of persistent viral infection is not known but it seems justifiable at present to regard B hepatitis as potentially precancerous in the hope that successful prevention may reduce the incidence of hepatic cancer (Zuckerman 1982).

Nodular hyperplasia

Hepatocyte hyperplasia associated with a loss of normal vascular relationships (nodular hyperplasia) may involve only a limited region of liver substance, in which case the condition is termed focal nodular hyperplasia, or it may affect a substantial part of the liver, in which case the term 'diffuse nodular hyperplasia' is employed.

It is not known whether either of these conditions is pre-neoplastic, but the view has been canvassed that such hyperplastic conditions may have a neoplastic (sometimes malignant) counterpart (Peters 1976). Evidence to support this assertion is difficult to define and remains largely circumstantial in relation to lesions in man. Focal nodular hyperplasia has been described in children and in young and middle-aged adults of both sexes (Knowles and Wolfe 1976). In most instances, on morphological grounds it appears to be distinguishable from the hepatic adenoma associated with administration of oral contraceptives (Fechner 1977) but a few of the liver lesions observed in contraceptive pill-takers show characteristics of both nodular hyperplasia and hepatic adenoma (Klatskin 1977). Since it is known that occasionally the lesion associated with the oral contraceptive possesses malignant attributes (Davis *et al.* 1975), liver-cell adenomas in such patients have come to be regarded as representing a neoplasm which may develop invasive activity (Peters 1976). It is on this basis that focal nodular hyperplasia may be suspected of possessing a neoplastic potential, but no instance of clearly defined focal nodular hyperplasia has so far been reported as converting to a hepatocellular carcinoma—or even an unequivocal tumour.

Diffuse nodular hyperplasia is found with increased frequency in patients suffering from myeloproliferative conditions and dysgammaglobulinaemias (Wanless *et al.* 1981), but instances of conversion of this condition into a neoplastic state are difficult to define and to document. A variant of hepatocellular carcinoma—the polygonal-celled variety with lamellar fibrosis—is, however, reported as sometimes showing an association with nodular hyperplasia within the same liver and this finding has led to the suggestion that nodular hyperplasia may represent a precancerous state in man (Peters 1976).

In relation to the development of a benign neoplasm in a patient taking oral contraceptives, Thung and Gerber (1981) describe hepatic changes which preceded the development of the neoplasm. These resembled to some extent the changes noted in patients exposed to vinyl chloride monomer, and the authors stressed the findings of hepatocyte hyperplasia, hypertrophy of sinusoidal lining cells associated with an excess of reticulin fibres and sinusoidal dilatation 'leading to primary peliosis'. It is not clear whether such changes are common or specific.

Apart from these rather unusual examples, the evidence is not strong that the conditions designated as hyperplasia are truly pre-neoplastic.

The cases of hepatocellular carcinoma which have been associated with oral contraceptives probably represent malignant change in a pre-existing adenoma and a pre-neoplastic state has not been clearly identified (Davis *et al.* 1975).

Alpha-1-antitrypsin deficiency

The chronic liver disease associated with this deficiency is primarily cirrhosis of the liver, and the pathway to the cirrhosis is usually identified by the presence of PAS-positive cytoplasmic inclusions which shown localization of antibodies to alpha-1-antitrypsin. In several cases, there is striking bile-duct proliferation, the mechanism for which is not established. So far as can be gathered, the risk of development of neoplasm in such circumstances is no greater than that considered to be the risk in cirrhosis associated with other factors, although alpha-1-antitrypsin has been found in hepatocarcinoma (Palmer and Wolfe 1976). But of course, the association of cirrhosis and neoplastic disease is regarded as real and, in this respect, the alpha-1-antitrypsin deficiency lesion has certainly not been found to be less prone to this complication. There have been no reported cases of cholangiocarcinoma in patients with alpha-1-antitrypsin deficiency, which suggests that the ductal proliferation sometimes observed in this condition does not have a neoplastic connotation.

Metabolic diseases

An increased incidence of hepatocellular carcinoma is recognized in some forms of genetic metabolic diseases which affect the liver. This association has been reported particularly in patients who survive to adulthood with Type I glycogenosis, as well as with iron storage disease in which the relationship seems to be similar to that of cirrhosis and hepatocellular carcinoma. Long-term survival with these metabolic abnormalities usually implies a *forme fruste* of the condition, and it is therefore difficult to quantify the risk of neoplastic transformation. Nonetheless cases have been reported (Roe *et al.* 1979) but it may be via the pathway of cirrhosis which usually develops. No particular tendency to neoplastic development is reported in patients with Wilson's disease (Sternlieb 1978).

Biliary epithelial tumours

The current consensus view distinguishes hepatocellular carcinomas from cholangiocarcinomas on the basis of several structural and ultrastructural criteria, notably the ability of cholangiocarcinomas to synthesize mucin. This property is accepted as the definitive differentiating feature of cholangiocarcinoma, and mucin-secreting intrahepatic primary adenocarcinomas situated usually in the hilar region but sometimes deeper within the liver substance are regarded as cholangiocarcinomas even when the duct of origin cannot be identified (Klatskin 1965; Okuda *et al.* 1977).

Lesions of bile ducts, especially intrahepatic ducts, need to be carefully defined as a neoplastic potential is not recorded for all forms of ductal narrowing observed in various types of clinical studies. For example, long-standing purulent cholangitis secondary to some form of duct obstruction leads to fibrosis in adventitial tissue surrounding small ducts, with collagen sometimes replacing the duct wall. This is usually accompanied by the changes of chronic duct obstruction and cholangitis—notably proliferation of marginal ducts and much portal fibrosis, often with apparent linkage between portal tracts—but there is no association with cholangiocarcinoma. Other inflammatory and congenital ductal lesions are, however, sometimes considered to be precancerous.

Sclerosing cholangitis

The observation of Parker and Kendall (1954) that carcinoma of the liver is occasionally accompanied by long-standing ulcerative colitis was at first regarded as a chance association. Since that time these two conditions have been repeatedly observed in the same patient, and it appears that cholangiocarcinomas develop with a significantly increased frequency in patients with ulcerative colitis (Ross and Braasch 1973), but not in patients with Crohn's disease (Ritchie *et al.* 1974). The link between these seemingly unrelated diseases is considered to be sclerosing cholangitis. The incidence of this ill-defined entity varies in different reports, partly because of differences in diagnostic criteria required for its definition (Chapman *et al.* 1980). As the term implies, the main feature is increased formation of collagen in the walls of biliary channels (Fig. 9.1). The collagen replaces the mural structure of the bile duct and narrows the lumen, usually with destruction of the biliary epithelium. Sometimes the smaller ducts are completely replaced by a sphere of solid fibrous tissue with almost no characteristics identifiable as a former duct. Were it not for the accompanying hepatic artery, absence of an alternative ductal structure at the expected site, and other ducts showing different stages of development of the lesion, it seems possible that fibrous whorls might not be identified as former ductal structures. When the disease involves extrahepatic bile ducts and the gall bladder, the fibrosis is recognizable macroscopically. The biliary changes are demonstrable on cholangiography. Microscopical observations have not always been precise about the distinction between primary sclerotic changes and those secondary to cholangitis or lithiasis, and there is some vagueness about the distinction between sclerosing cholangitis and chronic pericholangitis. It seems convenient to regard lesions in which ducts show concentric collagenization with intact biliary epithelium and essentially normal lumina as 'pericholangitis' and the condition in which there is epithelial destruction and replacement by fibrosis and severe luminal compromise as 'sclerosing

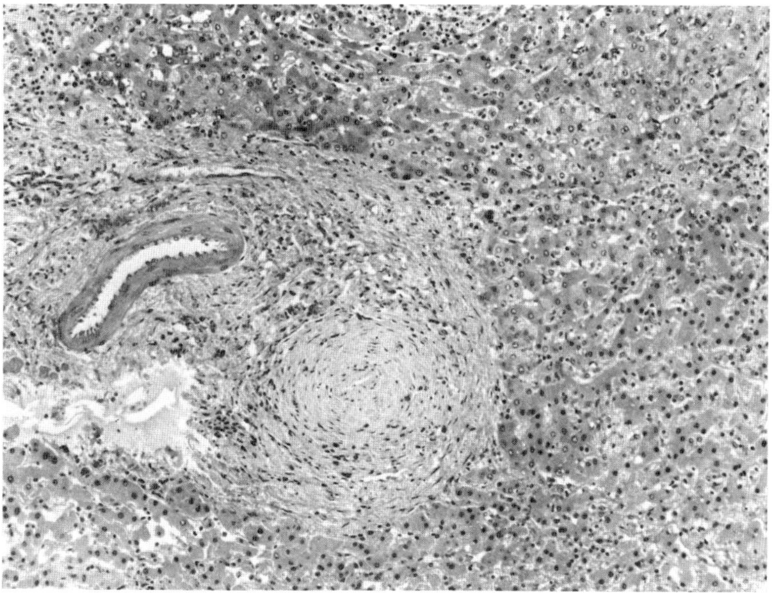

Fig. 9.1. Sclerosing cholangitis of intrahepatic bile duct. ×100. H & E.

cholangitis' or 'primary sclerosing cholangitis' (PSC). It is the latter condition that complicates ulcerative colitis in 5 per cent of cases and it is itself associated with the development of cholangiocarcinoma in approximately 10 per cent of instances (Converse *et al.* 1971).

The cholangiocarcinoma encountered in these circumstances usually affects patients younger than the mean age for cholangiocarcinoma and appears to carry a poor prognosis, although a patient of Ritchie *et al.* (1974) is reported to have survived four years after partial hepatectomy. The tumour is known to develop up to five years after total proctocolectomy for ulcerative colitis.

On epidemiological grounds PSC is a precancerous condition, but caution must be observed in reaching this conclusion in biopsy sections as there is no evidence that fibrosed bile ducts associated with long-standing obstruction and cholangitis and pericholangitis with intact ductal luminal epithelium carry a similar risk. The pathogenesis of the change from PSC to cholangiocarcinoma is not known. It is possible that PSC develops from pericholangitis. The pathogenesis of this periductal inflammatory change is not clear, but the effects of bacterial and metabolic products from the gut and undefined immunological reactions have been implicated (Kern 1976). The mean duration of the gut disease before development of PSC is approximately eight years with reports varying from 5 to 15 years (Ritchie *et al.* 1974). The definition of the condition is unclear clinically as indirect imaging and endoscopic observation indicate (at most) luminal narrowing and the possible absence of neoplatic disease, but provide no information about the possible mechanistic basis for the ductal occlusion.

Pericholangitis

This condition has a known association with chronic ulcerative colitis and, in general, is seen either as a periductal inflammatory exudate with separation of periductal adventitial connective tissue by oedema or as a distinct periductal concentric fibrosis. In view of the known association of pericholangitis with ulcerative colitis and because of the clinical oberservations that pericholangitis may be a reversible change (Wood and Cuschieri 1980), it seems reasonable to draw a distinction between the lesions of sclerosing cholangitis and pericholangitis even though it is possible that they may represent stages of one entity. So far there is no convincing evidence that pericholangitis is precancerous.

Parasitic infestation

Cholangiocarcinoma is found with increased incidence when there is infestation by the liver flukes *Clonorchis sinensis* and *Opisthorchis viverrini*, affecting populations in Hong Kong, South-East China, and Thailand (Gibson 1971). The mechanism by which neoplastic change is brought about is unknown as the epithelial changes encountered in affected bile ducts are mainly hyperplastic and similar to those found in other forms of intraductal inflammation. The association of cholangiocarcinoma with the particular parasites mentioned, and not with *Fasciola hepatica* or *Schistosoma* sp., suggests that infestation with the relevant flukes should be regarded as a precancerous state.

Non-parasitic cystic disease

Several varieties of congenital hepatic cysts are recognized. These vary in size and are found within the liver and involve also extrahepatic bile ducts.

Of the intrahepatic cysts, probably the most common lesion is polycystic disease. In this condition multiple thin-walled cysts, varying in size from one to tens of centimetres in diameter, are found throughout the liver; they consist of thin nearly translucent walls and contain almost colourless non-bile-stained fluid (Melnick 1955). In about 20 per cent of patients with polycystic disease of the liver there are small foci of confluent microscopical cysts enmeshed in fibrous tissue. The lining epithelium is flattened and these are referred to as microhamartomas or von Meyenburg complexes (von Meyenburg 1918). Such cystic lesions are usually not associated with the development of portal hypertension, but there is a raised incidence of polycystic kidneys (Dalgaard 1957). A condition in which small ducts are distorted and sometimes cystic and surrounded by mature fibrous tissue sharply demarcated from plates of hepatic parenchymal cells is recognized as congenital (Parker, 1956; Kerr *et al.* 1960) and referred to as congenital hepatic fibrosis. This condition is frequently associated with portal hypertension and with a peculiar form of renal disease known as distal tubular dilatation (Kerr *et al.* 1962; Murray-Lyon *et al.* 1973). A closely related condition is dilatation of the intrahepatic ducts (Caroli 1973). This condition is similar in some respects to congenital hepatic fibrosis, but, in addition to the typical microscopical changes and renal lesions of this condition, the ductal system shows varying degrees of dilatation.

Choledochal cysts are formed outside the liver and consist of cystic diverticula of the gall bladder or extrahepatic bile ducts. These appear to have no consistent associated lesion in the kidney and are encountered either as a cause of obstructive jaundice or as a cystic mass at surgery. Tumours are found with increased frequency in association with cyst formation (Fig. 9.2). The range is from 2 to 7 per cent, most often affecting congenital dilatation of bile ducts (Gallagher *et al.* 1972) and rather less frequently choledochal cysts (Cruickshank 1961; Kagawa *et al.* 1978). It is difficult to derive accurate estimates of the incidence of congenital cystic disease in the population as many cases are not reported and sometimes not even recorded in autopsy figures. When symptoms are associated with the various forms of cystic disease, the recognition of the cysts is recorded together with any symptom or sign-generating complications. Thus, although the figures for the incidence of neoplastic disease in these conditions may not be accurate, the existence of this complication seems well-established with the proviso that

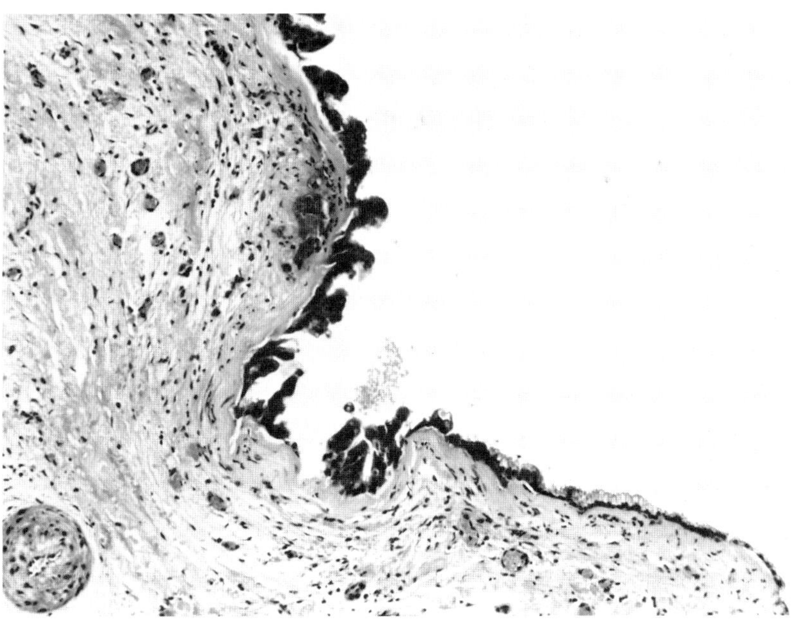

Fig. 9.2. Neoplastic change involving part of cyst wall. ×27. H & E.

the development of neoplastic change may be the factor which precipitates the recording of the cystic disease.

The possibility of neoplasms developing from von Meyenburg complexes was raised by Homer *et al.,* (1968) who reported four cases of micro-hamartoma (Von Meyenburg Complex, VMC); in two of the cases they described an adenomatous transformation and in a third case carcinomatous change. The conclusions in this paper are questionable, and it now seems clear that the three instances of neoplastic change in von Meyenburg complexes as reported by Homer and his colleagues are not supported by the authors' illustrations or reasoning. Microhamartomas are therefore not regarded as preneoplastic lesions, an important conclusion in view of the frequency of von Meyenburg complexes.

Intrahepatic congenital cysts are very rarely associated with neoplastic transformation. The cystic lesion described by Corrin (1962) as a cyst-adenoma probably arising from a bile duct is difficult to accept since the author notes without comment that part of the cyst was lined by epithelium of a simple variety, but in other areas there was multilayering of cells. It seems unreasonable to postulate that a tumour arising from a bile duct and then forming part of a cyst wall which had no detectable connexion with the bile duct should contain such normal non-neoplastic epithelium. A normal single-layered columnar epithelium is the usual lining of a hepatic cyst and the papillary granulations could clearly represent neoplastic transformation. Such cases are reported as showing neoplastic transformation in a cyst, including squamous carcinoma (Greenwood and Orr 1972). The distinction has been made between a cystadenoma which seems to be a cystic tumour *ab initio* and a neoplastic transformation within a cyst, which may therefore be interpreted as a pre-neoplastic lesion (Azizah and Paradinas 1980). The question is raised whether reports describing cystadenomas or cystadeno-carcinomas of the liver may include instances of confusion between a primarily cystic tumour and a tumour which has developed in an established cyst. On clinical grounds the distinction may be difficult as a space-occupying lesion detected in the liver may be a cyst or a cystic tumour. The sex incidence for both cysts and cystadenomas shows a predominance in females although this is not so for cystadenocarcinomas. Structural differences are described in the two groups. For the most part cystadenomas and cystadenocarcinomas (with one reported exception) are multilocular, and non-neoplastic cysts appear to be unilocular. The epithelial lining of cystadenomas even when acknowledged as being benign often shows pseudopapillary formations or infoldings, but these are not normally described in congenital cysts. The subepithelial stroma in the cases of tumours is compact and cellular and has been compared to ovarian stroma (Ishak 1977) whereas the epithelium of congenital cysts is usually surrounded by dense collagenous connective tissue sometimes containing smooth muscle and occasionally elastic fibres (Flanigan 1975). Intrahepatic cysts in which tumours are found are rarely reported as containing stones but stones were described in 25 per cent (6 of 24) of patients in whom neoplastic change was associated with extrahepatic bile duct cysts. It seems therefore that biliary cysts may show an increased tendency to neoplastic change especially if calculi are present.

The increased frequency of neoplastic change in Caroli's disease appears to be confirmed (Gallagher *et al.* 1972). What is not clear is whether the reported tumours arise in the walls of cysts or ductal dilatations, or whether the epithelium of the bile ducts is the site of origin of tumours. Although this matter is not resolved, it seems to be agreed that the risk of tumours of the biliary epithelium is increased in various forms of hepatic and biliary cysts, since the incidence of biliary carcinoma in non-cystic livers and bile ducts is only 0.0007 to 0.014 per cent of all hospital admissions (Converse *et al.* 1971).

Endothelial tumours

The main malignant tumour considered to arise from sinusoidal lining cells is the angiosarcoma which, because of its association with industrial hazards, has been examined at different times in workers who were at risk (Roth 1957; Creech and Johnson 1974). It is now clear that certain patients to whom thorium dioxide (thorotrast) was administered in the past also had an increased chance of developing this tumour (Battifora 1976). Such cohorts of exposed people have been examined after different periods of exposure and the possibility of identifying pre-neoplastic states for this tumour has been canvassed (Thomas *et al.* 1975). In liver biopsies from some workers engaged in the manufacture of polyvinyl chloride, focal portal and capsular fibrosis has been noted together with hyperplastic sinusoidal lining cells and an excess of reticulin fibres (Thomas *et al.* 1975). While it is true that focal fibrosis in portal and sub-capsular regions is often non-specific, the association with excessive sinusoidal fibres and hyperplasia of sinusoidal lining cells may be suggestive of developing angiosarcoma. In particular, these changes may be accompanied by hyperplasia of hepatocytes (Popper and Thomas 1975; Popper *et al.* 1978) and an increase of peri-sinusoidal fat-storing cells (Triche *et al.* 1975)—an overall combination of changes which suggests a pre-neoplastic condition.

Experimental tumours in animals

Considerations of experimentally induced preneoplastic states usually involve the reporting of early changes which develop in the livers of animals to which known carcinogens have been administered, and it is frequently difficult to identify which lesions will evolve into tumours and which will not (Bannasch *et al.* 1972).

During the development of neoplasms, several early changes are found which regress if carcinogen treatment is halted. These are generally regarded as having little to do with the carcinogenic process, and most early reversible alterations are taken to represent reactions to the toxic effects of the chemical compound. Putative pre-neoplastic changes which develop during exposure to carcinogens include almost all the alterations which are not interpreted as definitely neoplastic lesions (Bannasch 1980; Schauer and Kunze 1976). Thus many of the lesions so designated are not usually noted in livers other than those in which carcinogenesis is proceeding, but it is not usual for chronic liver conditions which are not considered to be neoplastic to be scrutinized for these changes. Lesions presumed to be pre-neoplastic are usually detectable after discontinuation of the carcinogen, but this period is often not stipulated (Teebor and Becker 1971; Farber 1980). In assessing stages of carcinogenesis, attention has been directed to possible different pathways of change depending on the cellular origin of tumours which develop in experimental circumstances (Bannasch 1968). The consensus view is that hepatocellular and cholangiocellular tumours probably arise from different cells of origin, as is considered to be the case for their human counterparts: it seems reasonable to accept that tumours designated 'cholangiocellular' often produce mucin and probably take origin from biliary epithelial cells and that tumours designated 'hepatocellular' do not synthesize mucin and arise from hepatic parenchymal cells.

The stages reported in experiments designed to study hepatocellular carcinogenesis are derived from observations on different treatment regimens (Miller 1978; Farber and Cameron 1980). The permutations employed in these procedures have a direct effect on the different sorts of phenotypes expressed by the affected cells and there is some difference of opinion as to the relative significance of these various features. In general, tissue alterations are found before the development of frank invasive carcinoma and most of the changes are confirmed. One difficulty here is that in most studies all experimental subjects are generally exposed to the offending compound and the changes which develop are assumed to be sequential steps in the carcinogenic process. But some of the changes observed may be due to non-carcinogenic effects of the test agent, and separation of the two sets of changes may be impossible.

With regard to the hepatocyte, some early reactions appear to be reversible during the period of administration of carcinogenic agents. These are generally regarded as not being pre-neoplastic and are usually part of a toxic, necrogenic or subnecrogenic effect or part of a compensatory hyperplastic phenomenon (Farber 1980). Morphological expression of such processes may be found in loss of glycogen, mitochondrial enlargement, cytoplasmic swelling, and disorganization of the rough endoplasmic reticulum as well as nuclear division. These changes do not usually persist for more than a month or so after beginning treatment with the carcinogen.

In general, the terminology employed in the discussion of cellular changes during exposure to carcinogenic agents has caused confusion in the past, but the consensus view about the nomenclature relates to the *size* of the lesion on the one hand and to its *supposed potential* on the other (Squire and Levitt 1975). A lesion smaller than a lobule is usually referred to as an altered *focus* (which does not disrupt architecture); one slightly larger than a lobule is described as an *area* (which is considered together with a focus); and the *neoplastic nodule*, which is the size of several lobules, compresses the surrounding liver parenchyma and is usually visible on naked-eye examination.

Persistent hepatocyte changes are sometimes correlated with the process of carcinogenesis, although the evidence on which this view is based is not always convincing. Hepatocellular glycogenosis or excessive cytoplasmic accumulation of glycogen is one feature considered by Bannasch (1980) to be of relevance (Fig. 9.3); he finds it to be a common alteration within hepatocytes, usually coupled with hypertrophy of the smooth endoplasmic reticulum. Accumulations of glycogen-rich hepatocytes are found as sharply demarcated nodules within the parenchyma which may persist for weeks or months even if the carcinogenic compound is withheld (Bannasch *et al.* 1972). Such lesions have developed even after single doses of diethylnitrosamine in rats (Scherer *et al.* 1972) and after repeated doses of other compounds (Kalengayi and Desmet 1973) and in other species (Vesselinovitch and Mikailovich 1967). Later nodules considered to be pre-neoplastic vary in their cellular glycogen content, although examples of both glycogenosis and proliferation of smooth endoplasmic reticulum are noted in later nodules currently referred to as neoplastic nodules. The early glycogen-rich

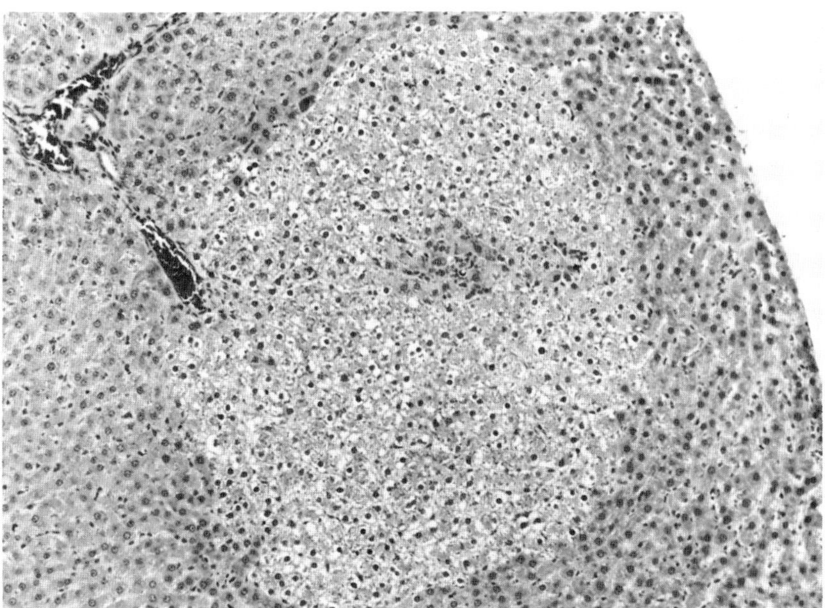

Fig. 9.3. Glycogen-rich nodule in rat liver. ×100. H & E.

nodules are considered to develop into more clearly defined neoplastic nodules (Reuber 1965; Farber 1973).

Before the development of macroscopically recognizable nodular lesions or even collections of hepatocytes showing evidence of expansive proliferation, foci of cells appear in which certain enzymes are altered in concentration or activity. Such enzyme deficiency or increase is demonstrable in sharply defined zones of the liver and can be detected after discontinuation of the carcinogen. These foci show a remarkable constancy in the range of enzymes affected: the activities of adenosine 5′-triphosphatase (Schauer and Kunze 1976), glucose 6-phosphatase (Gössner and Friedrich-Freksa 1968) and glucose 6-phosphate dehydrogenase (Kalengayi and Desmet 1974) are all decreased while the activity of gamma-glutamyl transpeptidase is strikingly increased (Kalengayi and Desmet 1978). Such foci show also increased nuclear incorporation of nucleic acid precursors and are consequently regarded as regions of probably increased growth activity (Rabes *et al.* 1972; Pugh and Goldfarb 1978). These various features are now well-recognized, but there are additional changes which also appear to distinguish putative pre-neoplastic foci from other liver tissue. Other enzymes are reported as showing reduced activity including β-glucuronidase and serine dehydratase (Katagawa and Pitot 1975), and increased enzyme activity has been recorded for DT-diaphorase (Schor *et al.* 1978) and arylesterase (Scherer and Emmelot 1976). Alpha-fetoprotein is also described as showing increased concentrations (Sell 1978). Certain alterations are noted in the physiological reactions of cells comprising these nodules: the hepatocytes appear to be unable to concentrate iron particles on iron-loading (Williams and Watanabe 1978), and the cytoplasmic glycogen is not labile on fasting (Bannasch 1980) whereas normal hepatocyte glycogen is not retained on fasting. Such parenchymal foci are frequently found in livers of several species (and especially studied in rats) during long-term exposure to known carcinogens: they have distinct and consistent morphological, histochemical, physiological, and proliferative properties and they are regarded by most workers as pre-neoplastic foci. The enzyme-deficient liver cells form islands, approximately 100-200 μm in diameter, which vary in position within the liver lobule according to time; up to six weeks, they usually occupy a position between portal tracts and hepatic venous radicles but by three months they are found in the perivenous regions (Emmelot and Scherer, 1980). The parenchymal islands provide a method of quantifying the effects of carcinogens and bear a relationship to the dose used, both in terms of their numbers and size. Increased numbers of islands result from the superimposition of partial hepatectomy on some carcinogenicity regimens but not on others (Craddock *et al.* 1978). Islands of ATPase-deficient liver cells were increased in number by performing partial hepatectomy in the case of DEN, DMN, and *N*-nitroso-*N*-ethylurea, but not for 2-acetyl-aminofluorene, methyl dimethylaminoazobenzene or aflatoxin (Emmelot and Scherer 1980). There is a suggestion that those compounds which produce more islands under the stimulus of partial hepatectomy also produce more tumours after this stimulus, and those islands which are not enhanced by partial hepatectomy are those which develop from administration of compounds which do not in fact produce a greater number of tumours with the resection. However data are not extensive and it must be recorded that in the case of 2-acetyl-aminofluorene, tumours appeared earlier if partial hepatectomy was added to carcinogen feeding (Laws 1959).

There is no strong evidence to support the view that all nodules simply transform into overt hepatocellular carcinoma, and Farber (1980) has reported regression of nodules with the appearance of normal liver structure being resumed. He has pointed out that, within the remodelled liver, normal-appearing liver cells persist which possess an antigen, probably the membrane-bound enzyme epoxide hydrase (Levin *et al.* 1978) which is found in some nodule cells and considered to be a pre-neoplastic marker. There is a distinct possibility that only certain cells within nodules may give rise to tumours, but the factors involved in the development of foci and nodules and what determines the production of neoplasms either within or outside the nodules are still obscure. Farber (1980) has proposed that certain cells from nodules may be selected and transformed into tumours, and others have postulated that nodules may not invariably be the precursor lesion (Bannasch 1980). An aspect of this problem which is difficult to analyse is the heterogeneity of various lesions which develop before frank neoplasm is observed. It is not clear, for example, whether the lesions which regress should be regarded as hyperplastic and those which do not appear to do so, as neoplastic. If these designations reflect the processes involved, then it might be assumed that the hyperplastic cells, the changes in which are reversible, develop from many hepatocytes while the neoplastic cells may be monoclonal. Markers of monoclonality may be of value in assessing nodules (Scherer and Hoffmann 1971).

Of the various models of chemical carcinogenesis which are employed by various workers, each appears to shed light on one or other aspect of the process (Peraino *et al.* 1971; Solt and Farber 1976; Williams 1980; Pitot 1977). But the question of interpreting changes in the carcinogenicity bioassay of the test compound is not yet resolved. At present, the lesions which are encountered at the end of a long and expensive assay are evaluated against controls. If early changes could be defined as definitely pre-neoplastic, then shorter assay times might become possible, but the varieties of tissue alterations are not clearly delineated as to which are part of the neoplastic process and which are not. Although particular experiments have indicated that some changes reverse during the course of the experiment, so far most of the lesions which have been described in the livers of animals receiving chemical carcinogens appear to be part of the same process.

References

Alpert, M.E. and Davidson, C.S. (1969). Mycotoxins. A possible cause of primary carcinoma of the liver. *Am. J. Med.* **46**, 325.

——, Hutt, M.S.R., and Davidson, C.S. (1969). Primary hepatoma in Uganda. A prospective clinical and epidemiological study of forty-six patients. *Am. J. Med.* **46**, 794.

Anthony, P.P. (1973). Liver cell dysplasia: a premalignant condition. *J. Pathol.* **110**, 37.

——, Vogel, C.L., and Barker, L.F. (1973). Liver cell dysplasia: a premalignant condition. *J. clin. Pathol.* **26**, 217.

Azizah, N. and Paradinas, F.J. (1980). Cholangiocarcinoma coexisting with developmental liver cysts: a distinct entity different from liver cystadenocarcinoma. *Histopathology* **4**, 391.

Bannasch, P. (1968). The cytoplasm of hepatocytes during carcinogenesis. *Rec. Res. Cancer Res.* **19**.

—— (1976). Cytology and cytogenesis of neoplastic (hyperplastic) hepatic nodules. *Cancer Res.* **36**, 2555.

—— (1980). Hepatocellular glycogenesis and hepatocarcinogenesis. *Biochim. Biophys. Acta* **605**, 217.

——, Papenburg, J., and Ross, W. (1972). Cytomorphologische und morphometrische Studien der Hepatocarcinogenese. I. Reversible und irreversible Veränderungen am cytoplasma der Leberparenchymzellen bei Nitromorpholin-vergifteten Ratten. *Z. Krebsforsch.* **77**, 108.

Bartók, I., Remenár, E., Toth, J., Duschanek, P., and Kanyar, B. (1981). Clinicopathological studies of liver cirrhosis and hepatocellular carcinoma in a general hospital. *Human Pathol.* **12**, 794.

Battifora, H.A. (1976). Thorotrast and tumors of the liver. In *Hepatocellular carcinoma* (ed. K. Okuda and R.L. Peters), p. 83. J. Wiley, London.

Blenkinsopp, W.K. and Haffenden, G.P. (1977). Aetiology of cirrhosis, hepatic fibrosis and hepatocellular carcinoma. *J. clin. Pathol.* **30**, 579.

Bras. G., Jelliffe, D.B., and Stuart, K.L. (1954). Veno-occlusive disease of liver with nonportal type of cirrhosis, occurring in Jamaica. *Arch. Pathol.* **57**, 285.

Caroli, J. (1973). Diseases of the intrahepatic biliary tree. *Clin. Gastroenterol.* **2**, 147.

Converse, C.F., Reagan, J.W., and De Cosse, J.J. (1971). Ulcerative colitis and carcinoma of the bile ducts. *Am. J. Surg.* **121**, 39.

Corrin, B. (1962). Cystadenoma of the liver. *J. Path. Bact.* **84**, 441.

Craddock, V.M., Henderson, A.R., and Ansley, C.M. (1976). Repair replication of DNA in the intact animal following treatment with dimethylnitrosamine and with methyl methanesulphonate, studied by fractionation of nuclei in a zonal centrifuge. *Biochim. Biophys. Acta* **447**, 53.

Creech, J.S. and Johnson, M.N. (1974). Angiosarcoma of liver in the manufacture of polyvinyl chloride. *J. occup. Med.* **16**, 150.

Cruickshank, A.H. (1961). The pathology of 111 cases of primary hepatic malignancy collected in the Liverpool region. *J. clin. Pathol.* **14**, 120.

Dalgaard, O.Z. (1957). Bilateral polycystic disease of the kidneys; a follow-up of two hundred and eighty-four patients and their families. *Acta Med. scand.* **158** (Suppl. 328), 1.

Daly, J.J. and Schiller, A.L. (1976). The liver in hereditary hemorrhagic telangiectasia (Osler-Weber-Rendu Disease). *Am. J. Med.* **60**, 723.

Dane, D.S., Cameron, C.H., and Briggs, M. (1970). Virus-like particles in serum of patients with Australia-antigen-associated hepatitis. *Lancet* **1**, 695.

Davis, M., Portmann, B., Searle, M., Wright, R., and Williams, R. (1975). Histological evidence of carcinoma in a hepatic tumour associated with oral contraceptives. *Brit. med. J.* **4**, 496.

Deodhar, K.P., Tapp, E., and Scheuer, P.J. (1975) Orcein staining of hepatitis B antigen in paraffin sections of liver biopsies. *J. clin. Pathol.* **28**, 66.

Edgington, T.S. and Chisari, F.V. (1975). Immunological aspects of hepatitis B virus infection. *Am. J. Sci.* **270**, 212.

Emmelot, P. and Scherer, E. (1980). The first relevant cell stage in rat liver carcinogenesis. A quantitative approach. *Biochim. Biophys. Acta* **605**, 247.

Farber, E. (1973). Proceedings: Experimental chemical carcinogenesis. *Proc. Nat. Cancer Conf.* **7**, 395.

—— (1980). The sequential analysis of liver cancer induction. *Biochim. Biophys. Acta* **605**, 149.

—— and Cameron, R. (1980). The sequential analysis of cancer development. *Adv. Cancer Res.* **31**, 125.

Fechner, R.E. (1977). Benign hepatic lesions and orally administered contraceptives. *Human Pathol.* **8**, 255.

Feizi, O. (1972). Hereditary hemorrhagic telangiectasia presenting with portal hypertension and cirrhosis of the liver. A case report. *Gastroenterology* **63**, 660.

Flanigan, P.D. (1975). Biliary cysts. *Ann. Surg.* **182**, 635.

Galambos, J.T. (1975). Classification of cirrhosis. *Am. J. Gastroenterol.* **64**, 437.

Gallagher, P.J., Millis, R.R., and Mitchinson, M.J. (1972). Congenital dilatation of the intrahepatic bile ducts with cholangiocarcinoma. *J. clin. Pathol.* **25**, 804.

Gibson, J.B. (1960). Chiari's disease and the Budd-Chiari syndrome. *J. Path. Bact.* **79**, 381.

—— (1971). Parasites, liver disease and liver cancer. In *Liver cancer*, p. 42. IARC Scientific Publications, Lyon.

Glassberg, A.B. and Rosenbaum, E.H. (1976). Oral contraceptives and malignant hepatoma. *Lancet* **1**, 479.

Gössner, W. and Friedrich-Freksa, H. (1964). Histochemische Untersuchungen über die Glucose 6-Phosphatase in der Rattenleber während der Kanzerisierung durch Nitrosamine. *Z. Naturforsch.* **B19**, 862.

Greenwood, N. and Orr, W. McN. (1972). Primary squamous-cell carcinoma arising in a solitary non-parasitic cyst of the liver. *J. Pathol.* **107**, 145.

Gudat, F., Bianchi, L., Sonnabend, W., Thiel, G., Genishaenslin, W., and Stalder, G.A. (1975). Pattern of core and surface expression in liver tissue reflects state of specific immune response in hepatitis B. *Lab. Invest.* **32**, 1.

Hann, H.L., London, W.T., Whitford, P., Kim, C.Y., and Blumberg, B.S. (1979). Hepatitis B virus and primary hepatocellular carcinoma: family studies in Korea. *Proc. Am. Soc. clin. Oncol.* **20** (c-588), 432.

Heyward, W.L., Bender, T.R., Lanier, A.P., Francis, D.P., McMahon, B.J., and Maynard, J.E. (1982). Serological markers of hepatitis B virus and alpha-fetoprotein levels preceding primary hepatocellular carcinoma in Alaskan eskimos. *Lancet* **ii**, 889.

Higginson, J. (1970). The epidemiology of primary carcinoma of the liver. In *Tumors of the liver* (ed. G.T. Pack and A.H. Islami) Chapter 4. Springer Verlag, Berlin.

Homer, L.W., White, H.J., and Read, R.C. (1968). Neoplastic transformation of v. Meyenburg complexes of the liver. *J. Path. Bact.* **96**, 499.

Ishak, K.G. (1977). Biliary cystadenoma. *Cancer* **40**, 2400.

Kagawa, Y., Kashihara, S., Kuramoto, S., and Maetani, S. (1978). Carcinoma arising in a congenitally dilated biliary tract. Report of a case and review of literature. *Gastroenterology* **74**, 1286.

Kalengayi, M.M.R. and Desmet, V.J. (1973). Sequential histological and histochemical study of the rat liver after single-dose aflatoxin B_1 intoxication. *Cancer Res.* **35**, 2836.

—— and —— (1978). Liver cell populations and histochemical patterns of adult and fetal type proteins during aflatoxin B_1 hepatocarcinogenesis. In *Primary liver tumors* (ed. H. Rummer, H.M. Bolt, P. Bannasch, and H. Popper), p. 467. MTP, Massachussetts.

Katagawa, T. and Pitot, H.C. (1975). The regulation of serine dehydratase and glucose 6-phosphatase in hyperplastic nodules of rat liver during diethylnitrosamine and N-2-fluorenylacetamide feeding. *Cancer Res.* **35**, 1075.

Kern, F. Jr. (1976). Hepatobiliary disorders in inflammatory bowel disease. In *Progress in liver disease* (ed. H. Popper and F. Schaffner), Vol. 5, pp. 575-89. Grune and Stratton, New York.

Kerr, D.N.S., Harrison, C.V., Sherlock, S., and Walker, R.M. (1961). Congenital hepatic fibrosis. *Quart. J. Med.* **30**, 91.

——, Warwick, C.K., and Hart-Mercer, J. (1962). A lesion resembling medullary sponge kidney in patients with congenital hepatic fibrosis. *Clin. Radiol.* (*Lond.*) **13**, 85.

Kew, M.C., Dos Santos, H.A., and Sherlock, S. (1971). Diagnosis of primary cancer of the liver. *Brit. med. J.* **4**, 408.

Klatskin, G. (1965). Adenocarcinoma of the hepatic duct at its bifurcation within the porta hepatis. An unusual tumor with distinctive and pathological features. *Am. J. Med.* **38**, 241.

—— (1977). Hepatic tumors: possible relationship to use of oral contraceptives. *Gastroenterology* **73**, 386.

Klemperer, P. (1928). Cavernomatous transformation of portal vein; its relation to Banti's disease. *Arch. Pathol.* **6**, 353.

Knowles, D.M. and Wolfe, M. (1976). Focal nodular hyperplasia of the liver. A clinicopathologic study and review of literature. *Human Pathol.* **7**, 533.

Larouze, B., Blumberg, B.S., London, W.T., Lustbader, E.D., Sankale, M., and Payet, M. (1977). Forecasting the development of primary hepatocellular carcinoma by the use of risk factors: studies in West Africa. *J. Nat. Cancer Inst.* **58**, 1557.

Laws, J.O. (1959). Tissue regeneration and tumour development. *Brit. J. Cancer* **13**, 669.

Lee, F.I. (1966). Cirrhosis and hepatoma in alcoholics. *Gut* **7**, 77.

Levin, W., Liu, A.Y.H., Thomas, P.E., Ryan, D., Kezir, D.E., and Griffin, M.J. (1978). Identification of epoxide hydrase as the preneoplastic antigen in rat liver hyperplastic nodules. *Proc. Nat. Acad. Sci. (USA)* **75**, 3240.

Macnab, G., Alexander, J., Lecatas, G. *et al.* (1976). Hepatitis B surface antigen produced by a human hepatoma cell line. *Br. J. Cancer* **34**, 509.

MacSween, R.N.M. (1974), A clinicopathological review of 100 cases of primary malignant tumours of the liver. *J. clin. Pathol.* **27**, 669.

——, and Scott, A.R. (1973). Hepatic cirrhosis: a clinicopathological review of 520 cases. *J. clin. Pathol.* **26**, 936.

Martini, G.A. (1959). Cirrhosis of the liver in hereditary haemorrhagic telangiectasia. In *Proc. 1st World Congress of Gastroenterology*, Vol. 2, p. 857. Williams and Wilkins, Baltimore.

Melnick, P.J. (1955). Polycystic liver; analysis of 70 cases. *Am. med. Ass. Arch. Pathol.* **59**, 162.

Miller, E.C. (1978). Some current perspectives on chemical carcinogenesis in humans and experimental animals: presidential address. *Cancer Res.* **38**, 1479.

Moore, T.A., Ferrante, W.D., and Crowson, T.D. (1976). Hepatoma occurring two decades after hepatic irradiation. *Gastroenterology* **71**, 128.

Murray-Lyon, I.M., Ockenden, B.G., and Williams, R. (1973). Congenital hepatic fibrosis—is it a single clinical entity? *Gastroenterology* **64**, 653.

Oettlé, A.G. (1965). The aetiology of primary carcinoma of the liver in Africa: a critical appraisal of previous ideas with an outline of the mycotoxin hypothesis. *S. Afr. med. J.* **39**, 817.

Okuda, K., Yusuhiko, K., Okazaki, N., Arishima, T., Hashimoto, M., Jinnouchi, S., Sawa, Y., Shimokawa, Y., Nakajima, Y., Noguchi, I., Nakano, M., Kojiro, M., and Nakashima, T. (1977). Clinical aspects of intrahepatic bile duct carcinoma including hilar carcinoma. *Cancer* **39**, 232.

Palmer, P.E. and Wolfe, H.J. (1976). Alpha-1-antitrypsin deposition in primary hepatic carcinomas. *Arch. Pathol.* **100**, 232.

Paradinas, F.J., Bull, T.B., Westaby, D., and Murray-Lyon, I.M. (1977). Hyperplasia and prolapse of hepatocytes into hepatic veins during longterm methyltesterone therapy: possible relationships of these changes to the development of peliosis hepatis and liver tumours. *Histopathology* **1**, 225.

Parker, R.G.F. (1956). Fibrosis of liver as congenital anomaly. *J. Path. Bact.* **71**, 359.

—— (1959). Occlusion of the hepatic veins in man. *Medicine (Baltimore)* **38**, 369.

—— and Kendall, E.J.C. (1954). Liver in ulcerative colitis. *Brit. med. J.* **2**, 1030.

Peraino, C., Fry, R.J.M., and Staffeldt, E. (1971). Reduction and enhancement by phenobarbital of hepatocarcinogenesis induced in the rat by 2-acetylaminofluorene. *Cancer Res.* **31**, 1506.

Peters, R.L. (1976). Pathology of hepatocellular carcinoma. In *Hepatocellular Carcinoma* (ed. K. Okuda and R.L. Peters) p. 107. John Wiley, London.

Pitot, H.C. (1977). The natural history of neoplasia. *Am. J. Pathol.* **89**, 401.

Popper, H. (1977). Pathologic aspects of cirrhosis (a review). *Am. J. Pathol.* **87**, 227.

—— and Thomas, L.B. (1975). Alterations of liver and spleen among workers exposed to vinyl chloride. *Ann. NY Acad. Sci.* **246**, 172.

—— ——, Telles, N.C., Falk, H., and Selikoff, I.J. (1978). Development of hepatic angiosarcoma in man induced by vinyl chloride, thorotrast and arsenic. Comparison with cases of unknown etiology. *Am. J. Pathol.* **92**, 349.

Prince, A.M. (1980). Evidence suggesting that hepatitis B virus is a tumor-inducing virus in man: an estimate of the risk of development of hepatocellular cancer in chronic HBsAg carriers and controls. In *The role of viruses in human cancer* (ed. G. Giraldo and E. Beth), p. 141. Elsevier/North Holland, New York.

Pugh, T.D. and Goldfarb, S. (1978). Quantitative histochemical and autoradiographic studies of hepatocarcinogenesis in rats fed 2-acetylaminofluorene followed by phenobarbital. *Cancer Res.* **38**, 4450.

Rabes, H.M., Scholze, P., and Jantsch, B. (1972). Growth kinetics of diethylnitrosamine-induced enzyme deficient "preneoplastic" liver cell populations in vivo and in vitro. *Cancer Res.* **32**, 2577.

Reed, G.B., Jr. and Cox, A.J., Jr. (1966). The human liver after radiation injury. A form of veno-occlusive disease. *Am. J. Pathol.* **48**, 597.

Reuber, M.D. (1965). Development of preneoplastic and neoplastic lesions of the liver in male rats given 0.025 percent N-2-fluorenyldiacetamide. *J. Nat. Cancer Inst.* **34**, 697.

Ritchie, J.K., Allan, R.N., Macartney, J., Thompson, H., Hawley, P.R., and Cooke, W.T. (1974). Biliary tract carcinoma associated with ulcerative colitis. *Quart. J. Med.* **43**, 263.

Roe, T.F., Kogut, M.D., Buckingham, B.A., Miller, J.H., Gates, G.F., and Landing, B.H. (1979). Hepatic tumours in glycogen storage disease (GSD) type I. *Pediatr. Res.* **13**, (abstr. no. 931), 481.

Ross, A.P. and Braasch, J.W. (1973). Ulcerative colitis and carcinoma of the proximal bile ducts. *Gut* **14**, 94.

Roth, F. (1957). Arsenic, liver and tumours; haemangioendothelioma. *Z. Krebsforsch.* **61**, 468-503.

Rubin, E., Krus, S., and Popper, H. (1962). Pathogenesis of postnecrotic cirrhosis in alcoholics. *Arch. Pathol. (Chicago)* **73**, 288.

Schauer, A. and Kunze, E. (1976). Tumours of the liver. In *Pathology of tumours in laboratory animals* (ed. V.S. Turusov), p. 41 IARC, Lyon.

Scherer, E. and Emmelot, P. (1976). Kinetics of induction and growth of enzyme deficient islands involved in hepatocarcinogenesis. *Cancer Res.* **36**, 2544.

—— and Hoffman, M. (1971). Probable clonal genesis of cellular islands induced in rat liver by diethylnitrosamine. *Eur. J. Cancer* **7**, 369.

—— ——, Emmelot, P., and Friedrich-Freksa, H. (1972). Quantitative study on foci of altered liver cells induced in the rat by a single dose of diethylnitrosamine and partial hepatectomy. *J. Nat. Cancer Inst.* **49**, 93.

Schoental, R. (1968). Toxicology and carcinogenic action of pyrrolizidine alkaloids. *Cancer Res.* **28**, 2237.

Schor, N., Ogawa, K., Lee, G., and Farber, E. (1978). The use of the D-T diaphorase for the detection of foci of early neoplastic transformation in rat liver. *Cancer Lett.* **5**, 167.

Sell, S. (1978). Distribution of alpha-fetoprotein and albumin-containing cells in the livers of Fisher rats fed four cycles of N-2 fluorenylacetamide. *Cancer Res.* **38**, 3107.

Shafritz, D.A. and Kew, M.C. (1981). Identification of integrated hepatitis B virus DNA sequences in human hepatocellular carcinomas. *Hepatology* **1**, 1.

Simson, I.W. and Middlecote, B.D. (1973). The Budd-Chiari syndrome in the Bantu. In *Liver* (ed. S.J. Saunders and J. Terblanche) p. 257. Pitman Medical, London.

Solt, D.B. and Farber, E. (1976). New principle for the analysis of chemical carcinogenesis. *Nature* **263**, 701.

Squire, R.A. and Levitt, M.H. (1975). Report of a workshop on classification of specific hepatocellular lesions in rats. *Cancer Res.* **35**, 3214.

Sternlieb, I. (1978). Diagnosis of Wilson's disease. *Gastroenterology* **74**, 787.

Summers, J., Smolec, J.M., and Snyder, R. (1978). A virus similar to human hepatitis B virus associated with hepatitis and hepatoma in woodchucks. *Proc. Nat. Acad. Sci. (USA)* **75**, 4533.

Sussman, E.B. and Sternberg, S.S. (1975). Hereditary haemorrhagic telangiectasia. A case with hepatocellular carcinoma and acquired hepatocerebral degeneration. *Arch. Pathol.* **99**, 95.

Takahashi, K., Akahane, Y., Gotanda, T., Mishiro, T., Imai, M., Miyakawa, Y., and Mayumi, M. (1979). Demonstration of hepatitis B e antigen in the core of Dane particles. *J. Immunol.* **122**, 275.

Takeuchi, J., Takada, A., Hasumura, Y., Matsuda, Y., and Ikegami, F. (1971). Budd-Chiari syndrome associated with obstruction of the inferior vena cava. A report of seven cases. *Am. J. Med.* **51**, 11.

Teebor, G.W. and Becker, F.F. (1971). Regression and persistence of hyperplastic hepatic nodules induced by N-2-fluorenylacetamide and their relationship to hepatocarcinogenesis. *Cancer Res.* **31**, 1.

Thomas, L.B., Popper, H., Berk, P.D., Selikoff, I., and Falk, H. (1975). Vinyl-chloride-induced liver disease. From idiopathic portal hypertension (Banti's syndrome) to angiosarcomas. *New Engl. J. Med.* **292**, 17.

Thung, S.N. and Gerber, M.A. (1981). Precursor stage of hepatocellular neoplasm following long exposure to orally administered contraceptives. *Human Pathol.* **12**, 472.

Triche, T., Nanba, K., Ishak, K., Wolkoff, A., and Berk, P.D. (1975). Hepatic ultrastructural changes in vinyl-chloride (VC) workers. *Clin. Res.* **23**, 259A.
Vesselinovitch, S.D. and Mihailovich, N. (1967). The effect of gonadectomy on the development of hepatomas induced by urethan. *Cancer Res.* **27**, 1788.
Vogel, C.L., Anthony, P.P., Mody, N., and Barker, L.F. (1970). Hepatitis-associated antigen in Ugandan patients with hepatocellular carcinoma. *Lancet* **2**, 621.
Von Meyenburg, H. (1918). Uber die Cystenleber. *Beitr. Path. Anat.* **64**, 477.
Wanless, I.R., Godwin, T.A., Allen, F., and Feder, A. (1980). Nodular regenerative hyperplasia of the liver in hematologic disorders: a possible response to obliterative portal venopathy. *Medicine* **59**, 367.
——, Solt, L.C., Kortan, P., Deck, J.H.N., Gardiner, G.W., and Prokipchuk, E.J. (1981). Nodular regenerative hyperplasia of the liver associated with macroglobulinemia. A clue to the pathogenesis. *Am. J. Med.* **70**, 1203.
Weinbren, K. (1978). Induction of liver nodules after portacaval anastomosis in rats. In *Primary liver tumours* (ed. H. Remmer, H. M. Bolt, P. Bannasch and H. Popper), p. 395. MTP Press, England.
—— and Washington, S.L.A. (1976). Hyperplastic nodules after portacaval anastomosis in rats. *Nature* **264**, 440.
Williams, G.M. (1980). The pathogenesis of rat liver cancer caused by chemical carcinogens. *Biochim. Biophys. Acta* **605**, 167.
—— and Watanabe, K. (1978). Quantitative kinetics of development of *N*-2-fluorenylacetamide-induced, altered (hyperplastic) hepatocellular foci resistant to iron accumulation and of their reversion or persistence following removal of carcinogen. *J. Nat. Cancer Inst.* **61**, 113.
Winkler, K. and Poulson, H. (1975). Liver disease with periportal sinusoidal dilatation. A possible complication to contraceptive steroids. *Scand. J. Gastroenterol.* **10**, 699.
Wogan, G.N. (1976). Aflatoxins and their relationship to hepatocellular carcinoma. In *Hepatocellular carcinoma* (ed. K. Okuda and R.L. Peters), p. 25. John Wiley, London.
Wood, R.A.B. and Cuschieri, A. (1980). Is sclerosing cholangitis complicating ulcerative colitis a reversible condition? *Lancet* **2**, 716.
Yanoff, M. and Rawson, A.J. (1964). Peliosis hepatis. An anatomic study with demonstration of two varieties. *Arch. Pathol. (Chicago)* **77**, 159.
Zuckerman, A.J. (1982). Developing synthetic vaccines. *Nature, Lond.* **295**, 98.

10 Precancerous and noninvasive lesions of the urinary bladder

S.M. Cohen, R.E. Greenfield, J.B. Jacobs, and G.H. Friedell

During the past thirty years, and particularly in the last fifteen, much has been learned about the pathogenesis of bladder cancer. While some of this knowledge has come from the study of patients with this disease, essential aspects have been clarified by the study of bladder cancer in experimental animals. In this review we summarize that information which pertains to the characterization of preneoplastic proliferative epithelial lesions of the bladder, we attempt to relate experimental findings to clinical problems, and we point out certain areas for further investigation.

Definitions

It is customary to begin with definitions, but this is still difficult for 'preneoplasia of the bladder' (Friedell 1976). Preneoplastic lesions lie in a continuum of morphological and biological entities between normal transitional bladder epithelium and invasive carcinoma. The term 'preneoplastic' does, however, imply that such lesion(s) can be recognized and distinguished from both normal and neoplastic epithelium, and that there is an obligate relationship between the presence of this lesion and the appearance of bladder cancer at some later time in that particular patient or experimental animal. With bladder cancers we still do not know whether the prefix 'pre' should be thought of as indicating that the particular lesion designated as 'preneoplastic' will *itself* evolve—given the right conditions—into an invasive carcinoma, or whether the prefix implies that the lesion in question is simply an indicator that there is a high statistical 'probability' that one of the cells in a field of atypical epithelium *somewhere in the bladder* will give rise to carcinoma. If, during treatment, a specific lesion is removed, the probability remains that cells in the atypical epithelium *elsewhere in the bladder* may progress to carcinoma.

The almost intractable difficulty of solving this problem short of performing large numbers of cystectomies and carefully examining all the bladder epithelium is reminiscent of the dilemma which surrounded the term 'carcinoma *in situ*' in the uterine cervix (Friedell *et al.* 1960; see also Chapter 12). The choice for the clinicians lay between either removing the entire cervix and examining it microscopically to exclude the presence of concurrent, invasive cancer; or leaving the cervix in the patient, after appropriate local treatment, and following all cases closely to see if the previously treated *in situ* lesion progressed.

Nevertheless, by defining carcinoma, carcinoma *in situ*, and preneoplasia of the bladder compared to normal epithelium we should at least be able to delimit the area on the continuum which we shall be discussing in the remainder of the chapter (Friedell 1965). Our definitions at this time will necessarily be based on light-microscopic findings and clinical correlations, and of necessity will be more qualitative than quantitative.

As more research is done the number of paramenters encompassed in our definitions will increase and biochemical, histochemical, ultrastructural, immunological, and other criteria will emerge from the laboratory for use in defining preneoplasia in the bladder (and at other sites).

Carcinoma—proliferation of epithelial cells with recognizable and characteristic histological and cytological abnormalities which invade subepithelial connective tissues, infiltrate the organ of origin and extend locally beyond it, and metastasize to distant sites. This progressive spread of tumour and its consequences reflect complex tumour-host interactions as well as the malignant capacity of the tumour itself (Friedell 1965).

Carcinoma in situ—proliferation of epithelial cells with histological and cytological features similar to those seen in carcinoma originating in the same organ, but without evidence of invasion of the subepithelial connective tissue. This lesion is related in space or time to carcinoma of the same histological type and, if untreated, will progress to an invasive neoplasm of the same histological type in a *significantly high percentage of cases.* It may not progress during the lifetime of the patient (although our assumption is that it would do so if the patient lived long enough), but only rarely does it spontaneously regress. Invasion will presumably be a function of the tumour-host interaction, as well as of the 'virulence' of the neoplastic epithelium (Friedell 1965, 1976).

Preneoplastic lesion—proliferation of epithelial cells with characteristic but non-neoplastic histological and cytological features associated in space or time with the development of *in situ* or invasive carcinoma of the same histological type. The constituent cells are atypical, but *individually and collectively they do not look like malignant cells.* The lesion, if not entirely removed by biopsy, *might persist* in this form or it *might progress* to *in situ* and/or invasive carcinoma (Friedell 1965, 1976).

Pathogenesis

Although multiple aetiological factors are undoubtedly involved in the pathogenesis of human bladder cancer, the net result of their interaction seems to be the development of a field of atypical proliferating bladder epithelium within which, in some cases, one or more areas of neoplastic epithelium appear. Foci of invasion develop within these areas of non-invasive carcinoma over a further period of time, and in some instances metastasis and death from bladder cancer follow. The process is not limited to the bladder as the mucosal surfaces at risk also include those of the urethra, the ureters, and the renal pelvicalycine system. The time-frame within which these events occur is variable, and with our present information we can make no definite statement about the likely time intervals between successive stages of the disease. But the disease can only be understood if the temporal element is remembered.

Some years ago, for example, it was thought that the demonstration of *in situ* carcinoma in biopsies of bladder epithelium meant that invasion was imminent and that cystectomy was mandatory (Melicow and Hollowell 1952; Farrow *et al.* 1976). More recently, however, in a clinical study where cases were detected by cytological studies, Farrow and his colleagues have shown that cases of carcinoma *in situ* may remain unchanged for eight years or more (Utz and Farrow 1980; Weinstein *et al.* 1980). Given a specific morphological picture, therefore, we cannot say how long it took to develop. This unpredictable and protracted period may reflect the extended, multistage process (i.e., initiation, promotion, and progression) of carcinogenesis suggested for bladder cancer by studies using animal models (Scribner and Suss 1978; Hicks and Chowaniec 1978; Hicks 1980).

Classification of bladder tumours

Macroscopically, bladder tumours may be exophytic or endophytic (Mostofi *et al.* 1973; Friedell *et al.* 1980, 1982). Most exophytic lesions are either papillary with narrow stalks, or sessile with a broad base. Endophytic (solid) tumours are more likely to be invasive, and the pattern of infiltration is generally tentacular. Papillary lesions, by contrast, are often superficial and when invasion is present it is often of the broad front variety. Both patterns of growth may be seen in one individual tumour.

Malignant epithelial tumours of the bladder are traditionally classified as transitional-cell, squamous, adenocarcinoma, or as undifferentiated carcinomas by generally accepted pathological criteria (Mostofi *et al.* 1973; Friedell *et al.* 1980, 1981). Within these categories further subdivision can be achieved by histological grading. The basic criteria for establishing the type and grade of bladder tumours were given in the WHO classification by Mostofi *et al.* in 1973 and were recently discussed by Friedell *et al.* (1980, 1981).

Transitional-cell carcinomas comprise the majority of invasive human bladder cancers in most countries. Both the depth of invasion, or stage, and the degree of anaplasia of the constituent tumour cells, or grade, are important prognostic factors. These two morphological features generally correlate quite closely: low-grade tumours, for example, are much less often invasive than higher-grade tumours, and when they do invade the low-grade tumours tend to be more superficial (Friedell *et al.* 1980).

The major element in grading transitional-cell carcinomas is the nuclear appearance. In grade-1 tumours the nuclei of the constituent cells are quite uniform with little variation in size, shape, or staining characteristics, and few mitoses (Fig. 10.1). These tumours may invade the subepithelial connective tissue, but they rarely extend as deep as the muscle coats. Metastases from such lesions are exceptional.

At the other end of the spectrum, grade-3 transitional-cell carcinomas (Fig. 10.3) are composed of cells which tend to be larger than normal basal or intermediate cells and exhibit much greater variation in size and shape than do those of grade-1 lesions. Their nuclei are far more pleomorphic with fairly numerous and often bizarre mitotic figures. Many large nuclei are characteristically present. The morphological appearances of grade-2 transitional-cell carcinomas (Fig. 10.2) are intermediate between those of grades 1 and 3. There is some variation of nuclear size and shape, but this is less prominent than in grade 3. Mitotic figures are fewer in number, though readily found, and the average nuclear diameter appears less than in grade-3 neoplastic epithelium.

Exfoliative cytology is an excellent way of monitoring the presence of grade-3 neoplastic transitional-cell epithelium in the bladder. Cells from this epithelium shed into urine or bladder washings are readily recognized by the cytopathologist, and the presence of malignant epithelium in the bladder is reported to the urologist. Cells from grade-2 transitional-cell carcinoma are

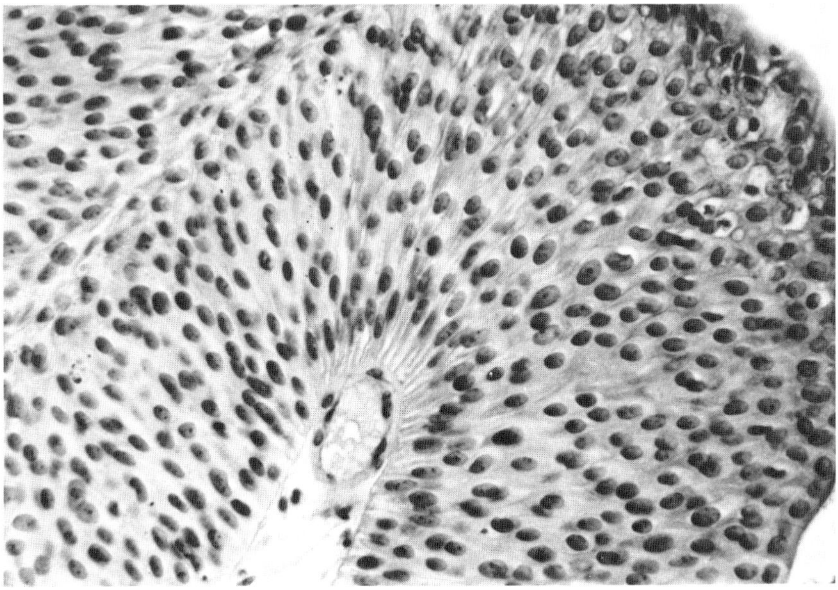

Fig. 10.1. Non-invasive, papillary transitional-cell carcinoma, grade 1. ×200. H & E.

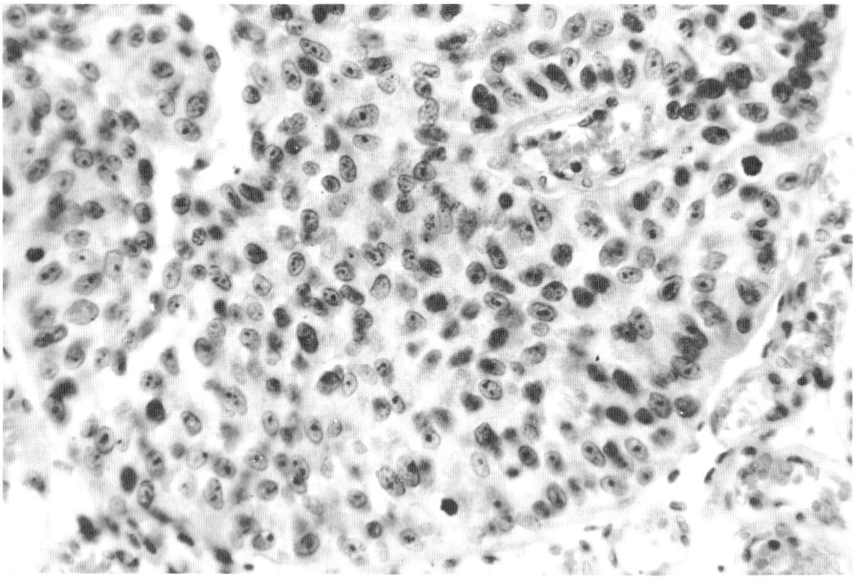

Fig. 10.2. Non-invasive, papillary transitional-cell carcinoma, grade 2. ×200. H & E.

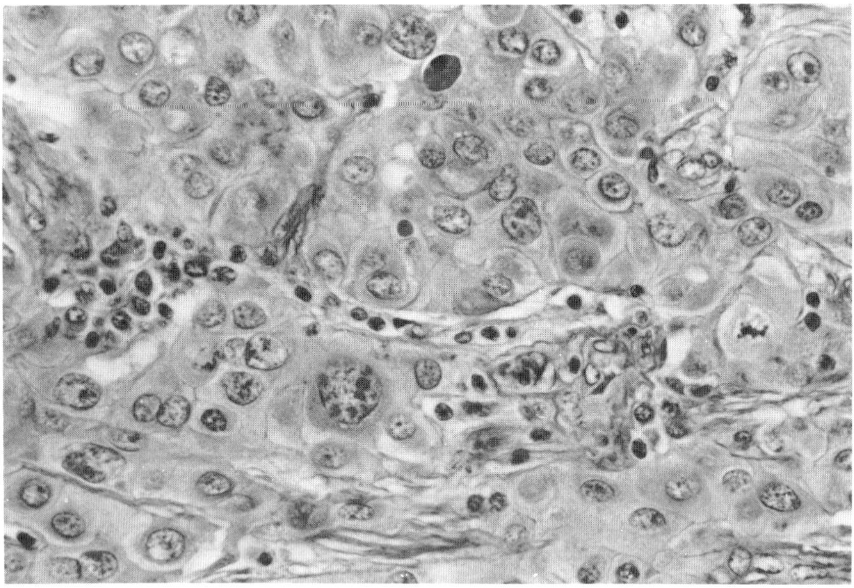

Fig. 10.3. Non-invasive, papillary transitional-cell carcinoma, grade 3. ×325. H & E.

less easily identified as neoplastic in nature as there is some overlap in appearance with cells originating in areas of marked chronic inflammation, but knowledgeable cytopathologists are increasingly able to make this distinction.

On the other hand, cells exfoliated from grade-1 papillary transitional-cell carcinomas cannot be distinguished from normal epithelial cells by currently used criteria of urothelial malignancy. Cystoscopy continues to be essential in the diagnosis and clinical management of bladder cancer patients. Scanning electron microscopy may provide us with more criteria for the recognition of exfoliated cells from grade-1 transitional-cell neoplasms, and this topic will be discussed later in the chapter.

Finally, with regard to the microscopic diagnosis of neoplastic bladder epithelial cells, either in cytological or histopathological preparations, it should be noted that the diagnostic criteria are the same regardless of whether the cell sample originated in an invasive or a non-invasive tumour. The application of the diagnostic terms 'neoplastic' or 'malignant' to exfoliated cells or to a tissue sample of epithelium implies that the tissue of origin has the potential to invade and metastasize whether or not it had done so at the time the sample was obtained.

Non-invasive carcinomas may be flat or papillary, and both may be found at the same time—or sequentially—in the bladder of an individual patient. The relationship between these two patterns of epithelial growth is not understood and it is not known if the aetiological factors are the same for each. Most of them are transitional-cell neoplasms, although some are squamous. Papillary lesions are much more common among the cases seen for the first time by the urologist. Perhaps one-third to one-half of non-invasive papillary transitional-cell carcinomas are grade-1 lesions, an equal or somewhat greater number are grade-2 lesions, and perhaps one-sixth are grade-3 lesions (Friedell 1980; Friedell *et al.* 1980, 1981). On the other hand, of the flat non-invasive carcinomas, none are grade-1, perhaps one-fifth are grade-2, and the rest are grade-3 lesions (Utz and Farrow 1980; Weinstein *et al.* 1980; Friedell *et al.* 1980; Friedell 1981).

Qualitative and quantitative epithelial abnormalities

The concept of a diagnostic threshold of bladder neoplasia based on the interaction of qualitative and quantitative abnormalities has been developed during the past few years by Friedell and has been recently discussed—see Friedell 1981. Expressed as a formula this interaction might be written as

$$K_{\text{malignancy}} = \text{qualitative abnormality} \times \text{quantitative abnormality}$$

where K_m represents the pathologist's diagnostic threshold for the histopathological diagnosis of non-invasive epithelial malignancy—that is, his subjective mental image of what a proliferative epithelial lesion of the bladder should look like in order to be recognized as cancer.

If a lesion of the bladder were a papillary one, the marked quantitative abnormality would immediately be evident and, if the constituent transitional epithelial cells showed even slight qualitative abnormality, use of the equation would result in the lesion being designated as a non-invasive papillary transitional-cell carcinoma, grade-1. The lesion in this example would have exceeded the diagnostic threshold of the pathologist, based on the interaction between the degrees of qualitative and quantitative abnormality. If there were *no* qualitative abnormality of the epithelium—the constitutent epithelial cells being entirely normal in appearance—K_m would be zero and the lesion would be designated as a 'papilloma' in our terminology. If there were moderate or marked qualitative abnormality of the papillary epithelium, then K_m would be easily exceeded.

On the other hand, in dealing with atypical proliferative lesions of the bladder with only minimal epithelial hyperplasia, i.e., without papillary projections, the lesions would have to show marked (or at least moderate) qualitative cellular and nuclear abnormalities before the diagnostic threshold (K_m) was reached. Thus, in most cases before pathologists would diagnose a flat proliferative epithelial lesion as carcinoma *in situ* the constituent epithelial cells would have to show marked nuclear abnormality in addition to some increase in the number of basal and/or intermediate cells (Fig. 10.4). It is possible that there may be a flat counterpart to the grade-1 non-invasive papillary transitional-cell carcinoma, but with currently used light-microscopic criteria the pathologist will not be able to make the diagnosis. For several years, however, Friedell and his associates have advanced the hypothesis that the nuclei of grade-1 transitional carcinoma cells

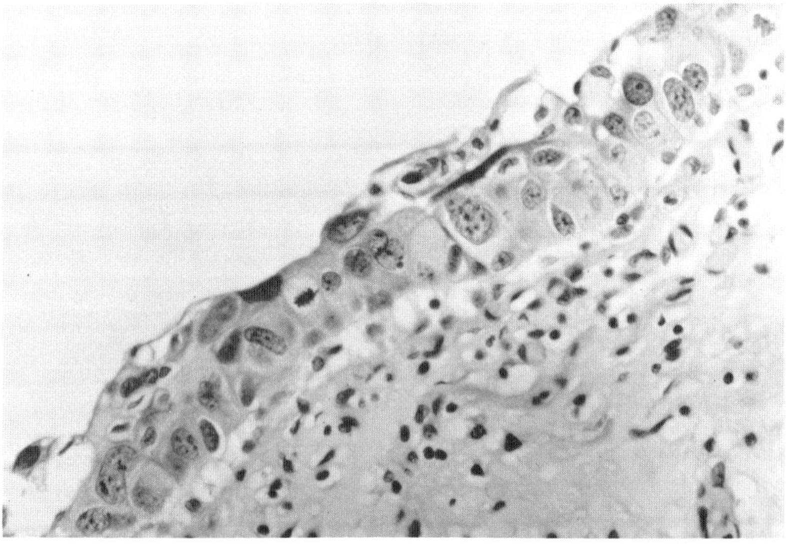

Fig. 10.4. Transitional-cell carcinoma *in situ*. ×200. H & E.

1. have a mean diameter greater than that of normal bladder epithelium;
2. have a relatively small standard deviation from the mean diameter when compared to that of nuclei of normal bladder epithelium (less variation in size);
3. have a mean nuclear diameter ± 2 standard deviation that lies within two standard deviations of the mean of the nuclei of normal bladder epithelium (size within the normal range).

This hypothesis, depicted in Fig. 10.5, was based on preliminary studies made by Friedell and Tiltman (unpublished observations), using ocular micrometers in light microscopes during a review of histopathological sections of transitional-cell carcinomas. The observations leave much to be desired, but with the advent of more precise methods of measuring, recording, and computing nuclear diameters or volumes in histological or cytological material, the possibility of testing these propositions has very much improved.

Dysplasia (morphological preneoplasias)

If the qualitative abnormality of basal or intermediate cells is slight or moderate and there is *no* appreciable increase in the number of these cells i.e., no significant *hyperplasia* in a flat lesion, the diagnosis would probably be some degree of *dysplasia* (Fig. 10.6), a term which is applied to non-papillary lesions. Slight or moderate qualitative cellular abnormality alone, without associated *marked* quantitative abnormality, is unlikely to exceed the diagnostic threshold of the pathologist for non-invasive epithelial malignancy (K_m). One of us has used the same principles in proposing a classification of lesions of the uterine cervix (Friedell 1965) but they are even more applicable to proliferative lesions of the bladder epithelium.

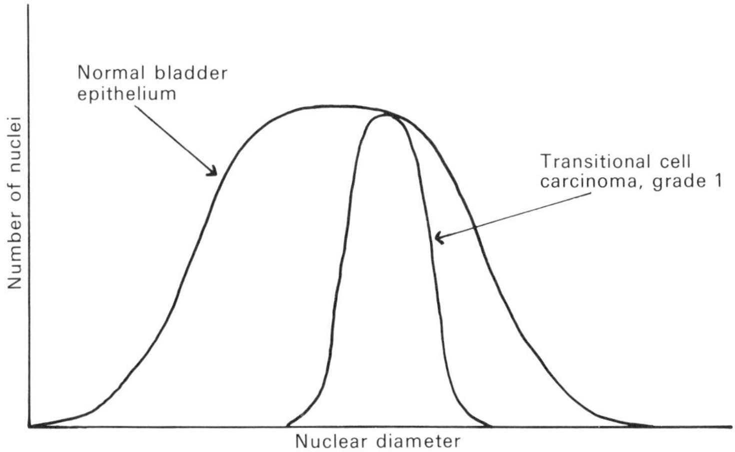

Fig. 10.5. Nuclear diameters of normal urothelial and grade-1 transitional-cell carcinoma cells.

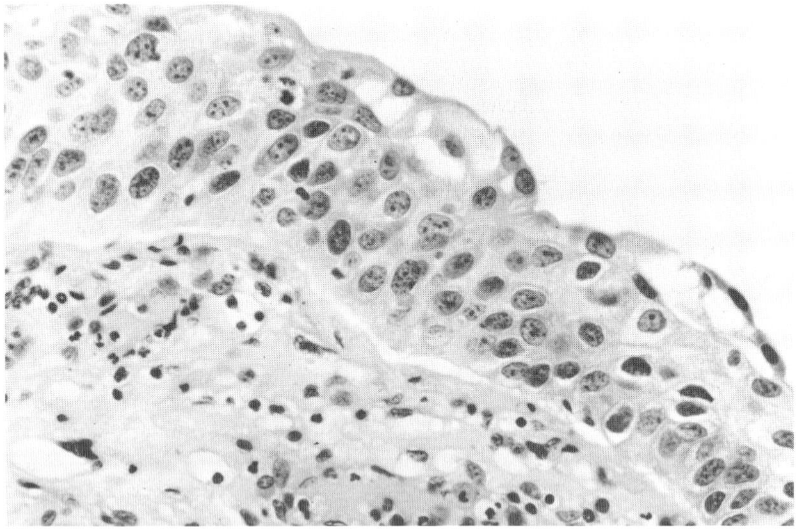

Fig. 10.6. Dysplasia of urinary bladder epithelium. ×200. H & E.

Cancers of other mucous membrane surfaces—the uterine cervix, the oral cavity, bronchus, and oesophagus (see Chapters 5-7, 12)—differ from bladder cancer insofar as the fate of the patient with carcinoma of the bladder is often determined less by the character of the lesion which is removed than by the neoplastic potential of the bladder epithelium remaining behind. This is particularly true when the tumour visible through the cystoscope—and removed transurethrally—is a small, superficial papillary lesion.

Whether or not agreement among pathologists can be achieved on the terminology for these lesions of the bladder remains to be seen. We are well on the way to doing so for invasive cancer, and this gives us some grounds for optimism in refining the diagnosis of *in situ* carcinoma. Agreement in the classification of preneoplastic lesions is a much more difficult problem, but a recent study reported by Nagy *et al.* (1981) suggests that such differences among pathologists can be resolved.

Benign proliferative lesions of the bladder

Von Brunn's nests, cystitis glandularis, and cystitis cystica are frequently present and have been collectively referred to as proliferative cystitis (Friedell *et al.* 1981). Although such lesions are composed of hyperplastic epithelium, mitoses are no more frequent than in the normal bladder mucosa. Some investigators have considered them to be precancerous since they are frequently present in bladders containing carcinoma, and they occasionally show marked atypia (dysplasia). But it would appear from recent studies mapping the presence of these abnormalities in bladders at autopsy that they are very common, increase in frequency with age, and are present focally in virtually all urinary bladders in people over the age of 50 (Wiener *et al.* 1979; N. Ito, personal communication). The presence of dysplasia is approximately as frequent in these lesions as in mucosa not involved by proliferative cystitis. These data indicate that such lesions are not precancerous and are of no predictive value clinically (Friedell *et al.* 1982).

Relationship between morphology and biology

The obvious major problem confronting the pathologist and the urologist is that the (morphological) diagnostic threshold of the pathologist may not coincide with the true biological threshold of malignancy. Some of the papillary lesions currently described as low-grade carcinomas by the pathologist may represent hyperplasia rather than neoplasia; conversely, some of the flat lesions with only moderate qualitative cellular abnormality may already be biologically committed neoplastic lesions rather than dysplasias. In these cases the epithelium does not look malignant though it does look abnormal, and the problem is to distinguish between epithelium which is a forerunner of cancer and that which is benign.

One approach is by longitudinal studies of patients who have had biopsies revealing non-neoplastic but abnormal bladder epithelium. Successive cystoscopic examinations together with selected-site mucosal biopsies and studies of cytological specimens obtained by bladder washings or from voided urine will permit sequential evaluation of epithelial morphology. This information can in turn be correlated with follow-up findings. The subsequent clinical course of the patient provides the only means currently available for assessing the malignant potential of the epithelium. A second approach is through the judicious use of information obtained from standardized animal models. The extrapolation of the more readily available animal data to man can be reasonably close if care is taken to ensure that all information used is carefully classified and that truly similar phenomena are being compared.

Ultrastructural changes related to malignancy

The ultrastructure of bladder cancer has been extensively examined in man and in experimental animals. A unique feature of the luminal border of the urothelium is the presence of asymmetric membrane composed of plaques (Hicks 1975; see Fig. 10.7). In species such as the rat, as much as 80 per cent of the luminal surface of the bladder can be covered by asymmetric membrane. It is obvious, however, that the asymmetric membrane is only part of the barrier to urine which the urothelium provides; symmetric interplaque membranes and the tight junctions between the cells are the remaining barrier components (Merk *et al.* 1977). In other species, including man, a relatively small proportion of superficial cells normally have asymmetric membrane and the proportion appears to decrease with age (Alroy *et al.* 1977). Bladder tumour cells in man and in animals do not produce asymmetric membrane (Ito 1976), but it is also absent in rapidly proliferating epithelial cells as in,

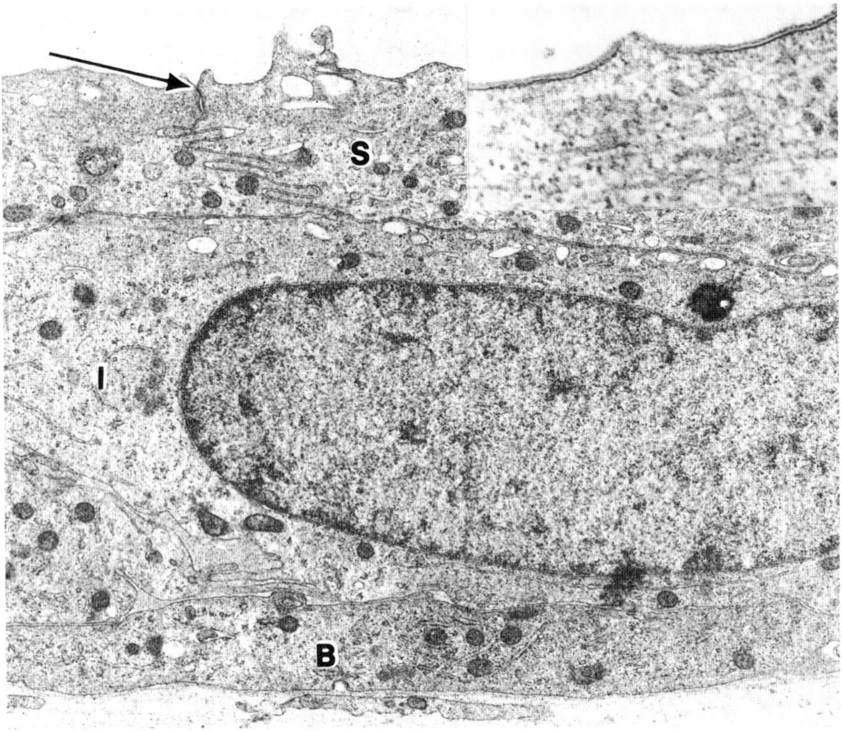

Fig. 10.7. Normal urinary bladder epithelium with characteristic asymmetric luminal membrane, fusiform vesicles, and junctional complex (arrow). The epithelium is composed of three cell layers, superficial (S), intermediate (I), and basal cells (B). ×3000. Insert (right upper corner): Asymmetric luminal membrane. ×7000.

for example, the mucosal repair associated with cystitis (Shirai *et al.* 1978; Fukushima *et al.* 1981). Thus, the absence of asymmetric membrane is not indicative of malignancy.

Additional studies with the transmission electron microscope, particularly in man, suggest that there are differences in the junctions between cells in normal bladder epithelium and those in transitional-cell carcinomas (Weinstein *et al.* 1976). Quantitative investigations have been reported determining the number of desmosomes and the proportion of cell membrane consisting of desmosomes (Pauli *et al.* 1978; Alroy *et al.* 1981). Initial studies indicated that high-grade transitional-cell carcinomas had fewer desmosomes per surface area of the cell membrane than normal epithelium or low-grade tumours. But when invasive and non-invasive tumours were compared, it became clear that the number of desmosomes was related to invasion and not to grade. High-grade papillary carcinomas which were non-invasive had increased numbers of desmosomes compared to normal epithelium, and low-grade invasive papillary carcinomas had decreased numbers of desmosomes.

In experimental bladder tumours, tight junctions become attenuated and the number of tight junctions decreases early in the carcinogenic process (Merk *et al.* 1977). They do not disappear, however, even in invasive cancer and they can occasionally be identified in deeply invasive tumours, both in experimental animals and in human patients (Weinstein *et al.* 1976; Merk *et al.* 1977). This change does not provide a basis for distinguishing between invasive and non-invasive neoplastic epithelium, but the attenuation and decreased numbers of tight junctions may form the basis for the increased permeability of the epithelium in bladder tumours compared to normal urothelium.

The surface of bladder tumour cells contains numerous microvilli covered with a thickened glycocalyx 'fuzz' (Hicks and Wakefield 1976; see Fig. 10.8). This material was initially thought to be characteristic of transitional-cell carcinomas but it has subsequently be found in normal bladders on the small microvilli occasionally seen on cells lining the luminal surface. It is also frequently seen on the microvilli which are present during regenerative hyperplasia, particularly in experimental animals (Hicks 1975; Koss 1967; Fukushima *et al.* 1981*a, b*; L.M. Franks personal communication).

With scanning electron microscopy (SEM), short microvilli which are uniform in size and shape are frequently seen on the luminal surface of the

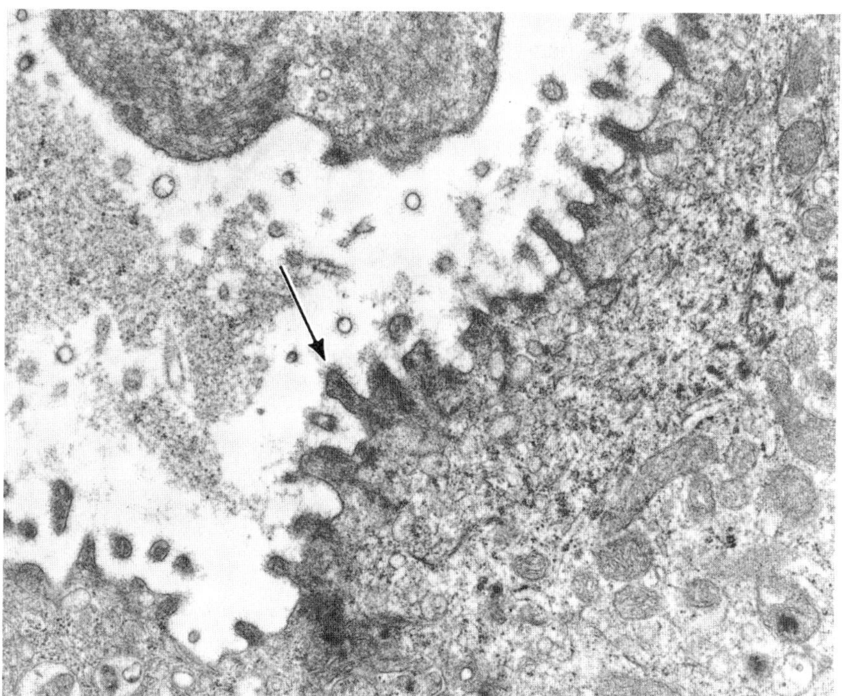

Fig. 10.8. Microvilli on the surface of a focus of transitional-cell carcinoma covered with a glycocalyx 'fuzz'. × 6500.

normal urinary bladder, particularly when intermediate cells are visualized before developing into large, superficial cells (Hicks 1975; Hicks and Wakefield 1976; Ito 1976; Weinstein *et al.* 1976; Jacobs *et al.* 1976*a,* 1977*a*; Merk *et al.* 1977; Alroy *et al.* 1977, 1981; Koss 1967; Hicks and Chowaniec 1978; Pauli *et al.* 1978; Fukushima *et al.* 1981*a*). By contrast, transitional-cell carcinomas (like carcinomas in general) have pleomorphic microvilli which vary in size and shape; pleomorphism increases with increasing grade of tumour (Jacobs *et al.* 1976*a*, 1977*a*; Hicks and Chowaniec 1978). Although pleomorphic microvilli were described on the surfaces of human bladder carcinoma cells by Fulker *et al.* in 1971, their significance was not appreciated until Jacobs and his colleagues investigated this change in an experimental system which involved the feeding of a carcinogen, N-[4-(5-nitro-2-furyl)-2-thiazolyl] formamide (FANFT), to rats for varying periods of time (Jacobs *et al.* 1976*a*, 1977*a*; Cohen *et al.* 1976).

During carcinogenesis induced with this agent, the epithelium passes through several morphological stages beginning with simple hyperplasia (Fig. 10.9) and progressing to nodular and papillary hyperplasia (Fig. 10.10), papilloma, non-invasive carcinoma (Fig. 10.11), and invasive carcinomas which occasionally metastasize (Jacobs *et al.* 1976*a,* 1977*a*; Cohen *et al.* 1976). The appearance of pleomorphic microvilli on the luminal surface of the urothelium of the urinary bladder closely correlated with the development of irreversible hyperplastic lesions at weeks 6-8 (Jacobs *et al.* 1976*a,* 1977*a*). In addition, pleomorphic microvilli were present on all transitional-cell carcinomas induced by this chemical. Subsequent studies with other carcinogens in the rat and other species (Arai *et al.* 1974; Shirai *et al.* 1977;

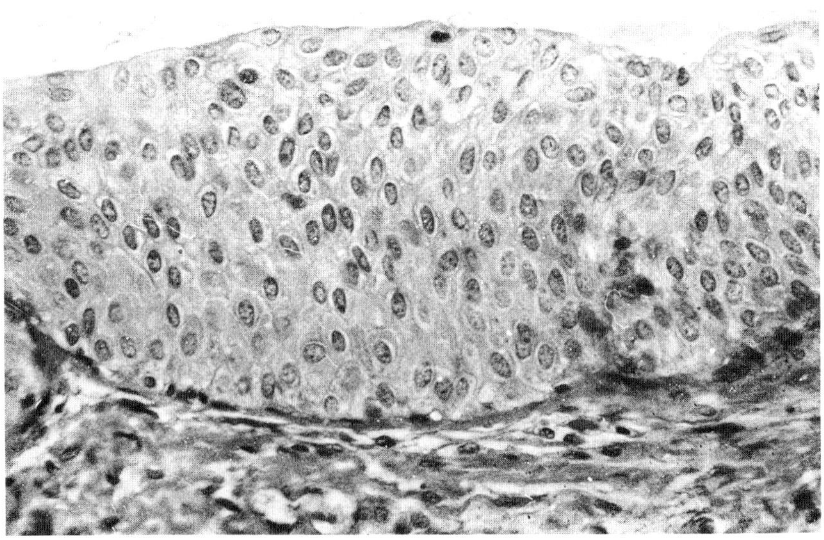

Fig. 10.9. Simple hyperplasia of the urinary bladder in a rat fed FANFT. ×200. H & E.

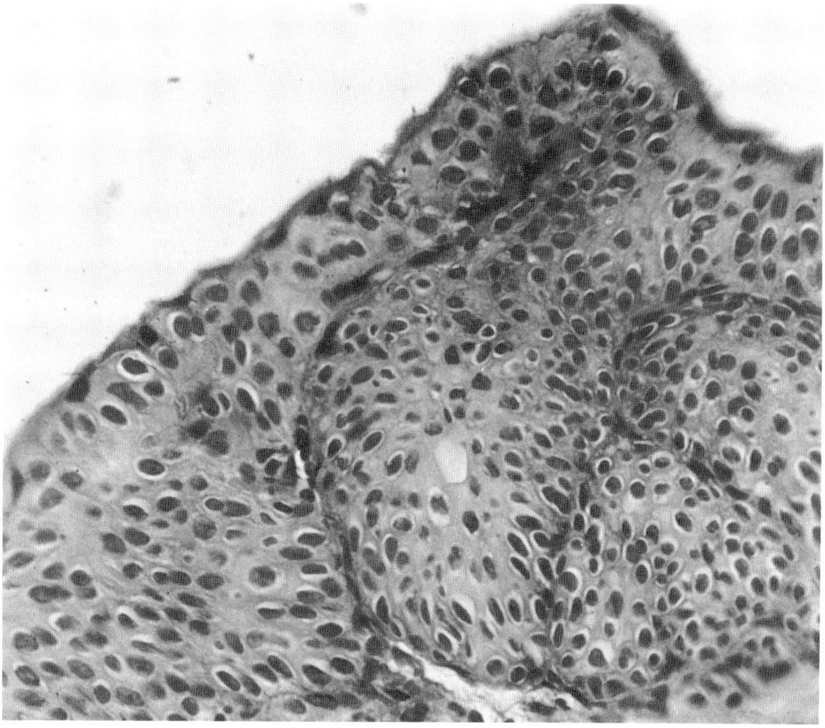

Fig.10.10. Nodular hyperplasia of the urinary bladder in a rat fed FANFT. ×200. H & E.

Hicks and Chowaniec 1978) indicated that pleomorphic microvilli were present on transitional-cell carcinomas in all species tested (Jacobs *et al.* 1976*a*) parallelling the same finding in human bladder cancer (Fulker *et al.* 1971; Jacobs *et al.* 1977*b*; Hicks and Chowaniec 1978; see Fig. 10.12 and Fig. 10.13).

In addition, cells could be obtained from the urine of animals with early preneoplastic lesions and observed by SEM (Jacobs *et al.* 1976*b*). Cells with pleomorphic microvilli were present very early during the course of carcinogenesis (week 10), long before clearly malignant cells were observable in cytological preparations by light microscopy (week 60).

Although pleomorphic microvilli are always present in transitional-cell carcinomas, they are not present on all carcinoma cells. They have not so far been reported on epithelial cells in the normal urinary bladder but it appears from recent studies that they are not specific for neoplasia (Fukushima *et al.* 1981*a,b*). Pleomorphic microvilli are occasionally present on the luminal surface of hyperplastic cells in the reversible lesions induced by cyclophosphamide, ulceration by freezing, surgical incisions, or by the instillation of formalin.

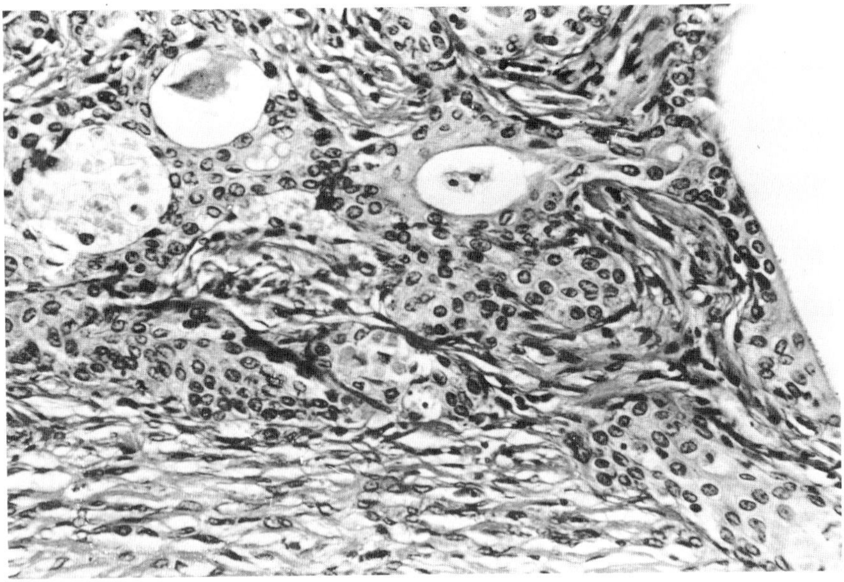

Fig. 10.11. Non-invasive transitional-cell carcinoma of the urinary bladder in a rat fed FANFT. ×200. H & E.

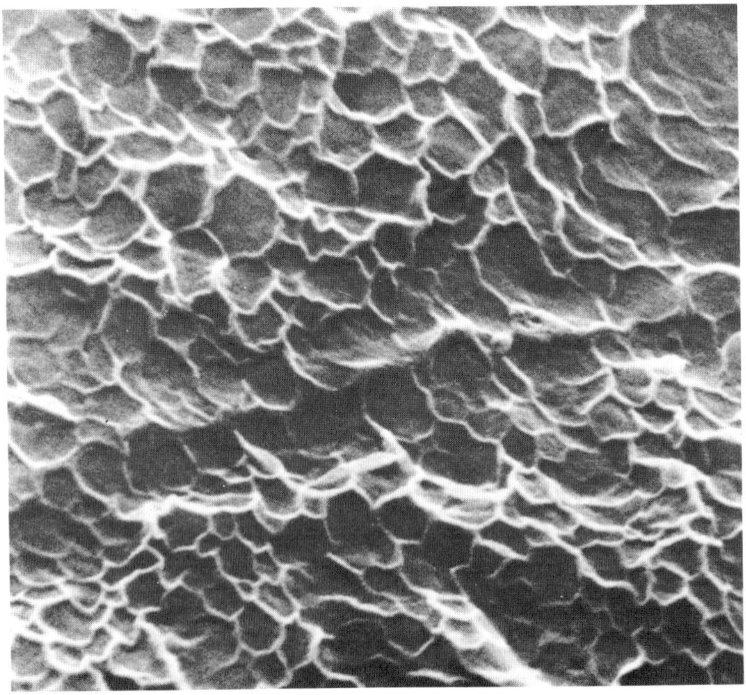

Fig. 10.12. The luminal surface of a superficial cell from the bladder of a normal rat. Micro-ridges formed from symmetric membrane 5 cm between areas of asymmetric membrane. ×14 000. (From J.B. Jacobs (1982).)

It has been suggested that there are quantitative, if not qualitative, differences between the pleomorphic microvilli on hyperplastic cells and those on tumour cells. For example, microvilli on the surfaces of hyperplastic cells induced by cyclophosphamide injection were frequently present in clusters rather than diffusely as seen in tumour cells (Fukushima *et al.* 1981*b*). Other features observed by scanning electron microscopy such as the degree of variation in cell size and shape, spaces between microvilli, and the distribution of microvilli appear to be different in tumour cells and in hyperplastic cells (Jacobs *et al.* 1981).

In this same study by Jacobs and his colleagues quantitation of SEM changes in human biopsy specimens was carried out. Cell surface patterns were classified into one normal and four abnormal categories. The most anaplastic cells on the luminal surface of the bladder were covered completely by pleomorphic microvilli (Fig. 10.13) or had smooth surfaces with intercellular seams which were markedly thickened and raised (Fig. 10.14). Predictably, grade-1 carcinomas tended to have cells that more nearly resembled cells seen in the normal bladder; grade-3 lesions had a greater

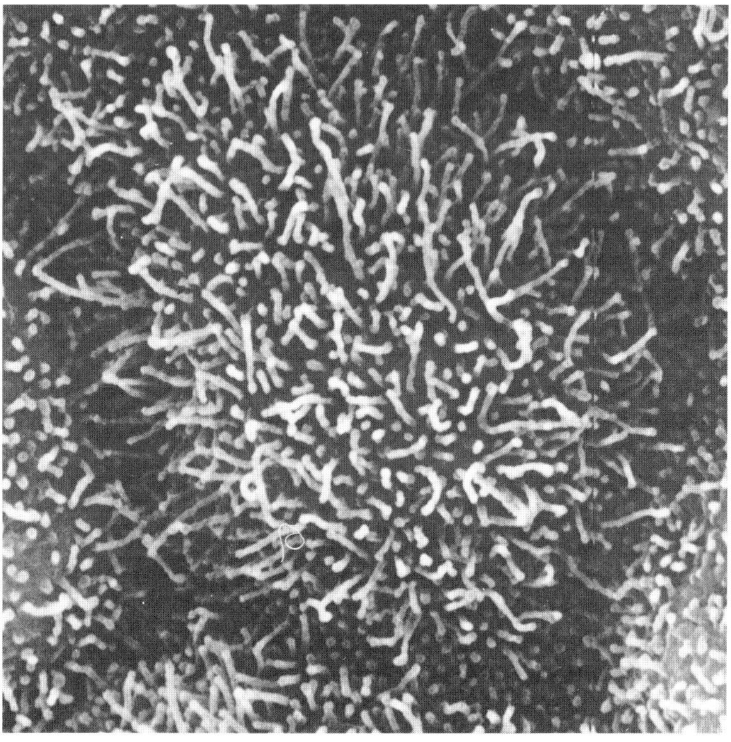

Fig. 10.13. Pleomorphic microvilli on the surface of a grade 3 transitional carcinoma in man. ×8600. (From Jacobs *et al.* (1981).)

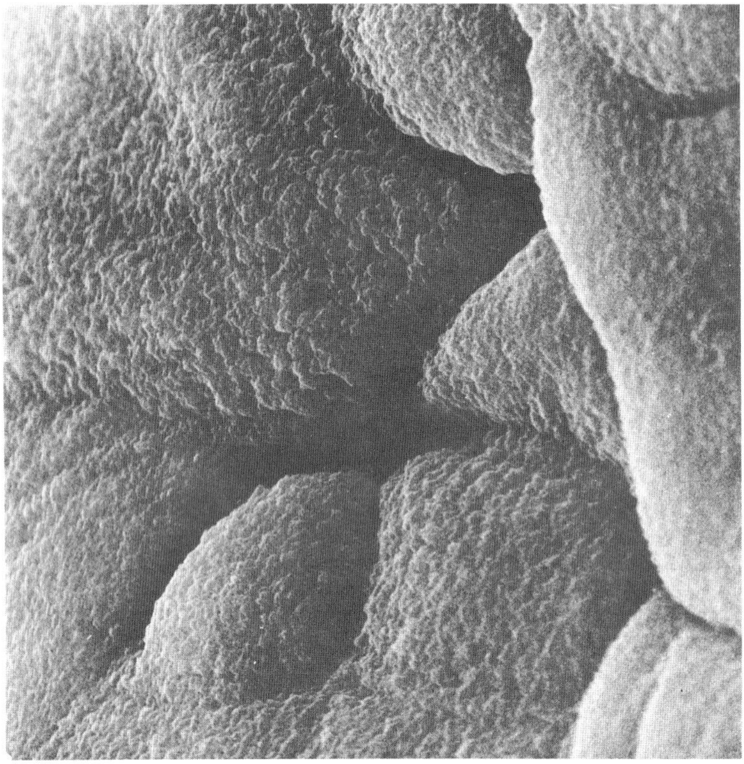

Fig. 10.14. Surface of a cell from a patient with grade 3 transitional cell carcinoma showing a bumpy, corrugated surface and thick seams between cells. ×5000. (From Jacobs *et al.* (1981).)

proportion of very abnormal cells, many cells with lesser abnormalities, and no normal cells.

Preliminary studies of cytological material from the human urinary tract carried out in our laboratory and others (Jacobs *et al.* 1977*b,* 1981; Domagala *et al.* 1979; Gilchrist *et al.* 1980) indicate that pleomorphic microvilli are present on exfoliated transitional-cell carcinoma cells (Fig. 10.15); they have not yet been observed in the urine of normal subjects or in cytological samples from patients with non-neoplastic epithelial proliferations. In 15 cases with histologically proven non-invasive papillary grade-1 or -2 transitional-cell carcinomas, light microscopic cytology showed malignant cells in six cases whereas SEM revealed cells with pleomorphic microvilli in twelve cases. In five cases with grade-3 carcinomas, pleomorphic microvilli were seen on cells in the cytological specimens from all cases. Urine specimens from 14 persons without urinary tract disease, ten patients with bacterial cystitis, and two patients with cyclophosphamide-induced haemorrhagic cystitis were negative in this regard. Patients with adenocarcinoma of the prostate occasionally had cells in the urine with pleomorphic microvilli (five of ten cases), but these cells were readily distinguishable from

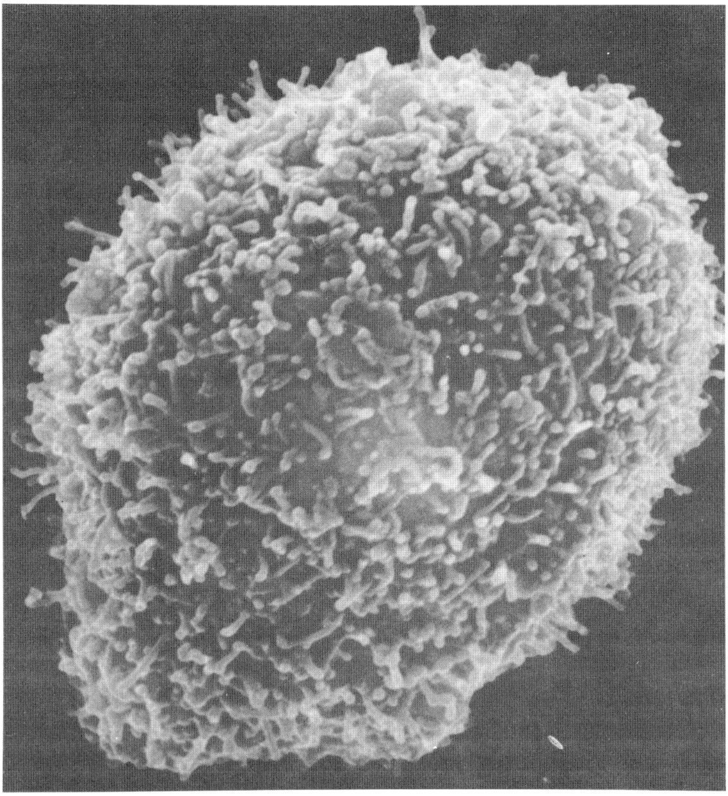

Fig. 10.15. Exfoliated cell in bladder washing of a patient with transitional cell carcinoma, grade 2, having numerous pleomorphic microvilli on its surface. ×3000. (From J.B. Jacobs (1982).)

transitional-cell carcinoma by their general shape. Similar results in small series of patients have also been reported by Domagala *et al.* (1979) and by Gilchrist *et al.* (1980).

SEM examination is also potentially useful in evaluating cytological specimens from patients who previously had bladder carcinoma—the population at highest risk for the development (or re-development) of bladder cancer. In preliminary studies by us (Jacobs *et al.*, unpublished observations), five of twelve patients being followed for possible recurrence of bladder carcinoma had cells with pleomorphic microvilli in bladder washings even though cystoscopy was negative. Although these might at first be considered as false-positive cases, two of these patients developed recurrent, cystoscopically visible, low-grade bladder carcinoma between one and six months after cells with pleomorphic microvilli were observed. Additional follow-up of the remaining cases and the study of additional patients will be necessary to determine the fuller significance of this finding.

The use of SEM cytological studies is also being evaluated (Jacobs *et al.* unpublished observations) as a means of detecting persistent or recurrent tumour in patients with bladder cancer treated by pelvic irradiation. Although changes in cell surface features due to radiotherapy are evident on normal cells, the response of normal cells to radiation was different from that of neoplastic cells. In a preliminary study of 30 bladder-cancer patients treated by radiation therapy, we found the presence of pleomorphic microvilli on cells related to the presence of tumour in these cases.

Finally, it should be noted that the SEM evaluation of urinary-tract cytological specimens from workers exposed to known or suspected chemical carcinogens may provide information regarding the significance of pleomorphic microvilli on exfoliated cells which do not have the light-microscopic characteristics of neoplasia. Such studies are in progress in our laboratory. The significance of positive findings is not yet known, but with prolonged follow-up this point should be clarified.

In summary, although SEM examination is impractical for all urinary-bladder biopsy and cytological specimens, there may be selected instances in which it will be of diagnostic or prognostic value in revealing the neoplastic 'committment' of cells and epithelia which, by light-microscopic criteria, would be classified as preneoplastic.

Other markers

Blood-group isoantigens

Several studies have been reported evaluating various immunological techniques for identifying antigens in bladder epithelium. Some appear promising as aids in the diagnosis or prognosis of bladder cancer. Detection of blood-group isoantigens A, B, and H using the specific red-cell adherence (SRCA) technique developed by Davidsohn and his colleagues (Kovarik *et al.* 1968) has shown the greatest potential as a prognostic indicator.

With the SRCA test, blood-group isoantigens were detected in normal epithelium, whereas untreated invasive carcinoma showed deletion of these antigens (Kay and Wallace 1961; Davidsohn 1973; Decenzo *et al.* 1975; Limas and Lange 1982). The antigens were present in some cases of non-invasive transitional-cell carcinoma and absent in others, but clinical correlation revealed that, when antigens were present, 95 per cent of the cases had no evidence of invasive cancer during a follow-up period of five years (Decenzo *et al.* 1975; Ramsey 1980). By contrast, approximately two-thirds of patients with non-invasive carcinomas showing deletion of the antigens subsequently developed invasive disease within five years. It is of interest that although the SRCA test had predictive significance concerning *invasion*, it failed to predict *recurrence* (Lange and Limas 1980).

It should also be noted that when using formalin-fixed, paraffin-embedded tissue in the procedure—something which makes this a practical procedure in the routine pathology laboratory—the test is reliable only if the patient has blood group A, B, or AB. It is not reliable for the H antigen in patients with blood group O (Lange and Limas 1980; Ramsey 1980) when paraffin-embedded material is used, and frozen sections of fresh material or formalin-fixed but non-paraffin-embedded tissue may be required.

Although initial reports of the SRCA test showed antigenic deletion in all invasive bladder carcinomas, subsequent studies reported the retention of antigens in some cases (Alroy *et al.* 1978). It was eventually discovered that those patients in whom antigen was present had been previously irradiated, and it became apparent that in some instances expression of the antigens in invasive carcinoma followed irradiation even if the antigens were absent before radiotherapy (Alroy *et al.* 1978). Other cases of invasive carcinoma reported to have blood-group isoantigens present may well have been irradiated (Kay and Wallace 1961).

In patients with carcinoma *in situ* of the bladder, isoantigens were usually deleted, not only in the obviously neoplastic areas of the bladder but also in regions of dysplasia and even in adjacent normal-appearing epithelium. This finding suggests a more pervasive abnormality than that revealed by routine light-microscopic examination (Weinstein *et al.* 1979).

Carcinoembryonic antigen

Carcinoembryonic antigen (CEA) is one of several oncofetal antigens associated with the presence of various malignancies and certain non-malignant conditions. Its presence in serum was originally considered specific for carcinomas of the digestive tract (Gold and Freedman 1965) but CEA has now been demonstrated in a variety of malignancies including bladder cancer (Reynoso *et al.* 1972; Zimmerman *et al.* 1980). As the sensitivity of the methods improved, it was also shown that people without cancer had measurable serum CEA levels and that the difference between normal individuals and patients with cancer was quantitative rather than qualitative.

Serum CEA levels have generally not been elevated in cases of bladder cancer except occasionally in patients with extensive metastases (Zimmerman *et al.* 1980). On the other hand, *urinary* levels of CEA are frequently raised in patients with bladder cancer (Reynoso *et al.* 1972: Zimmerman *et al.* 1980). The antigen has been demonstrated in neoplastic transitional cells, and these cells are presumably the principal source of the urinary CEA in these patients (Zimmerman *et al.* 1980). Normal transitional cells of the urothelium also contain CEA (Shevchuk *et al.* 1981), and positive urinary tests, even when significantly elevated, are far from specific; patients with bacterial cystitis have elevated urinary CEA in the same range as in cancer patients (Reynoso *et al.* 1972; Zimmerman *et al.* 1980; Shevchuk *et al.* 1981).

Urinary CEA levels are not related to the grade of the tumour (Zimmerman *et al.* 1980). They are generally higher in more advanced stages of the disease, and tend to decrease following therapy if the tumour is eradicated. Levels occasionally increase with recurrence or progression of the tumour. Whether or not CEA determinations will prove of value in identifying cases with 'committed' but microscopically non-neoplastic bladder epithelium remains to be seen, but urinary CEA determination does not appear to be helpful in general clinical practice.

Histochemical and biochemical markers

In addition to the ultrastructural and immunological techniques examined in a search for markers with diagnostic and/or prognostic value, biochemical and histochemical techniques have also been applied to bladder cancer. The most extensively studied histochemical marker in experimental bladder cancer has been the enzyme alkaline phosphatase (Stiller and Rauscher 1971; Kunze *et al.* 1975; Hicks and Chowaniec 1978). Normal urothelium contains relatively large amounts of this enzyme whereas transitional-cell carcinomas have considerably lower levels. Indeed, the enzyme often appears to be absent when measured with the histochemical assays in common use (Stiller and Rauscher 1971; Kunze *et al.* 1975). Similar losses of alkaline phosphatase activity are, however, seen in reversible regenerative hyperplasias of the bladder induced by various methods such as intraperitoneal cyclophosphamide injection or ulceration of the bladder by freezing (Athans and Cohen, unpublished observations). Alkaline phosphatase activity returns to normal levels as the hyperplastic epithelial changes resolve. Studies of β-glucuronidase demonstrate that, as for alkaline phosphatase, the levels decrease in reversible regenerative hyperplasia as well as in transitional-cell carcinomas (Athans and Cohen, unpublished observations).

Other markers involve differences in the distribution of concentration of sugar residues on cell surfaces. These residues comprise one component of the membrane surface and are partly responsible for cellular antigenicity. The blood-group isoantigens described earlier are examples of such antigenic-sugar residues. Several plant lectins have been identified which bind to specific sugar residues. Concanavalin A, which binds to mannose, has been shown to increase the agglutinability of dispersed bladder tumour cells (Kakizoe *et al.* 1979, 1980). Increased agglutinability was present very early in the course of the carcinogenic process but total binding, measured with fluorescent labelled concanavalin A, was similar for neoplastic and normal urothelial cells (Athans and Cohen, unpublished observations). These data suggest that the differences in agglutinability are due to aggregation of the concanavalin A receptors in one portion of the cell surface rather than to differences in the total number of receptors present.

Ricinus communis agglutinin, specific for galactose, also binds to neoplastic bladder cells in animal models. Unlike concanavalin A, it binds only weakly to the normal urothelium and to reversible hyperplastic lesions induced by cyclophosphamide or freeze ulceration (Daly *et al.* 1979); Athans and Cohen, unpublished observations). Preliminary studies with human tumours indicate that *Ricinus communis* agglutinin binds to transitional-cell carcinomas and not to non-neoplastic urothelium (Daly *et al.* 1979). Subsequent studies have, however, shown marked variability in the binding of tumour cells, even when the same tumour was evaluated on consecutive days (Cohen, unpublished observations).

In addition to sugar residues on the cell surface, cell membranes contain a number of sugar transferases. Galactosyl transferase has been shown to be elevated in several human tumours (Podolsky *et al.* 1978), particularly cancers of the pancreas and colon, but also in carcinomas of the urinary bladder (Plotkin *et al.* 1977, 1979, 1980; Hagen-Cook *et al.* 1978). Galactosyl transferase activity can be measured on cells exfoliated in the urine. Cells in normal urine have low levels of enzyme activity whereas neoplastic cells have elevated levels in experimental animals (Plotkin *et al.* 1979). Enzyme activity is not raised in animals with regenerative hyperplasia (Plotkin *et al.* 1980) but cystitis causes difficulty in interpretation in man because of the presence of galactosyl transferase in the non-cellular portion of urine which adheres to the cells during processing (Plotkin *et al.* 1979). The problem is compounded by the fact that the erythrocytes which frequently contaminate the urine in patients with cystitis and bladder tumours have very high levels of galactosyl transferase activity (Plotkin *et al.* 1980).

A few other enzymes have been studied as diagnostic aids for patients with bladder cancer. Such investigations have generally focused on urinary enzyme levels since few changes have been observed in the serum. Lactate dehydrogenase has been most extensively studied but, despite the use of isozyme analysis (Bredin *et al.* 1975), sensitivity and specificity have been inadequate for the test to be of clinical value.

Chromosomes

With the development of chromosome banding techniques and methods for chromosome analysis in cells from solid tumours, cytogenetic analysis of bladder carcinomas has become possible. Results so far indicate that such analyses are useful in identifying those patients with low-grade, low-stage papillary carcinomas which are likely to recur or progress (Falor 1971; Falor and Ward 1978; Sandberg 1980). In general these tumours have near-diploid chromosome numbers but chromosome markers, frequently chromosome No. 1, are present in approximately half the cases. It has been further demonstrated that marker chromosomes are often related to nuclear protrusions which can be detected with relatively simple light-microscopic techniques.

The presence of marker chromosomes has been closely correlated with the development of recurrence (Falor 1971; Falor and Ward 1978; Sandberg 1980). In one series, for example (Sandberg 1980), 42 of 78 patients with papillary carcinomas had marker chromosomes, and 21 of these 42 patients developed recurrences. Recurrent tumours generally had similar chromosome patterns to the original tumour although slight changes in chromosome number were observed. Only one of the 36 patients without marker chromosomes developed recurrent tumour.

Addendum: Bilharziasis and the evolution of bladder cancer

There is now considerable evidence that carcinoma of the bladder in man and experimental animals is a multistage process (Hicks 1980). Non-genotoxic agents which cause non-specific irritant effects on the urothelium can act as promoters in the carcinogenic process and recent work on *Schistosoma haematobium* infestations is of particular interest (Hicks *et al.* 1980; Hicks 1983). Studies in young Egyptian men living in a high-risk area of Bilharziasis-associated bladder cancer have shown a high incidence of combined *S. haematobium* infestation and mixed bacterial infections in the urinary tract. Elevated levels of N-nitroso compounds were demonstrated in the urine and could be broadly correlated with the numbers of nitrate-reducing bacteria. Urine-borne N-nitroso compounds may thus act as the initial genotoxic carcinogen in these individuals while *S. haematobium* infestations act at a later stage. Results of experiments with baboons (*Papio* sp) are consistent with this suggested sequence of events (Hicks *et al.* 1980). The animals were infested with *S. haematobium* and then dosed intermittently with N-butyl-N-(4-hydroxybutyl) nitrosamine (BBN) throughout the experiment, simulating the human situation. Control animals treated with BBN alone did not develop tumours. Control animals infested with *S. haematobium* alone showed chronic urinary tract inflammation with mucosal hyperplasia but no neoplasms. Test animals infested with parasites and also exposed to BBN developed gross abnormalities of the lower urinary tract and a high incidence of carcinoma.

References

Alroy, J., Pauli, B.U., Weinstein, R.S., and Merk, F.B. (1977). Association of asymmetric unit membrane plaque formation in the urinary bladder of adult humans with therapeutic radiation. *Experientia* **33**, 1645.

——, Teramura, K., Miller, A.W., III, Pauli, B.U., Gottesman, J.E., Flanagan, M., Davidsohn, I., and Weinstein, R.S. (1978). Isoantigens A, B and H in urinary bladder carcinomas following radiotherapy. *Cancer* **41**, 1739.

——, Pauli, B.U., and Weinstein, R.S. (1981). Correlation between numbers of desmosomes and the aggressiveness of transitional cell carcinoma in human urinary bladder. *Cancer* **47**, 104.

Arai, M., Kani, T., Sugihara, S., Matsumura, K., Miyata, Y., Shinohara, Y., and Ito, N. (1974). Scanning and transmission electron microscopy of changes in the urinary bladder in rats treated with N-butyl-N- (4-hydroxybutylnitrosamine). *Gann* **65**, 529.

Bredin, H.C., Daly, J.J., and Prout, G.R., Jr. (1975). Lactic dehydrogenase isoenzymes in human bladder cancer. *J. Urol.* **113**, 487.

Cohen, S.M., Jacobs, J.B., Arai, M., Johansson, S., and Friedell, G.H. (1976). Early lesions in experimental bladder cancer: Experimental design and light microscopic findings. *Cancer Res.* **36**, 2508.

Daly, J.J., Prout, G.R., Jr., Hagen K., Lin, J.C., Kamali, H.M., Plotkin, G.M., and Wolf, G. (1979). Identification of malignant transitional cells by their binding of fluorescein-labelled lectin. *Surg. Forum* **30**, 565.

Davidsohn, I. (1973). Isoantigen test for bladder carcinoma. *Med. World News* **14**, 31.

Decenzo, J.M., Howard, P., and Irish, C.E. (1975). Antigenic deletion and prognosis of patients with stage A transitional cell bladder carcinoma. *J. Urol.* **114**, 874.

Domagala, W., Kahan, A.V., and Koss, L.G. (1979). The ultrastructure of surfaces of positively identified cells in the human urinary sediment. A correlative light and scanning electron microscopic study. *Acta Cytologica* **23**, 147.

Falor, W.H. (1971). Chromosomes in non-invasive papillary carcinoma of the bladder, *J. Amer. Med. Assoc.* **216**, 791.

——, Ward, R.M. (1978). Prognosis in early carcinoma of the bladder based on chromosomal analysis. *J. Urol.* **119**, 44.

Farrow, G.M., Utz, D.C., and Rife, C.C. (1976). Morphological and clinical observations of patients with early bladder cancer treated with total cystectomy. *Cancer Res.* **36**, 2495.

Friedell, G.H. (1965). Terminology for epithelial abnormalities of the uterine cervix. *Amer. J. clin. Pathol.* **44**, 280.

—— (1976). Carcinoma, carcinoma *in situ*, and 'early lesions' of the uterine cervix and the urinary bladder. Introduction and definitions. *Cancer Res.* **36**, 2482.

—— (1981). Precancerous lesions of the urinary bladder. *Acta Endoscopica.* **11**, 53.

——, Hertig, A.T., and Younge, P.A. (1960). *Carcinoma in situ of the uterine cervix.* Charles C. Thomas, Springfield, Illinois.

——, Parija, G.C., Nagy, G.K., and Soto, E.A. (1980). The pathology of human bladder cancer. *Cancer* **45**, 1823.

——, Soto, E.A., Parija, G.C., and Nagy, G.K. (1982). The renal pelves, ureters, urinary bladder, and uretha. In *Principles and practice of surgical pathology* (ed. S.G. Silverberg).

Fukushima, S., Arai, M., Cohen, S.M., Jacobs, J.B., and Friedell, G.H. (1981*a*). Scanning electron microscopy of cyclophosphamide-induced hyperplasia of the rat urinary bladder. *Lab. Invest.* **44**, 89.

——, Cohen, S.M., Arai, M., Jacobs, J.B., and Friedell, G.H. (1981*b*). Scanning electron microscopy of reversible hyperplasia of the rat urinary bladder. *Amer. J. Pathol.* **102**, 373.

Fulker, M.J., Cooper, E.H., and Tanaka, T. (1971). Proliferation and ultrastructure of papillary transitional cell carcinoma of the human bladder. *Cancer* **27**, 71.

Gilchrist, K.W., Benson, R.C., Jr., and Kutchera, A.R. (1980). Pleomorphic microvilli and low-grade human urothelial cancer. *Urology* **15**, 69.

Gold, P. and Freedman, S.D. (1965). Specific carcinoembryonic antigens of the human digestive system. *J. exp. Med.* **122**, 467.

Hagen-Cook, K., Prout, G.R., Jr., Plotkin, G.M., Gilbert, S.L., and Wolf, G. (1978). Galactosyl transferase in benign and neoplastic human bladder mucosa. *Surg. Forum* **29**, 627.

Hicks, R.M. (1975). The mammalian urinary bladder: An accommodating organ. *Biol. Rev.* **50**, 215.

—— (1980). Multistage carcinogenesis in the urinary bladder. *Br. med. Bull.* **36**, 39.

—— (1983). The canopic worm: role of bilharziasis in the aetiology of human bladder cancer. *J. R. Soc. Med.* **76**, 16.

——, and Wakefield, J. St. J. (1976). Membrane changes during urothelial hyperplasia and neoplasia. *Cancer Res.* **36**, 2502.

——, and Chowaniec, J. (1978). Experimental induction, histology, and ultrastructure of hyperplasia and neoplasia of the urinary bladder epithelium. *Int. Rev. exp. Pathol.* **18**, 199.

——, James, C., and Webbe, G. (1980). Effect of *Schistosoma haematobium* and N-butyl-N-(4-hydroxylbutyl) nitrosamine on the development of urothelial neoplasia in the baboon. *Br. J. Cancer* **42**, 730.

Ito, N. (1976). Early changes caused by N-butyl-N-(4-hydroxybutyl) nitrosamine in the bladder epithelium of different animal species. *Cancer Res.* **36**, 2528.

Jacobs, J.B. (1982). The potential of scanning electron microscopic (SEM) exfoliative cytology in the clinical management of bladder cancer. In *Bladder cancer* (ed. W.W. Bonney). Williams and Wilkins.

——, Arai, M., Cohen, S.M., and Friedell, G.H. (1976*a*). Early lesions in experimental bladder cancer: scanning electron microscopy of cell surface markers. *Cancer Res.* **36**, 2512.

—— —— —— —— (1976*b*). Light and scanning electron microscopy of exfoliated bladder epithelial cells in rats fed N-(4-(5-nitro-2-furyl)-2-thiazolyl) formamide. *J. Nat. Cancer Inst.* **57**, 63.

—— —— —— —— (1977*a*). A long-term study of reversible and progressive urinary bladder cancer lesions in rats fed N-4-(5-nitro-2-furyl)-2-thiazolyl formamide. *Cancer Res.* **37**, 2817.

——, Cohen, S.M., Arai, M., and Friedell, G.H. (1977*b*). SEM on bladder cells. *Acta Cytologica* **21**, 3.

—— ——, Farrow, G.M., and Friedell, G.H. (1981). Scanning electron microscopic features of human urinary bladder cancer. *Cancer* **48**, 1399.

Kakizoe, T., Kawachi, T., and Sugimura, T. (1979). Agglutination of bladder cells by concanavalin A during the early phase of treatment of rats with N-butyl-N-(4-hydroxybutyl) nitrosamine. *Cancer Res.* **39**, 3353.

——, Komatsu, H., Niijima, T., Kawachi, T., and Sugimura, T. (1980). Increased agglutinability of bladder cells by concanavalin A after administration of carcinogens. *Cancer Res.* **40**, 2006.

Kay, H.E. and Wallace, D.M. (1961). A and B antigens of tumors arising from urinary epithelium. *J. Nat. Cancer Inst.* **26**, 1349.

Koss, L.G. (1967). A light and electron microscopic study of the effect of a single dose of cyclophosphamide on various organs of the rat. 1. The urinary bladder. *Lab. Invest.* **16**, 44.

Kovarik, S., Davidsohn, I., and Stejskal, R. (1968). ABO antigens in cancer. Detection with the mixed cell agglutination reaction. *Arch. Pathol.* **86**, 12.

Kunze, E., Schauer, A., and Krusmann, G. (1975). Focal loss of alkaline phosphatase and increase in proliferation in preneoplastic areas of the rat urothelium after administration of N-butyl-N-(4-hydroxybutyl)-nitrosamine and N-(4-(5-nitro-2-furyl)-2-thiazolyl) formamide. *Z. Krebsforsch.* **84**, 143.

Lange, P.N. and Limas, C. (1980). Tissue blood group antigen testing in transitional cell carcinoma of the bladder. *J. Urol.* **124**, 304.

Limas, C. and Lange, P.N. (1982). A, B, H antigen detectability in normal and neoplastic urothelium. *Cancer* **49**, 2476.

Melicow, M.M. and Hollowell, J.W. (1952). Intra-urothelial cancer: carcinoma *in situ*, Bowen's disease of the urinary system; discussion of thirty cases. *J. Urol.* **68**, 763.

Merk, F.B., Pauli, B.U., Jacobs, J.B., Alroy, J., Friedell, G.H., and Weinstein, R.S. (1977). Malignant transformation of urinary bladder in humans and in N-(4-(5-nitro-2-furyl)-2-thiazolyl) formamide-exposed Fischer rats. Ultrastructure of the major components of the permeability barrier. *Cancer Res.* **37**, 2843.

Mostofi, F.K., Sobin, L.H., and Torloni, J. (Eds.) (1973). *Histological typing of urinary bladder tumors.* World Health Organization, Geneva.

Nagy, G.K., Frable, W.J., and Murphy, W.M. (1981). Classification of premalignant urothelial abnormalities: a Delphi study of the National Bladder Cancer Collaborative Group A. *Pathol. Ann.* **17**(1), 219.

Pauli, B.U., Cohen, S.M., Alroy, J., and Weinstein, R.S. (1978). Desmosome ultrastructure and the biological behaviour of chemical carcinogen-induced urinary bladder carcinomas. *Cancer Res.* **38**, 3276.

Plotkin, G.M., Brigham, S.C., Wolf, G., Jacobs, J.B., and Arai, M. (1977). Uridine 5′-diphosphate galactose: glycoprotein galactosyl transferase activity in exfoliated bladder epithelial cells in rats fed N-(-4-(5-nitro-2-furyl)-2-thiazolyl) formamide. *Cancer Biochem. Biophys.* **2**, 59.

——, Wides, R.J., Gilbert, S.L., Wolf, G., Hagen, I.K., and Prout, G.R., Jr. (1979). Galactosyl transferase activity in human transitional cell carcinoma lines and in benign and neoplastic human bladder epithelium. *Cancer Res.* **39**, 3856.

——, Gilbert, S.L., Wides, R.J., Wolf, G., Cohen, S.M., and Fukushima, S. (1980). Galactosyl transferase activity in rat bladder transitional cell carcinoma lines and in exfoliated cells in urine during carcinogenesis and reversible hyperplasia. *Cancer Biochem. Biophys.* **4**, 251.

Podolsky, D.K., Weiser, M.M., Isselbacher, K.J., and Cohen, A.M. (1978). A cancer-associated galactosyltransferase isoenzyme. *New Engl. J. Med.* **299**, 703.

Ramsey, E.W. (1980). Specific red cell adherence technique. *J. Urol.* **124**, 304.

Reynoso, G., Chu, T.M., Guinan, P., and Murphy, G.P. (1972). Carcinoembryonic antigen in patients with tumors of the urogenital tract. *Cancer* **30**, 1.

Sandberg, A.A. (1980). Chromosomes in human bladder tumors. *National Bladder Cancer Project Investigators Workshop,* p. 46. (Abstract).

Scribner, J.D. and Suss, R. (1978). Tumor initiation and promotion. *Int. Rev. exp. Pathol.* **18**, 137.

Shevchuk, M.M., Fenoglio, C.M., and Richart, R.M. (1981). Carcinoembryonic antigen localization in benign and malignant transitional epithelium. *Cancer* **47**, 899.

Shirai, T., Murasaki, G., Tatematsu, M., Tauda, H., Fukushima, S., and Ito, N. (1977). Early surface changes of the urinary bladder epithelium of different animal species induced by N-butyl-(4-hydroxybutyl) nitrosamine. *Gann* **68**, 203.

Stiller, D. and Rauscher, J. (1971). Irreversible preneoplastic defect in alkaline phosphatase in cancerization of transitional epithelium. *Exp. Pathol.* **5**, 255.

Utz, D.C. and Farrow G.M. (1980). Management of carcinoma *in situ* of the bladder; the case for surgical management: *Urol. Clinics. N. America* **7**, 533.

Weinstein, R.S., Merk, F.B., and Alroy, J. (1976). The structure and function of intercellular junctions in cancer. *Adv. Cancer Res.* **23**, 23.

——, Alroy, J., Farrow, G.M., Miller, A.W., III, and Davidsohn, I. (1979). Blood group isoantigen deletion in carcinoma *in situ* of the urinary bladder. *Cancer* **43**, 661.

——, Miller, A.W., III, and Pauli, B.U. (1980). Carcinoma *in situ*: comments on the pathobiology of a paradox. *Urol. Clinics N. America* **7**, 523.

Wiener, D.P., Koss, L.G., Sablay, B., and Freed, S.Z. (1979). The prevalence and significance of Brunn's nests, cystitis cystica and squamous metaplasia in normal bladders. *J. Urol.* **122**, 317.

Zimmerman, R., Wahren, B., and Edsmyr, F. (1980). Assessment of serial CEA determinations in urine of patients with bladder carcinoma. *Cancer* **46**, 1802.

11 Precancerous lesions of the prostate

F.K. Mostofi

It is generally agreed that precancerous lesions, unless eradicated, will progress towards malignancy and that a variable proportion will evolve into tumours which are invasive and (usually) metastasize. Given that the great majority of malignant tumours of the prostate are epithelial in origin, the end-stage of prostatic premalignancy will be the development of carcinoma. Although no precancerous lesions have been conclusively demonstrated in the prostate, certain morphological changes in the gland parenchyma appear to have the potentiality to progress towards malignancy. These lesions are discussed here, together with incidental and latent carcinomas of the prostate. Particular emphasis is given to the difficulties of categorizing dysplastic epithelium in the prostate—a continuing problem which urgently needs to be solved.

Hyperplasia and its variants: 'The dysplasia problem'

Many years ago Motz and Perearnau first called attention to the fact that hyperplasia in the prostate arose from mucosal and submucosal glands, and Young observed in 1918 that the most common site of prostatic carcinomas was the posterior subcapsular stratum. These findings have often been confirmed, and there is general agreement that hyperplasia and carcinoma do not occur in the same nodule and that prostatic hyperplasia does not constitute a premalignant change. Most patients beyond the age of 70 show hyperplasia of the prostate and about 30 per cent of these patients also have latent prostatic carcinoma. Although the majority of these latent carcinomas develop in the peripheral subcapsular zone of the prostate, a number are intermingled with hyperplastic glands; the same association is seen in incidental carcinomas. Armenian *et al.* (1974) claim that patients with benign prostatic hyperplasia have a threefold higher risk of carcinoma and postulate some kind of association between prostatic hyperplasia and carcinoma, but a definite histogenetic or causal relationship has not so far been established between these two lesions (see also Chapter 1).

Although the two extremes—typical prostatic hyperplasia and poorly differentiated and anaplastic carcinomas—are clearly defined, a number of lesions have been observed which have been categorized as atypia, atypical hyperplasia, atypical glandular hyperplasia, atypical epithelial hyperplasia, and atypical adenomatous hyperplasia with varying degrees of relationship to carcinoma. There is considerable confusion as to what is meant by these terms and the published descriptions and illustrations from different reports record a bewildering variety of changes—a group of closely packed acini, interacinar hyperplasia with papillary or cribriform growth patterns, secondary or post-atrophic hyperplasia, basal-cell hyperplasia, or transitional-cell metaplasia. The illustrations in some papers even suggest a well-differentiated carcinoma. In reviewing the problem, Kastendieck and his colleagues (Kastendieck and Altenahr 1976; Kastendieck *et al.* 1976; Kastendieck 1980) proposed the term dysplasia. This was defined in Kastendieck's 1980 paper as 'unusual or atypical proliferation in glands, cytological atypia of proliferating epithelium and disorganization of morphologic unity between glandular epithelium and fibromuscular stroma (i.e., disorganization of epithelial-stromal junctions)'. Since the potential significance of these alterations was not exactly known Kastendieck aimed to separate dysplasia from terms such as early cancer or carcinoma *in situ,* but what precisely was meant by these criteria is difficult to understand. How, for example, is dysplasia to be distinguished from well-differentiated carcinoma? Confusion may also be encountered with inflammation of the prostate, particularly granulomatous prostatitis, which is sometimes associated with distinct cytological atypia; previously Kastendieck *et al.* (1976) had considered that in such cases '. . . the epithelial changes should be called dysplasia'. A fundamental objection is that it is not made clear whether all three of Kastendieck's criteria have to be satisfied for a diagnosis of dysplasia to be made. According to the author (Kastendieck *et al.* 1976), a very important feature of dysplasia is 'the morphological disintegration of the normally intact relationship between glandular epithelium and fibromuscular stroma, with displacement and sometimes even disorganization of the stroma'—but does this not mean invasion of the stroma, and how do the two differ? In his 1980 paper, Kastendieck has wisely minimized the use of the term 'dysplasia', substituting atypical primary hyperplasia instead. The term 'dysplasia' is confusing in many contexts such as the uterine cervix and urinary bladder, and its application to prostatic glandular and epithelial elements would seem to be best avoided at the present time. Kastendieck defined atypical primary hyperplasia as irregular architecture of glands lined by atypical cells together with focal, indistinct demarcation of glandular epithelium and stroma. The atypical cells have lost their polarity and appear moderately enlarged with pleomorphic nuclei containing chromatin of variable density. This definition is also identical to Mostofi and Price's description of cellular changes in otherwise atypical hyperplasia, which was designated as carcinoma originating from hyperplasia (see Mostofi and Price 1973).

Kastendieck (1980) found evidence of atypical hyperplasia in 106 out of 180 patients with carcinoma of the prostate. Early stages of carcinoma were associated with atypical primary hyperplasia in 83.3 per cent. Small volume tumours showed a much higher percentage of coincidental atypical hyperplasia than larger neoplasms (85.7 compared to 19.5 per cent). These hyperplastic lesions were more common in multifocal tumours than in neoplasms confined to a single focus, and were more frequently seen in association with well differentiated carcinomas.

Helpap (1980) investigated the distribution of atypical hyperplasia in transurethral resections and biopsy material of the prostate with or without carcinoma, and performed autoradiographic investigations using tritiated (^{3}H) thymidine. He compared typical hyperplasia with atypical hyperplasia and with carcinoma. He found 122 cases of atypical hyperplasia with microglandular, papillary, clear-cell, or adenomatous intraglandular cribriform growth patterns. Slight cellular atypia was seen in 37.9 per cent, moderate atypia in 35.7 per cent, and marked cellular and structural atypia in 13.9 per cent. 12.4 per cent showed a transition from severe atypia to carcinoma in material examined by serial sectioning. Among 524 prostatic carcinomas, 49.4 per cent co-existed with atypical hyperplasia. Differentiated adenocarcinomas were most frequently associated with slight or moderate microglandular, clear-cell, or papillary atypical hyperplasia. On the other hand, there was a high coincidence of severe atypical hyperplasia with a predominantly cribriform growth pattern and anaplastic and cribriform carcinomas. The average labelling index in 65 cases of simple glandular hyperplasia was 0.49 ± 0.4 per cent. In 11 cases of prostatic hyperplasia with cellular atypia but without carcinoma, an average labelling index of 1.60 ± 0.8 per cent was calculated. In atypical primary hyperplasia with pronounced cellular and structural atypia in the vicinity of adenocarcinoma, the labelling index was 1.50 ± 0.84 per cent. Single values ranged from 0.2 to 4.1 per cent. This range of labelling indices was comparable to that of poorly differentiated adenocarcinomas (0.2-2.4 per cent) and cribriform carcinomas (0.4-5.7 per cent). Helpap's illustrated examples of atypical primary hyperplasia with moderate and severe atypia are histologically and cytologically indistinguishable from well differentiated carcinoma, and it is hardly suprising that they have the same labelling index as carcinomas.

In this rather detailed discussion of the work from Kastendieck and Helpap and their associates, it is not our intention to criticize the contributions that these investigators have made, but rather to emphasize the complexity of the problem and the need for further studies to clarify an immensely confused situation.

We follow a simpler working approach in which two categories of hyperplastic epithelium are recognized—with and without cellular anaplasia. We defined anaplastic cells as those that are more cuboidal and show a loss of cell polarity and/or piling up of the epithelium. The nuclei are large and pleomorphic with coarse chromatin, varying amounts of nuclear vacuolization, and an irregularly outlined but prominent and distinct nucleolus.

Hyperplasia without cellular anaplasia

In a brief reference to prostatic hyperplasia, the authors of the WHO text on the histological typing of prostatic tumours (Mostofi *et al.* 1980) distinguished between *nodular* hyperplasia as hyperplasia of varying proportions of glandular and stromal tissues of the prostate, and *lobular* hyperplasia as a proliferation of acini of uniform appearance surrounding a duct or acinus. Atrophy-associated hyperplasia (*postatrophic* hyperplasia) was described as a proliferation of small irregularly-shaped and -distributed acini around a central atrophic duct; cellular atypia is sometimes seen in this condition which occurs in the peripheral zones of the prostate and has been associated with carcinoma of small acinar type. Focal intra-acinar hyperplasia (*secondary* hyperplasia) was categorized as focal intra-acinar proliferation of epithelium forming plaques and papillary projections in a cystic acinus, otherwise lined by flattened involuted cells. Interpreted as representing renewed secondary hyperplastic activity after involution, it may occur in any part of the prostate. *Basal-cell* hyperplasia was defined as an intra-acinar proliferation of small basophilic cells with ovoid nuclei and scant cytoplasm, sometimes obliterating the lumen. There is usually maturation of epithelium toward the centre and the stroma is commonly hyperplastic.

All these variant lesions are frequently seen in prostatic tumours containing carcinoma where their presence would seem to indicate increased activity of prostatic epithelium, but with the exception of some cases of post-atrophic hyperplasia (see later) their premalignant potential has not been established.

Hyperplasia with cellular anaplasia

A definition of anaplastic cells was given earlier, and some examples are illustrated in Figs. 11.1-11.3. The crucial question here is: What is the significance of cellular anaplasia of this kind when it is confined to a group of glands without apparent invasion and/or the architectural disturbances of typical carcinoma? We believe that such lesions are at least precancerous if not early carcinomas. The basis for this view is that we have seen these changes at the margins of fully developed carcinomas and transitions from them to frank carcinomas. When such zones are incidentally found in specimens from transurethral resections for clinically benign prostates, the urological surgeon should be alerted to the possible presence of a carcinoma elsewhere in the gland. It should be emphasized, however, that it has not been possible to establish the natural history of these lesions because they are discovered only after the affected tissue has been surgically removed and processed for histological examination. It is essential that certain points are borne in mind when discussing these lesions. Post-atrophic hyperplasia, intra-acinar hyperplasia, and basal-cell hyperplasia *without* cellular anaplasia must be recognized as such and not labelled as atypia or dysplasia. When anaplastic cells are seen (notably in post-atrophic hyperplasia) which are

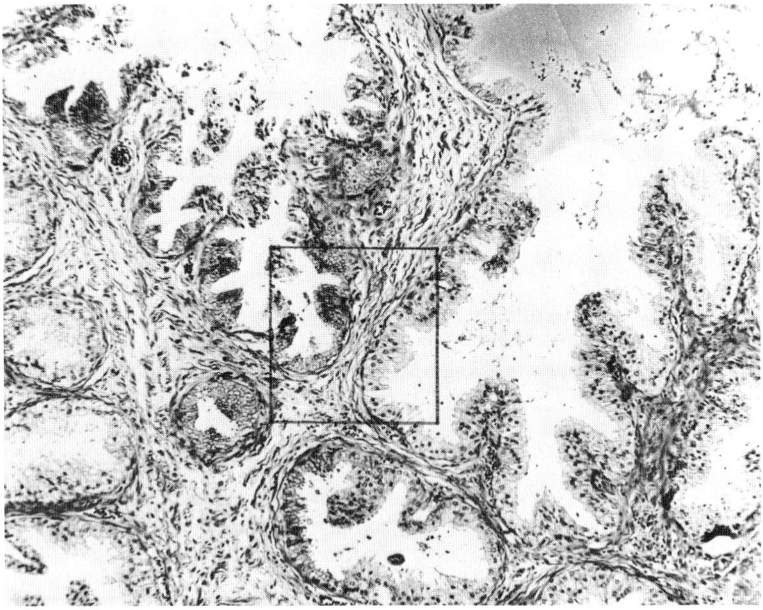

Fig. 11.1. Carcinoma arising in a hyperplastic gland. Parts of two hyperplastic glands are seen with foci of heaped-up epithelium. AFIP Neg. 68-9113 ×72. H & E.

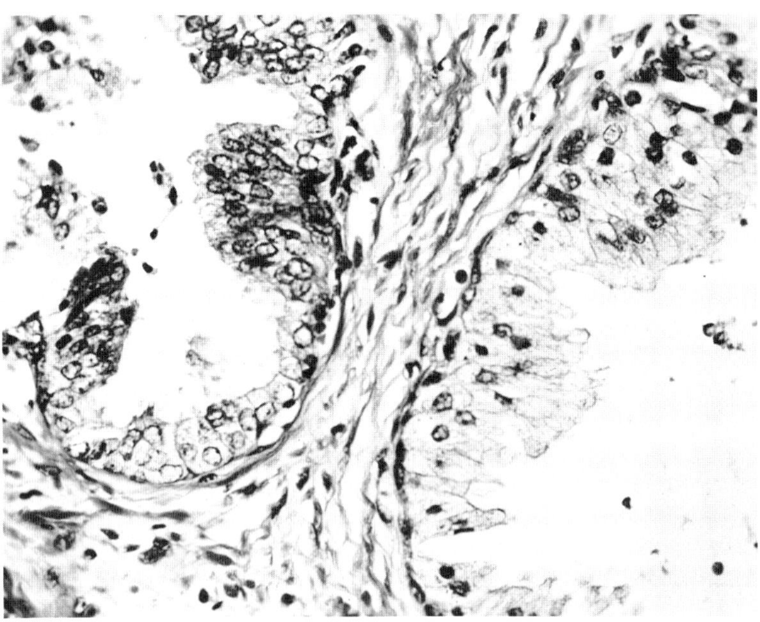

Fig. 11.2. Higher magnification of the area enclosed in a box in Fig. 11.1. The hyperplastic gland on the right contains a double layer of tall secretory cells with small regular nuclei. The basal cells have small dark-staining nuclei. In contrast, the cells of the neoplastic acinus on the left are more cuboidal, the nuclei are vacuolated and they vary moderately in size. There is condensation of nuclei in three areas. AFIP Neg. 68-9114 × 350. H & E.

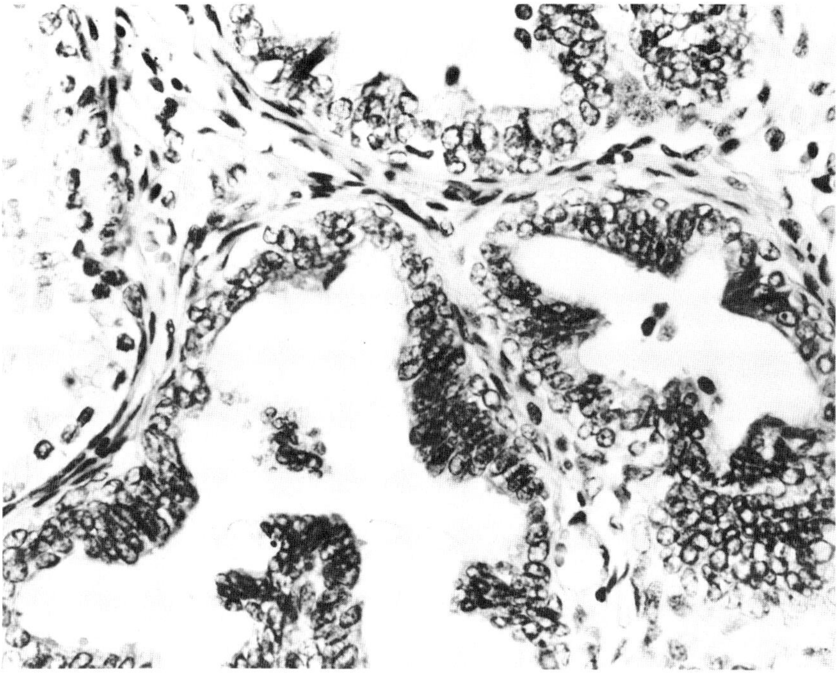

Fig. 11.3. Parts of four acini are seen in the field. The acinus on the left is hyperplastic. The other three maintain a hyperplastic growth pattern but are lined by disorganized cells with nuclei that vary in size and shape and are vacuolated. AFIP Neg. 81-17980 ×160. H & E.

identical to those seen in carcinoma of the prostate, the change is designated as carcinoma rather than atypia or dysplasia. If 'disorganization of morphologic unity between glands and stroma' is seen, then the changes are those of early invasive carcinoma rather than dysplasia or atypia.

The term 'atypia' should be reserved for two categories of change: (1) when the growth pattern is disturbing but not typical of carcinoma, and (2) when the nuclear changes are abnormal but do not fulfil the criteria for a diagnosis of carcinoma. Thus the distribution of the glands may suggest invasion but appearances are not definitely diagnostic; or the individual cells are abnormal but there is a question as to whether such changes are truly neoplastic or reactive. The nucleoli, if present, are not large or irregular in outline (Fig. 11.4).

Atrophy

For many years it has been known that most prostatic carcinomas originate in the peripheral horseshoe-shaped portion of the prostate (the male prostate), that in older individuals this region is often atrophic, and that carcinoma often follows atrophy. The term 'atrophy', although descriptive of the light microscopic appearance of the acini, does not adequately characterize the constituent cells which are low cuboidal with darkly staining nuclei

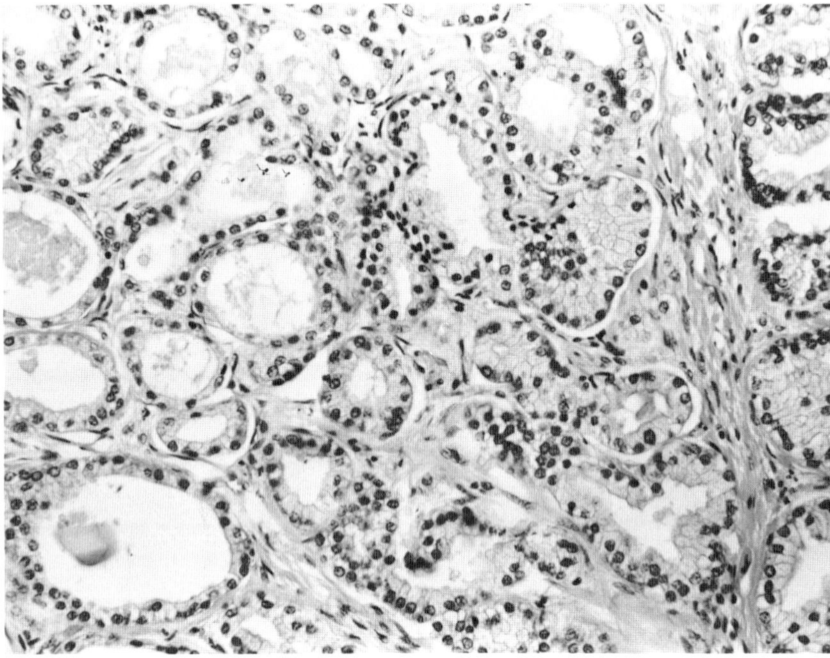

Fig. 11.4. Atypical hyperplasia. A small focus is seen consisting of closely packed glands lined by a single layer of cells. The nuclei are small and uniform and show no evidence of anaplasia. AFIP Neg. 82-5154 ×100. H & E.

arranged in a single row. 'Dormant' is a better characterization of these acini and their lining epithelium.

Liavag (1968) studied the relationship of atrophy, small alveolar proliferation, and carcinoma of the prostate in 340 consecutive autopsies in men aged 40 years or more. Atrophy was classified as slight, moderate, or marked. Atrophy was found in all prostates containing carcinoma while in non-cancerous prostates 90.3 per cent showed atrophy. Liavag observed small alveolar proliferations connected with atrophic glands which appeared to originate from active-looking cell aggregates or buds in the atrophic glands. He considered these as evidence of regeneration, representing replacement growth taking place from survivors of cells in atrophic glands. Significant correlations between atrophy, small alveolar proliferation, and eventually frank carcinomas were observed.

Some years ago in a study of total prostatectomy specimens removed for early carcinoma, we described certain changes in 'atrophic' acini which indicated malignant transformation (Figs. 11.5-11.9). The earliest manifestations of such transformation are nuclear swelling and vacuolation. The nuclei enlarge and the cytoplasm becomes more prominent and eosinophilic, but the cells still retain their cuboidal shape. In the earliest stages these carcinomas consist of small glands lined by cuboidal cells. The basement

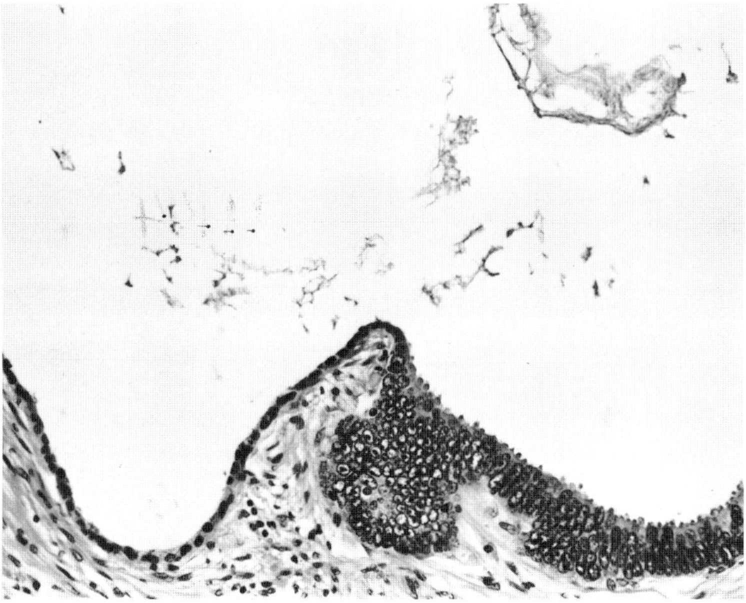

Fig. 11.5. Carcinoma arising in an atrophic gland. A cystically dilated gland is lined partly by low cuboidal epithelium with small regular nuclei, and partly by piled-up epithelial cells with crowding of nuclei that show vacuolization. AFIP Neg. 82-5486 ×90. H & E.

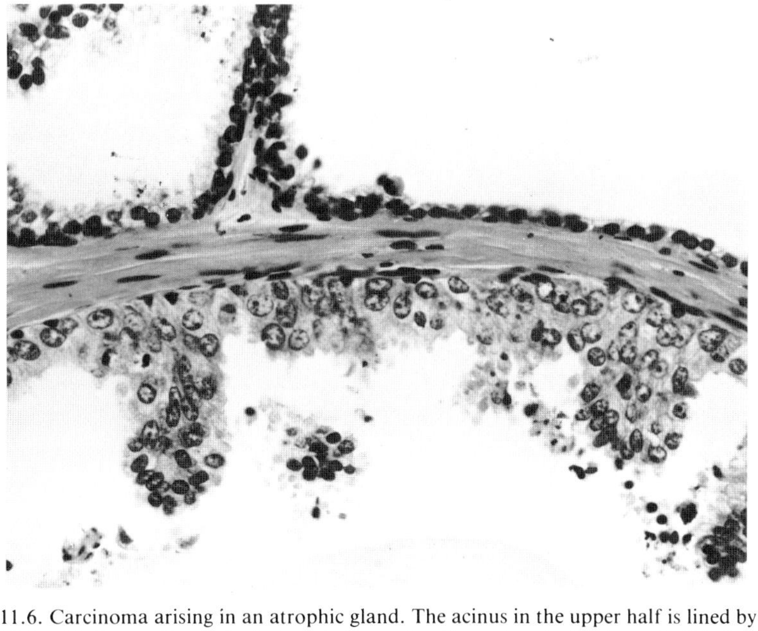

Fig. 11.6. Carcinoma arising in an atrophic gland. The acinus in the upper half is lined by low cuboidal epithelium with small, dark-staining nuclei. The acinus in the lower half is lined by piled-up cells with moderate variation in nuclear size, shape and staining; many nuclei are vacuolated. AFIP Neg. 81-17979 ×144. H & E.

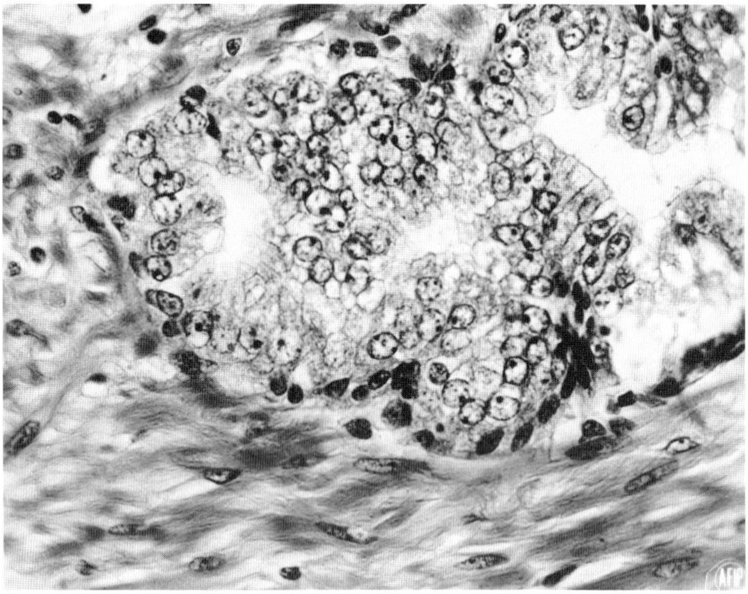

Fig. 11.7. Carcinoma arising in an atrophic acinus. On the right, the epithelial cells are low cuboidal with dark-staining nuclei. On the left, the nuclei vary considerably in size and shape; they are vacuolated and contain ill-defined but prominent nucleoli. AFIP Neg. 66-3588 ×428. H & E.

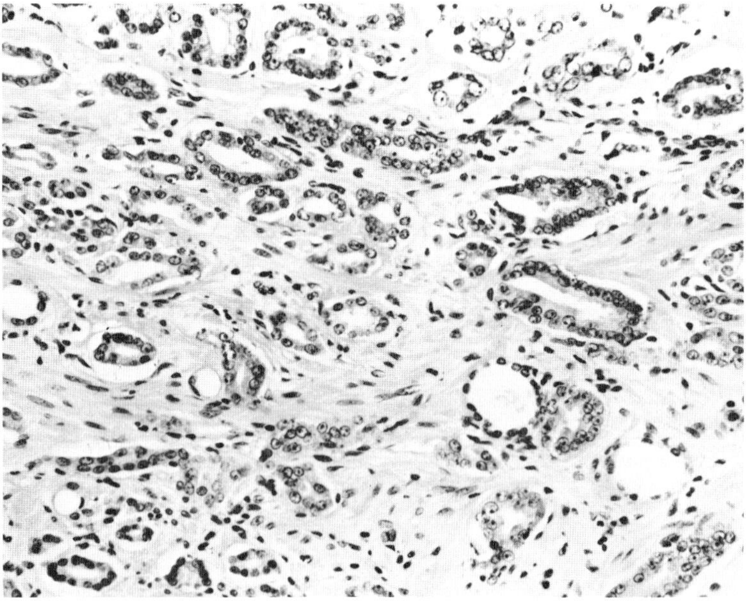

Fig. 11.8. Carcinoma arising in atrophic acini. The stroma is hyalinized and the acini are small. A new acini are lined by low cuboidal or flattened cells. The majority are lined by a single layer of cuboidal cells. The nuclei vary in size, shape and staining. Many are vacuolated and contain a prominent nucleolus. AFIP Neg. 82-5323 ×90. H & E.

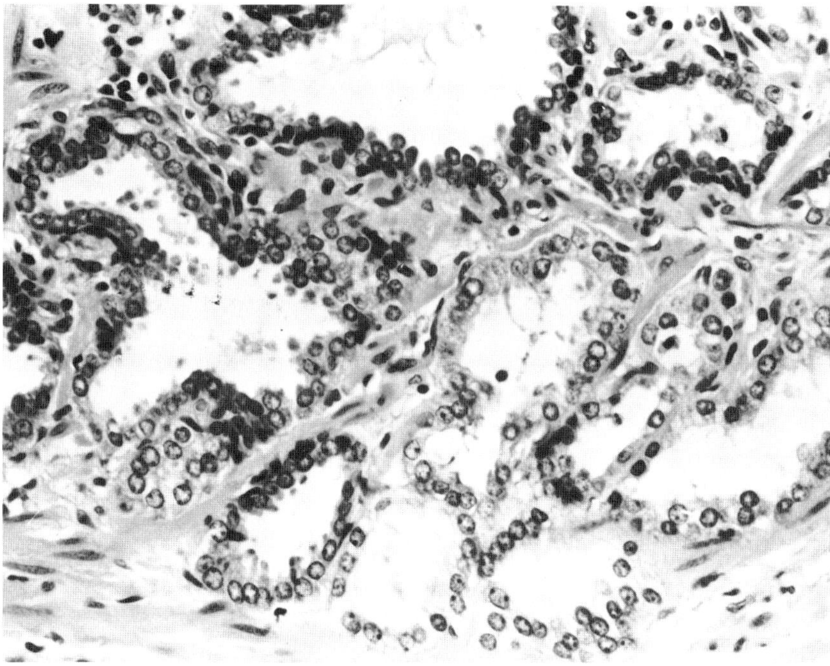

Fig. 11.9. Post-atrophic hyperplasia with early carcinomatous change. Four acini in the upper portion of the field are lined by small cells with dark-staining nuclei. Some of the nuclei, however, are vacuolated and pleomorphic. In one area a clone of cells appears to have invaded the stroma. The acini on the lower right-hand side are lined by similar nuclei. AFIP Neg. 81-17975 ×160. H & E.

membrane seems to be broken and the cells appear to stream out into the surrounding fibromuscular tissue. Thus small acini, columns of cells, or large acini may be seen side by side populated by cells whose nuclei present the characteristic features of prostatic carcinoma. Stromal and perineural invasion provide further support for the diagnosis of malignant transformation of these cells and the proposed premalignant categorization of some 'atrophic' glands.

Incidental carcinoma

In 6-20 per cent of prostates removed for clinically benign enlargement of the gland, pathological examination of the tissue reveals histological carcinoma. Such cases constitute between 22 per cent (blacks) and 25.8 per cent (whites) of all prostatic carcinomas (Murphy 1981). These carcinomas usually consist of a group of small acini lined by a single layer of fairly uniform cells. The cytoplasm is amphophilic, basophilic, or vacuolated. The nuclei are homogeneously pale staining, vacuolated, or dark staining and contain prominent nucleoli. There is some irregularity of size and shape of the cells and nuclei. Sometimes the lesion has a cribriform or fused glandular pattern or shows more than one pattern. The lesion may be focal or diffuse, confined to one area or extensive.

Some pathologists label such areas as atypia and dysplasia; others, although recognizing the lesions as carcinoma, still dismiss them as *clinically* benign. We regard these lesions as carcinoma and endeavour to evaluate their malignant potential in terms of the amount of the tumour and the degree of glandular differentiation and cellular anaplasia. Some incidental carcinomas have a poor prognosis, and the adverse features to be noted are multifocal or diffuse origin and moderate-to-poor histological differentiation with moderate-to-marked cellular anaplasia. We have seen a number of patients whose well-differentiated incidental carcinomas were missed on initial pathological examination of the tissue, returning years later with metastatic carcinoma, but the frequency with which this occurs is unknown.

The recent introduction of staging techniques has demonstrated that, at the time of their discovery, 5-10 per cent of these incidental carcinomas have already metastasized to regional lymph nodes. Lymph-node metastases are seen in 25 per cent of diffuse or multifocal carcinomas (Golimbu *et al.* 1978). These observations suggest that, although many incidental carcinomas are biologically inactive, at least some of them have the potential to progress to clinical carcinoma, as manifested by local extension and metastases.

Latent carcinoma

Latent carcinoma has been defined as carcinoma that is demonstrated by the pathologist in prostatic tissue from a patient who has died from some causes other than carcinoma of the prostate. Beginning with Albarran and Holle in 1898, many investigators have reported varying incidence rates but rising with age to 80 per cent in the ninth decade (for references see Muir 1934; Rich 1935; Moore 1935; Gaynor 1938; Baron and Angrist 1941; Hirst and Bergman 1954; Franks 1954; Butler *et al.* 1959; Karube 1961; Oota 1961; Halpert *et al.* 1963; Liavag 1968; Scott *et al.* 1969; Lundberg and Berg 1970; Wynder *et al.* 1971; Gyorkey 1974; Hohbach and Dhom 1972; Owen 1976; Tulinius 1977).

Age and geography seem to have an important bearing on the incidence of these carcinomas. Breslow *et al.* (1977) reported a world-wide comparative study of frequency and characteristics of latent carcinoma of the prostate in seven areas. They found 350 such carcinomas in 1327 autopsies. Two Chinese populations (Hong Kong and Singapore) showed a low frequency in contrast to the high frequency among Western Europeans (Sweden and the German Federal Republic) and Negroes from Jamaica, with an intermediate incidence for Israelis and black Ugandans. These carcinomas were divided into small (those that occupied 1 or 2 octants), medium (3-8 octants), and large (9-17 octants).*

* Microscopic study of cancers involving three octants showed that the actual volume could range from 65 to 530 mm.

Small carcinomas occurred in 12.3 per cent of prostates and there was no statistically significant variation in this figure by age or area. In contrast, the frequency of medium and large carcinomas increased steadily with age (from 4.6 per cent in the youngest group to 28.7 per cent in the oldest). Geography also seemed to play a significant role in the variation in size of the tumour. The frequency of larger carcinomas was low in Hong Kong, Singapore, and Israel (6.9, 5.0, and 5.6 per cent, respectively), while Jamaica, the German Federal Republic and Sweden all had relatively high frequencies (18.5, 17.9, and 26.8 per cent respectively).

These observations are interesting by themselves but they become especially intriguing when it is realized that the frequency of latent carcinoma for each of the areas in the present study has virtually the same ranking as that of mortality from clinical cancer of the prostate. This at once suggests that in the high-incidence areas some environmental factor may stimulate latent carcinomas to progress to clinical carcinoma. While a large majority of latent carcinomas remain small and confined to the gland, occasionally such tumours may be quite extensive and invade the capsule.

The proportion of clinical cancers of the prostate which originates from such latent carcinomas is unknown but at least some do. More certain is the fact that these latent carcinomas are the source of all occult carcinomas (prostatic carcinomas that are discovered by their metastases before any clinical evidence implicates the prostate itself). These observations strongly suggest that incidental and latent carcinomas represent the initiating phase of prostatic carcinogenesis awaiting the promoting phase to progress to clinical cancer.

References

Albarran, J. and Holle, N. (1898). Hypertrophie et néoplasies épitheliales de la prostate. *Ann. de mal. d'org. genito-urin.* **16**, 797.

Armenian, H.K., Lilienfeld, A.M., Diamond, E.L., and Bross, I.D.J. (1974). Relation between benign prostatic hyperplasia and cancer of the prostate. *Lancet* **ii**, 115.

Baron, E. and Angrist, A. (1941). Incidence of occult adenocarcinoma of the prostate after fifty years of age. *Arch. Pathol.* **32**, 787.

Breslow, N., Chan, C.W., Dhom, G., Drury, R.A.B., Franks, L.M., Gellei, B., Lee, Y.S., Lunberg, S., Sparke, B., Sternby, W.H., and Tulinius, H. (1977). Latent carcinoma of prostate at autopsy in seven areas. *Int. J. Cancer* **20**, 680.

Butler, J., Braunstein, H., Freiman, D.G. and Gall, E.A. (1959). Incidence, distribution and enzymic activity of carcinoma of the prostate gland. *Arch. Pathol.* **68**, 243.

Byar, D.P. and Mostofi, F.K. (1972). Cancer of the prostate: prognostic evidence of certain pathological features in 208 radical prostatectomies. *Cancer.* **30**, 5.

Dhom, G. (1979). Frühie neoplastische Veränderungen der Prostata. *Verh. Dtsch Ges. Pathol.* **63**, 218.

Franks, L.M. (1954). Latent carcinoma of the prostate. *J. Pathol. Bact.* **68**, 603.

Gaynor, E.P. (1938). Zür Frage des Prostatakrebses. *Virchow's Arch. (Pathol. Anat.).* **301**, 602.

Golimbu, M., Schinella, R., Morales, P., and Kurusu, S. (1978). Differences in pathological characteristics and prognosis of clinical A_2 prostatic cancer from A_1 and B disease. *J. Urol.* **119**, 618.

Gyorkey, F. (1974). Some aspects of cancer of the prostate gland. In *Methods in cancer research* (ed. Harris Busch), Vol. 10, p. 279. Academic Press, New York.

Halpert, B., Sheehan, E.E., Schmalhorst, W.R. and Scott, R. (1963). Cancer of the prostate: a survey of 5000 autopsies. *Cancer* **16**, 737.

Helpap, B. (1980). The biological significance of atypical hyperplasia of the prostate. *Virchow's Arch. (Pathol. Anat.).* **387**, 307.

Hirst, A.E., Jr. and Bergman, R.T. (1954). Cancer of the prostate in men 80 or more years old. *Cancer* **7**, 136.

Hohbach, M. and Dhom, G. (1972). Aktuelle Probleme des Prostatakarzinoms. *Munch. med. Wschr.* **114**, 45.

Karube, K. (1961). Study of latent carcinomas of the prostate in the Japanese based on autopsy material. *Tohoku J. Exp. Med.* **74**, 265.

Kastendieck, H. (1980). Correlation between atypical primary hyperplasia and carcinoma of the prostate. A histological study of 180 total prostatectomies. *Path. Res. Pract.* **169**, 366.

—— and Altenahr, E. (1976). Cyto- and histomorphogenesis of the prostatc carcinoma. A comparative light and electron microscopic study. *Virchow's Arch. (Path. Anat.)* **370**, 207.

—— ——, Hussduann, H., and Bressel, M. (1976). Carcinoma and dysplastic lesions of the prostate. *Z. Krebs Forsch* **88**, 33.

Liavag, I. (1968). Atrophy and regeneration in pathogenesis of prostatic carcinoma. *Acta Path. Microbiol. Scand.* **73**, 338.

Lundberg, S. and Berg, T. (1970). Prostatic carcinoma. An autopsy study. *Scand. J. Urol. Nephrol.* **4**, 93.

Moore, R.A. (1935). The morphology of small prostatic carcinoma. *J. Urol.* **33**, 224.

Mostofi, F.K. and Price, E.B., Jr. (1973). Tumors of the male genital system. (Fasc. 8). *Atlas of tumor pathology, 2nd series,* Armed Forces Institute of Pathology, Washington, DC.

——, Sesterhenn, I., and Sobin, L.H. (1980). *Histological typing of prostate tumors.* WHO, Geneva.

Muir, E.G. (1934). Carcinoma of the prostate. *Lancet* **i**, 667.

Murphy, G.P. (1981). Prostate cancer—continuing progress. *Cancer J. Clinicians* **31**, 96.

Oota, K. (1961). Latent carcinoma of the prostate among the Japanese. *Acta Un. Int. Cancer* **17**, 952.

Owen, W.L. (1976). Carcinoma of the prostate: a literature review. *J. chron. Dis.* **29**, 89.

Rich, A.R. (1935). On the frequency of occurrence of occult carcinoma of the prostate. *J. Urol.* **33**, 215.

Scott, R., Jr., Mutchnik, D.L., Laskowski, T.Z., and Schmalhorst, W.R. (1969). Carcinoma of the prostate in elderly men: incidence, growth, characteristics and clinical significance. *J. Urol.* **101**, 602.

Tulinius, H. (1977). Tumours of the male genital system. In *Recent results in cancer research* (ed. E. Grundmann and W. Vahlensieck), Vol. 60, p. 3. Springer Verlag, Berlin, Heidelberg, New York.

Wynder, E.K., Mabuchi, K., and Whitmore, W.F. Jr. (1971). Epidemiology of cancer of the prostate. *Cancer* **28**, 344.

12 Precancerous states of the cervix uteri

A.I. Spriggs

Of all the organs of the human body in which cancer develops, by far the most extensively studied is the cervix uteri. This is because of the introduction of population-screening programmes specifically intended to detect cervical precancerous states by means of cytology. These programmes have made available to medical science a vast body of data about the precursors of cervical cancer which are now diagnosed daily in many centres throughout much of the world.

History

In the first third of this century, most pathologists would have agreed that the essential criterion for a diagnosis of cancer is the demonstration of infiltration or metastasis. The existence of histologically identifiable precancerous states of the cervix has only been recognized within living memory.

Cullen, in his treatise *Cancer of the uterus* (1900), described the technique of cervical biopsy, and illustrated what he called 'suspicious changes' at the margin of invasive carcinoma (Fig. 12.1). A more explicit description of what became known as 'carcinoma *in situ*' was given by Schauenstein (1908), and Fig. 12.2 shows one of his drawings. Further beautiful coloured drawings from those days can be found in the monograph by Schottlaender and Kermauner (1912). These 'incipient cancers' continued to be observed and published. In 1933 Walter Schiller did not hesitate to call them cancer, in spite of the absence of invasion, because they resembled cancer in all other respects, and Broders (1932) helped to make 'carcinoma *in situ*' a respectable diagnosis. Unfortunately, this tendentious name has caused endless subsequent confusion which was not resolved by replacing it with 'Stage 0 carcinoma' (Kottmeier 1959).

The common-sense inference that these are pre-invasive stages of cancer was reinforced during the 1940s and 1950s by numerous case reports in which clinical carcinoma of the cervix was preceded, often many years before, by punch biopsies showing lesions of this type. Some of the most convincing evidence of a long precancerous stage was provided by Jones *et al.* (1957). They examined the notes of all available cases of clinical cervical carcinoma to find any in which cervical biopsies had been performed in previous years.

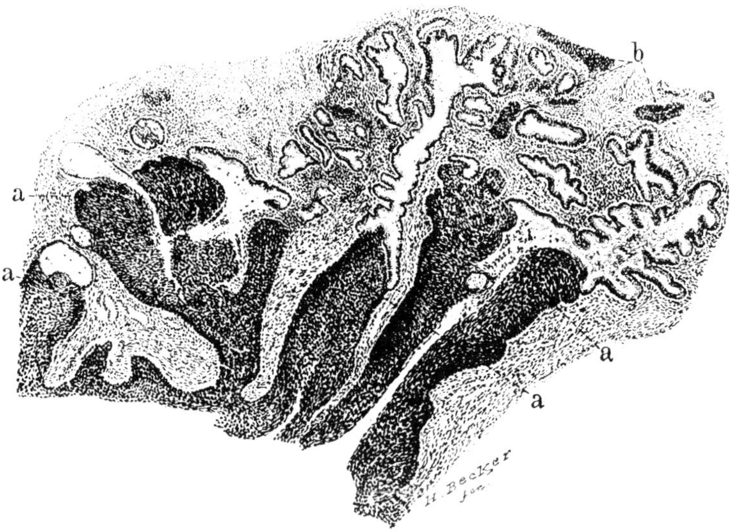

FIG. 56.—PARTIAL OBLITERATION OF THE CERVICAL GLANDS IN SQUAMOUS-CELL CARCINOMA OF THE CERVIX. (40 diameters.)

Gyn.-Path. No. 173. At *a* the squamous cells of the new growth are extending into and rapidly choking the normal cervical glands. Note the intense stain of the squamous cells, and how closely packed together they are. *b* indicates cell-nests of the growth in the depth of the cervix.

Fig. 12.1. Drawing and caption from Cullen (1900), showing a Grade-III lesion ('carcinoma *in situ*') involving cervical glands, and possibly showing microinvasion (at (b)).

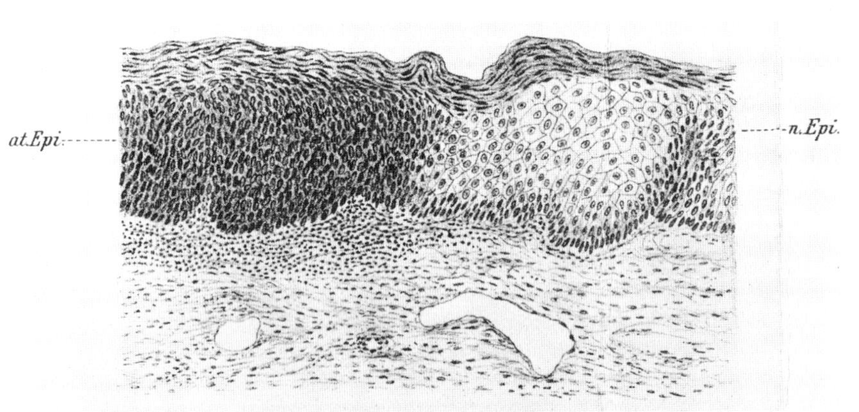

Fig. 12.2. Drawing from Schauenstein (1908), illustrating the junction between 'normal epithelium' on right and 'atypical epithelium' on left. The latter would now be regarded as a Grade-III lesion ('severe dysplasia').

Twenty-four cases were traced, and the histology was reviewed; all had been originally reported at a time when the diagnosis of 'carcinoma *in situ*' had not been entertained. The results of the review are shown in Table 12.1. The shorter intervals are not to be taken as evidence for a brief duration; they simply result from the accident that biopsy was performed a relatively short time before clinical presentation. The long durations, on the other hand, have to be accepted as evidence that the recognizable development of the disease may at least take up to 20 years.

The main objection to this type of evidence is that the biopsies were taken at gynaecological consultations, presumably on account of symptoms; therefore some of these patients may have had invasive cancer already, the biopsy having just missed the invasive part of the lesion. A similar objection applies to prospective studies undertaken around the same time, in which women with biopsies showing a supposedly precancerous state were followed (by biopsy at intervals) without any treatment. The best known of such series is that of Petersen (1955), and Fig. 12.3 shows his curve of the cumulative proportion of cases developing invasive cervical cancer with the passage of time. Taken at face value, it appears that the curve flattens out at about

Table 12.1. *Data of Jones, Galvin and Te Linde (1957)*

Case no.	Original biopsy	Interval: Years	Interval: Months
1	Carcinoma *in situ*	1	0
2	Carcinoma *in situ*	1	5
3	B.C.H.	1	11
4	B.C.H.	2	6
5	Carcinoma *in situ*	3	4
6	Carcinoma *in situ*	3	5
7	Carcinoma *in situ*	3	6
8	Carcinoma *in situ*	4	7
9	B.C.H.	4	10
10	No abnormality	4	11
11	Carcinoma *in situ*	5	8
12	No abnormality	5	11
13	Carcinoma *in situ*	6	2
14	Carcinoma *in situ*	7	0
15	Carcinoma *in situ*	7	9
16	Carcinoma *in situ*	9	11
17	Carcinoma *in situ*	11	0
18	No abnormality	12	7
19	Carcinoma *in situ*	13	10
20	Carcinoma *in situ*	13	2
21	Carcinoma *in situ*	14	10
22	Carcinoma *in situ*	16	8
23	No abnormality	18	0
24	Carcinoma *in situ*	20	2

In all cases given above the final biopsy indicated invasive carcinoma.
BCH, basal cell hyperplasia (see p. 336).

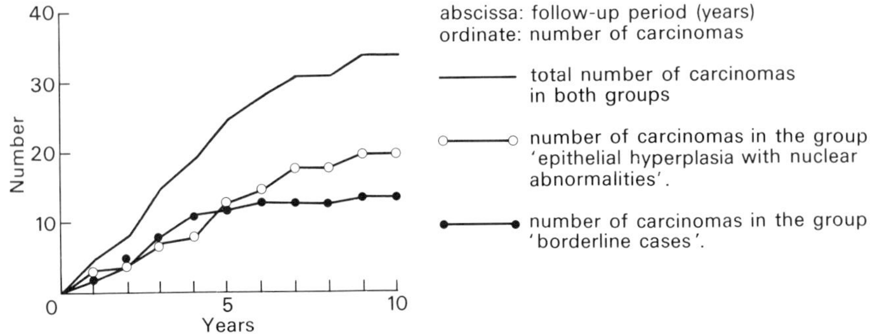

Fig. 12.3. Cumulative curve of development of invasive cervical carcinoma from precancerous states. The results were not expressed in life-table form, but evidently at least a third of these cases progressed to invasion. (From Petersen (1955).)

30-40 per cent. Since the remaining cases after about ten years no longer have positive biopsies, the lesions are presumed to have regressed or else been nibbled away piecemeal at repeated follow-up attendances.

Evidence of this kind was widely accepted as proving that 'carcinoma *in situ*' was the usual precursor of invasive cervical cancer, which could, in principle, be prevented by finding and treating the pre-invasive lesion. This was now possible as a result of the Papanicolaou smear. Papanicolaou and Traut had written in 1943, 'It is hoped that study of early lesions, discovered by means of the vaginal smear, will lead to further knowledge and a better understanding of the primary chapters in the life history of the disease process.' As a result of this breakthrough, massive projects for population screening by the vaginal or cervical smear were initiated in the 1950s, in the hope that cervical cancer would be eliminated.

Nomenclature

With the introduction of large-scale screening, it became apparent that lesions of the carcinoma *in situ* type were common, usually about five per thousand. At the same time it was realized that abnormal cervical smears revealed about five times as many lesser abnormalities, and histopathologists were called upon more and more frequently to make a decision whether to diagnose carcinoma *in situ* or to apply some other name suggesting a lesser abnormality, for instance 'dysplasia' (Reagan *et al.* 1953).

Anyone coming new to the literature of this subject needs to know that authors have differed greatly in their use of histopathological terms. Usually they have given no definitions and, when they have done so, they have been lax in adhering to them. Consequently the literature, which in any case is voluminous and of varying quality, is also extremely confusing. Particularly misleading is the use of the word 'cancer', which in many statistics and tables of results is used to include 'carcinoma *in situ*'.

The cytological terminology has been equally inconsistent. Papanicolaou

(1954) introduced the word 'dyskaryosis' to describe the nuclear changes seen in cells coming from carcinoma *in situ* and from less advanced lesions, and only spoke of 'malignant cells' in the context of invasive carcinoma. Subsequently many (probably most) authorities on diagnostic cytology have used the term 'malignant cell' or 'cancer cell' to include cells shed from any supposedly precancerous lesions. A common solution to this difficulty is to avoid naming the cells at all, but to guess the probable underlying histology from the whole smear (Riotton and Christopherson 1973). This system is generally recommended in America, while the recent British recommendation is to retain Papanicolaou's usage for communication between cytologists (Spriggs *et al.* 1978).

The histological dividing line between 'carcinoma *in situ*' and 'dysplasia' was defined in 1961 at an international Congress in Vienna (Bettinger and Reagan, 1962) as follows:

> Only those cases should be classified as carcinoma *in situ* which, in the absence of invasion, show as surface lining an epithelium in which, throughout the whole thickness, no differentiation takes place. The process may involve the lining of the cervical glands without thereby creating a new group. It is recognized that the cells of the uppermost layers may show some slight flattening. The very rare case of an otherwise characteristic carcinoma *in situ* that shows a greater degree of differentiation belongs to the exceptions for which no classification can provide. All other disturbances of differentiation of the squamous epithelial lining of surface and glands are to be classified as dysplasia.

A British committee (Govan *et al.* 1969) continued to insist on lack of surface differentiation as the deciding characteristic of carcinoma *in situ*, but many pathologists (perhaps most) departed from this, and so did Poulsen and Taylor (1975) in the *International Histological Classification of Tumours.* They define carcinoma *in situ* as a lesion in which *all or most* of the epithelium shows the cellular features of carcinoma. They say that a keratinizing form occurs, and that 'dysplasia and carcinoma *in situ* may at times be almost indistinguishable'.

With this degree of vagueness and confusion, it seems best to discard altogether the name 'carcinoma *in situ*', which carries a built-in unverifiable prognostic assumption (Smith 1978).

Richart and Barron (1969), later supported by Koss (1978), propose dividing all these lesions into three grades of 'cervical intraepithelial neoplasia' (CIN), called CIN I, II, and III. Even if the expression CIN is eventually replaced by another (and I would prefer the word 'dysplasia'), the division into three grades can be maintained. Grade I corresponds to 'mild dysplasia' and probably includes lesions produced by wart virus. Grade III corresponds to 'carcinoma *in situ*' and 'severe dysplasia' lumped together. Grade II is the intermediate grade which is humanly necessary when a continuous series is to be divided subjectively into the smallest possible number of parts. Figs. 12.4-12.7 show these grades according to Nelson *et al.* (1975),

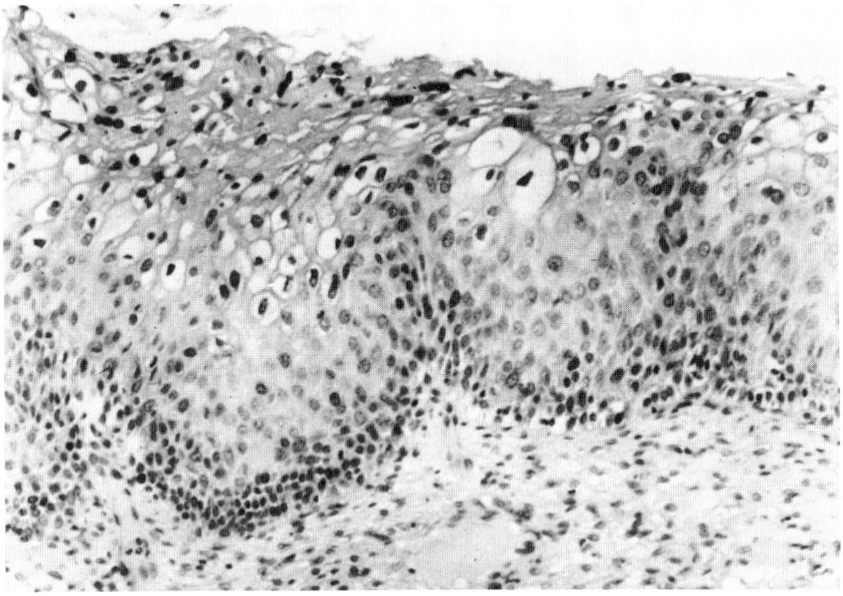

Fig. 12.4. Slight dysplasia or CIN Grade 1. Undifferentiated neoplastic cells form up to one-third of the thickness of the epithelium. (Reproduced from Nelson *et al.* (1975) by courtesy of Dr R.M. Richart.)

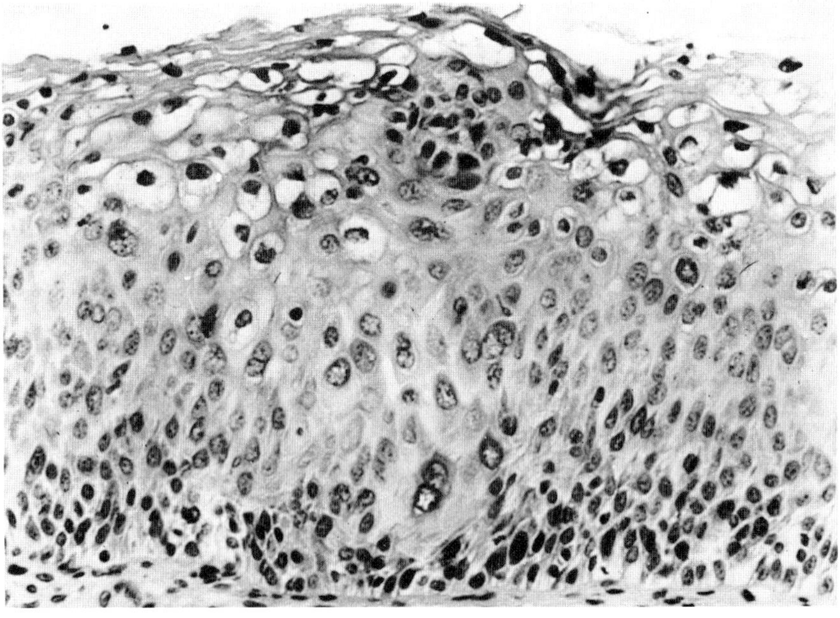

Fig. 12.5. Moderate dysplasia or CIN Grade 2. One-third to two-thirds of the thickness of the epithelium is occupied by undifferentiated neoplastic cells. (Reproduced from Nelson *et al.* (1975) by courtesy of Dr R.M. Richart.)

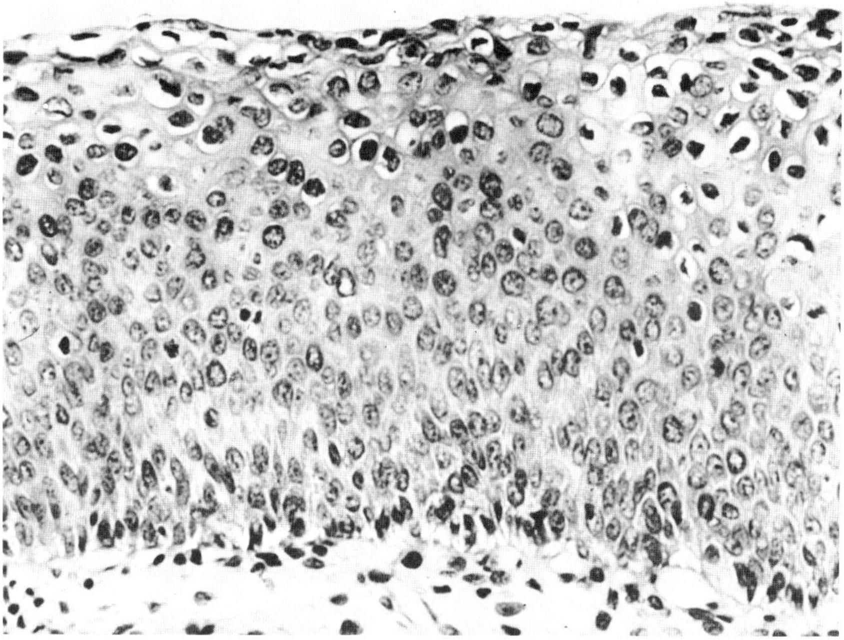

Fig. 12.6. Severe dysplasia or CIN Grade 3. Over two-thirds of the thickness of the epithelium is occupied by undifferentiated neoplastic cells. (Reproduced from Nelson *et al.* (1975) by courtesy of Dr R.M. Richart.)

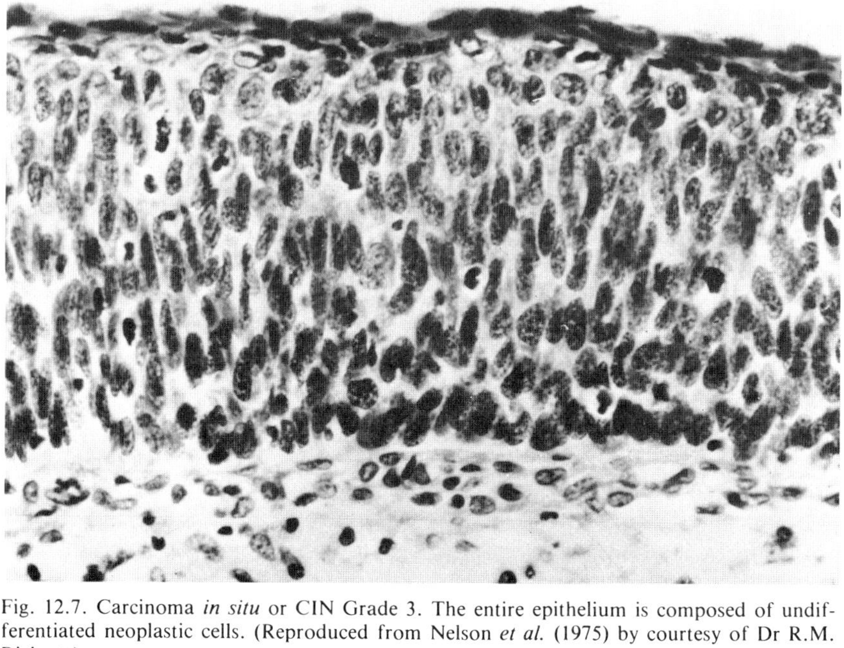

Fig. 12.7. Carcinoma *in situ* or CIN Grade 3. The entire epithelium is composed of undifferentiated neoplastic cells. (Reproduced from Nelson *et al.* (1975) by courtesy of Dr R.M. Richart.)

and some different examples have been published by Buckley *et al.* (1982). This system, though not internationally agreed, will be used in the rest of the chapter.

Anatomy and histology

Normal

The vagina and the ectocervix are covered by a flat epithelium which is histologically of squamous type, but without keratinization. The endocervical canal is covered by an epithelium which under low magnification with the colposcope shows delicate grapelike villi, translucent enough to cause a red colour to the naked eye. Microscopically this is a simple columnar mucus-secreting epithelium, and it extends into clefts and tunnels several millimetres deep from the surface (Fluhmann 1961).

To the naked eye, in some but not all cervices, the os is surrounded by a red area of 'ectopic' endocervical epithelium, and this may be seen even in neonates (Gruenagel 1957). Its extent is inconstant and it is subject to the process of squamous metaplasia, often occurring quite irregularly and particularly accelerated during first pregnancy (Coppleson and Reid 1967).

The normal squamo-columnar junction is sharp, even as seen microscopically; the columnar epithelium ends and native squamous epithelium begins. A more complex relationship exists when squamous metaplasia is occurring, and in most cervices there is a whole area, the *Umwandlungszone* or transformation zone, in which there is a dynamic process producing new and older squamous metaplastic epithelium overlying endocervical glands (which themselves may have undergone metaplasia), bordered by native endocervical columnar epithelium in the canal and native squamous epithelium on the ectocervix. Seen colposcopically, squamous metaplasia begins by the endocervical villi fusing together, and the new squamous epithelium is flat, but punctuated by gland openings. Some of these may become obstructed and form macroscopically visible cysts ('Nabothian follicles'). Many illustrations of this process can be found in Coppleson *et al.* (1978) and in Kolstad and Stafl (1977).

Squamous metaplasia is believed to arise by squamous differentiation of proliferated reserve cells (Langley and Crompton 1973). Reserve cells are not often visible in histological sections of normal cervix, but are presumed to be present in small numbers. They can multiply to form one and then several layers of small cells without much cytoplasm, beneath the layer of columnar cells. Reserve cell hyperplasia may be found in the absence of any squamous differentiation, but often the more superficial reserve cell layers begin to develop squamous-cell features even while columnar cells are still in position at the surface (Fig. 12.8). In other cases after the columnar cells are shed the immature metaplastic epithelium may be mistaken for an early neoplastic process because of the lack of differentiation. It then becomes

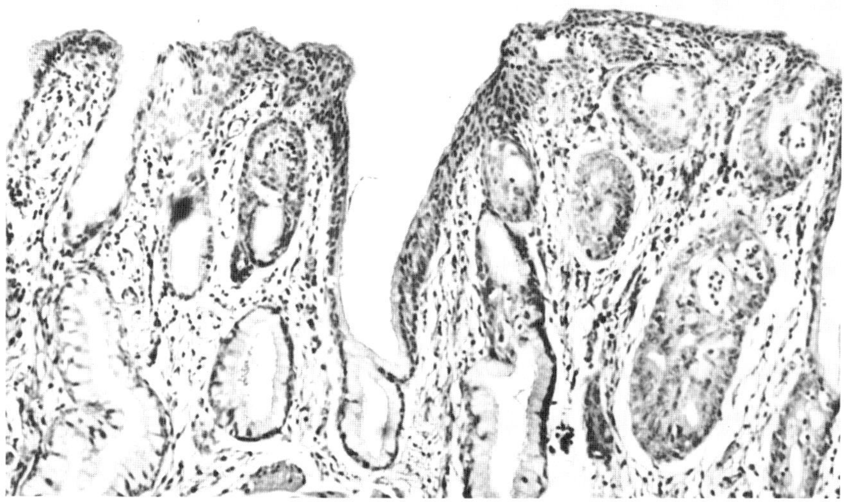

Fig. 12.8. Squamous metaplasia in the transformation zone. Endocervical columnar epithelium, still visible in some of the glands, is being replaced by squamous metaplasia. In places columnar epithelial cells remain on the surface of metaplastic epithelium. × 150. H & E.

more mature and finally may be hard to distinguish from native squamous epithelium except that it overlies endocervical glands.

Seen in cervical smears, the surface cells of immature metaplastic squamous epithelium resemble the surface cells of atrophic ectocervical or vaginal epithelium (in Papanicolaou's terminology, 'parabasal cells'), as in prepubertal or postmenopausal women. With further maturation the epithelial cells come to resemble those of ordinary native squamous epithelium, with flattened but usually non-glycogenated 'intermediate' cells.

Walter Schiller (1933) introduced the test which bears his name, in which the living cervix is painted with Lugol's iodine. Native squamous epithelium stains on account of its glycogen content, whereas the transformation zone with squamous metaplastic epithelium and the endocervical columnar epithelium (as well as any areas of CIN) remain unstained. This test is still in use, and in the absence of a colposcope will quickly display to the surgeon the outline of the original squamocolumnar junction. (For further details of the histochemistry of this region see Blackwell and Markham 1976).

Cervical intraepithelial neoplasia

The transformation zone is the area where CIN develops. The colposcopist observes mainly changes in the vascular pattern, particularly punctation (formerly called *Grund* or 'ground') and the net-like pattern called 'mosaic' (Fig. 12.9). These colposcopic appearances do not correspond exactly to any histological entity, but they serve to reveal the extent and outline of abnormal areas which are completely invisible to the unaided eye.

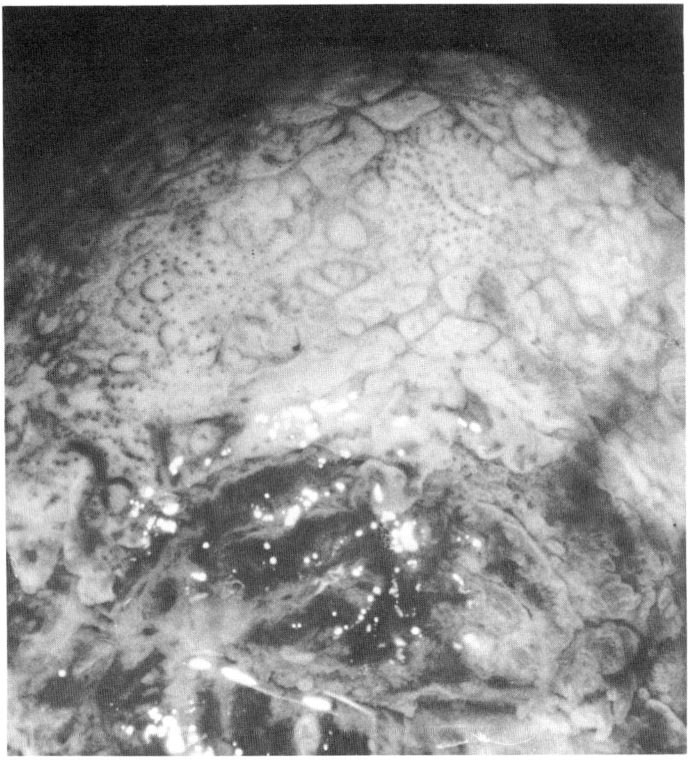

Fig.12.9. Colposcopic view of an atypical transformation zone. Below is the os cervicis, surrounded by normal endocervical epithelium. The white area above is entirely new epithelium of the transformation zone, showing 'punctation' and 'mosaic' corresponding to a Grade-III lesion. (From Coppleson *et al.* (1978) by courtesy of Dr M. Coppleson.)

Histologically, a whole gradation of alterations may be found in this area, from the simple squamous metaplasia already described through minor grades of atypia with nuclear irregularity but with good surface maturation (grades I-II), through forms with more severe atypia and sometimes complete loss of stratification (grade III). Examples have been shown in Figs. 12.4-12.7. Most writers on the subject believe, with Richart (1963), that these are stages in the same process analogous to the successive stages seen in the mouse cervix treated with carcinogens (for literature see Langley and Crompton 1973; Foulds 1975), but an unknown proportion of the milder lesions (grades I and II) may be reversible manifestations of wart virus infection (Meisels *et al.* 1981). There is an enormous range of appearances, and the interested reader should consult the monograph of Burghardt (1973).

Many of these lesions, particularly the more severe ones, appear to arise from abnormal reserve-cell proliferations (Johnson *et al.* 1964; Christopherson 1977; Patten 1978) while the classical small-celled type of 'carcinoma *in situ*' may originate in reserve-cell hyperplasia without any sign of squamous maturation (Reagan and Hicks 1953; Christopherson 1969; Beyer-Boon and Verdonk 1978; Spriggs and Boddington 1980).

Most of these lesions are detected by cytological examination of smears. The presence of cells with nuclear enlargement, irregularity, hyperchromasia, and, in the severer grades, a failure of cytoplasmic maturation can provide a fairly reliable estimate of the corresponding histological lesion (Patten 1978; Briggs 1979).

The different degrees of CIN are marked histologically by the loss of orderly stratification, and by the nuclear aberrations which occur with cervical neoplasia in general—nuclear enlargement, irregularity of outline, hyperchromasia, anisonucleosis, and mitosis occurring above the parabasal level. In the cases answering the former strict definition of carcinoma *in situ*, the nuclei have lost their polarity and are distributed apparently haphazardly through the thickness of the epithelium with perhaps only a layer or two of flattened surface cells, still with enlarged and hyperchromatic nuclei (Fig. 12.7). Endocervical glands may be filled with epithelium of this type.

Grade III also includes many cases not fulfilling the strict criteria for carcinoma *in situ* but given that name by the majority of pathologists (Koss 1979) while others describe it as severe dysplasia. The whole epithelial thickness is disordered, with mitotic activity extending beyond the parabasal layer but with more or less surface maturation (Fig. 12.6).

A striking feature of Grade-III lesions is the occurrence of mitoses at levels normally occupied by end cells, sometimes throughout the epithelial thickness. Abnormal mitotic figures are common, particularly the '3-group metaphase' (Fig. 12.10) in which some chromosomes fail to align on the metaphase plate and are seen on each side (Parmentier and Dustin 1951; Moricard and Papatheodorou 1953). The presence of this abnormality has been used as one of the criteria for attaching the label 'carcinoma *in situ*' (Kirkland *et al.* 1967). Not uncommonly, one also sees nuclei with chromosome condensation within an intact nuclear membrane. Some of these are telophases but others are nuclei in which endomitosis is occurring (Fig. 12.11).

Microcarcinoma, microinvasive carcinoma

In some cases, in an area of Grade III, the histologist sees pointed or frayed prongs of neoplastic epithelium apparently creeping into the subepithelial connective tissue. This is the so-called microcarcinoma (microinvasive foci). The cells which are beginning or attempting to invade are often *more* differentiated than the epithelium from which they arise (Fig. 12.12) and there may be a lymphocytic reaction around them. The words microinvasion and microcarcinoma are also applied to clearly invasive lesions not more than 5 mm deep (Ng and Reagan 1969). Therefore, if these terms are used, it is necessary to define them first. In any case, the prognosis following any standard surgical treatment is the same for invasive lesions up to 5mm deep as it is for grade III without invasion, in that subsequent death from

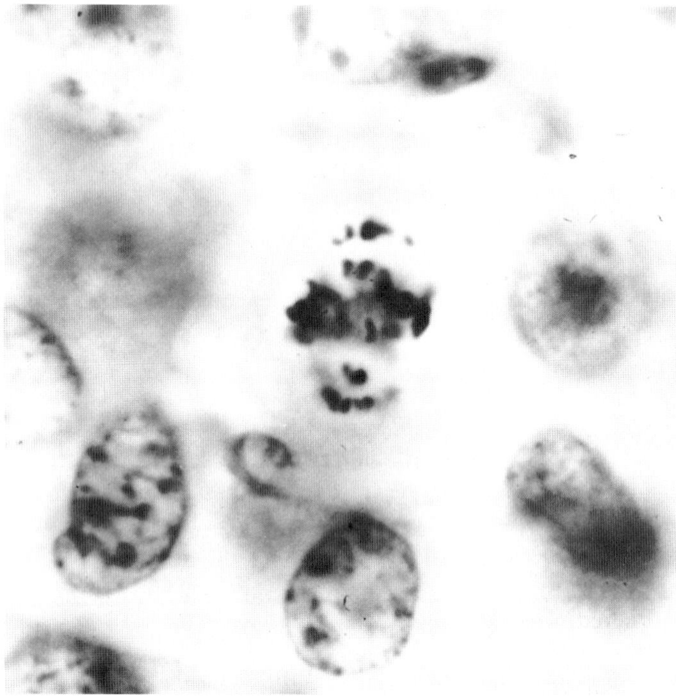

Fig. 12.10. '3-group metaphase'. In this abnormality of cell division, which is common in Grade-III lesions, some of the chromosomes are seen round the outside of the mitotic spindle, even near the poles. This must result in unequal distribution of chromatids to the daughter nuclei. (From a cervical smear: ×1800. Papanicolaou.)

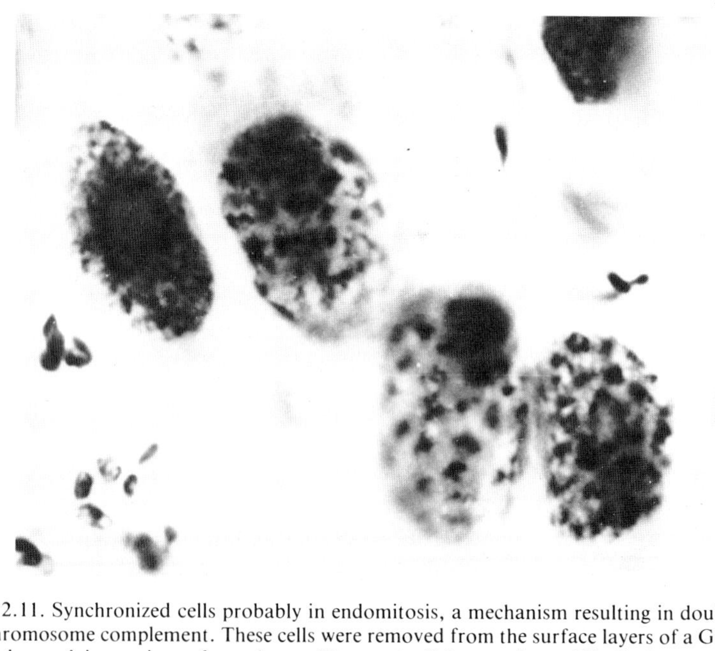

Fig. 12.11. Synchronized cells probably in endomitosis, a mechanism resulting in doubling of the chromosome complement. These cells were removed from the surface layers of a Grade-III lesion by applying a piece of membrane filter to the living cervix. ×600. Feulgen.

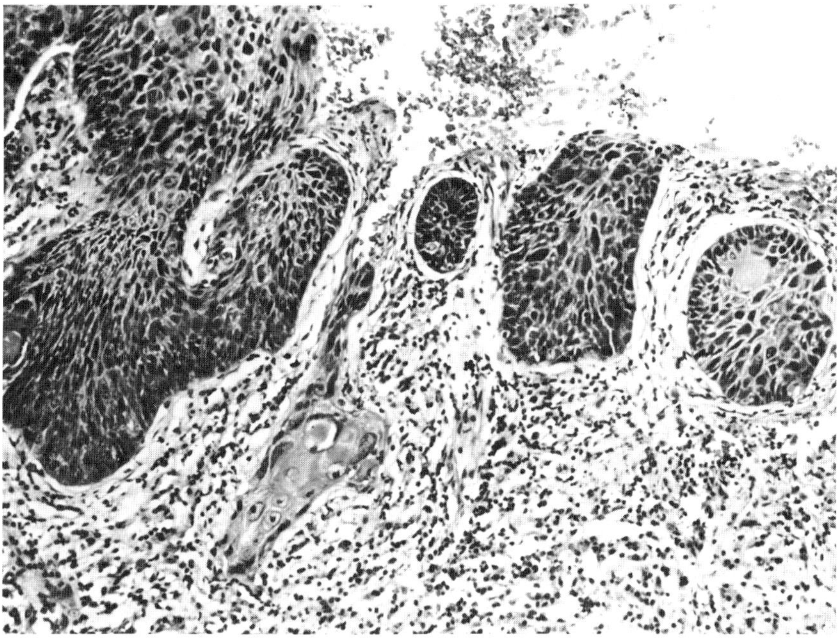

Fig. 12.12. 'Microcarcinoma'. Cervical glands are filled by abnormal epithelium (Grade III). At left of centre, a tongue of more differentiated squamous epithelium is invading the stroma. ×140. H & E.

carcinoma of the cervix has hardly ever been reported (Ng and Reagan 1969; Boyes *et al.* 1970; Coppleson 1976; Christopherson 1977). It cannot even be assumed for certain that all such lesions are necessarily irreversible since, according to Wentz (1962), in the mouse cervix treated with methylcholanthrene the removal of the carcinogen may be followed by regression of early invasive lesions. (This does not seem to have been observed by other experimenters; for literature see Langley and Crompton 1973.)

The onset of 'microinvasion' cannot be reliably determined from cervical smears (Koss 1979) although some authors maintain that subtle changes are visible, particularly an increase in the proportion of cells with distinct or enlarged nucleoli (Patten 1978). The tendency of invasive epithelium to appear more differentiated than the 'carcinoma *in situ*' from which it arose is sometimes manifested in the smear by the presence of small distorted forms of squamous cells with variable cornification. Another distinctive appearance is that of fusiform, even fibre-shaped cells (Fig. 12.13). Evidently the cells of carcinoma *in situ*, although their genome is altered, can still retain part of their programme for making keratin and this becomes depressed when invasion occurs; but the capacity to produce flat hexagonal squames is lost, either because of genetic loss by the clone or because of the scrambling of the vertical columns of epithelial cells with consequent loss of signals from the cells which should be adjacent.

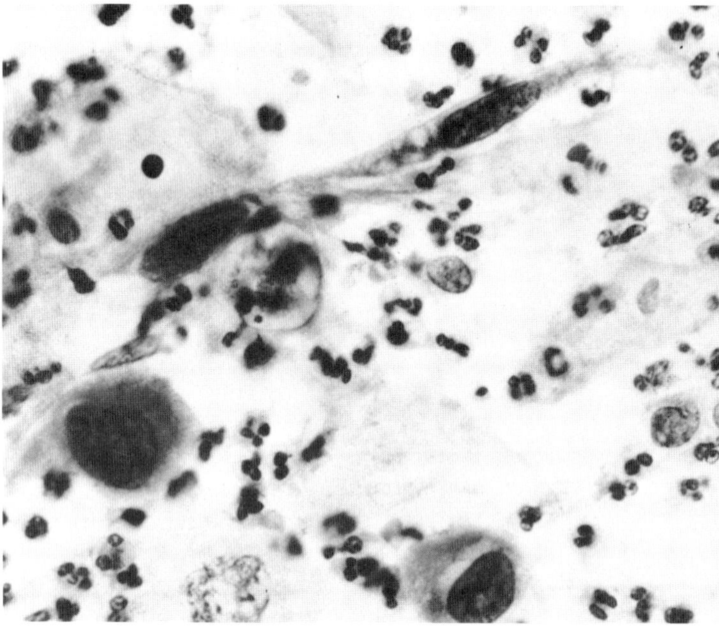

Fig. 12.13. Cervical smear from an early invasive squamous carcinoma. The rounded epithelial cells could equally come for a pre-invasive lesion. The spindle-shaped cells, however, would rarely be found in the absence of an invasive carcinoma. ×600. Papanicolaou.

Electron microscopy

As in so many other areas of pathology, the electron microscope has extended the description already made from light microscopy, but produced no diagnostic or prognostic breakthrough.

Shingleton *et al.* (1968) published a useful study of the ultrastructure of CIN lesions. As expected, dedifferentiation was marked by increased nucleocytoplasmic ratio, nuclear irregularity, nucleolar enlargement, reduction in cell attachments, fewer tonofibrils, less glycogen, and more free ribosomes. Extensive spaces between the cells were often occupied by villous processes, a feature which has also been found in reserve cell hyperplasia (Laguens *et al.* 1971). In general, the ultrastructural features support the idea that these lesions are neoplastic, in that the changes are similar to those found in invasive carcinoma. These findings have been repeatedly confirmed (Kraus 1973).

One area in which transmission electron microscopy has recently made an interesting contribution is in the demonstration that some cervical lesions of Grade I (mild dysplasia) are manifestations of wart virus infection. In these 'flat condylomas', a small proportion of the squamous cells may contain arrays of typical virus particles (Laverty *et al.* 1978).

Jordan and Williams (1971) applied scanning electron microscopy to CIN lesions and observed that squamous cells of the native ectocervical epithelium were covered with ridges, while those of CIN were covered with blunt microvilli. However, a study of the normal transformation zone by Ferenczy and Richart (1973) showed that the same difference in surface features was seen between mature squamous cells and the immature surface cells of squamous metaplasia, and the presence of microvilli is by no means confined to precancerous conditions. Scanning electron microscopy provides the most beautiful demonstration of cell arrangement and relationships, but no new insight into the nature of CIN has so far appeared.

Immunohistochemistry

A start has been made with the application of immunochemical staining procedures to cervical lesions, using antibodies with more or less specificity for neoplastic tissue. For instance, it has been found that an antibody against 'epithelial membrane antigen', prepared by immunizing rabbits against defatted human milk globules, reacts strongly with various carcinomas (Sloane and Ormerod 1981; Sloane *et al.* 1982). The normal cervical squamous epithelium was found to be negative, but staining was found in carcinoma *in situ* and in the adjacent morphologically normal epithelium.

The monoclonal antibody Ca 1 made by H. Harris and his colleagues has been found to have considerable, though not complete, specificity for the cells of human neoplasms (McGee *et al.* 1982), but its application to precancerous states of the cervix has not yet been reported at the time of writing.

Cell growth and kinetics

Squamous epithelia are normally generated from the layers near to the base, and cells which are no longer capable of mitotic division rise towards the surface in regular columns, maturing as they rise, and are finally shed at the surface (Allen and Potten 1976). The histopathological and cytopathological literature contains descriptions of epithelia in which a neoplastic lesion is supposed to involve the basal but not the superficial layers or *vice versa.* This is not, of course, possible according to any standard theory of how neoplasms grow, and whatever visual impression is received it must be accepted that at least whole vertical sections are involved, or else it is not a neoplasm. In the case of a clonal proliferation with mitosis occurring at different levels, proliferation in lateral directions must also have occurred and one does frequently see sharp divisions where (probably) one clone abuts upon another. Some of these sharp divisions represent the margins of the transformation zone where it meets native squamous or columnar epithelium, but junctions between two abnormal epithelia are also seen. It is also true that gradual transitions are seen between an undifferentiated area and a partially differentiated one.

The kinetics of cell renewal in the human cervix have been studied by *in vitro* labelling of small biopsies (Richart 1963) and by local injection of

^{3}H-thymidine *in vivo* with subsequent biopsy examination (Averette *et al.* 1970).

From the latter study it appears that cell renewal normally takes place in one or two parabasal layers, the basal layer serving as a reserve compartment. The mean cell cycle time is about three days, but by oestrogen stimulation this can be reduced to about 1½ days. The transit time from labelling to surface desquamation is at least four days. Estimates made by the *in vitro* method from a number of different centres have been tabulated by Langley and Crompton (1973), but usually the basal and parabasal layers have not been distinguished.

Although not studied in much detail, it appears that in CIN the cell cycle time is considerably shortened, even to as little as 12 hours (Richart 1963; Fettig and Sievers 1966; Feit and Staniček 1967), and this is consistent with the visible high mitotic activity, particularly in grade-III lesions. It has been pointed out, however, that most of the dividing cells are in metaphase and this stage may be abnormally prolonged (Timonen 1955). Evidently the classical 'carcinoma *in situ*' actively produces abnormal cells which continue to be shed into the vagina in large numbers over a period of many years, even decades, and it is these abundant exfoliated 'malignant cells' which permitted the diagnosis to be made so readily by the original aspirated vaginal smear method of Papanicolaou and Traut (1943).

Tissue culture

In culture, the epithelial cells of CIN are said to behave similarly to the 'transformed' cells which have occasionally been observed to arise in cultured normal cervices; their independence and capacity to overlap their fellows is like that of neoplastic cells in general (Wilbanks and Fink 1976).

Field theory versus clonal theory

It is sometimes suggested that there are two mutually exclusive possibilities; (a) cancer (for example of the cervix) begins from a whole abnormal 'field' of induced epithelium; or (b) it arises from a single mutated cell. There are good reasons for thinking that these two hypotheses are simultaneously right (Foulds 1975).

In a small proportion of cases, precancerous states and invasive carcinomas are found simultaneously or successively in the cervix, vagina, and vulva (Marcus 1960), and the conclusion is unavoidable that a whole area has in some way been predisposed, as occurs so frequently with urothelial neoplasia. Even in these rare cases, only a few growths arise out of many billions of cells exposed to the same factors; hence it is almost certain that we are dealing with a multi-hit process—a sequence of successive changes in the genetic material, each with a low probability. Presumably in the above cases large numbers of cells have undergone the first change or changes, and successively smaller numbers have undergone subsequent ones. In the commonest situation, where only a part of the cervix is involved, Richart (1967) found most CIN lesions to be unifocal; and when followed colposcopically without treatment, they were seen to grow by peripheral expansion, replacing the normal epithelium.

Given that the final invasive tumour is clonal (and the evidence about to be described supports this) and given that carcinoma of the cervix develops from CIN, does an area of CIN arise from a single altered cell? Two methods have been developed which can throw light on this question.

Evidence from lyonization

In women heterozygous for the isoenzymes of glucose-6-phosphate dehydrogenase, biopsies from normal tissues will show both types (A and B), one being expressed by cells with an active paternal X chromosome, the other by those with an active maternal X. If a whole biopsy consists of a clone of cells descended from a single cell subsequent to fetal life (when lyonization of the X chromosome occurs), it will contain only the A or only the B isoenzyme, not both. For this method to succeed, the cells in question must not be mixed with any different extraneous cells, such as associated blood or connective tissue. This is difficult to achieve, so that evidence of nonclonality does not carry the same conviction as evidence of single-cell origin.

Park and Jones (1968) applied this method to cervical cancer, and found that of eight invasive cervical carcinomas, five had a single isoenzyme and three had both. Smith *et al.* (1971), however, found single bands in all of six cases with CIN, and in four of seven with invasion.

There seems to have been no recent confirmation of these findings, probably because of dissatisfaction with the purity of the epithelial samples. Moreover, we do not know the size of the original patches of epithelial cells in the uterine cervix which would be expected to express the same isoenzyme. For skin it has been estimated at about 1500 cells (Friedman and Fialkow 1976).

Cytogenetic evidence

In the 1960s a considerable literature arose concerning the chromosomal changes in CIN. Most of the writers on this subject were not particularly concerned with the question of single-cell origin, but rather with the presence or absence of abnormal karyotypes and their relationship, if any, to prognosis.

A fairly complete account of this work can be found elsewhere (Spriggs 1974) but, to summarize, it can be said that all workers agree that invasive carcinomas of the cervix consist of cells with abnormal karyotypes, usually with either hypodiploid or hypertriploid counts. Grade-III lesions also have abnormal chromosome counts, often near to 46 or somewhat below 92. Grade-I lesions seldom show enough mitotic activity for counts to be possible, but in a few cases they have been normal and in fewer still were probably tetraploid.

Single-cell origin can be inferred if all the analysable cells have similar abnormal karyotypes—similar enough to rule out their separate appearance by chance. Direct preparations are necessary, since a single abnormal cell can give rise to a clone in culture. Because of the difficulty of making good direct chromosome preparations from solid tissues, the most convincing evidence comes from cases with marker chromosomes, i.e. chromosomes which differ morphologically from any in the normal set. Because of the known occurrence of non-random translocations producing a similar marker in different cases of neoplastic disease (for example, the one found regularly in chronic granulocytic leukaemia), it cannot be pronounced as a general law that several cells with the same marker belong to the same clone; but in the context of CIN and carcinoma of the cervix uteri, in which each case seems to have a different complex abnormality, the evidence from markers is acceptable.

Established invasive cervical cancer seems, from cytogenetic evidence, to consist of a clone (as is general in malignant tumours). In Grade-III lesions associated with dubious or incipient invasion, the same markers have been found in all or most of the cells from the anterior and posterior lips of the cervix, indicating that the lesion consists of a clone which has encircled the cervix by lateral spread. In two cases the marker was a ring chromosome and anaphase bridges identified the probable distribution of the ring in histological sections (Spriggs and Cowdell 1972). In Grade-III without micro-invasion the evidence is less compelling, but paired samples from anterior and posterior lips usually show concordant chromosome counts, and the same markers have sometimes been demonstrated (Spriggs *et al.* 1971). It has to be said also that the scatter of counts is often wider than can easily be explained by technical error, and it would seem that a 'field' exists in which a number of aneuploid clones are probably competing. This 'clonal selection' concept is expressed diagrammatically in Fig. 12.14.

If histograms are constructed showing the frequency of modal chromosome counts as reported in the literature, there appears to be a clear difference between invasive carcinoma and lesions of Grades II and III (Spriggs 1974). The precancerous stages show a markedly bimodal distribution with peaks around the diploid level and at 80-9, with very few in the 50-69 region. Invasive cancers are more frequently hypodiploid, counts between 50 and 69 are relatively common, and the second peak is at 70-9. In other words the distribution is shifted downwards, and this may reflect systematic chromosome loss in the course of progression.

Microdensitometry of Feulgen-stained nuclei

DNA estimations performed on cell populations by Feulgen microdensitometry represent a less exact but (in this context) more easily applicable

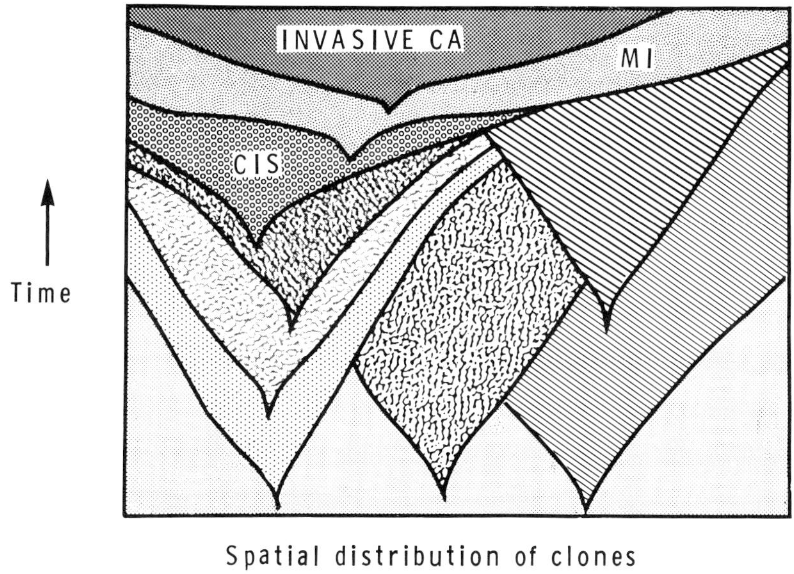

Fig.12.14. Clonal selection concept. A carcinogenic stimulus has caused three cells to escape from normal controls sufficiently to overgrow their neighbours. New cell lines emerge from two of these populations, and further ones from that on the left; later the whole represented area is occupied by a 'microinvasive' clone and from this a fully invasive carcinoma develops.

method of revealing deviations from the normal karyotype. There have been many quite extensive studies, but unfortunately most authors have paid no attention to the systematic errors which cause cells with larger nuclear areas to register higher readings, even in normal samples in which it is reasonably believed that, in G_1 or G_0 cells, the DNA is constant.

DNA histograms made from Feulgen-stained sections or smears of CIN lesions show a wide scatter of values with modal peaks at abnormal levels (Sandritter and Fischer 1962; Atkin 1969; Wagner *et al.* 1976), and the existence of these peaks is presumably due to the proliferation of aneuploid clones. It would be of particular interest to be able to separate lesions which are clearly aneuploid from those in which the scatter of values is only due to cells in the S phase and to polyploidy. Wagner *et al.* (1972) examined 17 cases of CIN, and while the more severe lesions showed evidence of aneuploidy, those with mild and moderate dysplasia were thought to show polyploidy only. Subsequently, Wagner *et al.* (1976), performing measurements on smears, distinguished presumably harmless 'suspicious' cells showing polyploidy from presumably precancerous aneuploid ones. However, Sachs and Schittko (1975) found aneuploid peaks in even the mildest lesions.

Nasiell *et al.* (1979) measured the DNA in cells from 'dysplasia' which had been followed without treatment and had either regressed to normal or progressed to a higher grade (carcinoma *in situ*). Both groups showed a scatter of abnormal values, without clear peaks at $2n$, $4n$, $8n$, and they concluded that this method did not distinguish between a progressive neoplastic type of dysplasia and a harmless type which mimics it.

It has to be admitted that the methods so far used do not really permit a reliable distinction, partly because of technical problems and also because these lesions contain cells in the process of DNA synthesis. A possible solution to the latter problem is the use of a membrane filter to remove a single layer of surface cells from the living cervix (Burn *et al.* 1974). Except in a few cases of classical carcinoma *in situ* these will be end- cells and, in principle, it should be possible to determine whether the readings are consistent with multiples of the normal $2n$ value or not. This would be of particular interest in Grade I, many of which may be lesions produced by wart virus and destined to resolve spontaneously.

Progression and regression

There is a twofold difficulty in studying the natural history of this disease. First, the course of the disease is apt to be changed by the means used to investigate it. Secondly, doctors have an obligation to treat patients, especially if neoplastic disease is in question.

There are two main types of study which shed light on this problem:

1. Prospective follow-up of untreated women following the discovery of a putative precancerous lesion.
2. Epidemiological study of the incidence of the putative precancerous stages compared with that of clinical invasive carcinoma; their relative numbers and age distributions.

Follow-up without treatment

There is a large volume of published data concerning cases followed without definitive treatment, mostly incompletely recorded. The changes should of course be given as proportions per unit time but this has rarely been done—indeed most authors do not seem to have considered the time-scale important.

Results from the major series are shown in Tables 12.2-12.4. Table 12.2 shows series of cases diagnosed by small biopsies as dysplasia, or its obsolete names anaplasia (Boston) and basal cell hyperplasia (Baltimore). Table 12.3 shows those followed by smears only. In these two sets of data, because of ethical considerations, carcinoma *in situ* was taken as the end-point. Consequently any cases progressing to invasive carcinoma are only accidentally included.

Table 12.4 shows the series of cases recorded in the literature in which patients with cervical lesions diagnosed as carcinoma *in situ* (i.e. Grade-III lesions) were followed without definitive treatment. A few substantial series are excluded because the data are not presented so as to make the relevant information available.

Two series deserve separate mention, those of Stern and Neely (1964) and Richart and Barron (1969), particularly as their evidence appears to conflict.

Table 12.2. *Untreated 'dysplasia' followed up after diagnosis by biopsy*

Reference	Number of cases	Interval	Regressed (per cent)	Progressed to CIS (per cent)	Progressed to invasion (per cent)
Glatthaar (1950)	36		22	64	
Galvin *et al.* (1955)					
Grades of 'basal cell					
hyperplasia I	93		54	2	
II	63	2 m-4 y	44	13	
III	35		17	66	
Peckham and Greene (1957)					
Atypical BCH	133		50	6	
Equivocal CIS	109	58 per cent <1 y	29	16	
McKay *et al.* (1959)	129	mean 3.7 y	20		
		mean 2.5 y		4	0.8
Simon and Sheehan (1962)	44	1-10 y	55	5	
Scott and Ballard (1962)	223	<9 y	50	8	
Koss *et al.* (1963)	26	6 m-10 y	38	42	0.25
Johnson *et al.* (1968)	141	<5 y	50	1.4	
Kern and Nolens (1969)	106	2-9 y	33	37	3
Christopherson (1969)	'over 200'	1-13 y	≏30	≏20	1.3
Sedlis *et al.* (1970)	168	<5 y	42	18	6
Villa Santa (1971)	63	<9 y	48	16	21
Nasiell *et al.* (1976)[a]					
grades of dysplasia					
mild	555	mean 2.1 y	65	11	
moderate	892	mean 4.6 y	54	25	
severe	265	mean 4.1 y	43	38	

[a] Some followed without biopsy BCH, basal cell hyperplasia; CIS, carcinoma *in situ*

Table 12.3. *Untreated 'dysplasia' diagnosed by cytology. Followed up without any biopsy*

Reference	Number of cases	Interval	% Regressed	% Progressed to CIS	% Progressed to invasion
Scott and Ballard 1962	120	<9y	60	1.7	
Patten (1966)					
slight	218		72		
moderate	102	9m–2y	44	?	
marked	44		16		
Fox (1967) (mild and moderate)	278	<11y	31	60 (SD + CIS)	0.7
Patten (1978)					
slight	3299			0.5	
moderate	661	5y	?	2.4	
marked	125			9.6	0.8
Jordan *et al.* (1981)					
slight	545	mean 2y for regression	75	0	
moderate	144		80	1.4	
severe	41	mean 3.5y for progression	66	17	

SD, severe dysplasia; CIS, carcinoma *in situ*

Table 12.4. '*Carcinoma* in situ' *followed without treatment*

Reference	Number of cases	Biopsy or not	Interval (years)	Regressed	Progressed to invasion
Carson and Gall (1954)	4	yes	2–12 (mean 7.5)	?	3 (75%)
Petersen (1955)	127	yes	3–17 (mean 7.4)	30 (24%)	34 (26%)
Masterson (1957)	25	yes	1– 5	1 (4%)	7 (28%)
Lange (1960)	100	yes	5–13	30 (30%)	24 (24%)
Kottmeier (1961)	31	yes	>12	?	22 (71%)
Fox (1967)	33	no	1– 7	? 0	0
Kern and Nolens (1969)	106	? yes	2– 9	35 (33%)	3 (3%)
Christopherson (1969)	29	yes	1– 5	0	10 (34%)
Gad (1976)	11	yes	1– 8 (mean 4.6)	0	6 (54%)

Stern and Neely studied 130 women with the biopsy diagnosis of cervical dysplasia at fixed intervals, in order to estimate the incidence rates of regression and of progression to carcinoma *in situ.* The progression rate per year was 64 per thousand (compared with 0.04 per thousand in women without dysplasia). Regression to negative smear occurred at the rate of 32 per cent per year, regardless of whether further biopsies were taken, but these 'recurred' to dysplasia again at the rate of 33 per cent per year. The temporary regressions to a normal smear may, of course, be explained by 'false negative' tests but the authors postulate that most are genuine and that recurrence is due to 'continuing environmental effects'.

Richart and Barron's series (1969) consisted of 557 cases diagnosed by cytology as dysplasia, and followed (mostly for short periods) without any interference by biopsy procedures. They claimed an accuracy of 95 per cent in predicting the histology from smear examination, and stated that the false negative rate was less than 5 per cent. Regression was only observed in six of the 462 cases with 'mild' dysplasia, and never in those with more severe lesions. Median transit times were calculated between four grades of abnormality of which the final one was carcinoma *in situ.* For severe dysplasia, the median transit time to carcinoma *in situ* was one year, but for very mild dysplasia it was about seven years. Three patients developed invasive carcinoma while under observation.

The findings in this series therefore differ considerably from the rest of the data in Table 12.2 in respect of the rate of regression, and the authors attribute this to the effect of biopsy. They differ also, however, from the data of Stern and Neely (1964) and the other series shown in Table 12.3 in which initial biopsy was not performed. This may be due to the initial selection of relatively severe and persistent lesions.

In Tables 12.2 and 12.3, the proportion of 'progressions' is artificially increased by a fallacy which is not mentioned by any of the authors concerned. This is, that the same cervix commonly harbours both dysplasia and carcinoma *in situ* (by whatever criteria are used to distinguish them). When a small biopsy is taken from such a cervix, if it samples an area of carcinoma *in situ*, the patient will receive treatment and will not enter the series. If, on the other hand, only dysplasia is seen on the biopsy, the case will be followed and will subsequently 'progress' to carcinoma *in situ.*

In any case, Tables 12.2-12.4 show a trend which is consistent with most clinical opinion—that is, that group-I lesions (which are particularly common in the young) regress spontaneously in most cases and that group-III lesions may persist for many years but often finally result in invasive carcinoma.

Kinlen and Spriggs (1978) tried to circumvent the ethical dilemma by collecting, from all over the United Kingdom, cases with unsuspected positive smears in which no biopsy or treatment had been undertaken for at least two years, because of default, change of address, or other failures of a personal or administrative nature. 'Positive' was taken to cover all abnormal smears which were considered to deserve referral for biopsy and included various grades of disease, but all would have been treated if they had not escaped. Table 12.5 shows the results. Evidently it is true that spontaneous regression is common (19 out of 60 re-examined), and also that fatal invasive carcinoma (six† in this series) can result from failure to act on positive cytological evidence.

Table 12.5. *Follow-up of cases with unsuspected 'positive' cervical smears, left untreated at least two years against advice. Mean follow-up period five years. (Data from Kinlen and Spriggs (1978))*

Untraced	31	Smear still abnormal, no biopsy	8
Refuses further smears	8	Smear negative ('regression')	19
Died, no PM	1	CIS or dysplasia	20
Hysterectomy, no histological study	1	'Microinvasive carcinoma'	3
		Invasive carcinoma	10*
Total unusable	41	Total with information	60

* Six deaths.

Spriggs and Boddington (1980) reviewed all the available original smears from the above series, in which either regression or progression to invasion were observed; and they also added other cases with abnormal smears and a known outcome in the absence of any treatment. There is a clear relationship between the severity of the cytological abnormality and the final outcome. No example was seen of progression to invasive carcinoma among those with only 'superficial dyskaryosis' or other cytological appearances usually associated with Grade-I lesions. Of those with smears suggesting Grade-III lesions, four examples were seen of spontaneous regression, but the majority were among those progressing to invasive carcinoma.

As a result of reviewing all the available original cervical smears from the series of Kinlen and Spriggs (1978), I have constructed a chart (Fig. 12.15) showing the course over time, assuming that any observed change occurred fairly rapidly at the central point between the initial cytological observations and the biopsy, which is taken as the end-point. The cases are classified into grades (this involves a good deal of subjective judgement made from smears of varying technical quality and preservation of staining). In each case the starting point is that of first detection, not of course the onset of disease.

† One more patient has died since the paper of Kinlen and Spriggs (1978) was published.

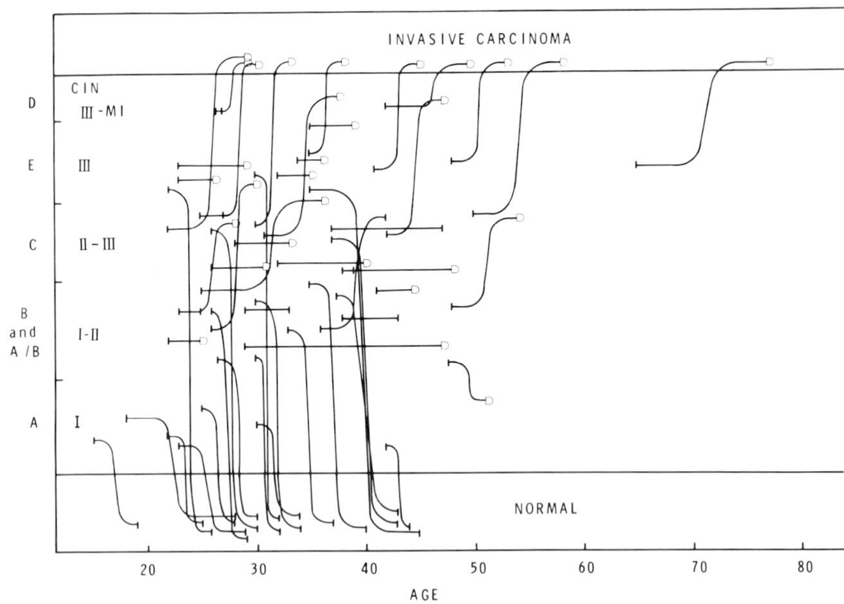

Fig. 12.15. Cases from the 'defaulters' series of Kinlen and Spriggs (1977), classified into five categories according to the estimated severity of the initial cervical smears. In each case there are at least two observed points, before and after an interval without surgical interference. Any change in status is deemed to have occurred at the mid-point of the interval. Final status indicated thus: ——┤ cervical smear only; ——○ biopsy, or clinical presentation with carcinoma. Note that the first point is that of discovery, not of the onset of disease, which may have been many years earlier. The lettering on the left refers to the cytological notation of Spriggs and Boddington (1980). These grades are expected to correspond with the CIN grades as shown.

Epidemiological evidence

There is a large body of data from population screening which, in principle, should provide figures for age-specific incidence and prevalence of the different grades, and hence (if they are indeed stages of the same disease) a picture of the natural history, as proposed more than 25 years ago by Dunn (1953). Unfortunately there are large errors introduced by the occurrence of 'false negative' tests (Briggs 1979); these may form a small proportion of all significant lesions but they certainly account for a substantial proportion of conversions from negative to positive in successive annual tests, and it is upon those that the figures for age-specific incidence are based.

Calculations based on age-specific incidence and prevalence of carcinoma *in situ* result in a calculated duration of less than ten years (Dunn and Martin 1967; Barron *et al.* 1977), but because of the uncertainties in the data this is not dependable. As was pointed out in the Walton report (1976) the modal age of incidence of CIN II-III is 25·9 years, and of clinical invasive carcinoma 60·4 years, giving a duration of 35 years for the detectable disease.

This is even longer than the 20 years derived by Stern (1959) in a similar way. This conclusion could be wrong on account of a changing pattern of disease in different cohorts, but evidently the modal duration is measured in decades.

Causation

For many years there have been convincing epidemiological grounds for supposing that a necessary causal factor for cervical cancer is transmitted by sexual intercourse. More recent studies have failed to confirm certain earlier ideas, for instance that protection is conferred by circumcision of the partner. Even the well-known association between cervical neoplasia and an early age of first coitus has been found by Harris *et al.* (1980) to disappear when correction is made for the number of sexual partners. This careful study has demonstrated that different grades of CIN and invasive cervical cancer all share similar epidemiological characteristics, and that there is a strong correlation with multiple sex partners and a less strong one with the use of oral contraceptives and with smoking. An important factor is likely to be promiscuity of the male partner (Buckley *et al.* 1982; Skegg *et al.* 1982).

Apart from the obvious inference that there may be an infective cause, another idea has been propagated by Bevan Reid and his colleagues (Reid 1964). This is that the heads of spermatozoa themselves carry a 'mutagen' to the DNA of cervical epithelial cells. Reid's view of the activities of DNA are idiosyncratic and, although nuclei of spermatozoa can certainly in some circumstances fuse with those of epithelial cells (Bendich *et al.* 1976), there is so far no evidence that this is related to carcinoma of the cervix.

Most authorities feel that an infective agent is implicated, and look towards the viruses. Two of these are considered possible candidates at the time of writing—Herpes simplex and human wart virus.

Herpes simplex virus (HSV)

The genital strain of HSV (Type 2) is a common, venereally transmitted, infective agent which produces characteristic cytological changes visible in smears. Women who have been infected are identifiable subsequently by serology, but unfortunately there is cross-reaction with the universal HSV type I and kinetic neutralization tests are necessary to separate them.

Naib (1966) found unusually large numbers of cases of CIN following HSV 2 infection, and suggested that there might be a connection. Rawls *et al.* (1969) demonstrated an association between HSV 2 antibodies and cervical carcinoma, in that 78 per cent of 41 patients with the cancer had serological evidence of past infection, while this was only found in 22 per cent of matched controls. Corresponding figures for 'dysplasia' and 'carcinoma *in situ*' were 24 and 35 per cent, which offered weak support for a causal connection if CIN is an early stage of the same disease.

This was followed by a series of studies from different parts of the world, some showing a strong association between the virus and cervical carcinoma and/or CIN, but others showing only weak association (for literature, see Skinner, 1976; Thiry, 1976; Kessler 1981). Some of the milder dysplasias, without evidence of HSV 2 infection, may represent a separate condition which is not precancerous (Thomas and Rawls 1978).

Frenkel *et al.* (1972) published a report indicating that viral DNA corresponding to part of the HSV 2 genome could be demonstrated in the nuclei of cells from cervical carcinoma. Other workers failed to confirm this, but more recently there have been reports of the detection of HSV 2 RNA by *in situ* hybridization using frozen sections (McDougall *et al.* 1980; Eglin *et al.* 1981). The group in Baltimore have continued to produce evidence that the cells of CIN and cervical carcinoma contain HSV 2, as demonstrated by staining with labelled antibodies to antigens of HSV 2. This group claims that these reactions are specific for patients with either active HSV 2 infection or else CIN or invasive cervical carcinoma, and consequently could be applied to automated screening of smears (Aurelian *et al.* 1979, 1981). Further evidence of this type is reviewed by Galloway and McDougall (1983). It is also reported that specific antibodies can be eluted from cervical carcinoma tissue (Seth and Balachandran 1980). Finally, Wentz *et al.* (1981) have produced carcinoma of the cervix in mice, using inactivated herpes virus. Although the Baltimore investigators consider that 'the viral agent of the disease is clearly established' (Kessler 1981), the hypothesis that the genital herpes virus is causal in man must still remain *sub judice.*

Human wart virus

A more recent candidate for the role of cervical carcinogen is the virus of genital warts (condylomata acuminata). It has been known for many years that visible cervical infective warts produce a particular, cytological picture, which is characterized by enlarged and hyperchromatic nuclei surrounded by a clear area ('koilocytotic atypia'; Koss and Durfee 1956). In the last few years it has been realized that many of the lesions formerly called mild dysplasia or CIN I are in fact flat condylomata (Meisels *et al.* 1977, 1981; Purola and Savia 1977). This has been established by finding the wart virus particles in electron micrographs (Laverty *et al.* 1978; Reid *et al.* 1980) and by the immunoperoxidase method with antibody prepared against papilloma virus (Shah *et al.* 1980). Figs. 12.16 and 12.17 show corresponding cytological and histological appearances and Fig. 12.18, from a different case, shows an electron micrograph of the virus believed to be responsible.

Since many Grade-I lesions are known to regress spontaneously, this information may be thought to explain why many cervical smears in the past were 'false positive', but not to throw any light on the causation of cervical carcinoma. However, zur Hausen (1976) has marshalled the evidence for supposing that this virus may be oncogenic and referred to the reports in the literature of carcinoma arising in genital condylomata; moreover, Reid *et al.* (1982) found 91 per cent of women with cervical carcinoma or

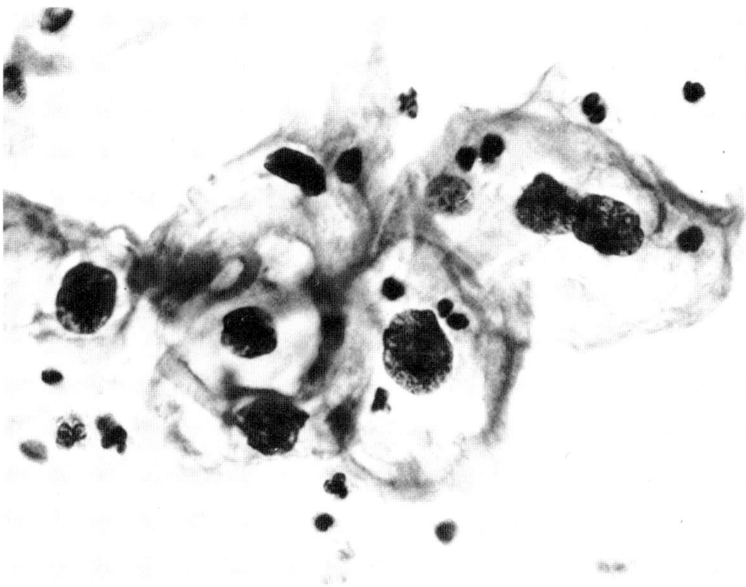

Fig. 12.16. Cervical smear showing epithelial cells with markedly enlarged, irregular, and hyperchromatic nuclei, surrounded by clear 'haloes'. This appearance is believed to be commonly produced by genital wart virus infection. ×600. Papanicolaou.

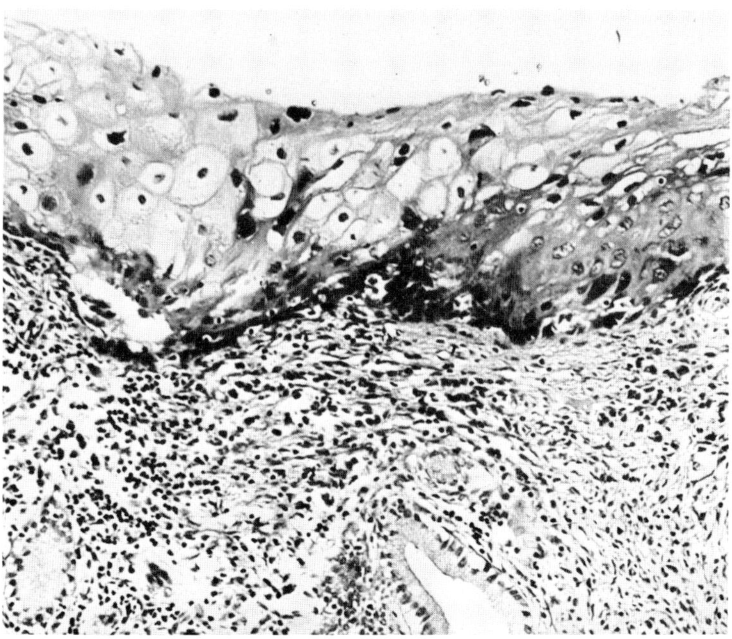

Fig. 12.17. Histological section of cervical biopsy from the same case as Fig. 12.15. There were no actual cervical warts, but this type of 'dysplasia' is probably produced by human wart virus. ×150. H & E.

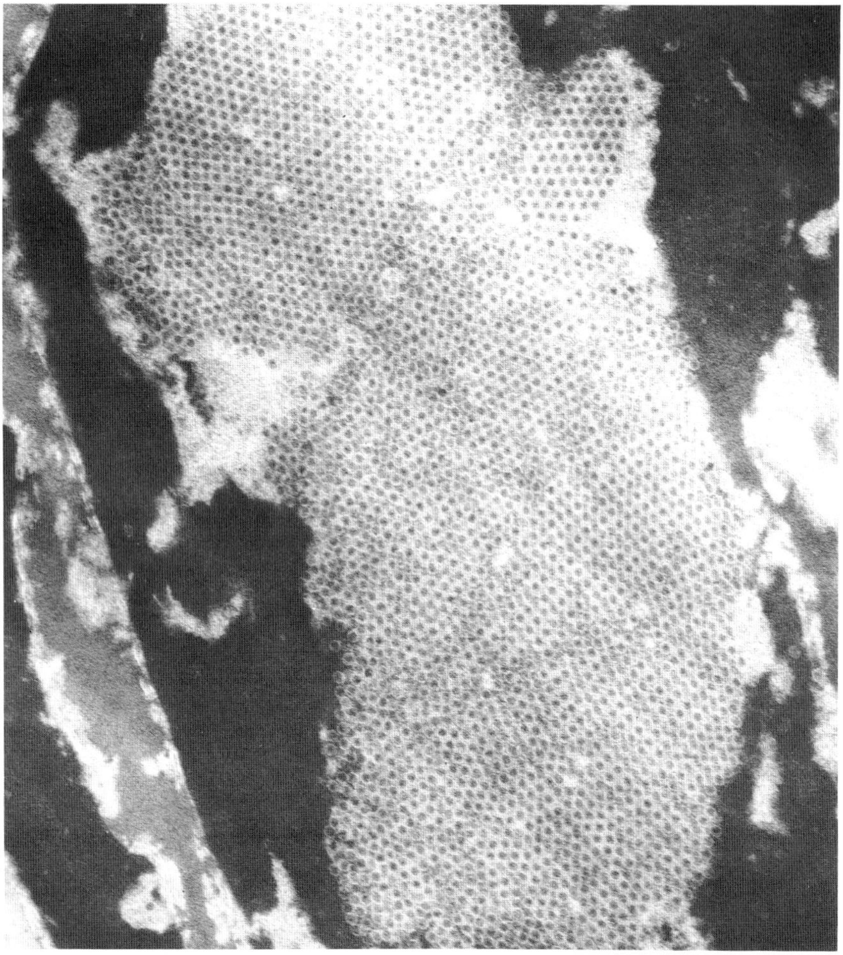

Fig. 12.18. Electron micrograph showing genital wart virus particles in the nucleus of a squamous epithelial cell from the human cervix. ×14 350. (By courtesy of Dr Dulcie V. Coleman.)

CIN to have associated histological evidence of wart virus infection. Some genital condylomata are reported to contain aneuploid cells, as determined by Feulgen microdensitometry (Jagella and Stegner 1974), though most are probably polyploid (Shevchuk and Richart 1982). It appears that genital warts are polyclonal (Friedman and Fialkow 1976), but this does not exclude the proposition that cancer may develop in the virus-infected cells. As we have seen, many authors have observed 'progression' of untreated dysplasia to the stage of carcinoma *in situ,* and some of these were of 'mild' type which could well have been flat condylomas (Galvin *et al.* 1955; Peckham and Greene 1957; Richart and Barron 1969). Certainly the microsopic appearance of the nuclei in these cases bears a much closer resemblance to cancer than does the nuclear lesion of herpes simplex, and, if we posulate a developmental period of 20-30 years—much longer than the periods of observation generally recorded in the literature—it is possible that the wart virus is a common or even necessary cause of cervical cancer. Sero-epidemiiological studies may help to resolve this question (Baird 1983).

Efficacy of screening programmes

Regular screening of symptomless women by the cervical (originally vaginal) smear was introduced on a large scale without any properly designed controlled trial, and this is now ethically and politically impossible. For many years epidemiologists felt considerable doubt about the efficacy of cervical screening, because there was no dramatic fall in mortality from cervical cancer—only a continuation of the gradual fall which was occurring before screening was introduced. Recently the data from several countries such as Finland and Iceland (Hakama *et al.* 1975; Johannesson *et al.* 1978) as well as a comparison between Canadian districts with different screening rates (Miller *et al.* 1976) have convinced most remaining sceptics that the lesions which are detected and removed would, if left untouched, have contributed substantially to the mortality (for discussion see Guzick (1978) and Berget (1979)).

There is, however, a continuing debate about the age limits and the frequency to be recommended for testing (Eddy 1981). Knox (1976) first put this on a logical foundation. He pointed out that, if the duration of the detectable disease before it becomes incurable is x years, then this is theoretically the optimum interval. Therefore, if the duration is 20 years, tests performed at intervals of 15, 10, 5 or 1 year should all be equally effective in prevention. Allowing for a variety of different 'natural histories' and also for the false negative error, he calculated that 5-year intervals would have a nearly maximal effect on mortality. He also pointed out that the same calculations, based on age-specific deaths from cervical cancer in the early-1970s, gave no support to the practice of performing multiple smears on women aged under 30.

Contrary to the above opinion many gynaecologists and cytopathologists, particularly in the United States, strongly advise women to have annual tests. Even more widespread is the recommendation that cervical smear testing should be performed regularly in young women from the onset of sexual activity, so as to find and remove CIN lesions at the earliest possible moment. The Canadian 'task force' (Walton 1976), and a British working party (Draper 1982) have given different recommendations about this matter, which remains at present an unresolved question of cost-benefit; it is made more difficult by an apparently changing pattern of disease, with increasing frequency in the young. Annual testing, at whatever age, is certainly extravagant of skilled manpower and, in many countries, of public money.

Adenocarcinoma

Endocervical adenocarcinomas are much less common than squamous carcinomas, accounting for about 5 per cent of cervical cancers. They show a variety of histological patterns and are sometimes difficult to distinguish from endometrial carcinoma (see Chapter 13). Adenocarcinoma appears to be relatively commoner in unmarried women and in nulliparae, compared with squamous carcinoma (Korhonen 1980).

Like squamous carcinoma, cervical adenocarcinoma passes through recognizable precancerous or incipient stages (see the illustrations of Burghardt 1973). Foci are seen in which crowded atypical glandular cells with hyperchromatic nuclei are associated with anomalies of architecture, such as the budding of solid cords. It is sometimes associated with squamous CIN (Qizilbash 1975; Christopherson *et al.* 1979). In cervical smears, sheets of endocervical cells are seen in which normal polarity is disturbed, usually without much nuclear pleomorphism (Qizilbash 1975; Bousfield *et al.* 1980). Because benign endocervical-cell hyperplasia and hypertrophy are so common, the cytological diagnosis of early adenocarcinoma is very easily missed, and indeed the distinction is a subtle one giving rise to many false-positive and false-negative errors.

Very little is known about the natural history of this condition. As a result of reviewing 'negative' smears taken before the development of cervical adenocarcinoma (Boddington *et al.* 1976), it is clear that abnormal cells were already present in some cases, even eight years before clinical presentation. In one case in which the lesion was still *in situ* at the time of biopsy, smears taken seven years previously contained neoplastic cells on review. Similarly, Boon *et al.* (1981) reviewed 18 'negative' endocervical biopsies taken 3-7 years before presentation of adenocarcinoma, and in five of these they found areas of adenocarcinoma *in situ.* It can therefore be assumed that adenocarcinoma of the endocervix, like most other cancers, has a prolonged pre-invasive stage and that this is identifiable (sometimes with difficulty) by the cervical smear.

Conclusion

At the beginning of this chapter it was stated that carcinoma of the cervix had been more thoroughly studied than any other human cancer. We know how the squamous type could, theoretically, be prevented (by premarital celibacy and bilateral marital fidelity); we know how to detect it when it is practically 100 per cent curable (by cytology). We still do not know its cause, but that is not necessary for prevention and control. When this disease kills, it does so in spite of our knowlege, not because of our ignorance.

References

Allen, T.D. and Potten, C.S. (1976). Significance of cell shape in tissue architecture. *Nature* **264**, 545.

Atkin, N.B. (1969). The use of microspectrophotometry. *Obstet. Gynec. Survey* **24**, 794.

Aurelian, L., Gupta, P.K., Frost, J.K., Rosenshein, N.B., Smith, C.C., Tyrer, H.W., Mantione, J.M., and Albright, C.D. (1979). Fluorescence-activated separation of cervical abnormal cells using Herpesvirus antigenic markers. *Anal. quant. Cytol.* **1**, 89.

——, Manak, M.M., McKinlay, M., Smith, C.C., Klacsmann, K.T., and Gupta, P.K. (1981). 'The herpes virus hypothesis'—are Koch's postulates satisfied? *Gynaecol. Oncol.* **12**, S56.

Averette, H.E., Weinstein, G.D., and Frost, P. (1970). Autoradiographic analysis of cell proliferation kinetics in human genital tissues. *Amer. J. Obstet. Gynec.* **108**, 8.

Baird, P.J. (1983). Serological evidence for the association of papillomavirus and cervical neoplasia. *Lancet* **ii**, 17.

Barron, B.A., Cahill, M.C., and Richart, R.M. (1978). A statistical model of the natural history of cervical neoplastic disease. *Gynec. Oncol.* **6**, 196.

Bendich, A., Borenfreund, E., Witkin, S.S., Beju, D., and Higgins, P.J. (1976). Information transfer and sperm uptake by mammalian somatic cells. *Progr. nucleic Acid Res. Mol. Biol.* **17**, 43.

Berget, A. (1979). Screening for cervical neoplasia. *Dan. med. Bull.* **26**, 313.

Bettinger, H.F. and Reagan, J.W. (Chairmen) (1962). Proceedings of the International Committee on Histological Terminology for lesions of the uterine cervix. In *Proc. 1st Int. Congr. Exfol. Cytol. (Vienna 1961),* p. 283. Lippincott, Philadelphia.

Beyer-Boon, M.E. and Verdonk, G.W. (1978). The identification of atypical reserve cells in smears of patients with premalignant and malignant changes in the squamous and glandular epithelium of the uterine cervix. *Acta. Cytol.* **22**, 305.

Blackwell, P. and Markham, R. (1976). The histochemistry of the cervical epithelium. In *The cervix* (ed. J.A. Jordan and A. Singer), p. 61. Saunders, London.

Boddington, M.M., Spriggs, A.I., and Cowdell, R.H. (1976). Adenocarcinoma of the uterine cervix: cytological evidence of a long preclinical evolution. *Brit. J. Obstet. Gynaec.* **83**, 900.

Boon, M.E., Baak, J.P.A., Kurver, P.J.H., Overdiep, S.H., and Verdonk, G.W. (1981). Adenocarcinoma *in situ* of the cervix: an underdiagnosed lesion. *Cancer* **48**, 768.

Bousfield, L., Pacey, F., Young, Q., Krumins, I., and Osborn, R. (1980). Expanded cytologic criteria for the diagnosis of adenocarcinoma *in situ* of the cervix and related lesions. *Acta. Cytol.* **24**, 283.

Boyes, D.A., Worth, A.J., and Fidler, H.K. (1970). The results of treatment of 4389 cases of pre-clinical cervical squamous carcinoma. *Brit. J. Obstet. Gynaec.* **77**, 769.

Briggs, R.M. (1979). Dysplasia and early neoplasia of the uterine cervix. *Obstet. Gynec. Survey* **34**, 70.

Broders, A.C. (1932). Carcinoma *in situ* contrasted with benign penetrating epithelium. *J. Amer. med. Assoc.* **99**, 1670.

Buckley, C.H., Butler, E.B., and Fox, H. (1982). Cervical intraepithelial neoplasia. *J. clin. Pathol.* **35**, 1.

Buckley, J.D., Harris, R.W.C., Doll, R., Vessey, M.P., and Williams, P.T. (1981). Case-control study of the husbands of women with dysplasia or carcinoma of the cervix uteri. *Lancet* **2**, 1010.

Burghardt, E. (1973). *Early histological diagnosis of cervical cancer.* Saunders, Philadelphia.

Burn, G.P., Singer, A., and Spriggs, A.I. (1974). A membrane filter method for correlating colposcopic, histological, and cytological pictures: The application to nuclear DNA measurements. *J. clin. Pathol.* **27**, 542.

Carson, R.P. and Gall, E.A. (1954). Preinvasive carcinoma and precancerous metaplasia of the cervix. A serial block survey. *Amer. J. Pathol.* **30**, 15.

Christopherson, W.M. (1969). Concepts of genesis and development in early cervical neoplasia. *Obstet. Gynec. Survey* **24**, 842.

—— (1977). Dysplasia, carcinoma *in situ*, and microinvasive carcinoma of the uterine cervix. *Human Pathol.* **8**, 489.

——, Nealon, N., and Gray, L.A. (1979). Noninvasive precursor lesions of adenocarcinoma and mixed adenosquamous carcinoma of the cervix uteri. *Cancer* **44**, 975.

Coppleson, M. (1976). Management of preclinical carcinoma of the cervix. In *The cervix* (ed. J.A. Jordan and A. Singer), p. 453. Saunders, London.

—— and Reid, B. (1967). *Preclinical carcinoma of the cervix uteri.* Pergamon, Oxford.

——, Pixley, E., and Reid, B.L. (1978). *Colposcopy.* 2nd edn. Thomas, Springfield.

Cullen, T.S. (1900). *Cancer of the Uterus.* Kimpton, London.

Draper, G.J. (1982). Screening for cervical cancer: revised policy. The recommendations of the DHSS Committee on Gynaecological Cytology. *Hlth. Trends* **14**, 37.

—— and Martin, P.L. (1967). Morphogenesis of cervical cancer. *Cancer* **20**, 1899.

Dunn, J.E. (1953). The relationship between carcinoma *in situ* and invasive cervical carcinoma. *Cancer* **6**, 873.

Eddy, D.M. (1981). Appropriateness of cervical cancer screening. *Gynecol. Oncol.* **12**, S168.

Eglin, R.P., Sharp, F., Cordiner, J.W., *et al.* (1981). The association between herpes virus and human cervical squamous cell neoplasms: latency of the virus in uterosacral ligaments and transcription of the genome in neoplastic cells. *4th World Cong. Int. Fed. Cervical Pathology and Colposcopy,* London 13-17 October, Paper 9.

Feit, J. and Staniček, J. (1967). Histoautoradiographical investigation of DNA synthesis in precancerous states and carcinomas of the uterine cervix in bioptical material. *Neoplasma* **14**, 499.

Ferenczy, A. and Richart, R.M. (1973). Scanning electron microscopy of the cervical transformation zone. *Amer. J. Obstet. Gynec.* **115**, 151.

Fettig, O. and Sievers, R. (1966). ^{3}H-Index und mittlere Generationszeit des menschlichen Portiokarzinoms und seiner Vorstufen. *Beitr. path. Anat.* **133**, 83.

Fluhmann, C.F. (1961). *The cervix uteri and its diseases.* Saunders, Philadelphia.

Foulds, L. (1975). *Neoplastic development,* Vol. 2, Chapter 3, Academic Press, London.

Fox, C.H. (1967). Biologic behavior of dysplasia and carcinoma *in situ. Amer. J. Obstet. Gynec.* **99**, 960.

Frenkel, N., Roizman, B., Cassai, E., and Nahmias, A.J. (1972). A DNA fragment of Herpes simplex 2 and its transcription in human cervical cancer tissue. *Proc. Nat. Acad. Sci.* **69**, 3784.

Friedman, J.M. and Fialkow, P.J. (1976). Viral 'tumorigenesis' in man: cell markers in *condylomata acuminata. Int. J. Cancer* **17**, 57.

Gad, C. (1976). The management and natural history of severe dysplasia and carcinoma *in situ* of the uterine cervix. *Brit. J. Obstet. Gynaec.* **83**, 554.

Galloway, D.A. and McDougall, J.K. (1983). The oncogenic potential of herpes simplex viruses: evidence for a 'hit & run' mechanism. *Nature, Lond.* **302**, 21.

Galvin, G.A., Jones, H.W., and Te Linde, R.W. (1955). The significance of basal-cell hyperactivity in cervical biopsies. *Amer. J. Obstet. Gynec.* **70**, 808.

Glatthaar, E. (1950). *Studien über die Morphogenese des Plattenepithelkarzinoms der Portio vaginalis uteri.* Karger, Basle.

Govan, A.D.T., Haines, R.M., Langley, F.A., Taylor, C.W., and Woodcock, A.S. (1969). The histology and cytology of changes in the epithelium of the cervix uteri. *J. clin. Path.* **22**, 383.

Gruenagel, H.H. (1957). Die Plattenepithel-Zylinderepithelgrenze an der Portio vaginalis uteri bei unreifen und reifen Neugeborenen, Säuglingen und Kindern bis zu neun Jahren. *Frankf. Zeitschr. Path.* **68**, 465.

Guzick, D.S. (1978). Efficacy of screening for cervical cancer: A review. *Amer. J. Publ. Hlth.* **68**, 125.

Hakama, M., Joutsenlahti, U., Virtanen, A., and Räsänen-Virtanen, U. (1975). Mass screenings for cervical cancer in Finland 1963-71. *Ann. clin. Res.* **7**, 101.

Harris, R.W.C., Brinton, L.A., Cowdell, R.H., Skegg, D.C.G., Smith, P.G., Vessey, M.P., and Droll, R. (1980). Characteristics of women with dysplasia or carcinoma *in situ* of the cervix uteri. *Brit. J. Cancer* **42**, 359.

Hausen, H., zur (1976). Condylomata acuminata and human genital cancer. *Cancer Res.* **36**, 794.

Jagella, H.P. and Stegner, H.E. (1974). Zur Dignität der Condylomata acuminata. *Arch. Gynäk.* **216**, 119.

Johannesson, G., Geirsson, G., and Day, N. (1978). The effect of mass screening in Iceland, 1965-74, on the incidence and mortality of cervical carcinoma. *Int. J. Cancer* **21**, 418.

Johnson, L.D. Easterday, C.L., Gore, H., and Hertig, A.T. (1964). The histogenesis of carcinoma *in situ* of the uterine cervix. *Cancer* **17**, 213.

——, Nickerson, R.J., Easterday, C.L., Stuart, R.S. and Hertig, A.T. (1968). Epidemiological evidence for the spectrum of change from dysplasia through carcinoma *in situ* to invasive cancer. *Cancer* **22**, 901.

Jones, H.W., Galvin, G.A., and te Linde, R.W. (1957). Re-examination of biopsies taken prior to the development of invasive carcinoma of the cervix. In *Proc. 3rd Nat. Cancer Conf.*, p. 678. Lippincott, Philadelphia.

Jordan, J.A. and Williams, A.E. (1971). Scanning electron microscopy in the study of cervical neoplasia. *J. Obstet. Gynaecol.* **78**, 940.

Jordan, S.W., Smith, M.L., and Dike, L.S. (1981). The significance of cervical cytologic dysplasia. *Acta Cytol.* **25**, 237.

Kern, G. and Nolens, J.P. (1969). Langzeitbeobachtungen von dysplastischen und gesteigert atypischem Epithel. *Arch. Gynäk.* **207**, 342.

Kessler, I.I. (1981). Etiological concepts in cervical carcinogenesis. *Gynecol. Oncol.* **12**, 57.

Kinlen, L.J. and Spriggs, A.I. (1978). Women with positive cervical smears but without surgical intervention. *Lancet* **2**, 463.

Kirkland, J.A., Stanley, M.A., and Cellier, K.M. (1967). Comparative study of histologic and chromosomal abnormalities in cervical neoplasia. *Cancer* **20**, 1934.

Knox, E. (1976). Ages and frequencies for cervical cancer screening. *Brit. J. Cancer* **34**, 444.

Kolstad, P. and Stafl, A. (1977). *Atlas of colposcopy* (2nd edn). University Park Press, Baltimore.

Korhonen, M.O. (1980). Epidemiological differences between adenocarcinoma and squamous cell carcinoma of the uterine cervix. *Gynecol. Oncol.* **10**, 312.

Koss, L.G. (1978). Dysplasia. A real concept or a misnomer? *Obstet. Gynecol.* **51**, 374.

—— (1979). *Diagnostic cytology and its histopathologic bases* (3rd edn). Lippincott, Philadelphia.

—— and Durfee, G.R. (1956). Unusual patterns of squamous epithelium of the uterine cervix; cytologic and pathologic study of koilocytotic atypia. *Ann. NY Acad. Sci.* **63**, 1245.

——, Stewart, F.W., Foote, F.W., Jordan, M.J., Bader, G.M., and Day, E. (1963). Some histological aspects of behavior of epidermoid carcinoma *in situ* and related lesions of the uterine cervix. *Cancer* **16,** 1160.
Kottmeier, H.L. (1959). Carcinoma of the cervix. *Acta. Obstet. Gynec. Scand.* **38,** 522.
—— (1961). Évolution et traitement des épithéliomas. *Rev. franç. Gynéc. Obstét.* **56,** 821.
Kraus, F.T. (1973). The biology of carcinoma *in situ* and microinvasive carcinoma of the cervix. In *The uterus* (ed. H.J. Norris, A.T. Hertig, and M.R. Abell), p. 348. Williams and Wilkins, Baltimore.
Laguens, R.P., Lagrutta, J., and Quijano, F. (1971). Fine structure of reserve cell hyperplasia and incomplete squamous metaplasia of the uterine cervix. *Int. J. Gynec. Obstet.* **9,** 41.
Lange, P. (1960). Clinical and histological studies on cervical carcinoma. *Acta path. microbiol. Scand.* **50,** Suppl. 143.
Langley, F.A. and Crompton, A.C. (1973). *Epithelial abnormalities of the cervix uteri.* Springer, Berlin.
Laverty, C.R., Russell, P., Hills, E., and Booth, N. (1978). The significance of noncondylomatous wart virus infection of the cervical transformation zone. A review with discussion of two illustrative cases. *Acta Cytol.* **22,** 195.
Marcus, S.L. (1960). Multiple squamous cell carcinomas involving the cervix, vagina, and vulva: the theory of multicentric origin. *Amer. J. Obstet. Gynec.* **80,** 802.
Masterson, J.G. (1957). An analysis of untreated intra-epithelial carcinoma of the cervix. *Proc. 3rd Nat. Cancer Conf,* p. 671. Lippincott, Philadelphia.
McDougall, J.K., Galloway, D.A., and Fenoglio, C.M. (1980). Cervical carcinoma: detection of herpes simplex virus RNA in cells undergoing neoplastic change. *Int. J. Cancer* **25,** 1.
McGee, J.O'D., Woods, J.C., Ashall, F., Bramwell, M.E., and Harris, H. (1982). A new marker for human cancer cells. 2, Immunohistological detection of the Ca antigen in human tissues with the Ca 1 antibody. *Lancet* **2,** 7.
McKay, D.G., Terjanian, B., Poschyachinda, D., Younge, P.A., and Hertig, A.T., (1959). Clinical and pathologic significance of anaplasia (atypical hyperplasia) of the cervix uteri. *Obstet. Gynec.* **13,** 2.
Meisels, A., Fortin, R., and Roy, M. (1977). Condylomatous lesions of the cervix. II Cytologic, colposcopic and histopathologic study. *Acta Cytol.* **21,** 379.
——, Roy, M., Fortier, M., Morin, C., Casas-Cordero, M., Shah, K.V., and Turgeon, H. (1981). Human papillomavirus infection of the cervix. The atypical condyloma. *Acta Cytol.* **25,** 7.
Miller, A.B., Lindsay, J., and Hill, G.B. (1976). Mortality from cancer of the uterus in Canada and its relationship to screening for cancer of the cervix. *Int. J. Cancer* **17,** 602.
Moricard, R. and Papatheodorou, B. (1953). Les anomalies de nombre et de position des chromosomes comme nouvelle méthode de diagnostic des épithéliomas intra-épithéliaux pavimenteux du col utérin en dehors de la gestation. *Gynec. Obstet.* **52,** 251.
Murray, R.F., Hobbs, J. and Payne, B. (1971). Possible clonal origin of common warts (Verruca vulgaris). *Nature* **232,** 51.
Naib, Z.M. (1966). Exfoliative cytology of viral cervico-vaginitis. *Acta Cytol.* **10,** 126.
Nasiell, K., Auer, G., Nasiell, M., and Zetterberg, A. (1979). Retrospective DNA analyses in cervical dysplasia as related to neoplastic progression or regression. *Anal. quant. Cytol.* **1,** 103.

——, Nasiell, M., Václavinkova, V., Roger, V., and Hjerpe, A. (1976). In *Health control in detection of cancer.* (ed. H. Boström, T. Larsson and N. Ljungstedt), p. 244. Almqvist and Wiksell, Stockholm.

Nelson, J.H., Averette, H.E., and Richart, R.M. (1975). *Detection, diagnostic evaluation and treatment of dysplasia and early carcinoma of the cervix.* Professional Education Publication, American Cancer Society.

Ng, A.B.P. and Reagan, J.W. (1969). Microinvasive carcinoma of the uterine cervix. *Amer. J. clin. Path.* **52**, 511.

Papanicolaou, G.N. (1954). *Atlas of exfoliative cytology.* Commonwealth Fund, Harvard University Press, Cambridge, Massachusetts.

—— and Traut, H.F. (1943). *Diagnosis of uterine cancer by the vaginal smear.* Commonwealth Fund, New York.

Park, I-J. and Jones, H.W. (1968). Glucose-6-phosphate dehydrogenase and the histogenesis of epidermoid carcinoma of the cervix. *Amer. J. Obstet. Gynec.* **102**, 106.

Parmentier, R. and Dustin, P. (1951). Reproduction expérimentale d'une anomalie particulière de la métaphase des cellules malignes (métaphase 'à trois groupes'). *Caryologia* **4**, 98.

Patten, S.F. (1966). Dysplasia of the uterine cervix. In *New concepts in gynecologic oncology* (ed. G.C. Lewis, W.B. Wentz, and R.M. Jaffe), p. 33. Davis, Philadelphia.

—— (1978). *Diagnostic cytopathology of the uterine cervix* (2nd edn). Karger, Basle.

Peckham, B. and Greene, R.R. (1957). Follow-up on cervical epithelial abnormalities. *Amer. J. Obstet. Gynec.* **74**, 804.

Petersen, O. (1955). Precancerous changes of the cervical epithelium. *Acta. Radiol. (Stockholm),* Suppl. 127.

Poulsen, H.E. and Taylor, C.W. (1975). *International histological typing of genital tract tumors.* World Health Organization, Geneva.

Purola, E. and Savia, E. (1977). Cytology of gynecologic condyloma acuminatum. *Acta Cytol.* **21**, 26.

Qizilbash, A.H. (1975). *In-situ* and microinvasive adenocarcinoma of the uterine cervix. *Amer. J. clin. Pathol.* **64**, 155.

Rawls, W.E., Tomkins, W.A.F., and Melnick, J.L. (1969). The association of herpesvirus Type 2 and carcinoma of the uterine cervix. *Amer. J. Epidemiol.* **89**, 547.

Reagan, J.W. and Hicks, D.J. (1953). A study of *in situ* and squamous-cell cancer of the uterine cervix. *Cancer* **6**, 1200.

——, Seidemann, I.L., and Saracusa, Y. (1953). The cellular morphology of carcinoma *in situ* and dysplasia or atypical hyperplasia of the uterine cervix. *Cancer* **6**, 224.

Reid, B.L. (1964). The behaviour of human sperm toward cultured fragments of human cervix uteri. *Lancet* **1**, 21.

Reid, R., Laverty, C.R., Coppleson, M., Isarangkul, W., and Hills, E. (1980). Non-condylomatous cervical wart virus infection. *Obstet. Gynecol.* **55**, 476.

Reid, R., Stanhope, R., Herschman, B.R., Booth, E., Phibbs, G.D., and Smith, J.P. (1982). Genital warts and cervical cancer. I. Evidence of an association between subclinical papilloma virus infection and cervical malignancy. *Cancer* **50**, 377.

Richart, R.M. (1963). A radioautographic analysis of cellular proliferation in dysplasia and carcinoma *in situ* of the uterine cervix. *Amer. J. Obstet. Gynec.* **86**, 925.

—— (1967). Natural history of cervical intraepithelial neoplasia. *Clinical Obstet. Gynecol.* **10**, 748.
—— and Barron, B.A. (1969). A follow-up study of patients with cervical dysplasia. *Amer. J. Obstet. Gynec.* **105**, 386.
Riotton, G. and Christopherson, W.M. (ed.) (1973). *Cytology of the female genital tract.* Int. Histological Classification of Tumours, No. 8. World Health Organization, Geneva.
Sachs, H. and Schittko, G. (1975). Zytofotometrisch ermittlelte DNS-Muster in präkanzerösen Dysplasien der Cervix uteri. *Arch. Gynäk.* **218**, 95.
Sandritter, W. and Fischer, R. (1962). Der DNS-Gehalt des normalen Plattenepithels, des Carcinoma *in situ* und des invasion Carcinoms der Portio. In *Proc. 1st Int. Congr. Exfol. Cytol.* (*Vienna 1961*), p. 189. Lippincott, Philadelphia.
Schauenstein, W. (1908). Histologische Untersuchungen über atypisches Plattenepithel an der Portio und an der Innenfläche der Cervix uteri. *Arch. Gynäk.* **85**, 576.
Schiller, W. (1933). Early diagnosis of carcinoma of cervix. *Surg. Gynecol. Obstet.* **56**, 210.
Schottlaender, J. and Kermauner, F. (1912). *Zur Kenntnis des Uteruskarzinoms.* Karger, Berlin.
Scott, R.B. and Ballard, L.A. (1962). Problems of cervical biopsy. *Ann. NY Acad. Sci.* **97**, 767.
Sedlis, A., Cohen, A., and Sall, S. (1970). The fate of cervical dysplasia. *Amer. J. Obstet. Gynec.* **107**, 1065.
Seth, P. and Balachandran, N. (1980). Elution of herpes simplex virus-specific cytotoxic antibodies from squamous cell carcinoma of the uterine cervix. *Nature* **286**, 613.
Shah, K.H., Lewis, M.G., Jenson, A.B. *et al.* (1980). Papillomavirus and cervical dysplasia. *Lancet* **2**, 1190.
Shevchuk, M.M. and Richart, R.M. (1982). DNA content of condyloma acuminatum. *Cancer* **49**, 489.
Shingleton, H.M., Richart, R.M., Wiener, J., and Spiro, D. (1968). Human cervical intraepithelial neoplasia. Fine structure of dysplasia and carcinoma *in situ. Cancer Res.* **28**, 695.
Simon, T.R. and Sheehan, J.F. (1962). Reversible atypia of cervical epithelium. In *Proc. 1st Int. Congr. Exfol. Cytol. (Vienna 1961),* p. 116. Lippincott, Philadelphia.
Skegg, D.C.G., Corwin, P.A., Paul, C., and Doll, R. (1982). Importance of the male factor in cancer of the cervix. *Lancet* **2**, 581.
Skinner, G. (1976). Viral infections. In *The cervix* (ed. J.A. Jordan and A. Singer), p. 269. Saunders, London.
Sloane, J.P. and Ormerod, M.G. (1981). Distribution of epithelial membrane antigen in normal and neoplastic tissues and its value in diagnostic tumour pathology. *Cancer* **47**, 1786.
—— ——, Carter, R.L., Gusterson, B.A., and Foster, C.S. (1982). An immunocytochemical study of the distribution of epithelial membrane antigen in normal and disordered squamous epithelium. *Diag. Histopathol.* **5**, 11.
Smith, C. (1978). Carcinoma *in situ. Human Pathol.* **9**, 373.
Smith, J.W., Townsend, D.E., and Sparkes, R.S. (1971). Genetic variants of glucose-6-phosphate dehydrogenase in the study of carcinoma of the cervix. *Cancer* **28**, 529.
Spriggs, A.I. (1974). Cytogenetics of cancer and precancerous states of the cervix uteri. In *Chromosomes and cancer* (ed. J. German), p. 423. Wiley, New York.
——, Bowey, C.E., and Cowdell, R.H. (1971). Chromosomes of precancerous lesions of the cervix uteri. *Cancer* **27**, 1239.

—— and Cowdell, R.H. (1972). Ring chromosomes in carcinoma *in situ* of the cervix as evidence of clonal growth. *J. Obstet. Gynaec. Brit. Cwlth.* **79**, 833.
——, Butler, E.B., Evans, D.M.D., Grubb, C., Husain, O.A.N., and Wachtel, G.E. (1978). Problems of cell nomenclature in cervical cytology smears. *J. clin. Pathol.* **31**, 1226.
—— and Boddington, M.M. (1980). Progression and regression of cervical lesions. *J. clin. Pathol.* **33**, 517.
Stern, E. (1959). Rate, stage and patient age in cervical cancer. *Cancer* **12**, 933.
—— and Neely, P.M. (1964). Dysplasia of the uterine cervix. Incidence of regression, recurrence and cancer. *Cancer* **17**, 508.
Thiry, L. (1976). Herpes simplex virus and carcinoma of the cervix. *Eur. J. Cancer* **12**, 851.
Thomas, D.B. and Rawls, W.E. (1978). Relationship of Herpes simplex virus Type-2 antibodies and squamous dysplasia to cervical carcinoma *in situ. Cancer* **42**, 2716.
Timonen, S. (1955). Prophase index in the diagnosis of gynaecological cancer. *Ann. chir. gynaec. Fenn.* **4**, 222.
Villa Santa, U. (1971). Diagnosis and prognosis of cervical dysplasia. *Obset. Gynecol.* **38**, 811.
Wagner, D., Sprenger, E., and Blank, M.H. (1972). DNA-content of dysplastic cells of the uterine cervix. *Acta. Cytol.* **16**, 517.
—— ——, and Merkle, D. (1976). Cytophotometric studies in suspicious cervical smears. *Acta Cytol.* **20**, 366.
Walton, R.J. (Chairman) (1976). Cervical cancer screening programs. The Walton Report. *Can. med. Assoc. J.* **114**, 1003.
Wentz, W.B. (1962). The significance of mucosal lesions antedating mouse cervical cancer. *Amer. J. Obstet. Gynecol.* **84**, 1506.
——, Reagan, J.W., Fu, Y-S., Heggie, A.D., and Anthony, D.D. (1981). Experimental studies of carcinogenesis of the uterine cervix in mice. *Gynecol. Oncol.* **12**, S90.
Wilbanks, G.D. and Fink, C.G. (1976). Tissue and organ culture of cervical epithelium—physiological and preinvasive. In *The cervix* (ed. J.A. Jordan and A. Singer). p. 429. Saunders, London.

13 Endometrial hyperplasia and endometrial carcinoma: morphological and pathogenic considerations

Alex Ferenczy and Morrie M. Gelfand

Issues of major interest in the field of endometrial cancer centre on the pathologist's ability to distinguish between early carcinoma and adenomatous hyperplasia, its presumed precursor, and on the precise pathogenic relationship between these abnormal endometrial proliferations and ovarian hormonal influences. Morphological distinction between early endometrial neoplasia and florid hyperplasia is difficult, partly because of the complex histological configuration of endometrial glands and partly because of the inconspicuous cytological alterations which may accompany early malignancy. These problems lead to the use of subjective rather than objective morphological criteria for pre-invasive neoplasms of the endometrium and have resulted in a variety of ill-defined terms such as adenomatous hyperplasia, atypical adenomatous hyperplasia, dysplasia, and carcinoma *in situ*. Confusion is compounded by the fact that many benign endometrial conditions as well as normal endometrium in various phases of the menstrual cycle may be misinterpreted as hyperplasia or even as well-differentiated adenocarcinoma. The lack of adequate long-term follow-up data on women with (putative) precursor lesions of endometrial carcinoma provides another reason for our fragmentary knowledge and understanding of the natural history of endometrial hyperplasia and carcinoma. The available prospective studies suffer from poor diagnostic ascertainment, small numbers of cases, and short follow-up periods which preclude adequate statistical analysis (Ferenczy 1978). There are no obvious ways to improve prospective documentation of precursor lesions because, once discovered, they will be treated with progestogens or by curettage with or without subsequent hysterectomy. As a result, long-term follow-up of a large number of undisturbed precursor lesions cannot be carried out. Because of these inescapable limitations of clinical studies, investigators have turned to laboratory studies to gain insight into the morphology and biological significance of early carcinoma and its precursors.

In recent years, a series of comparative ultrastructural (Ferenczy 1977, 1980*b*), kinetic (Ferenczy 1979, 1980*b*; Ferenczy *et al.* 1979), and sex-steroid receptor analyses (Ferenczy 1980*b*; King 1978; Vihko *et al.* 1978) have been carried out in normal, hyperplastic, and neoplastic endometrial tissues. The specific aims of this work were to provide objective histologic criteria for distinguishing between early endometrial neoplasia and its presumed precursors, and to assess whether the development of such lesions is related to hormonal influences. Since disease states represent exaggeration of or deviation from normal biological events, a thorough knowledge of the normal endometrium is essential for any evaluation of pathological endometrial tissues. In the following account we review the results so far obtained from examining over 200 specimens of normal and abnormal endometria together with findings obtained from Feulgen-DNA microspectrophotometry (Hustin 1976; Wagner *et al.* 1967), histochemistry (Dallenbach-Hellweg 1971; Henzl *et al.* 1972; Prianishnikov 1978), and blood steroid biochemistry (Hutton *et al.* 1979; King 1978; MacDonald *et al.* 1978). Epidemiological observations are also discussed (Gusberg 1980; Hulka *et al.* 1980; Lucas 1974; Silverberg and Major 1978).

Endometrial cytodynamics

Normal endometrium

Endometrium prior to ovulation is a proliferating tissue with a diploid-to-tetraploid nuclear DNA content (Wagner *et al.* 1967), elevated labelling index (Fig. 13.1(a); Table 13.1), and numerous mitoses in the nuclei of gland cells, stromal fibroblasts, and vascular endothelium (Ferenczy *et al.* 1979). In the transmission electron microscope (Ferenczy 1977), the cytoplasm of the gland cells is seen to contain abundant free and bound ribosomes, Golgi, mitochondria, primary lysosomes rich in acid phophatase (Henzl *et al.* 1972), and microfilaments which presumably help to support their tall cytoplasmic substance. Proliferating gland cells have low monoamine oxidase and high alkaline phosphatase activity (Prianishnikov 1978). The formation of cilia and surface microvilli is prominent in proliferative endometrial glandular epithelium and is well demonstrated by scanning electron microscopy (Ferenczy 1977; see Fig. 13.1(b)). Cilia are considerably reduced in gland cells during the progestational phase of the menstrual cycle as well as in castrated women or animals, and they reappear when exogenous oestrogens are administered: their development is thus regarded as one of the most sensitive morphological indicators of endometrial response to oestrogenic stimulation (Ferenczy 1977). Receptors for oestradiol and progesterone are elevated (Table 13.2), particularly in late proliferative endometrium (Ferenczy 1980*b*; King 1978; Vihko *et al.* 1978). All these alterations are presumably produced by oestradiol (E_2)-stimulated, DNA-dependent RNA synthesis (Vihko *et al.* 1978). During the proliferative phase of the menstrual cycle, plasma oestradiol-17β (E_2) and, to a lesser degree, oestrone (E_1) are elevated (Hutton *et al.* 1979; King 1978).

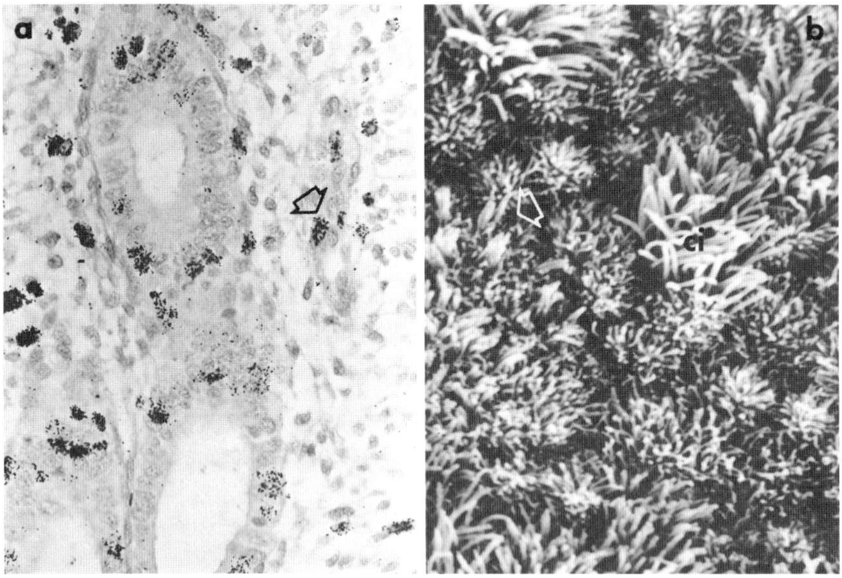

Fig. 13.1. Proliferative endometrium, cycle days 8-10. (a) Historadioautograph of heavily labelled nuclei of gland cells, stromal fibroblasts, and vascular endothelium (arrow). ×188. H & E. (b) Scanning electron micrograph of surface epithelium with numerous ciliated cells (ci) mixed with nonciliated microvillous cells. Arrow points to cell in early phase of ciliogenesis. ×2250.

In early secretory-phase endometrium, the effects of progesterone are manifest in the gland cells by the appearance of intraepithelial glycogen-containing vacuoles in a subnuclear location. Ultrastructually, the mitochondria assume giant forms and the nuclei and nucleoli contain basket-like channel systems (Ferenczy 1977); see Fig. 13.2(a)). The latter are unique to the post-ovulatory human endometrium but their significance is unknown. By day 19 of the cycle, the epithelial cells are engaged in glycoprotein synthesis which involves the ergastoplasm-glycogen-mitochondria-Golgi complex; monoamine oxidase and steroid-17β-dehydrogenase activities are elevated as well as enzymes related to oxidative phosphorylation (Prianishnikov 1978). Coinciding with intraluminal gland secretion, DNA synthesis declines and mitotic figures are no longer seen (Ferenczy *et al.* 1979), Fig. 13.2(b)). Surface microvilli become shorter and fewer and ciliated cells are limited almost exclusively to the endometrial surface epithelium (Ferenczy 1977). From day 25 onwards, the blastocyst-free endometrium undergoes gradual involution and dehiscence, a process mediated by lysosomal enzymes (Henzl *et al.* 1972). Progesterone is a potent membrane stabilizer of E_2-produced primary lysosomes. Coinciding with the premenstrual fall of plasma progesterone, lysosomal membrane integrity is impaired and release of acid hydrolases is stimulated. This results in the enzymatic digestion and destruction of the glandular epithelium, predecidual stromal cells, and local

Table 13.1. *Ultrastructural characteristics of normal and abnormal endometrium*

Glandular epithelium	Cyclic proliferative	APPEM	CGH	AH	AAH	CIS	AC
Organelles	2+	4+	3+	3+	Increasingly pleomorphic		
Microfilaments	1+	2+	2+	3+	Increasingly disorganized		
Primary lysosomes	2+	4+	3+	3+	2+	1+	1+
Autophagocytosis	0/1+	1+	1+	1+	1-2+	2+	3+
Ciliogenesis	2+	4+	3+	3+	2-3+	2+	1+
Microvillogenesis	1+	4+	3+	3+	2-3+	1+	1+
Nuclear membrane	Regular			Slightly irregular	Increasingly irregular		
Plasma membrane	Regular to slightly convoluted			Slightly convoluted	Increasingly convoluted		

Abbreviations. APPEM, anovulatory persistent proliferative endometrium; CGH, cystic glandular hyperplasia; AH, adenomatous hyperplasia; AAH, adenomatous hyperplasia with severe cytological atypia; CIS, carcinoma *in situ*; AC, invasive adenocarcinoma.

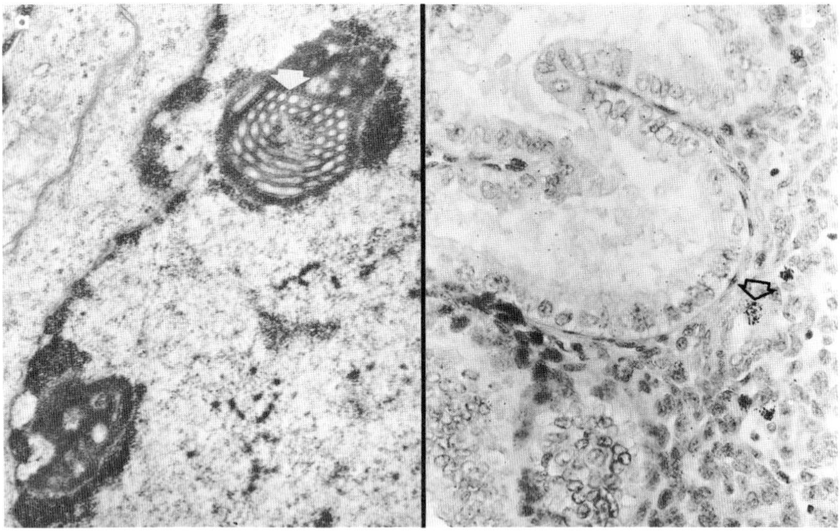

Fig. 13.2. Secretory endometrium, cycle day 19. (a) Interanastomosing hollow tubules of nuclear membrane origin form the so-called nucleolar channel system seen in one of the nucleoli (arrow) of a gland cell. ×6400. (b) Historadioautograph of secretory gland cells devoid of nuclear labelling. Incorporated radiothymidine in nuclei of vascular endothelial cells (arrow) ×160. H & E.

blood vessels (Ferenczy 1977; Ferenczy 1980*a*; Henzl *et al.* 1972). Low progesterone levels, injury to endothelial membranes, and acute inflammation in the late secretory-phase endometrium are likely to promote prostaglandin-mediated vascular contraction and thrombosis, leading to local tissue anoxia and necrosis. In summary, progesterone promotes secretory differentiation of oestrogen-primed proliferative endometrium and inhibits DNA synthesis and mitotic activity—presumably by lengthening the DNA-synthesis phase and by eventually inducing the epithelial cells to enter the G_0, non-dividing stage of cell cycle (Ferenczy 1980*a*). The anti-proliferative effect of progesterone in the human is in agreement with experimental observations. In the animal model, secretory differentiation of the endometrium is associated with arrest of cell growth followed by death of tissue (Epifanova 1971).

Hyperplastic endometrium

Hyperplastic endometria have been examined by conventional histology (Dallenbach-Hellweg 1971; Ferenczy 1980*b*; Welch and Scully, 1977) and by the more specialized techniques of transmission- and scanning-electron microscopy (Ferenczy 1977), Feulgen-DNA-microspectrophotometry (Wagner *et al.* 1967), short-term incubation *in vitro* DNA historadioautography (Ferenczy 1979), 1980*b*), and specific receptor binding of E_2 and progesterone (Ferenczy 1980*b*; King 1978; Vihko *et al.* 1978). The overall results of these studies indicate that (in women who are presumed to be genetically predisposed to abnormal endometrial growth) endometrial hyperplasia represents a spectrum of changes that are intermediate between cyclic proliferative endometrium and carcinoma. Both cytodynamically and biologically, the development of endometrial hyperplasia may be subdivided into two phases: a proliferative, oestrogen-sensitive phase followed by a remodelling, relatively oestrogen-refractory phase (Ferenczy 1980*b*). The first proliferative phase consists of an absolute increase in the volume of endometrial mucosa including glandular and vascular elements as well as stromal fibroblasts. The general organization of such endometrium shows minimal architectural deviation from normal, pre-ovulatory endometrium and the changes are commonly referred to as anovulatory, persistent, proliferative endometrium (APPEM) (see Fig. 13.3(a)-(d)). Other workers prefer the term simple glandular hyperplasia (Silverberg and Major 1978). In the transmission electron microscope, there is an increase in intracytoplasmic organelles, cilia, and alkaline phosphatase-rich microvilli (Fig. 13.4(a),(b)) compared to normal proliferative endometrium (Table 13.1). Mitotic activity is conspicuous (Fig. 13.3(d)) and the nuclei of gland cells, stromal fibroblasts, and vascular endometrium avidly incorporate the nucleoprotein precursor tritiated (^{3}H)-thymidine (Fig. 13.5(a),(b)). The DNA-S phase of the cell cycle and the potential doubling time in APPEM are considerably shortened (Table 13.2). These structural and kinetic modifications are consistent with an exaggerated response of the endometrium to E_2 stimulation, and the demonstration of raised concentrations of E_2 and progesterone receptors—particularly the latter—supports this view (see Table 13.2).

APPEM may show focal or less frequently diffuse glandular dilatation leading to focal or diffuse cystic glandular hyperplasia (Fig. 13.6). In cystic glandular hyperplasia, the epithelial cells lining *non-dilated* glands and stromal fibroblasts both show ultrastructural, biochemical, and kinetic alterations which are similar to those of APPEM (Ferenczy 1977, 1980*b*). By contrast, the epithelium lining the cystically dilated glands demonstrates comparatively fewer active proliferative features so that the overall morphobiochemical characteristics of cystic glandular hyperplasia are somewhat reduced compared to APPEM (Tables 13.1 and 13.2).

The proliferative phase of endometrial hyperplasia is clinically unstable and it is not considered to be a direct precursor of endometrial carcinoma. Most symptomatic lesions revert to normal following a thorough curettage whereas the asymptomatic (and thus untreated) variant gradually regresses to atrophy. Such lesions are recognized in hysterectomy or autopsy specimens as regions of thickened, polypoid endometrium in which the stroma is hyalinized and the cystically dilated glands are lined by atrophic epithelium (personal observation). McBride (1955) followed 544 premenopausal women with cystic glandular hyperplasia prospectively over a 24-year period and reported an incidence of endometrial carcinoma of 0.4 per cent, a rate closely similar to that of the general postmenopausal population. On the

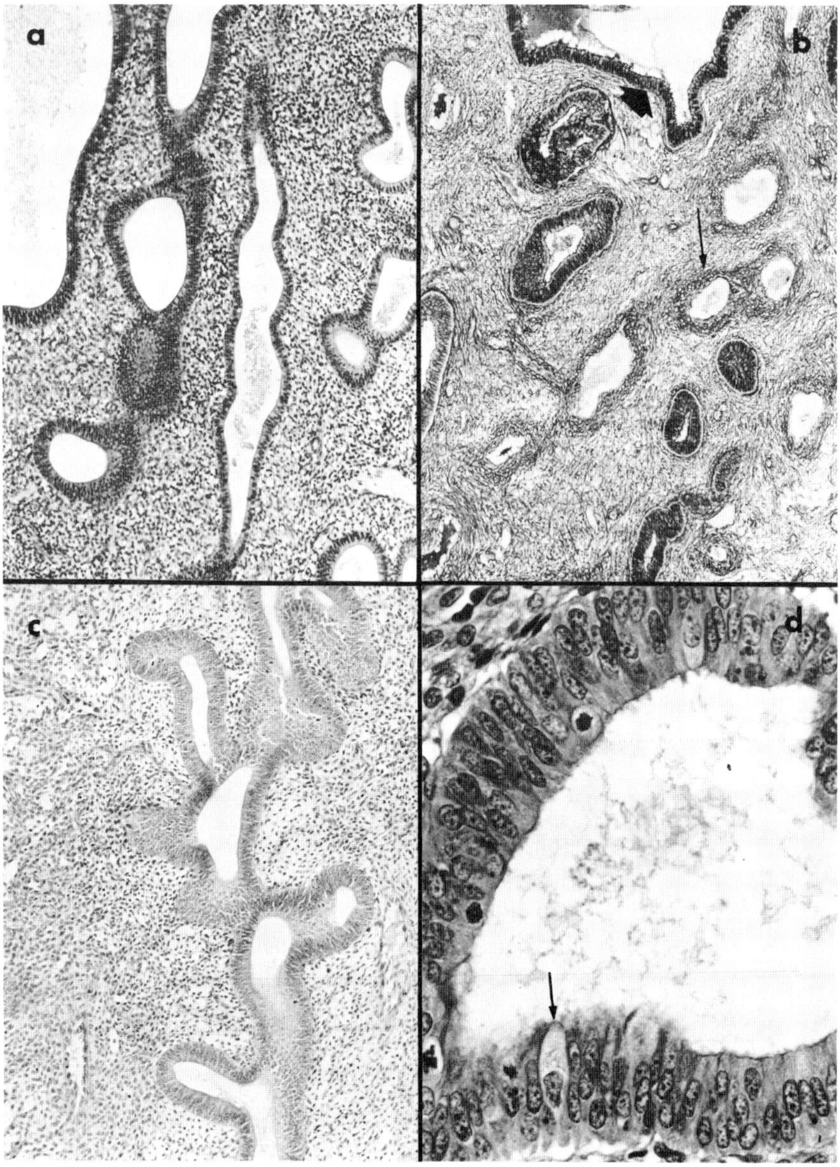

Fig. 13.3. Anovulatory persistent proliferative endometrium. (a) Thickened endometrial mucosa with voluminous glands and compact stroma. In these cases biopsy or curettage yield uniformly abundant tissue. The gland-stroma ratio is normal and architectural alterations in the glands are minimal. ×75. H & E. (b) Cystic dilatation of glands (large arrow) in focal areas (involving less than 15 per cent of endometrial mucosa). Perivascular (pericytic) thickening (fine arrow) and vascular ectasia are often seen in APPEM. ×75. Weigert. (c) Note lateral buddings into stroma. ×112. H & E. (d) Gland cells are taller and the nuclei more pseudostratified than their cyclic, proliferative counterparts. But the pencil-shaped nuclear pattern, finely granular and evenly distributed chromatin, and inconspicuous nucleoli are features similar to nuclei from normal proliferative endometrial glands. Mitoses and ciliated cell precursors with clear cytoplasm (arrow) are frequently seen. ×262. H & E.

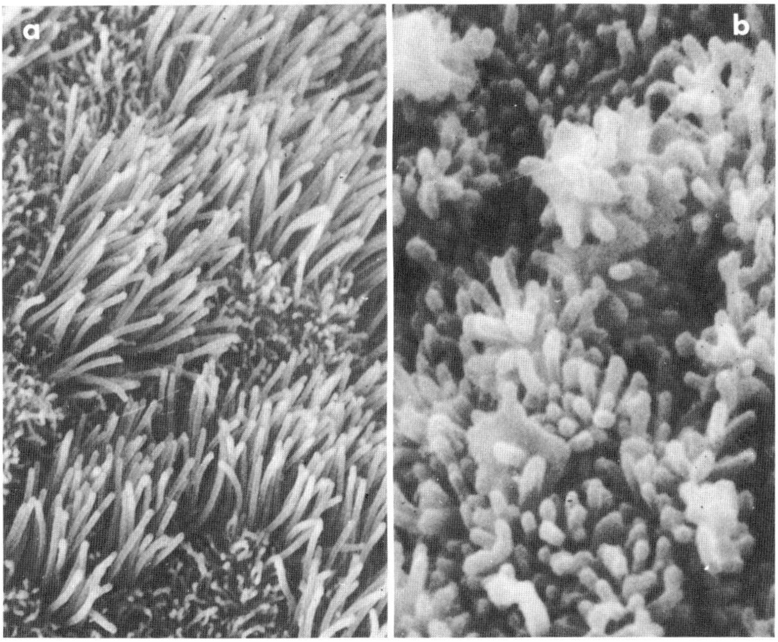

Fig. 13.4. Anovulatory persistent proliferative endometrium. (a) Ciliated cells are increased compared to cyclic proliferative endometrium ×3500. (b) Hair-like surface microvilli are more abundant, taller, and interbranching than in cyclic proliferative endometrium. ×14 000.

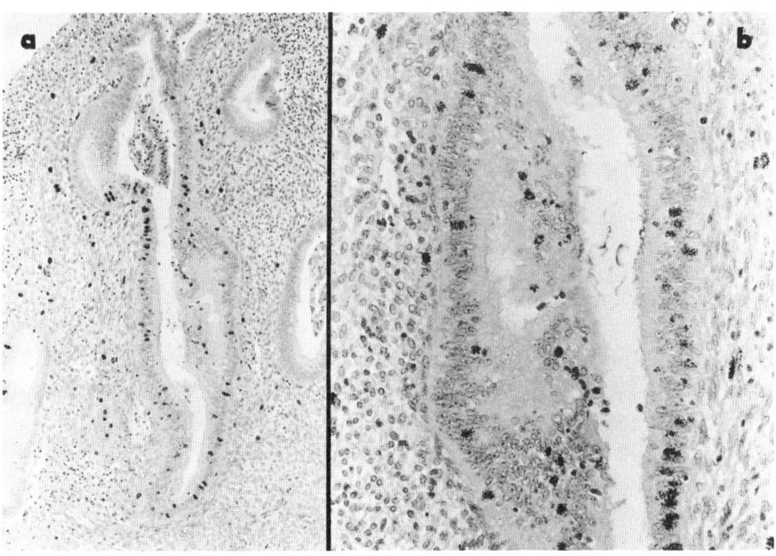

Fig. 13.5. Anovulatory persistent proliferative endometrium. (a) Historadioautograph of voluminous glands lined by columnar cells with heavily labelled nuclei. ×70. H & E. (b) Higher magnification of radiothymidine-labelled nuclei of gland cells and stromal fibroblasts. ×140. H & E.

Table 13.2. *Mean proliferation kinetics and sex-steroid receptor concentrations of normal and abnormal endometrium*

Histology	Kinetics			Progesterone receptors[a] (Fmoles/mg protein)
	LI (per cent)	DNA-S PHASE (hr)	$TpD = \frac{\lambda S}{LI}$ (hr)	
Proliferative (18)	7.5±3.5	7.9±2.3	94.6±15	1131±206
APPEM (11)	8.0±2.1	4.7±1.1	41.1± 7	1180±260
CGH (4)	6.8±2.3	5.3±2.6	59.7±11	900±230
AH (8)	3.8±1.9	6.5±3.0	119.7±14	609±185
AAH (6)	7.7±3.8	8.5±3.5	77.2±10	300±105
CIS (6)	7.4±3.0	12.8±5.1	121.0±19	300±105
AC (39)	7.9±2.5	13.2±5.0	116.9±23	308± 94

LI, labelling index; ±, mean standard errors; TpD, potential doubling time; λ, growth constant 1.0 for normal and 0.7 for hyperplastic-neoplastic tissue; Fmoles, femtomoles; brackets contain number of cases; other abbreviations as in Table 13.1.

[a]Progesterone receptors were measured by Dr G. Shymala, Lady Davis Institute for Medical Research, Montreal using dextran-coated charcoal-binding assays and R5020 as the ligand.

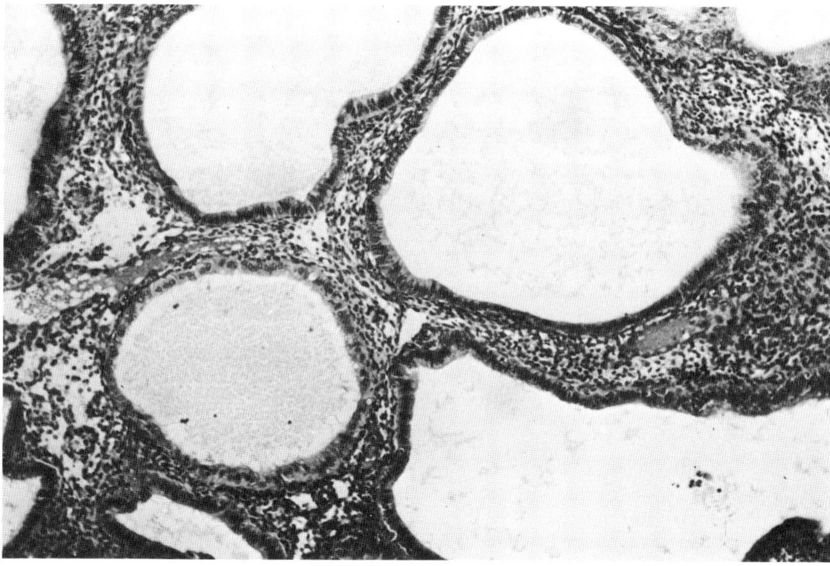

Fig. 13.6. Cystic glandular hyperplasia. The glands are cystically dilated and the intervening stroma is compact. ×70. H & E.

other hand, a definite, but as yet imprecisely defined, proportion of APPEM and cystic glandular hyperplasia may persist, or recur, or progress to the second (remodelling) phase of endometrial hyperplasia. In this phase, architectural changes develop in the glands, cytonuclear atypia is seen in their lining epithelium, and the volume of endometrial stroma gradually decreases in favour of the glands. Such hyperplastic endometrium tends to persist rather than regress and occasionally it progresses to carcinoma. Although standard terminology for this stage of endometrial hyperplasia has not yet been adopted, the changes range from adenomatous hyperplasia without atypia to adenomatous hyperplasias with increasing cytological and architectural abnormalities.

Light- (Welsh *et al.* 1977) and electron-microscopic (Ferenczy 1977, 1980*b*) studies of adenomatous hyperplasia show a spectrum of cytonuclear and histological abnormalities. In adenomatous hyperplasia, the glands are voluminous and convoluted with epithelial extensions into the adjacent stroma. In many instances they assume a Y-shaped configuration (Fig. 13.7 (a)). In adenomatous hyperplasia without significant cytological atypia, the cells are tall columnar with pseudostratified, pencil-shaped nuclei (Fig. 13.7(b)). The resulting appearance of nuclear hyperchromasia is apparent rather than real: the nuclear chromatin is finely granular and evenly distributed with a normal diploid-to-tetraploid DNA content (Wagner *et al.* 1967). Ciliated cells are generally numerous. Clusters of foam cells can be found in the stroma (Ferenczy 1977), the significance of which is unclear. According to certain investigators (Dallenbach-Hellweg 1971), oestrogenic

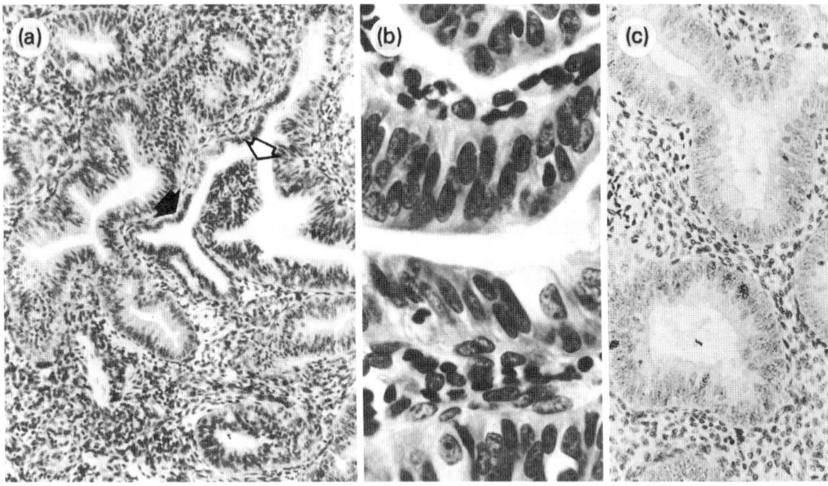

Fig.13.7 Adenomatous hyperplasia (AH) without cytologic atypia. (a) Glands with complex epithelial buddings into stroma (solid arrow) and lumen (empty arrow). Note that such growth pattern produces a Y-shaped configuration of glands. The gland-stroma ratio is in favour of glands. Despite architectural atypia, the lining cells and nuclei are closely similar to those of APPEM. ×32. H & E. (b) Detailed view of nuclei devoid of significant atypia. Nucleoli are slightly larger than in APPEM. ×256. H & E. (c) Radioisotope uptake is reduced compared to APPEM or normal proliferative endometrium. ×160. H & E.

influence unopposed by progesterone may lead to accumulation of cholesterol-containing lipid bodies within endometrial stromal fibroblasts. ^{3}H-thymidine uptake is significantly reduced in adenomatous hyperplasia (Table 13.2) compared to APPEM and cystic glandular hyperplasia, and so are mitotic figures (Fig. 13.7(c)). The DNA-S phase and the potential doubling time both last longer in adenomatous hyperplasia than in APPEM (Table 13.2). At the ultrastructural level, E_2-related changes are similar to those seen in cystic glandular hyperplasia but they appear slightly decreased compared to APPEM. The nuclear and plasma membranes show increased convolutions (Table 13.1). The relative decrease in DNA synthesis and mitotic activity together with lower concentrations of progesterone receptors (Table 13.2) in adenomatous hyperplasia without atypia, compared with APPEM and cystic glandular hyperplasia, suggest diminished oestrogenic responsiveness of this type of hyperplastic endometrium compared to the normal proliferative phase of endometrial hyperplasia or to APPEM.

A certain proportion of adenomatous hyperplasias, particularly in older women, present with considerable architectural and cytonuclear atypia. Such lesions are characterized histologically by extensive extraglandular and intraglandular epithelial budding and crowding of voluminous glands (Fig. 13.8(a)). The height of the lining epithelium is decreased and the diameter of cells is larger compared to adenomatous hyperplasia without atypia, APPEM, or cystic glandular hyperplasia. There is rounding and pleomorphism of nuclei, the nuclear chromatin is coarse, and the nucleoli are larger (Fig. 13.8(b)). Microabscesses in the tips of intraglandular epithelial proliferations may be encountered. Mitoses may be numerous, particularly in women on oestrogen replacement therapy. Ciliated cells are fewer than in hyperplastic endometrial glands devoid of atypia. Since it is *cytological* rather than architectural alterations that are believed to be significant in evaluating progression to carcinoma (Ferenczy 1978), subdivision of these alterations into mild, moderate, and severe (Table 13.3) may be pertinent. Such subdivision is, however, difficult and may be biased by the quality of fixation and sectioning of endometrial samples as well as by the cytologic interpretation of gland cells in histological sections. (In our laboratory, endometrial biopsies and curettings are fixed in Bouin's or Zenker's solution, both of which enhance preservation of cytological details; fixation in 10 per cent formalin solution gives less satisfactory results.) Morphological interpretation including the grading of atypia is confined to the functionalis layer (the upper two-third) of the body or fundus endometrium which contains at least ten hyperplastic glands. To achieve reproducibility, grading atypia is based on the quantitative evaluation of gland cells containing the greatest degree of cytological abnormality. On an arbitrary basis, adenomatous hyperplasia with mild, moderate, and severe atypia contains respectively less than 15, 30, and over 30 per cent of glands lined partly or

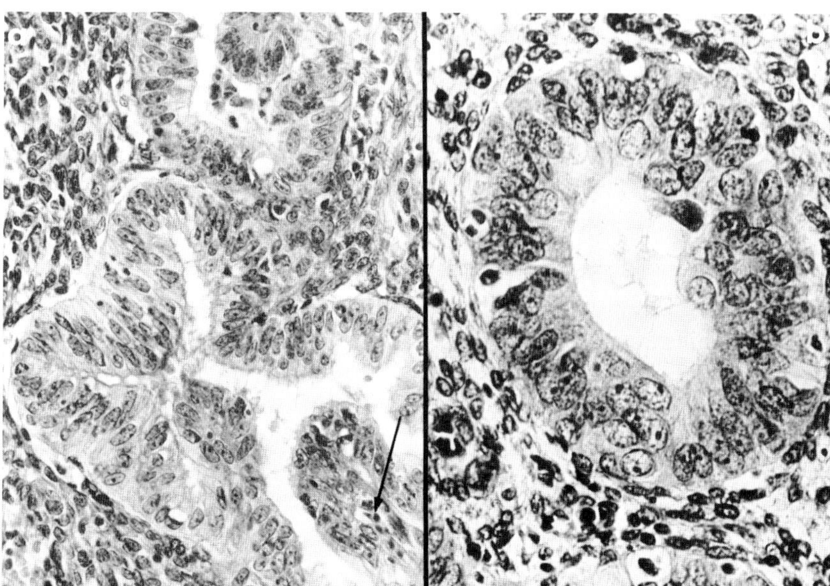

Fig. 13.8. Adenomatous hyperplasia with severe cytological atypia. (a) In contrast to the appearances in carcinoma *in situ*, intraluminal epithelial papillary projections are supported by fine stromal cores (arrows). ×195. H & E. (b) Note rounding of nuclei, disturbed nuclear cohesion and organization, coarse, granular chromatin, and enlarged nucleoli. ×350. H & E.

Table 13.3. *Pathogenic classification of endometrial hyperplasia*[a]

Anovulatory persistent proliferative endometrium (simple hyperplasia)
Cystic glandular hyperplasia
Adenomatous hyperplasia
Adenomatous hyperplasia with cytological atypia
Mild
Moderate
Severe
Polyp

[a] All forms may be focal or diffuse, or mixed, or contain squamous metaplasia, or show retrogressive or atrophic features, or evidence of glycogenization.

completely by atypical cells (Fig. 13.8(b)). Although precise correlation between the varying degrees of atypia and the biological behaviour of adenomatous hyperplasia is not yet available, our preliminary results (Ferenczy 1980*a*) and estimates by others (Gusberg 1980; Silverberg and Major 1978) suggest that the greater the atypia, the greater the progression rate to carcinoma; persistence and recurrence rates following curettage and/or progestogen treatment are also increased. The histological alterations of adenomatous hyperplasia with atypia are accompanied by significant ultrastructural abnormalities (Table 13.1). Compared to APPEM, cystic glandular hyperplasia, and adenomatous hyperplasia without significant atypia, the DNA-S phase is prolonged and the concentrations of progesterone receptors are reduced (Table 13.2). Indeed, the cytological, ultrastructural, and kinetic characteristics of adenomatous hyperplasia with severe cytological atypia appear intermediate between adenomatous hyperplasia without atypia and carcinoma *in situ.* Intermediate duration of DNA-S phase has been reported in other precursor lesions in sites such as the gastrointestinal tract and skin (Cavasto *et al.* 1971). These observations support the view that adenomatous hyperplasia with atypia is a precursor of *in situ* carcinoma and thus a significant risk factor in endometrial carcinoma (Gusberg 1980).

The available literature on prospective studies reveals that between 10 per cent (Ferenczy 1978) and 30 per cent (Gusberg 1980) of women with untreated adenomatous hyperplasia with atypia may progress to carcinoma. The finding of 17 to 43 per cent of endometrial carcinomas in association with cystic glandular hyperplasia, adenomatous hyperplasia, adenomatous hyperplasia with atypia, and carcinoma *in situ* (Ferenczy 1978) also supports a pathogenic interrelationship. The remaining adenocarcinomas are either diffuse, devoid of adjacent intact endometrium, or associated with atrophic endometrium. In the latter instances, however, thorough sampling of the uterus frequently reveals foci of remote hyperplastic endometrium and/or polyps with regressive atrophic features (Fig. 13.9). It is thus conceivable

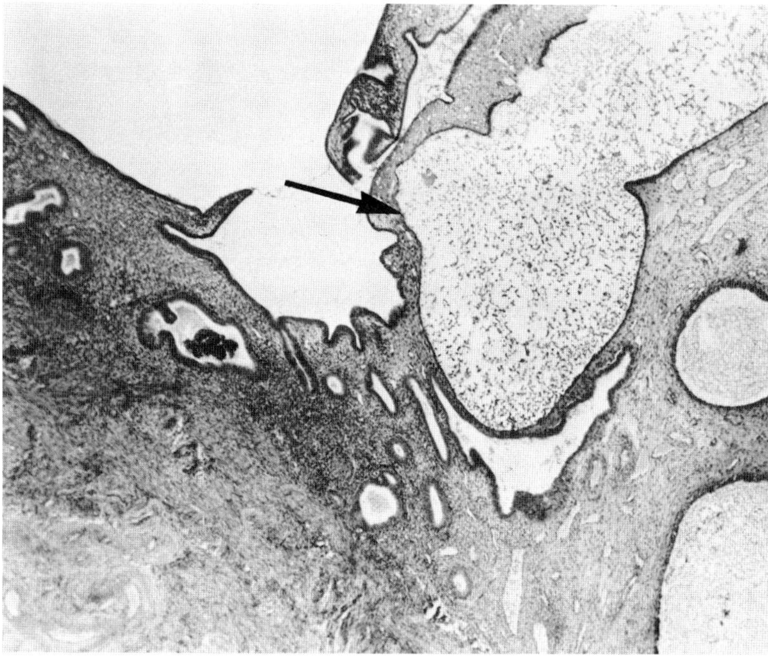

Fig.13.9. Polypoid endometrium with retrogressive atrophic features. Arrow points to thickened mucosa with hyalinized stroma. The cystically dilated glands are lined by atrophic epithelium. Such findings are consistent with remote focal hyperplasia or polyp. The adjacent endometrium is thin and atrophic. A bulky carcinoma, not shown in the photomicrograph, occupied the fundus of the uterus. ×100. H & E.

that such carcinomas arose in a hyperplastic focus which was then obliterated by neoplastic growth.

All forms of endometrial hyperplasia may present as a distinct focal polypoid growth containing hyperplastic changes similar to those in the adjacent endometrium. Polyps *per se* are not considered to be precursors of corpus carcinoma. A classification of endometrial hyperplasias based on the morphological and biological characteristics that have been outlined here is presented in Table 13.3.

Neoplastic endometrium

Since the original description of carcinoma *in situ* of the endometrium by Hertig *et al.* in 1949, its existence has remained highly controversial. The current data obtained from modern investigations confirm its existence and provide objective criteria for its histological recognition. Endometrial carcinoma *in situ* is characterized by large glands distended by extensive intraluminal projections; many of them fuse to produce the so-called 'gland in gland' or 'cribriform' pattern according to whether fusion is partial or involves the entire glandular apparatus (Fig. 13.10(a),(b)). These architectural alterations are the most distinctive histological features of the lesion.

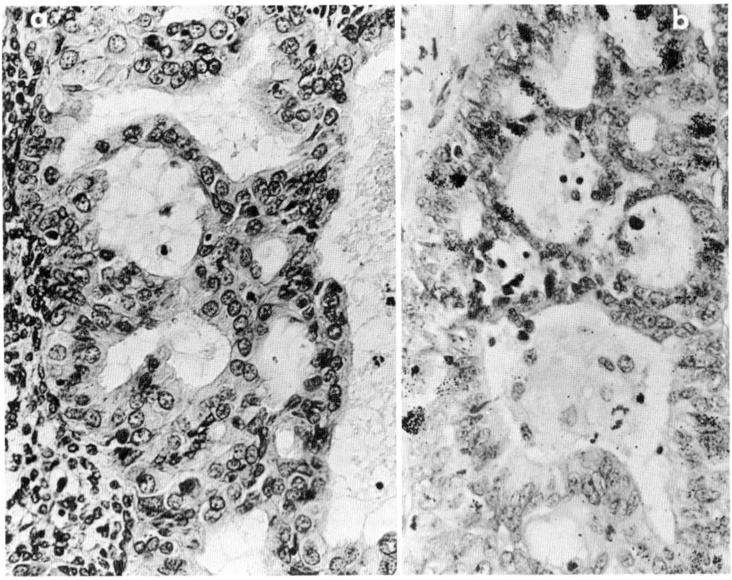

Fig. 13.10. Carcinoma *in situ* of endometrium. (a) Cribriform glandular pattern associated with large round nuclei. Pseudostratification is reduced and irregular, and the cytoplasmic substance is pale. Note peripheral aggregation of coarse nuclear chromatin and loss of cellular cohesion. ×210. H & E. (b) Cribriform glandular pattern and cytonuclear atypia are associated with heavy nuclear labelling of radioisotope. ×175. H & E.

The cells lining such glands have abundant, often pale cytoplasm and round nuclei with irregular membranes and often prominent nucleoli. The nuclei characteristically appear hypo- rather than hyperchromatic, but the chromatin is coarse and granular when examined at high magnification (Fig. 13.10 (a)). Hypochromasia in many instances is only relative and is presumably due to enlargement of the nuclear mass. The DNA content is aneuploid with stem lines often near the diploid or tetraploid DNA values (Wagner *et al.* 1967). Nuclear aneuploidy is a characteristic feature of noninvasive and invasive malignant cells in general and corresponds to significant mitotic defects; these in turn are associated with abnormal gains or losses in chromosome numbers.

The nuclear hypochromasia found in *in situ* carcinomas and in well-differentiated invasive adenocarcinomas in premenopausal anovular women (polycystic ovary syndrome) and in postmenopausal women on oestrogen replacement therapy may correspond to a normal diploid-tetraploid DNA content by Feulgen-DNA microspectrophotometry (Hustin 1976). The significance of this unusual phenomenon is unclear but similar DNA contents are found in a certain proportion of early, well-differentiated carcinomas arising in other endocrine target organs such as the breast, thyroid, and prostate. Despite 'normal' DNA content, the nuclei are grossly abnormal in their size, contour, and orientation which provide the clues for their correct interpretation. At higher magnification, the peripherally marginated nuclear chromatin is characteristically coarse.

The presence of intervening stroma between glands lined by neoplastic cells, together with the preservation of the general architecture and organization of the glands, are considered circumstantial evidence for the intraglandular origin of *in situ* carcinoma. Compared to cells from a region of adenomatous hyperplasia, the neoplastic cells have fewer oestrogen-related ultrastructural features such as cilia and microvilli (Ferenczy 1977), greater pleomorphism, and an abnormal distribution of intracytoplasmic organelles and microfilaments (Table 13.1) Virtually identical ultrastructural changes are seen in cells from well-differentiated adenocarcinomas which are invading the myometrium (Ferenczy 1977), strengthening the conclusions based on light microscopy that the cells in *in situ* carcinomas are indeed neoplastic and malignant (Fig. 13.11(a)-(d)). Further evidence for the existence of *in situ* carcinoma of the endometrium is derived from *in vitro* DNA-historadioautography (Ferenczy 1979, 1980*b*) in which a significant prolongation of the DNA-S phase is found in cells from both *in situ* and invasive adenocarcinomas compared with cells from adjacent hyperplastic or atrophic endometrium (Table 13.2). A prolonged DNA-S phase, such as nuclear aneuploidy, is a characteristic feature of invasive and pre-invasive malignant cells in several contexts (Cavasto *et al.* 1971). Labelling indices and concentrations of progesterone receptors are similar in *in situ* and in early invasive endometrial adenocarcinomas (Table 13.2).

The correct morphological recognition of various forms of endometrial hyperplasia as well as *in situ* carcinoma not only provides insight into their pathogenic relationships but also improves diagnostic accuracy in routine pathological practice. Endometrial hyperplasia and carcinoma *in situ* are often confused with benign endometrial conditions leading to overtreatment. Late-proliferative-early-secretory endometrium with compression artefacts of the glands, presumably sustained during handling of the specimen, may be reported as adenomatous hyperplasia. The glands in such cases show a 'back to back' pattern but they are devoid of other architectural or cytological alterations (Fig. 13.12(a)). Voluminous glands with compact stroma may be seen in the basal layer of the endometrium (Fig. 13.12(b)) masquerading as adenomatous hyperplasia, and the pathologist should not attempt to interpret endometrium which lacks surface epithelium. The latter is used as an indicator of the upper functionalis layer of the endometrial mucosa. The following conditions are often mistaken for endometrial neoplasia: menstrual endometrium; APPEM with focal coagulation necrosis and haemorrhage corresponding to 'oestrogen breakthrough bleeding' (Fig. 13.12(c)); adenomatous hyperplasia with benign squamous metaplasia (confused with adenoacanthoma) (Fig. 13.12(d)); gestational hypersecretory endometrium; and the Arias-Stella reaction. The common feature in all

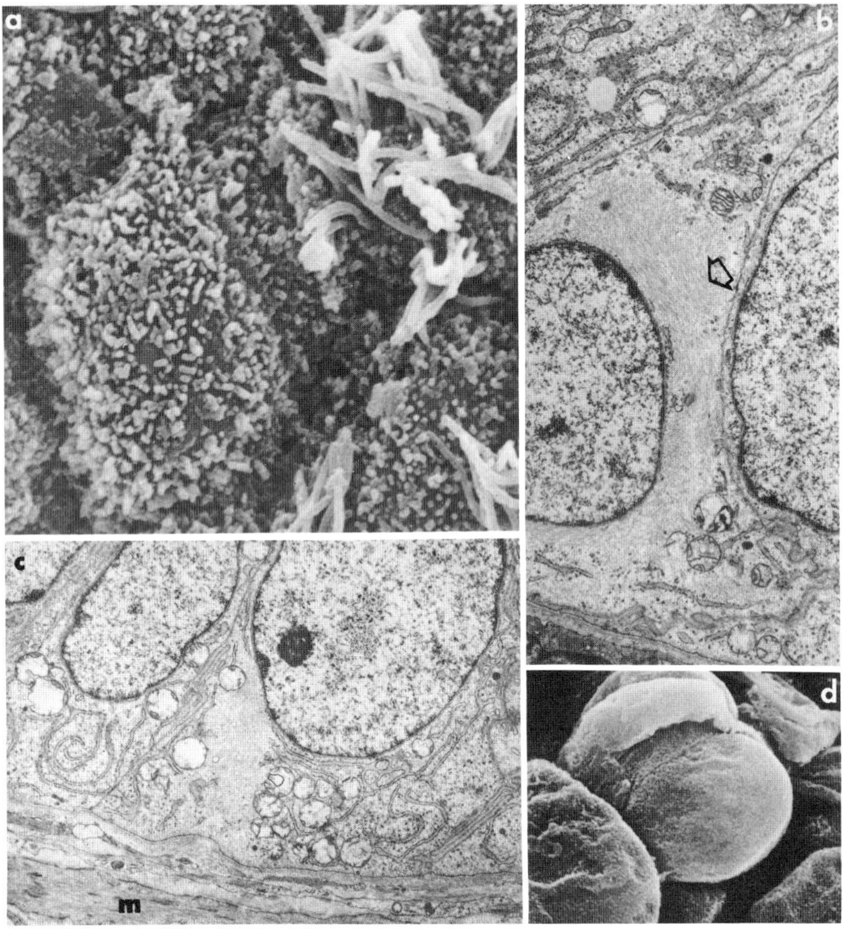

Fig. 13.11. Carcinoma *in situ* of endometrium. (a) Ciliated cells are decreased, cellular pleomorphism increased, and surface microvilli are shorter and fewer in number than in adenomatous hyperplasia, with or without cytological atypia. ×4900. (b) Transmission electron microscopy of cells from carcinoma *in situ*, showing pleomorphic mitochondria, convoluted membranes of granular endoplasmic reticulum and perinuclear distribution of microfilaments (arrow). Free ribosomes are sparse. ×4550. (c) Well-differentiated adenocarcinoma cells with invasion of myometrial cells (m). The invading tumour cells show the same fine structure as their intraepithelial counterparts. ×4340. (d) Poorly differentiated adenocarcinoma with severe pleomorphism lacks ciliated cells. ×1400.

these conditions is that the cells lack the cytological alterations that are found in endometrial adenocarcinoma.

Pathogenic relationship between endometrial hyperplasia, endometrial neoplasia, and the hormonal environment

We have seen earlier that the normal endometrium responds to cyclic stimulation by E_2 and progesterone by a sequence of proliferation and secretory

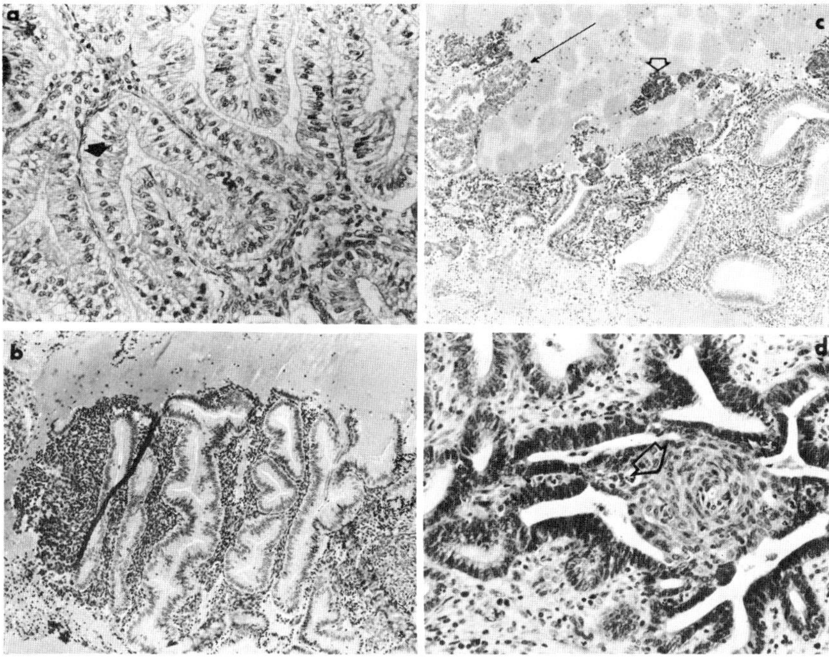

Fig. 13.12. Pseudohyperplasia and neoplasia of endometrium. (a) 18th day secretory endometrium. The glands are compressed, producing the 'back to back' pattern seen in hyperplasia. However, palisading of regular nuclei (arrow) is associated with sub- and supranuclear vacuolization and intraluminal secretions, features characteristic of 18th day secretory endometrium. ×145. H & E. (b) Basalis endometrium. Voluminous glands with compact stroma resembling hyperplasia. Note lack of surface epithelium of endometrium. The material represents denuded basal endometrium between the third and fourth day of the menstrual period. ×58. H & E. (c) Anovulatory persistent proliferative endometrium. Disrupted glands (long arrow) and aggregated stromal cells (short arrow) mixed with blood and acute inflammatory exudate may simulate carcinoma. Note intact endometrium of the anovulatory type (right) adjacent to necrotic zone. The changes are consistent with anovulatory cycles and 'oestrogen breakthrough' bleeding associated with early hyperplasia. ×58. H & E. (d) Adenomatous hyperplasia with squamous metaplasia should not be confused with adenoacanthoma. Although squamous metaplastic morules (arrow) may produce a 'gland-in-gland' neoplastic pattern, the gland cells are devoid of features of malignancy. ×145. H & E.

differentiation. Secretory activity is associated with arrest of growth. Such interplay implies that, in the vast majority of cyclic endometrial cells, the steroid hormone-receptor mechanism is intact and that the cells are highly sensitive to E_2. It has been suggested that an abnormal hormonal environment, particularly oestrogenic stimulation in the absence of progesterone, may lead to abnormal endometrial growth (Dallenbach-Hellweg 1971; Ferenczy 1980*b*; Gusberg 1980; Hulka *et al.* 1980; King 1978; Lucas 1974; Prianishnikov 1978). An association of this kind can be examined by measuring (first) the levels of circulating sex-steroid hormones in women with hyperplastic and neoplastic endometria and (second) those features that indicate endometrial reponsiveness to E_2. Although oestrogens are not necessarily grossly elevated in women with endometrial hyperplasia and carcinoma, these patients characteristically do not ovulate and they have circulating oestrogens in the absence of biologically effective progesterone (Hutton *et al.* 1979; King 1978; Lucas 1974; MacDonald *et al.* 1978). Such hormonal alterations are a reflection of certain metabolic abnormalities (Lucas 1974; MacDonald *et al.* 1978): These include:

1. Increased availability of the oestrone precursor, adrenocortical 1-4-androstenedione (Δ-4-A) which is found in anovulatory premenopausal women with polycystic ovary disease or with functional ovarian tumours;
2. Increased peripheral conversion of Δ-4-A to oestrone (E_1) in obese, elderly, postmenopausal women, a process which may take place in fat depots, the gastrointestinal tract and the endometrium itself;
3. Exogenous oestrogen replacement therapy of thin, postmenopausal women (Hulka *et al.* 1980; Hutton *et al.* 1979; Lucas 1974; MacDonald *et al.* 1978).

Excess E_1 is presumably converted to E_2 (MacDonald *et al.* 1978) at the level of the endometrial target cell, producing a biologically potent oestrogenic environment unopposed by progesterone. More recently, elevated circulating free E_2 (unattached to sex-hormone binding globulin) has been found in women with endometrial carcinoma and its precursors (Siiteri 1981) thus providing another source of relative hyperoestrogenism. Increased amounts of free E_2 in the plasma of these women are associated with low levels of sex-hormone-binding globulins, which in turn are presumably related to obesity. The concept of oestrogen-mediated abnormal endometrial growth is also supported by experimental data. CBA-strain mice are particularly resistant to spontaneous tumours, but treatment with E_2 or E_1 produces endometrial hyperplasia and occasionally early neoplasia. The spectrum of histological and ultrastructural changes is analogous to that seen in women (Papadaki *et al.* 1979). It is interesting that ageing in this animal model is accompanied by ovarian and endometrial atrophy and an anestrus state closely similar to the postmenopausal genital senescence found in women.

The precise pathobiological mechanisms responsible for hormone-induced abnormal endometrial growth are not clear. We have mentioned earlier that the first morphological evidence of E_2-related uterine proliferation is APPEM. It is speculated that the development of early endometrial hyperplasia is due to impaired control mechanisms of E_2-dependent uterine proliferation (Ferenczy 1980*b*) such as progesterone and (perhaps) the 'uterine chalone'. The latter is a tissue-specific antimitotic substance which is thought to control E_2-induced overgrowth of the uterus in the rat in the absence of progesterone (Gorski *et al.* 1977). An absence of progesterone and, more importantly, uterine chalone may thus lead to a loss of endometrial refractoriness to E_2. This results in E_2-stimulated endometrial overgrowth and the morphological appearances of APPEM. It is suspected that E_2-refractoriness is a genetically determined physiological property of normal endometrium, and impairment of this function would imply alterations in the genetic constitution of normal growth controls of the endometrium. Whether endometrial refractoriness is lost prior to the development of an abnormal hormonal environment or is a consequence of longstanding and continuous E_2-stimulation is not known, but clinical observations support a genetic predisposition for endometrial hyperplasia. Indeed, the vast majority of postmenopausal women with obesity and other risk factors for endometrial hyperplasia and carcinoma develop no other endometrial abnormalities (Ferenczy 1978). Similarly, only about 30 per cent of postmenopausal women treated with cyclic oestrogen replacement at a daily dose of 1.25 mg Premarin developed endometrial hyperplasia (Whitehead 1978).

Endometrial response to E_2 may be assessed by evaluating E_2-related morphological alterations, nuclear DNA activity, and progesterone receptor concentrations. Cilia are more numerous, DNA synthesis and progesterone receptor concentrations are enhanced, and the DNA-S phase and potential doubling time are significantly shorter in the early phases of endometrial hyperplasia—APPEM—than in normal proliferative endometrium and in advanced adenomatous hyperplasia and carcinoma (Tables 13.1 and 13.2). These findings reflect the maximum sensitivity of early endometrial hyperplasia to E_2 and a predominance of E_2-sensitive cells with an intact sex-steroid receptor mechanism (Ferenczy 1980*a,b*). Experimentally, E_2 accelerates DNA synthesis by stimulating cells in the G_0 resting phase to enter the DNA-S phase of the cell cycle and it shortens the duration of the DNA-S phase (Epifanova 1971). When exogenous gestagens such as medroxyprogesterone acetate (Provera) are given to postmenopausal women in combination with Premarin, the incidence of subsequent endometrial hyperplasia, particularly of the APPEM variety, is considerably reduced (3-6 per cent) compared to that following Premarin alone (Whitehead 1978). The slow decline in E_2-related morphological alterations, the lengthening of the DNA-S phase and the reduction in progesterone receptor content found in adenomatous hyperplasia without and with atypia, in carcinoma *in situ*, and in invasive carcinoma are all considered to be due to a gradual increase in E_2-*insensitive* (independent) cells at the expense of E_2-sensitive cells. The hormone-receptor mechanism in such cells is presumably reduced, impaired, or absent (Ferenczy 1980*b*). This shift in cell population is likely to represent an escape phenomenon by which endometrial refractoriness to unopposed oestrogenic stimulation is enhanced. It is possible that during this process cells escape to varying degrees from the normal growth control mechanisms. The concept of a gradual decrease in end-organ sensitivity to E_2 running parallel with increasing atypia in adenomatous hyperplasia and eventual carcinoma, is supported by various lines of indirect evidence. Despite elevated circulating oestrogens in many women with endometrial hyperplasia and carcinoma (Hutton *et al.* 1979; King 1978; Lucas 1974; MacDonald *et al.* 1978), the levels of E_2-induced progesterone receptors are lower in carcinomatous than in normal endometrial tissues, intermediate values being found in hyperplastic endometrium (Table 13.2). Despite the low content of progesterone receptors, the labelling index is elevated in adenomatous hyperplasia, carcinoma *in situ*, and early invasive carcinoma (Table 13.2). This dissociation between DNA synthesis and concentrations of progesterone receptors—both of which are profoundly affected by E_2 in the normal endometrium—strongly suggests E_2-independent autonomous growth in a population of endometrial cells composed of an increasing proportion of E_2-insensitive elements poor in progesterone receptors. Although a certain proportion of endometrial cells retain their E_2-sensitivity, their number decreases in parallel with histological and cytological dedifferentiation. E_2-sensitive cells with progesterone receptors are found more often, and at higher concentrations, in well-differentiated endometrial carcinomas than in poorly differentiated grade-3 tumours (Vihko *et al.* 1978). Finally, the therapeutic response of hyperplastic and neoplastic endometria to gestagens is at least partly influenced by a relative abundance of E_2-sensitive cells. Gestagens given in pharmacological doses may inhibit DNA synthesis and mitotic activity and transform hyperplastic or neoplastic cells into normal secretory cells (Ferenczy 1977, 1980*a*). The potential doubling time or the proliferative potential of such gestagen-suppressed endometria is considerably slowed (Ferenczy 1980*a*). Gestagen-induced effects are, however, more often produced (and are most marked) in early rather than advanced atypical hyperplasia and neoplasia of the endometrium (Ferenczy 1980*a*), and they are correlated with comparatively higher concentrations of E_2 and progesterone receptors (Ferenczy 1980*a*; Vihko *et al.* 1978). In carcinomas with negligible concentrations of progesterone receptors, E_2-sensitive cells are profoundly reduced or absent and gestagen-induced changes are not seen (Ferenczy, 1980*a*). Even in those carcinomas where gestagens produce redifferentiation of tumour cells which contain progesterone receptors, the morphological alterations are focal; the lesions recur when treatment stops (Ferenczy 1980*a*). The existence of heterogeneous subpopulations of E_2-sensitive and -insensitive cells in uterine carcinoma is also suggested by the regional variations in DNA-synthesis activity within a single tumour—and analogies may be seen here with human mammary carcinomas (Lee 1980) and with certain neoplasms in experimental animals (Fidler 1978).

Recent epidemiological studies have shown an association between oestrogen replacement therapy in postmenopausal women and the subsequent development of endometrial carcinoma. Women who have received exogenous oestrogens for more than three years are at an increased risk, variously estimated at between three- and fourteenfold according to the controls used, compared to women who did not have replacement therapy (Gusberg 1980;

Hulka *et al.* 1980). Most endometrial carcinomas associated with such treatment are Stage-I, grade-1, well-differentiated tumours with five year survival rates approaching 100 per cent (Robboy and Bradley 1979), and it has been suggested that they may constitute a distinct biological entity with a less aggressive course than the endometrial carcinomas that arise without such treatment. On the other hand, preliminary results from ultrastructural, kinetic, and sex-steroid receptor analyses of carcinomas arising in patients maintained on oestrogen replacement treatment for a minimum of two years show no significant differences when compared with endometrial carcinomas unassociated with previous replacement therapy, the two sets of tumours being matched for histological grade (Ferenczy 1980*b*). The findings of Robboy and Bradley (1979) of similar survival rates of women with uterine carcinomas, with and without a prior history of oestrogen replacement therapy but matched for histological differentiation, reinforce our own observations. It seems that the less aggressive behaviour of endometrial cancer associated with such treatment is a reflection of earlier diagnosis and (perhaps) accelerated promotion of the percursor stage of endometrial hyperplasia. Further studies of a large number of postmenopausal women with and without a history of oestrogen replacement therapy are in progress in our laboratory to validate our preliminary findings.

Conclusions

1. Normal endometrium consists mainly of E_2-positive cells which contain progesterone receptors. E_2 promotes their proliferation while progesterone promotes secretory differentiation.

2. Hyperplastic endometrium is induced by E_2 in the absence of biologically active progesterone (and the putative 'uterine chalone'). E_2-sensitive cells still predominate in the early stages of endometrial hyperplasia but, with increasing architectural and cytological atypia, the E_2-sensitive elements decrease and E_2-*insensitive* cells increase.

3. E_2-sensitive cells are reduced still further, or are absent, in endometrial carcinoma probably as a result of neoplastic dedifferentiation.

4. Current evidence supports the existence of *in situ* carcinoma of the endometrium which bridges the gap between adenomatous hyperplasia with severe cytological atypia and invasive carcinoma.

5. Endometrial carcinomas associated with oestrogen replacement therapy are not inherently different from tumours not associated with such treatment, provided they are matched for histological grade.

6. The data so far accumulated support the concept that oestrogens and particularly E_2 are not endometrial carcinogens. But in genetically predisposed individuals E_2 promotes the development of endometrial hyperplasia which may undergo malignant transformation, presumably during the process of acquiring refractory properties to longstanding, continuous E_2 stimulation unopposed by progesterone and the putative 'uterine chalone'.

References

Cavasto, F. and Pileri, A. (1971). Cell cycle of cancer cells in man. In *The cell cycle and cancer* (ed. R. Baserga), p. 99. Marcel Deckker, New York.

Dallenbach-Hellweg, G. (1978). *Histopathology of the endometrium.* Springer-Verlag, Berlin, New York.

Epifanova, O.T. (1971). Effects of hormones on the cell cycle. In *The cell cycle and cancer* (ed. R. Baserga), p. 145. Marcel Deckker, New York.

Ferenczy, A. (1977). Ultrastructural pathology of the uterus. In *Biology of the uterus* (ed. R.M. Wynn), p. 545. Plenum Press, New York.

—— (1978). The histogenesis and cytodynamics of endometrial hyperplasia and neoplasia. In *Hormonal biology of endometrial cancer* (ed. G.S. Richardson and D.T. MacLaughlin), p. 49. UICC Technical Report Series, Geneva.

—— (1979). Recent advances in endometrial neoplasia. *Exp. mol. Pathol.* **31**, 226.

—— (1980*a*). Morphological effects of exogenous gestagens on abnormal human endometrium. In *Functional morphological changes in female sex organs induced by exogenous hormones* (ed. G. Dallenbach-Hellweg), p. 101. Springer-Verlag, Berlin, Heidelberg, New York.

—— (1980*b*). Endometrial morphological response to endogenous and exogenous hormonal stimuli in health and disease: Normal endometrium during the menstrual cycle; endometrial hyperplasia and carcinoma. In *Hormones and cancer: progress in research and treatment* (ed. S. Iacobelli, R.J.B. King, H.R. Lindner, and M.E. Lipman), p. 489. Raven Press, New York.

——, Bertrand, G., and Gelfand, M.M. (1979). Proliferation kinetics of human endometrium during the normal menstrual cycle. *Amer. J. Obstet. Gynecol.* **133**, 859.

Fidler, I.J. (1978). Tumor heterogeneity and the biology of cancer invasion and metastasis. *Cancer Res.* **38**, 2651.

Gorski, J., Stormshak, F., Harris, J., and Wertz, N. (1977). Hormone regulation of growth: stimulatory and inhibitory influences of estrogens on DNA synthesis. *J. toxicol. Environ. Hlth.* **3**, 271.

Gusberg, S.B. (1980). Current concepts: the changing nature of endometrial cancer. *New Engl. J. Med.* **302**, 729.

Henzl, M.R., Smith, R.E., Boost, G., and Tyler, E.T. (1972). Lysosomal concept of menstrual bleeding in humans. *J. clin. Endocrinol. Metabol.* **34**, 860.

Hertig, A.T., Sommers, S.C., and Bengloff, H. (1949). Genesis of endometrial carcinoma: III carcinoma *in situ. Cancer* **2**, 964.

Hulka, B.S., Fowler, W.C., Kaufman, D.G., Grimson, R.C., Greenberg, B.G., Hogue, C.J.R., Berger, G.S., and Pulliam, C.C. (1980). Estrogen and endometrial cancer: cases and two control groups from North Carolina. *Amer. J. Obstet. Gynecol.* **137**, 92.

Hustin, J. (1976). Morphology and DNA content of endometrial cancer nuclei under progestogen treatment. *Acta Cytol.* **20**, 556.

Hutton, J.D., Jacobs, H.S., and James, V.H.T. (1979). Steroid endocrinology after the menopause: a review. *J. R. Soc. Med.* **72**, 835.

King, R.J.B. (1978). Estrogens, progestins and the production of endometrial hyperplasia and neoplasia. In *Hormonal biology of endometrial cancer* (ed. G.S. Richardson and D.T. MacLaughlin), p. 139. UICC Technical Report Series, Geneva.

Lee, S.H. (1980). Cellular estrogen and progesterone receptors in mammary carcinoma. *Amer. J. clin. Pathol.* **73**, 323.

Lucas, W.E. (1974). Causal relationships between endocrine-metabolic variables in patients with endometrial carcinoma. *Obstet. Gynecol. Surv.* **29**, 507.

MacDonald, P.C., Edman, C.D., Hemsell, D.L., Porter, J.C., and Siiteri, P.K. (1978). Effect of obesity on conversion of plasma androstenedione to estrone in postmenopausal women with and without endometrial cancer. *Amer. J. Obstet. Gynecol.* **130**, 448.

McBride, J.M. (1955). The functional activity of the genital tract in postmenopausal endometrial carcinoma. *J. Obstet. Gynaecol. Brit. Empire* **62**, 574.

Papadaki, L., Beilby, J.O.W., Chowaniec, J., Coulson, W.F., Darby, A.J., Newman, J., O'Shea, A., and Wykes, J.R. (1979). Hormone replacement therapy in the menopause: a suitable animal model. *J. Endocrinol.* **83**, 67.

Prianishnikov, V.S. (1978). A functional model of the structure of the epithelium of normal, hyperplastic and malignant human endometrium: a review. *Gynecol. Oncol.* **6**, 420.

Robboy, S.J. and Bradley, R. (1979). Changing trends and prognostic features in endometrial cancer associated with exogenous estrogen therapy. *Obstet. Gynecol.* **54**, 269.

Siiteri, P.K. (1981). Extraglandular oestrogen formation and serum binding of oestradiol: relationship to cancer. *J. Endocrinol.* **89**, 119.

Silverberg, S. and Major, F.J. (1978). *Estrogens and cancer.* John Wiley and Sons, New York.

Vihko, R., Robel, P., and Pollow, K. (1978). Estrogen and progestin receptors in endometrial hyperplasia and carcinoma. In *Hormonal biology of endometrial cancer* (ed. G.S. Richardson and D.T. MacLaughlin), p. 63. UICC Technical Report Series, Geneva.

Wagner, D., Richart, R.M., and Turner, J.Y. (1967). Deoxyribonucleic acid content of presumed precursors of endometrial carcinoma. *Cancer* **20**, 2067.

Welch, W.R. and Scully, R.E. (1977). Precancerous lesions of the endometrium. *Human Pathol.* **8**, 503.

Whitehead, M.I. (1978). The effects of estrogens and progestogens on the post-menopausal endometrium. *Maturitas* **1**, 87.

14 Some general clinical approaches to precancerous states

K.C. Calman

Several clinical aspects of precancerous states have been touched on in the preceding chapters, and the purpose of this final section is to consider some of the more general problems that they pose. It is self-evident that the clinician involved with the management of precancerous lesions is faced with a dual diagnostic and therapeutic challenge. The decisions taken may be of the greatest consequence to the individual patient since any therapeutic intervention may change the natural history of the disease. Inappropriate or inadequate therapy may be positively harmful, and it is particularly this latter aspect which makes the whole subject of premalignancy of such outstanding importance to the practising oncologist.

Precancerous lesions present to the clinician in several ways. In one instance, for example, a biopsy report provides histopathological evidence of a premalignant lesion. The clinical decisions here are whether further investigations will be required and whether treatment has been adequate. In another situation, a patient presents with the symptoms and signs of a disease known to have a defined premalignant potential, such as ulcerative colitis or—still more strikingly—familial polyposis coli. The clinical decisions here relate to the extent of investigation and screening and their frequency, and to the form of treatment to be used and its timing. A third context is illustrated by the desirability of screening asymptomatic patients and relatives of patients with a known malignancy which carries a familial association.

Recognition that a premalignant condition exists, or that a patient may have an increased risk of developing cancer, is perhaps the most important feature for the clinician. Information is not readily available as to the existence of precancerous lesions in all organs, and the oncologist may have difficulty in interpreting some clinical pictures. Further confusion may stem from the pathologist's nomenclature. It is essential, for example, that terms such are premalignancy, dysplasia, intraepithelial or *in situ* cancer, low-grade malignancy and early invasive cancer are used accurately and consistently by the pathologist and that their different implications are clearly understood by the clinician. Close and continuing contact must be maintained between clinician and pathologist, and both must be prepared jointly to review the diagnosis and to enlist specialist help where required. The versatility of endoscopy procedures and of diagnostic cytology have made the clinician aware that premalignant lesions can be identified at an increasing number of sites and that effective intervention is wholly realistic. But it must also be admitted that the use of newer investigative techniques and more frequent recourse to multiple sequential biopsies may on occasions compound, rather than solve, individual diagnostic problems. The pathologist is likely to be increasingly confronted with lesions that are unfamiliar and difficult to evaluate, and close follow-up over a long period of time is sometimes necessary before a decisive diagnosis can be reached.

The natural history of precancerous disease in relation to clinical decisions

One clear theme that has recurred in previous chapters is that the natural history of premalignant states is still imprecisely known. This uncertainty has obvious clinical and therapeutic implications, and two widely different clinical approaches have been adopted (Eddy 1980). Put crudely, biological determinists will question the independent existence of many precancerous states as distinct entities and will regard most of them as neoplastic *de novo*—an approach that was briefly discussed in the Introduction to this book. The alternative view, sometimes referred to as the *critical point hypothesis,* accepts that precancerous states do indeed represent (in many instances) an early stage in the development of what is ultimately likely to be a malignant tumour. Early diagnosis and treatment should prevent, or at least greatly reduce, the subsequent development of overt invasive cancer at the affected site. These two approaches are analysed in detail by Eddy (1980), but it would be fair to say that the critical point hypothesis reflects the predominant clinical view at the present time.

Investigation of patients with known precancerous disease and their follow-up

In spite of obtaining a histological diagnosis of precancerous disease, or of recognizing a condition known to be premalignant, it may be decided that no further investigations should be made. Depending on the clinical context provided by an individual patient, the oncologist will sometimes conclude that the risk of malignancy developing is low, that detailed investigations carry an unacceptable morbidity, and that the condition can be adequately assessed by regular observation. On the other hand, the recognition of a precancerous state may necessitate a whole series of investigations, some of which will need to be repeated at intervals. Some examples are discussed below.

Oesophagus

In areas of the world with a high incidence of oesophageal cancer, several screening programmes with endoscopy and brush cytology have been set up. The aim is to identify premalignant or early lesions so that effective treatment can be started without delay (Hishon *et al.* 1976; Dowlatshahi *et al.* 1978).

Stomach

Investigation and screening have been well studied in high-risk populations, particularly in Japan where the frequency of gastric cancer has stimulated extensive work on the early recognition of this tumour and its antecedent lesions (Hirayama 1978; Yoshida *et al.* 1983). The most usual methods of investigation involve a combination of endoscopy and double-contrast barium meals (Evans *et al.* 1978; Fielding *et al.* 1980). Minute mucosal lesions can be identified by these techniques and the histopathological appearances have been well described (see, for example, Nagayo 1971, 1977; also Chapter 7). Several attempts have been made to use gastric juice or gastric washings to follow patients or to screen high-risk groups by measuring various enzymes and mucopolysaccharides (Machado *et al.* 1977); none has so far proved suitable for general application.

Large intestine

The diagnostic problems here range from ulcerative colitis to adenoma of the colon and rectum. The investigative problems relate to viewing the complete length of the colon and rectum at regular intervals and to the diagnosis of small mucosal lesions. This may involve regular digital rectal examinations, sigmoidoscopy, double-contrast barium enemas, and colonoscopy. The last two procedures require adequate bowel preparation and clinical expertise, and would need to be performed annually in high-risk patients. They are not without morbidity, although it is small in experienced hands (Winawer *et al.* 1980*b*). It was initially hoped that measurements of plasma or serum carcinoembryonic antigen (CEA) would be useful in the follow-up of such patients, but current views indicate that serial estimations of CEA are of most value in patients with *overt* colorectal carcinomas as a means of early detection of metastatic disease developing after major surgery (Dhar *et al.* 1972; Chu and Murphy 1978; NIH Consensus Statement 1981). Simple examination of the stools for the presence of occult blood may be of value in detecting early malignant change (Winawer *et al.* 1980*a*; Winchester 1980; Hardcastle *et al.* 1983). Patient compliance is often poor, particularly among the older age groups who are at the greatest risk (de Jode 1982). All these investigations are designed to reveal small lesions (which may be multifocal) as early as possible so that treatment can be begun. The screening of asymptomatic patients or of high-risk groups for early bowel cancer or for premalignant lesions requires considerable resources and must be seen to be cost-efficient. Gilbertson and Nelms (1978) have shown that regular sigmoidoscopy is beneficial in carefully selected groups, and faecal occult blood testing may also prove useful (Winawer *et al.* 1980*a*).

Ovary

The clinical problem here is exemplified by the woman who presents with an ovarian lesion which the pathologist describes as borderline malignancy. The lesion may have been an incidental finding at laparotomy and a careful search for evidence of secondary spread or the taking of peritoneal washings may not have been carried out. The oncologist may decide to undertake no further investigations and merely follow the patient clinically, assuming that the lesion has been completely removed. Alternatively abdominal ultrasound, CT scan, and other isotope scans may be arranged although such procedures will only detect relatively gross disease. A 'second-look' laparotomy is occasionally indicated. More detailed follow-up with repeated abdominal ultrasound and CT scanning may be necessary. Blood markers such as carcinoembryonic antigen and α-fetoprotein are uninformative except in ovarian teratomas (Khoo *et al.* 1977).

Cervix uteri

The introduction of colposcopy has been an important development in the diagnosis and treatment of premalignant disease of the uterine cervix (Coppleson 1977). Various early lesions can be recognized and effectively treated by relatively simple methods. Routine cytology has long been used to identify abnormal cervical epithelia but the applications of conventional cytology to screening programmes have attracted some controversy. The value of such surveys has been questioned on the grounds that the incidence of overt cervical cancer was falling in several parts of the world at the time that such screening programmes were introduced. Recent epidemiological findings suggest, however, that the incidence of overt cervical cancer is tending to increase again and is affecting younger age groups; it may therefore be important to review the timing and age requirements for screening policies to take this disturbing trend into account (McGregor and Teper 1978; Clarke and Anderson 1979). Cordiner *et al.* (1980) have recently observed that patients requiring immunosuppressive treatment have a high incidence of intra-epithelial (noninvasive) cancer of the cervix, and regular follow-up of immunosuppressed patients may therefore be indicated.

Bladder

Premalignant states of the bladder are of particular interest as the entire mucosal surface can be readily seen at cystoscopy. Overt papillary and invasive tumours often coexist with other epithelial abnormalities, and repeat cystoscopy at regular intervals over prolonged periods of time is essential. Macroscopic abnormalities of the mucosa are biopsied and it may be appropriate to supplement standard histopathology with other morphological investigations (see Chapter 10).

Breast

Some of the general difficulties in defining precancerous states of the breast were discussed in Chapter 4, but certain more specifically clinical problems merit consideration. The first relates to the use of screening procedures for breast cancer. The subject is a difficult one (*Lancet* 1982; 1983) and attention here will be concentrated on what is perhaps the best-known of these programmes: the Breast Cancer Screening Project of the Health Insurance Plan of Greater New York (the H.I.P. Study). This trial was set up in 1963 to test whether periodic screening resulted in a reduced mortality from breast cancer. A total of 62 000 women aged between 40 and 64 were randomly allocated either to a group offered screening by physical examination and mammography in four successive years, or to a control group. After the first nine years (Shapiro 1977), 128 breast cancers were recorded in the control group of women, who continued to receive their usual medical care, compared with 91 in the study group. The benefits of the screening programme were confined to women aged 50 years or more. The risks resulting from radiation exposure incurred during mammography were thought to be outweighed by the advantages of screening. Shapiro concluded that the findings then available provided strong support for continuing periodic screening by clinical examination and mammography among women aged 50 or over. A review of results at 12-14 years was recently published (Shapiro *et al.* 1982). Forty four fewer deaths from breast cancer was found in the study group than among the controls, although the difference between them has inevitably narrowed: arithmetic gains due to screening have been maintained while the relative gains have shrunk. Once again, no clear advantages have been detected for women entering the screening programme below the age of 50. Several other population trials are now underway, notably in Sweden, the Netherlands, and the United Kingdom, and some of the outstanding problems may be resolved—notably the relative merits of mammography and palpation, agreement on optimal mammographic techniques, and the need to devise more effective screening procedures for women aged under 50.

A difficult related problem which may confront the clinician is the desirability of screening high-risk relatives of patients with breast cancer. The evidence so far available suggests that first-degree relatives of patients with breast cancer may be at higher risk of subsequently developing the disease, a risk which is increased if there is a strong family history (Lilienfeld 1963; Lynch *et al.* 1974). The decision to screen relatives routinely by clinical methods, mammography, and xeroradiography is not an easy one. It will almost inevitably cause stresses and strains in the women examined, and it may on occasions be counterproductive. The crucial question for the clinician is whether early diagnosis of breast cancer necessarily leads to a more favourable survival, and some supporting evidence is now becoming available (Shapiro 1977; NIH/ACS report 1979; Forrest and Roberts 1980; Miller and Bulbrook 1982; Shapiro *et al.* 1982).

A third clinical problem relates to the development of cancer in the *opposite* breast. In general terms, the risk is greater for lobular than ductal carcinomas (Robbins and Berg, 1964; Fischer 1977); the proportion of *in situ* and invasive lesions in the opposite breast varies in different accounts, almost certainly reflecting limitations in sampling and the difficulties of diagnosis, particularly of *in situ* lobular lesions (see Azzopardi 1979). At the time of surgery for a lobular carcinoma it is wise to take four quadrant biopsies from the contralateral breast and submit them to detailed histopathological examination—not frozen sections—in order to identify small lesions. The sampling error is unavoidably large. The indications for *prophylactic* removal of the opposite breast remain controversial.

Development of second tumours

In several clinical situations there is a possibility that the patient will develop a second tumour. These high-risk individuals may require regular screening. One such group consists of patients with a primary malignancy treated with immunosuppressive measures such as irradiation and/or cytotoxic drugs (Sieber 1975; Chabner 1977). Patients requiring immunosuppressive therapy following organ transplantation also have a higher risk of developing a malignant tumour, particularly of the brain and the cervix uteri (Penn and Starzl 1972; Hoover and Fraumeni 1973; Kinlen *et al.* 1979). Another important high-risk group is illustrated by patients with tumours at certain sites which are frequently either *multifocal* or *bilateral*. Examples include the bladder and colon, and the breast, ovary, and also the testis where *in situ* germ cell carcinomas have been reported in the contralateral testis of men with testicular tumours (Berthelsen *et al.* 1979). Regular review and follow-up of such patients should include screening for second tumours at the appropriate sites.

Treatment of precancerous lesions

For the clinician this is perhaps the most important and difficult decision to make. Should treatment, indeed, be undertaken at all? And if it is, how limited or how radical should such treatment be? There are no strict rules and, as the following examples show, considerable clinical judgement is required.

The patient with longstanding symptomatic ulcerative colitis is certainly at risk of developing colorectal carcinoma—a risk that is related to the extent of mucosal involvement, and the length of time that symptoms have been present (Lennard-Jones *et al.* 1977; Devroede and Taylor 1977). Panproctocolectomy may be required—a major procedure which is associated with significant morbidity and mortality. If the operation is carried out too early, the patient may not yet have developed malignant change. If the decision is postponed until a definite colonic cancer has been identified, major curative surgery may be too late. The morbidity of the procedure is partly related to removal of the rectum with the formation of an ileostomy. A case can be made for establishing an ileorectal anastomosis, though there is a chance that the rectal stump may be the site of recurrent colitis and ultimately of carcinoma (Baker *et al.* 1978).

The patient with a papillary tumour or an *in situ* carcinoma of the bladder is at a high risk of developing other lesions because of field change. Such lesions are usually managed conservatively by means of biopsy or diathermy. It is exceptional for cystectomy to be performed except when repeated lesions are found requiring regular treatment. The change from *in situ* carcinoma to an invasive lesion can be insidious and requires considerable clinical experience to recognize. Dysplasia and noninvasive carcinomas are sometimes widespread, and some investigators have advocated the use of cytotoxic drugs, either instilled directly into the bladder or given systemically (Koontz 1979; Soloway 1980). It is too early to assess the value of such a policy but the clinical dilemma is a particularly clear one; cyclophosphamide, for example, may *induce* invasive bladder cancer in man as well as (perhaps) prevent it.

The treatment of *in situ* carcinoma of the cervix has undergone a significant change following the wider use of colposcopy (Coppleson 1977) and the introduction of new techniques such as laser surgery. Small lesions may be readily visualized and treated locally by a variety of measures, and indications for more extensive surgery have been reduced.

General aspects: educational implications

Having recognized the lesion, undertaken the necessary investigations, and planned the appropriate treatment, the clinician must decide what to tell the patient. The simplest approach is to avoid any detailed discussion at all and to proceed without formally involving the patient. Following surgery the patient can then be told that the treatment has been successful, the danger removed, and that no further investigations or treatment will be required. This tactic clearly begs the question as to the nature of the premalignant state and the necessity for subsequent follow-up, but it may be entirely appropriate in certain situations. If, however, the patient has a high risk of developing a malignant lesion or if there is a chance that the risk is increased in the relatives, then more discussion is required. This may be very difficult; the niceties of pathological nomenclature will almost certainly be lost on the patient and considerable psychological stress may be engendered by the uncertainties which will inevitably be left in the patient's mind, especially when regular follow-up and investigation of asymptomatic relatives is required. A particular problem is the involvement of the patient in decisions regarding radical treatment, such as in the use of pan-procto-colectomy in ulcerative colitis.

Education in this extremely difficult field is required at all levels—for clinicians and pathologists as well as for patients, their relatives, and the general public. The implications in terms of possible cancer prevention are self-evident and the development of more accurate cost-effective screening procedures is an urgent need. Better use of existing screening systems is also necessary, and it is disconcerting to realize that the most important target groups for cervical cancer screening are still those very groups which are least likely to use the services now available (*British Medical Journal* 1980).

Premalignancy is one of the most stimulating areas in oncology. The clinical impact is only beginning to be recognized, but opportunities are becoming available to control potentially invasive lesions at an early stage. The clinician must become more fully involved in the area of premalignancy and, in collaboration with the pathologist and the epidemiologist, define more clearly the natural history of neoplastic diseases. He must begin to identify high-risk groups of patients and balance therapeutic intervention against possible morbidity. With clearer recognition of precancerous states, cancer therapy can at the same time become less destructive and more efficacious.

References

Azzopardi, J.G. (1979). *Problems in breast pathology.* W.B. Saunders, Philadelphia and Toronto.

Baker, W.N.W., Glass, R.E., Ritchie, J.K., and Aylett, S.O. (1978). Cancer of the rectum following colectomy and ileorectal anastomosis for ulcerative colitis. *Brit. J. Surg.* **65**, 862.

Berthelsen, J.G., Skakkebaek, N.E., Mogensen, P., and Sorensen, B.L. (1979). Incidence of carcinoma *in situ* of germ cells in contralateral testis of men with testicular tumours. *Brit. Med. J.* **2**, 363.

British Medical Journal (1980). High risk groups and cervical cancer. *Brit. med. J.* **2**, 629.

Chabner, B.A. (1977). Second neoplasm—a complication of cancer chemotherapy. *New Engl. J. Med.* **297**, 213.

Chu, T.M. and Murphy, G.D. (1978). Carcinoembryonic antigen evaluation of a screening assay in non-cancer clinics, *NY State J. Med.* **78**, 879.

Clarke, E.A. and Anderson, T.W. (1979). Does screening by "pap" smears help prevent cervical cancer: a case control study. *Lancet* **2**, 1.

Coppleson, M. (1977). Colposcopy. In *Recent advances in obstetrics and gynaecology* (ed. J. Stallworthy and G. Bourne, pp. 155-87. Churchill Livingstone, London.

Cordiner, J.W. Sharp, F., and Briggs, J.D. (1980). Cervical intraepithelial neoplasia in immunosuppressed women after renal transplantation. *Scott. med. J.* **25**, 275.

Devroede, G.J. and Taylor, W.F. (1976). On calculating cancer risk and survival of ulcerative colitis patients with the life table method. *Gastroenterol.* **71**, 509.

Dhar, P., Moore, T.L., Zamcheck, N., and Kupchik, H.Z. (1972). Carcino-embryonic antigen in colonic cancer. Use in pre- and post-operative diagnosis and prognosis. *J. Amer. Med. Assoc.* **221**, 31.

Dowlatshahi, K., Daneshbod, A., and Morbarhan, S. (1978). Early detection of cancer of oesophus along the caspian littoral. *Lancet* **2**, 125.

Eddy, D.M. (1980). *Screening for cancer: therapy analysis and design.* Prentice-Hall, Englewood Cliffs, New Jersey.

Evans, D.M.D., Craven, J.L., Murphy, F., and Cleary, B.K. (1978). Comparison of early gastric cancer in Britain and Japan *Gut* **19**, 1.

Fielding, J.W.L., Ellis, D.J., Jones, B.G., Paterson, J., Well, D.J., Waterhouse, J.A.H., and Brookes, V.S. (1980). The natural history of early gastric cancer: results of a 10 year study. *Brit. med. J.* **2**, 965.

Fisher, E.R. (1977). Pathology of breast cancer. In *Breast cancer, advances in research and treatment* (ed. W.L. McGuire). Churchill Livingstone, London.

Forrest, A.P.M. and Roberts, M.M. (1980). Screening for breast cancer. *Brit. J. hosp. Med.* **23**, 8.

Gilbertson, V.A. and Nelms, J.M. (1978). The prevention of invasive carcinoma of the rectum. *Cancer* **41**, 1137.

Hardcastle, J.D., Farrands, P.A., Balfour, T.W., Chamberlain, J., Amar, S.S., and Sheldon, M.G. (1983). Controlled trial of faecal occult blood testing in the detection of colorectal cancer. *Lancet* **ii**, 1.

Hirayama, T. (1978). Outline of stomach cancer screening in Japan. In *Screening in cancer: UICC Technical Report Series.* p. 264. UICC, Geneva.

Hishon, S., Smithies, A., Lovell, D., Shandon, H., Gummer, J.W.P., and Blendis, L.M. (1976). Cytology in the diagnosis of oesophageal cancer. *Lancet* **1**, 296.

Hoover, R. and Fraumeni, J.F. (1973). Risk of cancer in renal transplant recipients *Lancet* **2**, 55.

de Jode, L.R. (1982). Prospects in large bowel cancer. *J. roy. Soc. Med.* **75**, 301.

Khoo, S.K., Hill, R., and Mackay, E.V. (1977). Detection of CEA and AFP in serum ascitic fluid from patients with ovarian cancer. *Aust. N. Z. J. Obst. Gynaec.* **17**, 94.

Kinlen, L.J., Sheil, A.G.R., Peto, J., and Doll, R. (1979). Collaborative United Kingdom and Australian study of cancer patients treated with immunosuppressive drugs. *Brit. med. J.* **2**, 1461.

Koontz, W.W. (1979). Intravesical chemotherapy and chemoprevention and superficial low grade, low stage bladder tumors. *Seminar Oncol.* **6**, 217.

Lancet (1982). Editorial: screening for breast cancer. *Lancet* **i**, 1103.

—— (1983). Editorial: epidemiology of early breast neoplasia. *Lancet* **i**, 686.

Lennard-Jones, J.E., Morson, B.C., Richie, J.K., Shove, D.C., and Williams, C.B. (1977). Cancer in colitis: assessment of the individual risk by clinical and histological criteria. *Gastroenterol.* **73**, 1280.

Lilienfeld, A.M. (1963). The epidemiology of breast cancer. *Cancer Res.* **23**, 1503.

Lynch, H.T., Guirgis, H., Albert, S., and Brennan, M. (1974). Familial breast cancer in a normal population. *Cancer* **34**, 2080.

Machado, G., Clamp, J.R., and Read, A.E. (1977). Carbohydrate content of endoscopic gastric biopsies in carcinoma of the stomach, *Gut* **18**, 670.

McGregor, J.E. and Teper, S. (1978). Mortality from carcinoma of cervix uteri in Britain. *Lancet* **2**, 774.

Miller, A.B. and Bulbrook, R.D. (1982). Screening, detection and diagnosis of breast cancer. *Lancet* **1**, 1109.

Nagayo, T. (1971). Histological diagnosis of biopsied gastric mucosa with special reference to that of borderline lesions. *Gann Monogr. Cancer Res.* **11**, 245.

—— (1977). Precursors of human gastric cancer: their frequencies and histological characteristics. In *Pathophysiology of carcinogenesis in digestive organs* (ed. E. Farber), p. 151. University of Tokyo Press.

NIH/ACS Report of the working group of review the NCI/ACS breast cancer detection demonstration projects (1979). *J. Nat. Cancer Inst.* **62**, 699.

NIH Consensus statement (1981). Carcinoembryonic antigen: its role as a marker in the management of cancer. *Brit. Med. J.* **282**, 373.

Penn, S. and Starzl, T. (1972). Malignant tumors arising *de novo* in immunosuppressed organ transplant recipients. *Transplantation* **14**, 407.

Robbins, G.F. and Berg, J.W. (1964). Bilateral primary breast cancer. A prospective clinicopathological study. *Cancer* **17**, 1501.

Shapiro, S. (1977). Evidence on screening for breast cancer from a randomised trial. *Cancer* **39**, 2772.

——, Venet, W., Strax, P., Venet, L., and Roeser, R. (1982). Ten- to fourteen-year effect of screening on breast cancer mortality. *J. Nat. Cancer Inst.* **69**, 349.

Sieber, S.M. (1975). Cancer chemotherapeutic agents and carcinogenesis. *Cancer chemother. Rep.* **59**, 915.

Soloway, M.S. (1980). Rationale for intensive intravesical chemotherapy for superficial bladder cancer. *J. Urol.* **123**, 461.

Winchester, D.P. (1980). A mass screening programme for colorectal cancer using chemical testing for occult blood in the stool. *Cancer* **45**, 2955.

Winawer, S.J., Andrews, M., Flehinger, B., Sherlock, P., Schottenfeld, D., and Miller, D.G. (1980*a*). Progress report on controlled trial of fecal occult blood testing for the detection of colorectal neoplasia. *Cancer* **45**, 2959.

Winawer, S.J., Schottenfeld, D., and Sherlock, P. (1980*b*). *Colorectal cancer, prevention, epidemiology and screening,* Raven Press, New York.

Yoshida, Y., Yamaguchi, Y., Tebayashi, A., Arisue, T., Tamura, K., and Ichikawa, H. (1983). Precision in the first stage of the gastric carcinoma mass survey. *Int. J. cancer* **31**, 201.

Index